Parsons'
Diseases of the Eye

Stephen J.H. Miller KCVO, MD, FRCS

Consulting Ophthalmic Surgeon, St George's Hospital,
London; Moorfields Eye Hospital; The National Hospital for
Nervous Diseases, Queen Square

SEVENTEENTH EDITION

CHURCHILL LIVINGSTONE
EDINBURGH LONDON MELBOURNE AND NEW YORK 1984

CHURCHILL LIVINGSTONE
Medical Division of Longman Group Limited

Distributed in the United States of America by Churchill
Livingstone Inc., 1560 Broadway, New York, N.Y. 10036, and
by associated companies, branches and representatives
throughout the world.

First Edition 1907
Second Edition 1912
Third Edition 1918
Fourth Edition 1923
Fifth Edition 1926
Sixth Edition 1930
Seventh Edition 1934
Eighth Edition 1936
Ninth Edition 1938
Tenth Edition 1942
Eleventh Edition 1948
Twelfth Edition 1954
Thirteenth Edition 1959
Fourteenth Edition 1964
Fifteenth Edition 1970
Sixteenth Edition 1978
Seventeenth Edition 1984

ISBN 0 443 02114 7

British Library Cataloguing in Publication Data
Parsons, *Sir* John
    Parsons' diseases of the eye. — 17th ed.
    1. Eye — Diseases and defects
    I. Title   II. Miller, Stephen J.H.
    617.7   RE46

Library of Congress Cataloging in Publication Data
Parsons, John Herbert, Sir, 1868–1957.
    Parsons' Disease of the eye.
    Includes index.
    1. Ophthalmology. I. Miller, Stephen James
Hamilton. II. Title. III. Title: Diseases of the eye.
[DNLM: 1. Eye disease. WW 100 P268p]
RE46.P33 1983   617.7   82-14791

Printed in Hong Kong
by C & C Joint Printing Co., (H.K.) Ltd.

Preface

The seventeenth edition of this book attempts to demonstrate to the reader that ophthalmology in practice concerns the management of patients who present ocular problems many of which are due to lesions sited in the sphere of other specialties. Hence its breadth and depth of interest.

It should be of help to the postgraduate who wishes to become a consultant in providing a framework whereon to build. It is unlikely to interest the family doctor in the United Kingdom who is usually illiterate in ophthalmology thanks to our undergraduate deans who have yet to learn what a fund of teaching is ignored in every ophthalmic out-patient department where the young can see in detail exactly what they have been taught, for them a relatively rare and thrilling experience. Medical graduates in the Commonwealth, Ireland, the Continent of Europe and the United States of America are more fortunate in their training and general practitioners in these areas should have no difficulty in understanding the text and acquiring practical knowledge from reading its pages. The postgraduates of large areas of the Middle and Far East have found *Parsons' Diseases* most helpful (judging from their letters) and their needs have been kept in mind when planning the changes necessary to produce a new edition of this venerable treatise on a subject which is changing rapidly due to continuing advances in technology.

I am indebted to many authors both at home and abroad, and acknowledgements have been made in the text. I am particularly grateful to Merrill J Reeh and his co-authors for allowing me to reproduce diagrams from *Practical Ophthalmic Plastic and Reconstructive Surgery*, published by Lea and Febiger, Philadelphia, 1976.

London, 1984   S.J.H.M.

Contents

SECTION 1

Anatomy and physiology

Embryology and anatomy

EMBRYOLOGY

The central nervous system is developed from the neural groove which invaginates to form the neural tube running longitudinally down the dorsal surface of the embryo. At either side of the anterior portion of this structure a thickening appears at an early stage (the *optic plate*) which grows outwards towards the surface to form the *primary optic vesicle* (Fig. 1.1A and B). From this

pair of diverticula from the sides of the forebrain and the mesodermal and ectodermal structures in contact with it the two eyes develop.

After it meets the surface ectoderm, the primary optic vesicle invaginates from below (the *optic cup*), the line of invagination remaining open for some time as the embryonic fissure (Fig. 1.1C). The inner layer of the cup forms the main structure of the retina, the nerve fibres from which eventually grow backwards towards

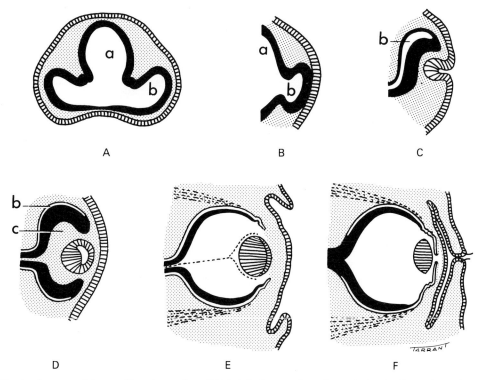

A B C

D E F

Fig. 1.1 The development of the eye. In each case the solid black is the neural ectoderm, the hatched layer the surface ectoderm and its derivatives, the dotted area is mesoderm: *a*, cavity of the forebrain; *b*, cavity of the optic vesicle; *c*, cavity of the optic cup (or secondary optic vesicle) formed by invagination. A. Transverse section through the anterior part of forebrain and optic vesicles of a 4-mm human embryo. B. The primary optic vesicle. C. The formation of the optic cup by invagination at the embryonic fissure, invagination of the surface epithelium. D. The optic cup and lens vesicle. E. The formation of the ciliary region and iris, the anterior chamber, the hyaloid artery and the lid folds. The lens is formed from the posterior cells of the lens vesicle. F. The completed eye

the brain. Its outer layer remains as a single layer of pigmentary epithelium; between the two lies a narrow space representing the original optic vesicle; and from its anterior border develop parts of the ciliary body and iris (Fig. 1.1E). Meantime, at the point where the neural ectoderm meets the surface ectoderm, the latter thickens to form the *lens plate*, invaginates to form the *lens vesicle*, and then separates to form the lens; and through the embryonic fissure the hyaloid artery enters the optic cup and grows forwards to meet the lens, bringing temporary nourishment to the developing structures before it eventually atrophies and disappears; as it does so, its place is taken by a clear jelly (the vitreous) largely secreted by the surrounding neural ectoderm. While these ectodermal events are happening, the mesoderm surrounding the optic cup differentiates to form the coats of the eye and the orbital structures; that between the lens and the surface ectoderm becomes hollowed to form the anterior chamber, lined by meso-

dermal condensations forming the anterior layers of the iris, the angle of the anterior chamber and the main structures of the cornea; while the surface ectoderm remains as the corneal and conjunctival epithelium. In the surrounding region folds grow over in front of the cornea, unite, and separate again to form the lids (Fig 1.1E and F).

ANATOMY

The wall of the globe is composed of a dense, imperfectly elastic supporting membrane (Fig. 1.2). The anterior part of the membrane is transparent — the cornea; the remainder is opaque — the sclera. The anterior part of the sclera is covered by mucous membrane — the conjunctiva — which is reflected from its surface onto the lids.

The *cornea* consists of three layers: the epithelium,

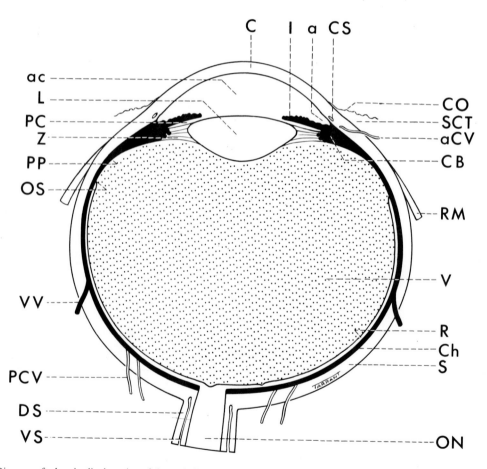

Fig. 1.2 Diagram of a longitudinal section of the eyeball: a, angle of anterior chamber; ac, anterior chamber; aCV, anterior ciliary vessel; C, cornea; CB, ciliary body; Ch, choroid; CO, ocular conjunctiva; CS, canal of Schlemm; DS, dural sheath; I, iris; L, lens; ON, optic nerve; OS, ora serrata; PC, posterior chamber; PCV, posterior ciliary vessel; PP, pars plana; R, retina; RM, rectus muscle; S, sclera; SCT, sub-conjunctival tissue; V, vitreous; VS, vaginal sheath; VV, vortex vein; Z, zonule

the substantia propria or stroma, and Descemet's membrane with its endothelium. The epithelium, which is stratified, may be regarded as the continuation of the conjunctiva over the cornea. Its basal cells lie on a lamina of the substantia propria, called Bowman's membrane. The substantia propria may be regarded as the continuation forwards of the sclera.

The stroma forming 90% of the total corneal thickness is composed of regularly arranged thin fibrils of collagen ensheathed by acidic muco-polysaccharides and set in a ground substance. They form ribbon-like bundles and give the stroma a laminated appearance. The collagen fibrils are circular in transverse section and are spaced equidistantly. They lie in staggered rows to form a hexagonal lattice.

Transparency of the cornea is related to the regularity of the stromal components. The lattice theory proposes that the stromal collagen fibrils are of regular diameter and arranged as a lattice with an inter-fibrillar spacing of less than a wave length of light so that tangential rows of fibres act as a diffraction grating resulting in destructive interference of scattered rays.

Descemet's membrane is a thin elastic membrane, covered on its posterior surface by endothelium. The primary mechanism controlling stromal hydration is a function of the corneal endothelium. Electrolytes are removed and water flows passively. The endothelium may be examined by the specular microscope at a magnification of (× 500). Endothelial cells become less in number with age and the individual cells enlarge to compensate.

The cornea is set into the sclera like a watch glass so that the latter overlaps the cornea all round the periphery; the junction of the two tissues is known as the *limbus*. The cornea is very richly supplied with nerve fibres derived from the trigeminal. It has no blood vessels with the exception of minute arcades, about 1 mm broad, at the limbus so that it is dependent for its nourishment upon diffusion of tissue-fluid from the vessels at its periphery.

Lining the inner aspect of the sclera are two structures: the highly vascular uveal tract concerned chiefly in the nutrition of the eye, and within this a nervous layer, the true visual nerve ending concerned in the reception and transformation of light stimuli, called the retina.

The uveal tract consists of three parts, of which the two posterior, the choroid and ciliary body, line the sclera while the anterior forms a free circular diaphragm, the iris. The plane of the iris is approximately coronal: the aperture of the diaphragm is the pupil. Situated behind the iris and in contact with the pupillary margin is the crystalline lens.

The *anterior chamber* is a space filled with fluid, the *aqueous humour*; it is bounded in front by the cornea, behind by the iris and the part of the anterior surface of the lens which is exposed in the pupil. Its peripheral recess is known as the *angle of the anterior chamber*, bounded posteriorly by the root of the iris and the ciliary body and anteriorly by the corneo-sclera (Fig. 1.3). In the inner layers of the sclera at this part there is a circular venous sinus, sometimes broken up into more than one lumen, called the *canal of Schlemm*, of great importance, in the drainage of the aqueous humour. At the periphery of the angle between the canal of

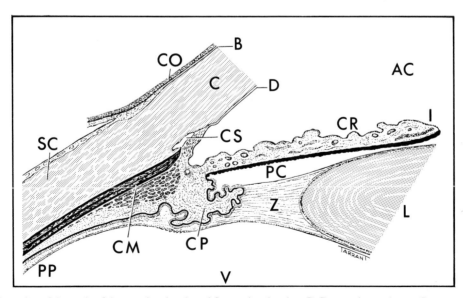

Fig. 1.3 The region of the angle of the anterior chamber: AC, anterior chamber; B, Bowman's membrane; C, cornea; CM, ciliary muscle, CO, corneal epithelium; CP, ciliary processes; CR, iris crypts; CS canal of Schlemm; D, Descemet's membrane; I, iris; L, lens; PC, posterior chamber; PP, pars plana of ciliary body; SC, sclera; V, vitreous; Z, zonule of Zinn

Schlemm and the recess of the anterior chamber there lies a loosely constructed meshwork of tissues, the *corneo-scleral trabeculae*. This has a general triangular shape, the apex arising from the termination of Descemet's membrane and the subjacent fibres of the corneal stroma and its base merging into the tissues of the ciliary body and the root of the iris. It is made up of circumferentially disposed flattened bands each perforated by numerous oval stomata through which tortuous passages exist between the anterior chamber and Schlemm's canal. The extracellular spaces contain both a coarse framework (collagen and elastic components) and a fine framework (muco-polysaccharides) of extracellular materials and they form the probable site of greatest resistance.

The endothelial cells of Schlemm's Canal are connected to each other by junctions which are not 'tight' but this intercellular pathway accounts for only 1% of drainage. The major outflow pathway is a series of transendothelial pores which are usually found in outpouchings of the endothelium called 'giant vacuoles' (Fig. 1.4A, B, C).

The anterior chamber is about 2.5 mm deep in the centre in the normal adult: it is shallower in very young children and also in old people.

The *iris* is thinnest at its attachment to the ciliary body, so that if torn it tends to give way in this region (Fig. 1.3). It is composed of a stroma containing branched connective tissue cells, usually pigmented but largely unpigmented in blue irides, and with a rich supply of blood vessels which run in a general radial direction. The tissue-spaces communicate directly with the anterior chamber through crypts found mainly near the ciliary border; this allows the easy transference of fluid between the iris and the anterior chamber. The stroma is covered on its posterior surface by two layers of pigmented epithelium, which developmentally are derived from the retina and are continuous with each other at the pupillary margin. The anterior layer consists of flattened cells, the posterior of cubical cells, and from the epithelial cells of the former two unstriped muscles are developed which control the movements of the pupil, the *sphincter pupillae*, a circular bundle running round the pupillary margin, and the *dilatator pupillae*, arranged radially near the root of the iris.

The anterior surface of the iris is covered with a single layer of endothelium, except at some minute depressions or crypts which are found mainly at the ciliary border; it usually atrophies in adult life.

The iris is richly supplied by sensory nerve fibres derived from the trigeminal. The sphincter pupillæ is supplied by motor nerve fibres derived from the oculomotor nerve, whilst the motor fibres of the dilatator muscle are derived from the cervical sympathetic chain.

The *ciliary body* in antero-posterior section is shaped roughly like an isosceles triangle, with the base forwards. The iris is attached about the middle of the base, so that a small portion of the ciliary body enters into the posterior boundary of the anterior chamber at the angle (Fig. 1.3). The chief mass of the ciliary body is composed of unstriped muscle fibres, the *ciliary muscle*. This consists of three parts with a common origin in the ciliary tendon, a structure which runs circumferentially round the globe blending with the 'spur' of the sclera and related to the corneo-scleral trabeculæ. The greater part of the muscle is composed of meridional fibres running antero-posteriorly on the inner aspect of the sclera to find a diffuse insertion into the suprachoroid. Most of

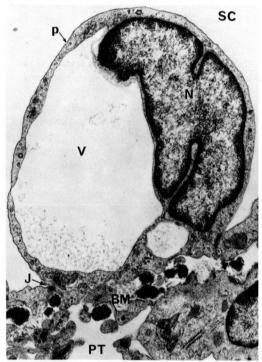

Fig. 1.4A Electron micrograph of a typical macrovacuolar configuration as seen normally in the endothelial cells lining the trabecular wall of Schlemm's canal. The vacuole, bound by a smooth unit membrane, is in fact formed by a basal invagination of the cell surface and eventually opens on the luminal aspect thus constituting a transient transcellular channel that allows the bulk outflow of the aqueous humour. Owing to the vacuolar configuration of the channel having small basal and apical openings, these openings are rarely encountered together in a single plane of section. The nucleus (N) is displaced to one side to accommodate the macrovacuole that contains aqueous humour. For comparison of the size of the macrovacuole, a micropinocytotic vesicle (100 nm) is denoted with p. J, junctional complex of lining endothelial cells; BM, patchy basal lamina seen beneath the endothelial lining of Schlemm's canal; PT, loosely organized pericanalicular tissue of the trabecular wall of Schlemm's canal (SC). × 18720

the remainder of the fibres run so obliquely in interdigitating V-shaped bundles as to give the impression of running in a circle round the ciliary body concentrically with the base of the iris. The third portion of the muscle is composed of a few tenuous iridic fibres arising most internally from the common origin and finding insertion in the root of the iris just anterior to the pigmentary epithelium in close relation to the dilatator muscle.

The inner surface of the ciliary body is divided into two regions; the anterior part is corrugated with a number of folds running in an antero-posterior direction while the posterior part is smooth. The anterior part is, therefore, called the pars plicata, the posterior, the pars plana. About 70 plications are visible around the circumference macroscopically, but if microscopical sec-

tions are examined, many smaller folds, the *ciliary processes*, will be seen between them. These contain no part of the ciliary muscle, but consist essentially of tufts of blood vessels, not unlike the glomeruli of the kidney. They are covered upon the inner surface by two layers of epithelium, which belong properly to the retina, and are continuous with the similar layers in the iris; the outer layer, corresponding to the anterior in the iris, consists of flattened cells, the inner of cubical cells, but unlike the condition in the iris, only the outer layer in the ciliary body is pigmented.

The ciliary body extends backwards as far as the *ora serrata*, at which point the retina proper begins abruptly; the transition from ciliary body to choroid, on the other hand, is gradual, although this line is conveniently

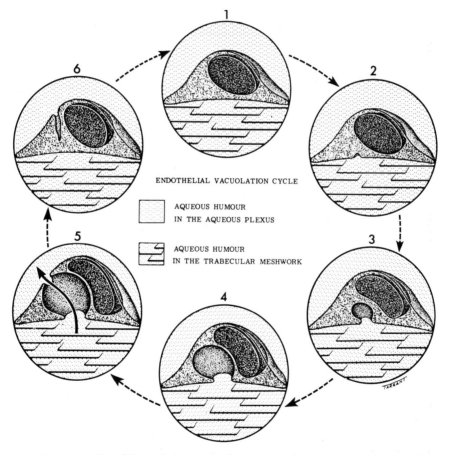

Fig. 1.4B Diagrammatic representation of the cyclical sequence of events in the formation of vacuolar transcellular channels that constitute a dynamic system of pores, and the mechanism of the bulk outflow of the aqueous humour across the endothelial barrier of Schlemm's canal. Initially, the vacuolar configuration is formed by a membranous depression or infolding on the basal aspect of the cell surface (stage 2). A progressive enlargement of this infolding leads to the formation of a macrovacuolar structure (stages 3 and 4) which eventually opens on the luminal aspect of the cell's surface (stage 5) thus forming a temporary vacuolar transcellular channel (continuous arrow). The bulk outflow of aqueous humor takes place down a pressure gradient (i.e., from the trabecular meshwork into the lumen of the canal of Schlemm) via such vacuolar transendothelial channels which also act as one-way valves. After a certain time interval, the basal infolding is occluded and the cell returns to its non-vacuolated state (stage 1)

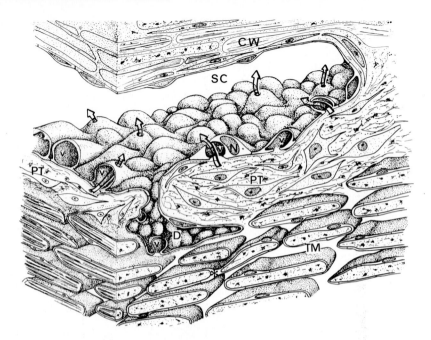

Fig. 1.4C Semi-diagrammatic representation of the walls of Schlemm's canal (SC) and adjacent trabecular meshwork in a composite sectional and three-dimensional view. The endothelial lining of the trabecular wall of Schlemm's canal is very irregular and normally the cells show luminal bulges corresponding to cell nuclei (N) and macrovacuolar configuration (V), the latter representing cellular invaginations beginning from the basal aspect and eventually opening on the apical aspect of the cell to form transcellular channels (arrows) through which aqueous humour flows down a pressure gradient. The sequence of events in this process is illustrated in B. A diverticula (D) on the inner wall of Schlemm's canal is seen with its endothelial lining being continuous with that of the canal and contains macrovacuolar configurations. Such blind, tortuous diverticulae course for a variable distance into the trabecular meshwork but remain separated from the open spaces of the meshwork by their continuous endothelial lining. The endothelial lining of the trabecular wall is supported by an interrupted, irregular basement membrane and a zone of pericanalicular connective tissue (PT) of variable thickness; the cellular element predominates in this zone and the fibrous elements, especially elastic fibers, are irregularly arranged in a net-like fashion, and the open spaces are narrower than the trabecular meshwork. The corneoscleral trabecular sheets show frequent branching and the endothelial covering (asterisk) may be shared between adjacent trabecular sheets. The corneoscleral wall (CW) of Schlemm's canal is more compact than the trabecular wall, with a predominance of lamellar arrangement of collagen and elastic tissue. (By courtesy of R. C. Tripathi.)

accepted as the limit of the two structures. The ora serrata thus circles the globe, but is slightly more anterior on the nasal than on the temporal side.

The ciliary body is richly supplied with sensory nerve fibres derived from the trigeminal. The ciliary muscle is supplied with motor fibres from the oculomotor and sympathetic nerves.

The *choroid* is an extremely vascular membrane in contact everywhere with the sclera, although not firmly adherent to it so that there is a potential space between the two structures — the *epichoroidal space* (Fig. 1.5). On the inner side, the choroid is covered by a thin elastic membrane, the *lamina vitrea*, or *membrane of Bruch*. The blood vessels of the choroid increase in size from within outwards, so that immediately beneath the membrane of Bruch there is a capillary plexus of fenestrated vessels, the *chorio-capillaris* (Fig. 1.6). Following upon this is the layer of medium-sized vessels, while most externally are the large vessels, the whole being held

together by a stroma consisting of branched pigmented connective tissue cells.

The choroid is supplied with sensory nerve fibres from the trigeminal as well as autonomic nerves presumably of vasomotor function.

The *retina* corresponds in extent to the choroid, which it lines, although the same embryological structure is continued forwards as a double layer of epithelium as far as the pupillary margin. If the two layers of epithelium are traced backwards, the anterior layer in the iris is found to be continuous with the outer layer in the ciliary body, and this again is continued into the pigment epithelium of the retina as a single layer of hexagonal cells lying immediately adjacent to the membrane of Bruch. Similarly, the posterior layer in the iris, although pigmented, passes into the inner unpigmented layer of the ciliary body, and this suddenly changes at the ora serrata into the highly complex visual retina.

The retina consists of a number of layers formed by

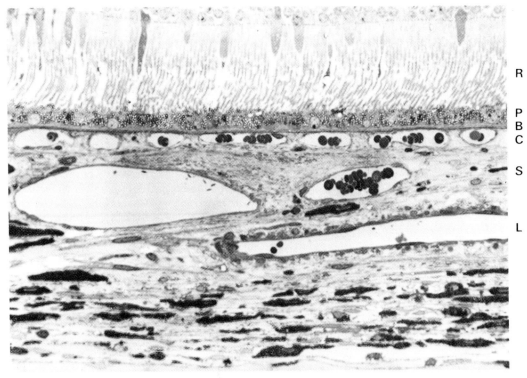

R
P
B
C
S
L

Fig. 1.5 Normal Choroid: R, rods and cones; P, pigment epithelium; B, Bruch's membrane; C, choriocapillaries; S, small vessels; L, large vessels (Garner)

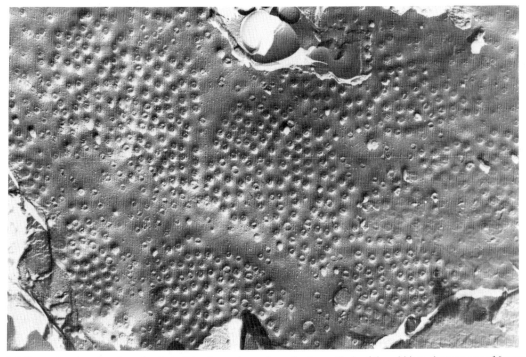

Fig. 1.6 Freeze-fractioned replica of endothelial cell membrane from chorio-capillaris of the rabbit to show groups of fenestrations separated by smooth cytoplasmic areas. (By courtesy of S. Melamed.)

three strata of cells and their synapses — the visual cells (lying externally), a relay layer of bipolar cells (lying intermedially), and a layer of ganglion cells (lying internally) and axons of which run into the central nervous system.

Most externally, in contact with the pigment epithelium, is a neural epithelium, the rods and cones which are the end-organs of vision (Fig. 1.8). The microanatomy of rods and cones reveals the transductive region (outer segment), a region for the maintenance of cellular homeostasis (inner segment), a nuclear region (outer nuclear layer), and a transmissive region (the outer plexiform or synaptic layer).

When rod outer segments are sectioned parallel to their long axis they are seen by the electron microscope to consist of a boundary or cell membrane which encloses a stack of membrane systems. The discs in rods of many species are continuously renewed throughout life. New discs are formed in the region of the inner segment and are progressively displaced towards the pigment epithelium. Rod discs have a limited life and are eventually lost to the pigment epithelium.

At the junction of the inner and outer segment the

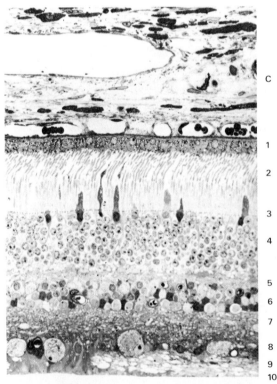

Fig. 1.7 Section of human retina: C, choroid; 1, pigment epithelium; 2, layer of rods and cones; 3, external limiting membrane; 4, outer nuclear layer; 5, outer plexiform layer; 6, inner nuclear layer; 7, inner plexiform layer; 8, ganglion cell layer; 9, optic nerve fibre layer; 10, internal limiting membrane. (By courtesy of Garner.)

cell body of both rods and cones constricts. The electron microscope reveals a connecting cilium which is always eccentric and provides the only link between the inner and outer segments.

The pigment epithelium consists of a single layer of hexagonal cells lying between the receptor outer segments and Bruch's membrane. They assist the metabolism of the retina by transporting selected substances to the receptor cells. Products of metabolism are freely exchanged between the receptor cells and the pigment epithelium.

The most striking inclusions in the pigment epithelium are the organelles responsible for its colour, the melanin granules. Most of the light which passes through the retina and is not absorbed by the photopigments in the receptor outer segments is absorbed by these granules. Phagosomes are known to be discarded rod discs that have been engulfed by the pigment epithelium. The phagocytic capacity of the pigment epithelium is demonstrated in the response of the retina to injury as by laser irradiation when the number of phagosomes in the underlying epithelial cells increases significantly (Fig. 1.7). Following this, in order from without inwards lie the outer nuclear layer (the nuclei of the rods and cones), the outer plexiform layer comprised of synapses, the inner nuclear layer (the nuclei of the bipolar cells), the inner plexiform layer (again synaptic), the ganglion cell layer, and finally (lying innermost), the nerve-fibre layer composed of the axons of ganglion cells running centrally into the optic nerve. These special nervous constituents are bound together by neuroglia, the better developed vertical cells being called the fibres of Müller, which in addition to acting as a supportive framework, have a nutritive function. The structure is completed by two limiting membranes, the outer perforated by the rods and cones, and the inner separating the retina from the vitreous.

To excite the rods and cones, incident light has to traverse the tissues of the retina but this arrangement allows these visual elements to approximate the (opaque) pigmented layer and form a functional unit, and their source of nourishment in the chorio-capillaris.

At the posterior pole of the eye, which is situated about 3 mm to the temporal side of the optic disc, a specially differentiated spot is found in the retina, the *fovea centralis*, a depression or pit, and here only cones are present in the neuroepithelial layer and the other layers are almost completely absent. The fovea is the most sensitive part of the retina, and it is surrounded by a small area, the *macula lutea*, or yellow spot which, although not so sensitive, is more so than other parts of the retina. It is here that the nuclear layers become gradually thinned out, while parts of the plexiform layers are especially in evidence: the ganglion cells too, instead of consisting of a single row of cells, are heaped up into

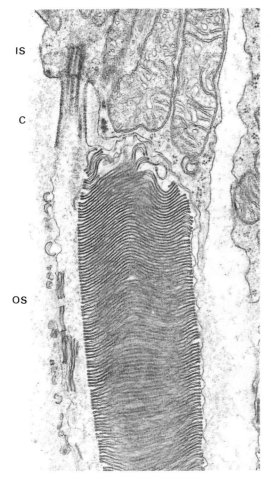

Fig. 1.8 Electron micrograph of a transverse section of a human rod cell at the junction of the inner and outer segment: OS, outer segment; IS, inner segment; C, cilium. (By courtesy of Marshall & Pedler.)

several layers. There are no blood vessels in the retina at the macula, so that its nourishment is entirely dependent upon the choroid.

At the optic disc the fibres of the nerve-fibre layer pass into the *optic nerve* (p. 165), the other layers of the retina stopping short abruptly at the edge of the aperture in the scleral canal. This is spanned by a transverse network of connective tissue fibres containing much elastic tissue, the *lamina cribrosa*, through the meshes of which the optic nerve fibres pass; on the posterior side they suddenly become surrounded by medullary sheaths. These fibres, the axons of the ganglion cells of the retina, are, of course, afferent or centripetal fibres, but the optic nerve also contains a few efferent or centrifugal fibres.

The *lens* is a biconvex mass of peculiarly differentiated epithelium. It is developed from an invagination of the epidermal epiblast of the fœtus, so that what was

originally the surface of the epithelium comes to lie in the centre of the lens, the peripheral cells corresponding to the basal cells of the epidermis. Just as the epidermis grows by the proliferation of the basal cells, the old superficial cells being cast off, so the lens grows by the proliferation of the peripheral cells. The old cells, however, cannot be cast off, but undergo changes (sclerosis) analogous to that in the stratum granulosum of the epidermis, and become massed together in the centre or nucleus: moreover, the newly formed cells elongate into fibres, the lens fibres, which have a complicated architectural form, being arranged in zones wherein the fibres growing from opposite directions meet in sutures. Without going into details, it is important to bear in mind that the central nucleus of the lens consists of the oldest cells and the periphery or cortex of the youngest (Fig. 1.9). The fibres of the central *embryonic nucleus* meet around Y-shaped sutures. Outside this embryonic nucleus, successive nuclear zones are laid down as development proceeds, called, depending on the period of formation *fetal nucleus* (corresponding to the lens at birth), the *infantile nucleus* (corresponding to the lens at puberty), the *adult nucleus* (corresponding to the lens in early adult life), and finally and most peripherally, the

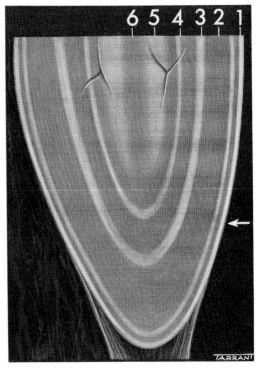

Fig. 1.9 The structure of the lens in an adult of 40 years, as shown in the optical beam of the slit-lamp: 1, anterior capsule; 2, cortex; 3, adult nucleus; 4, infantile nucleus; 5, fœtal nucleus; 6, embryonic nucleus

cortex comprised of the youngest fibres. In this part of the lens also the fibres meet along sutures with a general stellate arrangement. The mass of epithelium which constitutes the lens is surrounded by a hyaline membrane, the *lens capsule*, which is thicker over the anterior than over the posterior surface (p. 45); it is a cuticular deposit secreted by the epithelial cells having on the outside a thin membrane, the *zonular lamella*.

The lens in fetal life is almost spherical; it gradually becomes flattened so as to assume a biconvex shape. It is held in place by the *suspensory ligament* or *zonule of Zinn*. This is not a complete membrane, but consists of bundles of strands which pass from the surface of the ciliary body to the capsule where they join with the zonular lamella. The strands pass in various directions so that the bundles often cross one another. Thus the most posterior arise from the pars plana of the ciliary body almost as far back as the ora serrata; these lie in contact for a considerable distance with the ciliary body and then curve towards the equator of the lens to be inserted into the capsule slightly anterior to the equator. A second group of bundles springs from the summits and sides of the ciliary processes, i.e., far forwards, and passes backwards to be inserted into the lens capsule slightly posterior to the equator. A third group passes from the summits of the processes almost directly inwards to be inserted at the equator.

It will be noticed that there is a somewhat triangular space between the back of the iris and the anterior surface of the lens, having its apex at the point where the pupillary margin comes in contact with the lens; it is bounded on the outer side by the ciliary body. This is the *posterior chamber* and contains aqueous humour.

Behind the lens is the large vitreous chamber, containing the *vitreous humour*. This is a jelly-like material chemically of the nature of an inert gel containing a few cells and wandering leucocytes. As in other gels the concentration of the micellae on the surface gives rise to the appearance of a boundary membrane in sections — the so-called *hyaloid membrane*.

The *vitreous body* is attached anteriorly to the posterior lens surface by Wieger's Ligament. In the region of the ora the vitreous cortex is firmly attached to the retina and pars plana and this attachment is referred to as the vitreous base.

Posteriorly the vitreous body is attached to the margin of the optic disc and to the macula forming a ring around each structure. The primary vitreous is concentrated into the centre of the globe by the secondary vitreous and forms the canal of Cloquet which contains material less optically dense than the secondary vitreous.

The body of the vitreous has a loose fibrous framework of collagenous fibres whereas its cortex is made up of collagen-like fibres together with protein.

THE BLOOD SUPPLY OF THE EYE

The arteries of the eye in man are all derived from the ophthalmic artery, which is a branch of the internal carotid. The ophthalmic artery has few anastomoses, so that on the arterial side the ocular circulation is an offshoot of the intracranial circulation. This does not apply in so marked a degree to the venous outflow from the eye. In man most of the blood passes to the cavernous sinus by way of the ophthalmic veins, but they anastomose freely in the orbit, the superior ophthalmic vein communicating with the angular vein at the root of the nose, and the inferior ophthalmic vein with the pterygoid plexus.

The retina is supplied by the central artery, which enters the nerve on its lower surface, 15–20 mm behind the globe. The central artery divides on or slightly posterior to the surface of the disc into the main retinal trunks, which will be considered in detail later (Plate 1A). The retinal arteries are end-arteries and have no anastomoses at the ora serrata. The only place where the retinal system anastomoses with any other is in the neighbourhood of the lamina cribrosa. The veins of the retina do not accurately follow the course of the arteries, but they behave similarly at the disc, uniting on or slightly posterior to its surface to form the central vein of the retina, which follows the course of the corresponding artery.

The blood supply of the optic nerve head in the region of the *lamina cribrosa* is served by fine branches from the arterial circle of Zinn but mainly from the branches of the posterior ciliary arteries (Plate 7C). The central retinal artery of the retina makes no contribution to this region. The *prelaminar region* is supplied by centripetal branches from the peripapillary choroidal vessels with some contribution from the vessels in the lamina cribrosa region. The central artery of the retina does not contribute to this region. The surface layer of the *optic disc* contains the main retinal vessels and a large number of capillaries in addition to some small vessels. The capillaries on the surface of the disc are derived from branches of the retinal arterioles. In this part of the disc, vessels of choroidal origin derived from the adjacent prelaminar part of the disc may be seen usually in the temporal sector of the disc and one of them may enlarge to form a cilio-retinal artery. The capillaries on the surface of the disc are continuous with the capillaries of the peripapillary retina. These capillaries are mainly venous and drain into the central retinal vein. In the retro-laminar part of the optic nerve blood is supplied by the intraneural centrifugal branches of the central artery of the retina with centripetal contributions from the pial branches from the choroidal arteries, circle of Zinn, central artery of the retina and from the ophthalmic artery.

Venous drainage of the optic disc is mainly carried out by the central retinal vein. The prelaminar region also drains into the choroidal veins. There is no venous channel corresponding to the circle of Zinn. The central retinal vein communicates with the choroidal circulation in the prelaminar region.

The uveal tract is supplied by the ciliary arteries, which are divided into three groups — the short posterior, the long posterior and the anterior (Plates 1 and 2). The short posterior ciliary arteries, about 20 in number, pierce the sclera in a ring around the optic nerve, running perpendicularly through the sclera, to which fine branches are given off. The long posterior ciliary arteries, two in number, pierce the sclera slightly farther away from the nerve in the horizontal meridian, one on the nasal, the other on the temporal side. They traverse the sclera very obliquely, running in it for a distance of 4 mm. Both these groups are derived from the ophthalmic artery, while the anterior ciliary arteries are derived from the muscular branches of the ophthalmic artery to the four recti. They pierce the sclera 5 or 6 mm behind the limbus or corneo-scleral junction, giving off twigs to this region to the conjunctiva, the sclera and the anterior part of the uveal tract.

The ciliary veins also form three groups — the short posterior ciliary, the venæ vorticosæ, and the anterior ciliary. The short posterior ciliary veins are unimportant; they do not receive any blood from the choroid, but only from the sclera. The venæ vorticosæ are the most important, consisting usually of four large trunks which open into the ophthalmic veins. They enter the sclera slightly behind the equator of the globe, two above and two below, and pass very obliquely through this tissue. The anterior ciliary veins are smaller than the corresponding arteries, since they receive blood from only the outer part of the ciliary muscle.

Of these ciliary vessels the short posterior ciliary arteries supply the whole of the choroid, being reinforced anteriorly by anastomoses with recurrent branches from the ciliary body. The ciliary body and iris are supplied by the long posterior and anterior ciliary arteries. The blood from the whole of the uveal tract, with the exception of the outer part of the ciliary muscle, normally leaves the eye by the venæ vorticosæ only.

The two long posterior ciliary arteries pass forwards between the choroid and the sclera, without dividing, as far as the posterior part of the ciliary body. Here each divides into two branches (Plate 2): they run forward in the ciliary muscle, and at its anterior part bend round in a circular direction, anastomosing with each other and thus forming the *circulus arteriosus iridis major*. This is situated in the ciliary body at the base of the iris: from it the ciliary processes and iris are supplied. Other branches from the major arterial circle run radially through the iris, dividing dendritically and ending in

loops at the pupillary margin. A circular anastomosis takes place a little outside the pupillary margin, the *circulus arteriosus iridis minor*.

The tributaries of the vortex veins, which receive the whole of the blood from the choroid and iris, are arranged radially, the radii being bent, so as to give a whorled appearance — hence their name. The veins of the iris are collected into radial bundles which pass backwards through the ciliary body, receiving tributaries from the ciliary processes. Thus reinforced, they form an immense number of veins running backwards parallel to each other through the smooth part of the ciliary body. After reaching the choroid they converge to form the large anterior tributaries of the vortex veins.

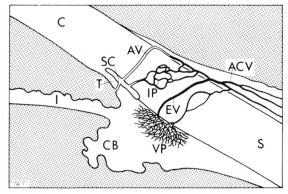

Fig. 1.10 The exit channels of the aqueous humour in man: C, cornea; S, sclera, I, iris; CB, ciliary body. The primitive drainage channels of lower animals are seen in VP, the ciliary venous plexus, draining by EV, the ciliary efferent veins into ACV, the anterior ciliary veins. Superimposed on this is the drainage system peculiar to primates, represented by T, the trabeculae, SC, the canal of Schlemm, IP, the intrascleral plexus and AV, an aqueous vein emptying into the anterior ciliary veins

The veins from the outer part of the ciliary body, on the other hand, pass forward and unite with others to form a plexus (the *ciliary venous plexus*) which drains into the anterior ciliary veins and the episcleral veins. These vessels communicate directly with the canal of Schlemm which is in intimate connection with the anterior chamber by means of numerous tortuous channels through the loose tissue of the trabeculæ (Fig. 1.3). From this canal the efferent channels form a complex system (Fig. 1.10); some of them drain into efferent ciliary veins in the sclera while others traverse the sclera and only join the venous system in the subconjunctival tissues (*aqueous veins*).

The marginal loops of the cornea and the conjunctival vessels are branches of the anterior ciliary vessels (Plate 2).

2

The physiology of the eye

THE NATURE AND FORMATION OF THE INTRA-OCULAR FLUID

For many years Leber's theory that it was a simple fil-tration from the blood was generally accepted. Chemi-cal analysis of the aqueous humour shows that such a simple hypothesis can not explain the facts; two mechan-isms are involved — ultrafiltration and secretion.

A two-way transference of fluid (tissue-fluid) occurs through the capillary walls in all the organs of the body; thereby nutriment is conveyed to the tissues and metabolites removed. The capillaries in different tissues vary considerably in their permeability to suit local needs. For optical purposes those in the retina (like those in the central nervous system) are relatively im-permeable so that practically no colloid molecules can pass into the cavity of the eye. Fluorescein in the blood stream is readily bound to albumen, making a larger molecular complex. The blood–retinal barrier by pre-venting dye leakage in the physiological state, results in a clear outline of retinal vessels of all calibres. In the choroidal circulation, fluorescein passes freely across the endothelium of capillaries to the extra-vascular spaces. There is, however, a physiological barrier to the passage of the dye from these spaces across Bruch's membrane and the intact retinal pigment epithelium into the sub-retinal space.

The system of semi-permeable membranes separating the blood from the ocular cavity is known as the *blood–aqueous barrier*, the composition of which is shown in Figure 2.1. It is formed in the posterior segment of the globe by the walls of the retinal capillaries which, like those of the central nervous system are very imper-meable and by Bruch's membrane and the retinal pigment epithelium. In the ciliary region it is formed by the two-layered ciliary epithelium which fluid must traverse before the posterior chamber is reached. In the iris it is formed by the walls of the capillaries in this tissue which are freely exposed to the anterior chamber through the crypts and spongy stroma.

The peculiar impermeability of the retinal capillaries and of the Bruch's membrane–pigment epithelial bar-

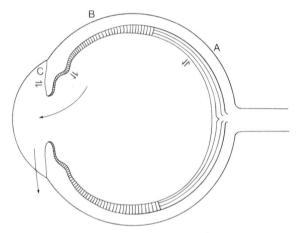

Fig. 2.1 The effective blood–aqueous barrier. A. In this zone the barrier is formed by retinal capillaries, Bruch's membrane and retinal pigment epithelium. B. In this zone the barrier consists of the ectodermal layer formed by the anterior part of the retina and its prolongation as the ciliary epithelium. C. In this zone the barrier is formed by the uveal capillaries only. The arrows indicate that in A and C, two-way traffic exists; in the ciliary region fluid traffic is essentially into the cavity of the eye, determining a circulation through the pupil and out at the angle of the anterior chamber

rier while necessary from the optical point of view, forbids the ready passage of large-sized molecules of any kind into the eye. Such therapeutic substances as penicillin when administered systemically are thus of little value in ocular therapeutics. Substances with a high lipoid-solubility, however, which easily penetrate living cells, traverse the barrier much more readily (sulphonamides, chloramphenicol, etc.).

It is obvious that if the permeability of the capillar-ies is increased, large molecules will be able to pass through their walls, so that a turbid fluid rich in pro-tein is formed — *plasmoid aqueous*. This increase in per-meability may be brought about by vasodilator drugs in inflammatory conditions such as iridocyclitis or choroidi-tis, and also if the capillary walls are mechanically stretched by suddenly lowering the intraocular pressure and removing their external support. This occurs when the globe is suddenly opened as by paracentesis or when the intra-ocular pressure is lowered by vigorous massage of the globe.

Such a two-way transference of fluid across the capillary walls would tend to stagnation. To it is added a secretory process conducted by the metabolic activity of the cells of the ciliary epithelium; it is probable that this accounts for some 95% of the total quantity of aqueous. The intimate mechanism is not understood, but it is known that a watery fluid rich in sodium and containing small quantities of ascorbic acid and other substances is secreted into the posterior chamber.

Having this dual origin, the aqueous humour thus consists of a dilute solution of all the diffusible constituents of the plasma, in addition to the substances specifically secreted. Since entry into the eye across the blood—aqueous barrier is difficult and exit through the drainage channels is easy, many of the constituents of the aqueous humour are in deficit in comparison with the blood with the exception of those secreted. There is, however, an incidental excess of lactic acid in the aqueous compared with the blood due to the formation of this substance as an end-product of the metabolism of the lens.

CIRCULATION OF THE AQUEOUS HUMOUR

Circulation is necessary both for metabolic purposes and to regulate the intra-ocular pressure. As the greater part of the fluid is formed in the ciliary region; it flows from the posterior chamber through the pupil into the anterior chamber and escapes through the drainage channels at the angle, and thence into the episcleral veins. In addition there is a second accessory exit (the *uveo-scleral outflow*) through the ciliary body into the choroid and suprachoroid and thence into the episcleral tissue; although a minor means of exit, this pathway may sometimes be of importance.

THE INTRA-OCULAR PRESSURE

Prolonged changes are essentially caused by two factors: (1) an alteration in the forces determining the formation of the aqueous, and (2) alterations in the resistance to its outflow. From the clinical point of view the latter is the more important. A rise in the intra-ocular pressure may be caused either by an increase in the pressure in the episcleral veins into which the aqueous drains or by any process which blocks the seepage of aqueous into the canal of Schlemm, such as sclerosis of the trabeculae or their obstruction by exudates or organized tissues. In either event glaucoma is the result. If the drainage channels to the canal of Schlemm are blocked, the intra-

ocular pressure does not rise indefinitely; it cannot rise above the mean blood pressure since at that point the circulation will cease; moreover, some drainage of intra-ocular fluid will take place through the uveo-scleral outflow.

While these are the principal factors determining prolonged changes in the intra-ocular pressure, other agencies can exert more temporary effects.

1. *Variations in the hydrostatic pressure in the capillaries.* It is obvious that the pressure in the eye will follow all such variations; thus it follows faithfully the pulse and respiratory rhythms.

2. *An increase in permeability of the capillaries*, allowing the formation of a plasmoid aqueous with a high protein content, will increase its osmotic pressure relatively to that of the blood and thus raise the pressure in the eye, a process accentuated if the drainage channels become clogged. This occurs particularly in inflammations.

3. *A change in the osmotic pressure of the blood* will be reflected in the intra-ocular pressure by altering the process of diffusion across the capillary walls, hypotonicity inducing a rise as in the water-drinking test and hypertonicity a fall. This can be demonstrated experimentally, and in clinical conditions such changes are induced by the use of glycerol by mouth or mannitol intravenously.

4. *Volumetric changes* within the globe should be immediately transformed into pressure changes owing to the indistensibility of the sclera; if extra fluid, for example, were forced into the eye its tension should rise abruptly.

5. *A blockage of the circulation of aqueous*, on the other hand, has a profound effect in raising the ocular tension. Such a block may occur in two places: (a) at the pupil where the flow of fluid from the posterior to the anterior chamber may be impeded, and (b) at the angle of the anterior chamber.

Obstruction in the first of these situations is usually due to one of two causes. The first arises in eyes with a shallow anterior chamber when the margin of the iris is firmly apposed to the anterior surface of the lens thus causing the condition of 'blockage of the pupil' wherein the aqueous becomes dammed in the posterior chamber; the iris is thus bellied forwards to reach the cornea and block the angle of the anterior chamber leading to an attack of primary closed-angle glaucoma. The second is due to organic changes when the iris becomes adherent to the anterior capsule of the lens in inflammatory conditions, when secondary glaucoma occurs. Inefficiency of the drainage channels, on the other hand, as we have seen, causes either a cumulative rise of pressure or transient increments.

The intra-ocular pressure within the eye normally varies from 10 to 20 mmHg. It is most accurately measured by a *manometer*, whereby a small cannula is inserted into the anterior chamber connected with a small-bored mercury or saline manometer. Such a technique is used experimentally on animals but its clinical application is obviously impossible. Since, however, the sclera is only very slightly elastic and is rendered tense by the internal pressure, a measurement of the degree to which it can be indented on the application of a standard weight or flattened by a measured pressure gives an indication of the ocular tension with considerable accuracy. Such a method is used clinically in *tonometry* (p. 78). The result thus obtained (usually given also as mmHg by standardization with a manometer on experimental animals) is referred to as the *ocular tension*.

THE METABOLISM OF THE OCULAR TISSUES

The vascularized tissues of the eye, particularly the uveal tract, differ in no respect in their general metabolism from other tissues in the body.

The non-vascularized tissues of the eye — the cornea and the lens — must obviously have a specialized metabolism, and so far as our present knowledge goes, they depend for their energy requirements essentially on carbohydrates which are utilized by phosphorylation and autoxidative mechanisms.

The *cornea* has few energy requirements which are necessary for the replacement of its tissues and the maintenance of transparency. The latter depends essentially on its state of relative dehydration which is maintained by an active transference of fluid outwards through the epithelium and endothelium, particularly the latter. A fall in metabolic activity or an increase in the permeability of its membranes thus leads to œdema and opacification. The essential physiological differences between the cornea and the sclera are that in the cornea the fibrils are arranged in a regular lattice-work in a ground-substance of mucopolysaccharide whereas the fibres of the sclera are irregularly arranged, and that the former tissue is bounded by cellular membranes by which its fluid-traffic is controlled.

The cornea derives its nutriment from three sources — oxygen directly from the air and solutes from the perilimbal capillaries and the aqueous humour. The first is an active process undertaken by the epithelium, and in an atmosphere of nitrogen, lactic acid collects rapidly in this layer of cells. The importance of diffusion from the limbal capillaries is seen clinically in the relative resistance of the peripheral parts of the cornea to de-generative changes, but at the same time, if these vessels are experimentally cut, corneal transparency is maintained. Similarly, if the aqueous is replaced by nitrogen, the cornea remains transparent; but it turns opaque if both these sources of nutrition are cut off. Metabolic activity which exhibits a high rate of aerobic glycolysis is maintained by the aid of enzyme systems, as occurs in the lens.

The *lens* derives its nourishment entirely from the aqueous humour in which it is immersed, the fluid-traffic being regulated by the semi-permeability of the capsule and the subcapsular epithelium. If this membrane is disrupted, the whole tissue, like the cornea, tends to adsorb fluid and turn opaque. Active transport takes place between the lens and the aqueous owing to the activity of the sub-capsular epithelium and the capsule itself is freely permeable to water and electrolytes as well as colloids of small molecular size, the posterior part being more permeable than the anterior. The permeability of the whole decreases with age.

The fact that the lens has a respiratory quotient (CO_2/O_2) of 1.0 shows that carbohydrate is its essential source of energy, a conclusion confirmed by the fact that the aqueous in the aphakic eye contains more glucose than in the normal eye. Chemical studies have shown that the initial stage in the break-down of the sugar is its combination with phosphates (phosphorylation) in the production of pyruvic acid; by experiments with radio-active tracers this has been found to occur particularly in the cortical layers. In all tissues this chemical process is effected by enzymes (such as hexokinase) which have been demonstrated in the lens; in this process oxygen is not required. For the further catabolism of pyruvate, oxygen is sometimes used. There is a small amount of oxygen in the aqueous derived from the blood, but by which enzymes it is used in the lens is not yet clear. The essential process is probably anaerobic and in the lens there is present a number of enzymes of the type whereby pyruvate is broken down to lactic acid and water. Lactic acid is found in considerable quantity in the aqueous humour when the lens is present; this is not so in the aphakic eye. Agents which appear to participate in this process are glutathione and ascorbic acid (vitamin C) which, reacting together, probably participate in an internal autoxidative system. The former, both as reduced and oxidized glutathione, occurs in very high concentration in the lens, particularly in the cortex; the latter is specially secreted by the ciliary body. Neither is present in cataract. Metabolic activity of the lens is largely confined to the cortex; the older nucleus is relatively inert.

3

The physiology of vision

When light falls upon the retina it acts as a stimulus to the rods and cones which serve as the sensory nerve endings. As contact of the skin with a foreign substance causes the sensation of touch, so stimulation of the retina by light causes visual sensations; upon these sensory cells the images of objects in the outside world are focused by the dioptric system of the eye. It follows that rays falling upon the optic disc give rise to no visual sensation and this is therefore called the *blind-spot* (of Mariotte). Light falling upon the retina, however, causes two essential reactions, photochemical and electrical.

The *photochemical changes* concern the pigments in the rods and cones. The most fully explored pigment is rhodopsin (visual purple), found in considerable quantity in the rods; several related pigments have recently been discovered in the rods of various types of animal, while it would seem that three different pigments are associated with the foveal cones. Rhodopsin is a chromoprotein, the molecule of which consists of a reactive part, a chromophore, responsible for the preferential absorption of light, attached to a protein which acts essentially as a support. The chromophore belongs to the family of the carotenoids and when exposed to light it is broken down through several intermediaries to the colourless vitamin A, a reaction which is reversible. It is this photochemical reaction which initiates the visual process and gives rise to the changes in electrical potential which are transmitted through the bipolar cells to the ganglion cells and along the fibres of the optic nerve to the brain. The pigments in the cones have not yet been fully elucidated, but it is likely that each reacts preferentially to different bands of wavelength in the spectrum which are perceived as red, green and blue.

The study of the *electrical responses* which follow has yielded results of great interest although all their implications are not yet clear. When the retina is stimulated, electrical variations (action-potentials) occur in the optic nerve fibres, presumably initiated by the photochemical changes in the rods and cones. These are of the same type as occur in all sensory nerves; they consist of biphasic variations always of the same amplitude (the all-or-none response) but varying in frequency with the intensity of the stimulation. In vertebrate eyes some fibres show a burst of activity at the onset of stimulation (the 'on-effect'), others show activity while the stimulus lasts, and others again show a burst of activity, presumably inhibitory in nature, when stimulation ceases (the 'off-effect'). Any single nerve fibre reacts when a considerable area of the retina is stimulated; this (the receptive field) varies in extent from a diameter of 0.5 to 1.0 mm and indicates the synaptic link-up of each ganglion cell with a number of receptor cells. Moreover, differences in the reaction resulting from stimulation by isolated wavebands of light show that a neural mechanism exists capable of colour discrimination. Reaching the occipital cortex some 124 msec after retinal stimulation, these impulses modify the electrical activity of the brain as recorded by the electroencephalogram. A somewhat crude additive record of the electrical changes in the retina can be obtained clinically in the electroretinogram, a technique which can be of diagnostic value in retinal disease.

VISUAL PERCEPTIONS

We are more concerned, however, with the sensations which result from stimulation of the retina with light. These are of four kinds, which are called the Light Sense, the Form Sense, Sense of Contrast and the Colour Sense.

Light sense

This is the faculty which permits us to perceive light, not only as such, but in all its gradations of intensity. If the light which is falling upon the retina is gradually reduced in intensity there comes a point when it is no longer perceived: this is called the *light minimum*. It varies greatly according to the amount of light which has been falling upon the retina before the observation is made (*adaptation*). We are all aware that if we go from bright sunshine into a dimly lit room we cannot perceive the objects in the room until some time has elapsed: the eyes have to become 'adapted' to the amount of illu-

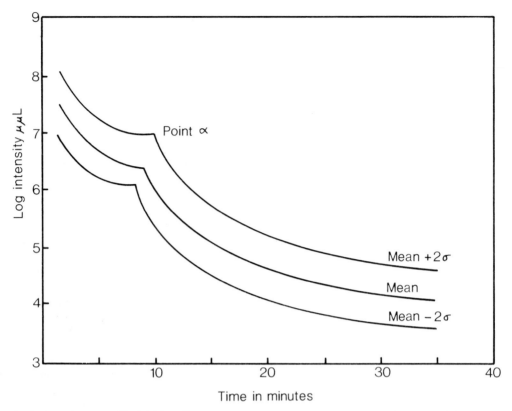

Fig. 3.1 Dark adaptation curve. The initial small symmetrical curve represents the adaptation of the cones. It is broken at a sharp knee (α) and the remainder of the curve represents the adaptation of the rods (after Sloan)

mination. Hence observations on the light minimum are only comparable when the eyes are in the same condition of dark adaptation as is obtained by excluding light from them for at least 20 to 30 minutes. The light minimum for the fovea is considerably higher than for the paracentral and peripheral parts of the retina, and retinal adaptation affects the macula relatively little (Fig. 3.1). It follows that in diseases which affect the rods particularly, much of the ability to adapt is lost and the patient is virtually night-blind.

The rods are much more sensitive to low illumination than the cones, so that in the dusk we see with our rods (*scotopic vision*); in bright illumination the cones come into play (*photopic vision*). Nocturnal animals, like the bat, have few or no cones; diurnal animals, like the squirrel, have no rods; man has an ample supply of both.

Form sense

This sense, which is next in importance, is the faculty which enables us to perceive the shape of objects in the outer world. Here the cones play the predominant part, and the form sense is most acute at the fovea, where they are most closely set and most highly differentiated.

It falls off very rapidly towards the periphery, as is shown in Figure 3.2, and it is noticeable that the curve agrees fairly well with the diminution in the number of cones. We are accustomed to speak of the ability to distinguish the shapes of objects as the *visual acuity*, and we mean by that the greatest acuity which it is possible to obtain. The acuity of vision, therefore, applies to central vision, or the vision of objects the images of which are formed at the fovea. The form sense is not a purely retinal function, for in the perception of composite forms — such as letters — it is largely psychological.

Sense of contrast

The ability to perceive slight changes in luminance between regions which are not separated by definite borders is just as important as the ability to perceive sharp outlines of relatively small objects. It is only the latter ability which is tested by means of the Snellen chart. In many diseases loss of contrast sensitivity is more important and disturbing to the patient than the loss of visual acuity (p. 102).

Colour sense

This is that faculty whereby we are enabled to distin-

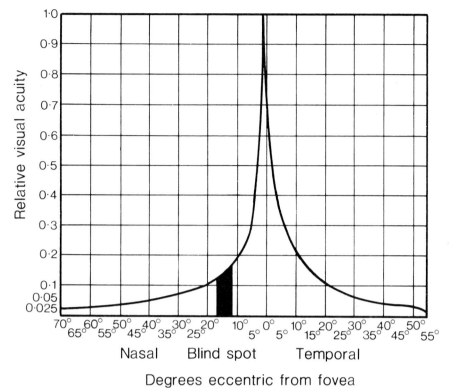

Fig. 3.2 The regional variations of the visual acuity in the retina

guish between different colours as excited by light of different wavelengths. The appreciation of colours is a function of the cones and therefore occurs only in photopic vision, that is, with lights of moderate or high intensity and with some degree of light adaptation of the retina. In very low intensities of illumination the dark-adapted eye sees no colour and all objects are seen as grey, differing somewhat in brightness.

In different cones there are three pigments which absorb preferentially wavelengths of light in the spectrum corresponding to the colours red, green and blue, and if these (or, indeed, any three colours sufficiently far apart in the spectrum) are chosen, all the other colours as well as white light can be formed by their combination in suitable proportions. Hence normal colour vision is called *trichromatic*. This is the basis of the Young–Helmholz theory of colour vision. In its original form this theory does not adequately explain all the phenomena associated with the appreciation of colour by normal individuals and in the colour-defective, but that there is a trichromatic stage in the visual process is undeniable.

4

The neurology of vision

THE VISUAL PATHWAYS

Comparison of the afferent tracts of common sensation with those of vision throws much light upon the latter.

The sensory impulse of common sensation in a limb is carried by a nerve fibre along the sensory nerve and the dorsal spinal root to the cord: it travels up in the posterior columns of the cord to the nucleus gracilis or the nucleus cuneatus as the case may be. The whole of this course is along the processes of a single cell or neurone, which has been called the neurone of the first order (I, Fig. 4.1A). The impulse is taken up in the nucleus gracilis or cuneatus by a second cell, and is carried along the nucleo-thalamic tract or medial lemniscus to the opposite thalamus. The cells in the nuclei gracilis and cuneatus are the neurones of the second order (II, Fig.

4.1A). A third cell, the neurone of the third order, situated in the thalamus, carries on the impulse to the cerebral cortex where the nervous impulse is transformed into a sensory perception.

Let us compare with this the visual afferent tracts (Fig. 4.1B). The end-organ is the neural epithelium of rods and cones. The first conducting nerve cell or neurone of the first order is the bipolar cell of the inner nuclear layer of the retina with its axon in the inner reticular layer. This microscopic cell corresponds morphologically to a dorsal root ganglion cell and its long processes stretching, in some cases, from the tip of the toe to the top of the spinal cord. The neurones of the second order are the ganglion cells in the retina the processes of which pass into the nerve fibre layer and along the optic nerve to the lateral geniculate body. Here a

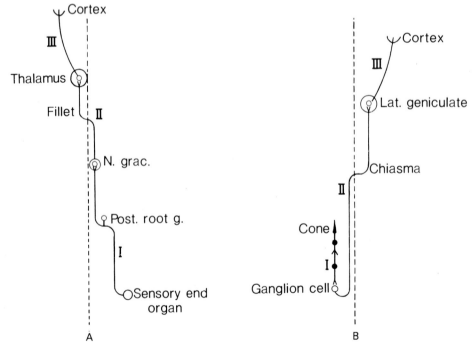

Fig. 4.1 A. The path of somæsthetic sensation. B. The visual path

new cell, the neurone of the third order, takes up the transmission of the impulse, travelling by way of the optic radiations to the cortex of the occipital lobe, which is the so-called *visual centre*.

The morphological identity of the two systems is apparent in spite of the great anatomical differences which specialization has brought about. The peripheral optic nerve proper corresponds to a bipolar cell in the inner nuclear and inner plexiform layers of the retina, while the so-called optic nerve is a part of the central nervous system homologous with the medial lemniscus in the medulla and pons.

The course of the fibres from the various parts of the retina is seen in Figure 4.2. In general it may be said that the fibres from peripheral parts enter the periphery of the optic nerve, while the fibres from parts of the retina near the optic disc enter the central parts of the nerve: they maintain this relative position as far back as the chiasma. The fibres from the macular region,

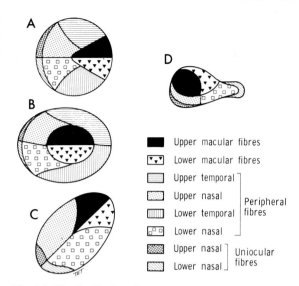

Upper macular fibres
Lower macular fibres
Upper temporal ⎤
Upper nasal ⎟ Peripheral
Lower temporal ⎟ fibres
Lower nasal ⎦
Upper nasal ⎤ Uniocular
Lower nasal ⎦ fibres

Fig. 4.3 The distribution of the fibres in the lower visual neurone of the right side: A, distal portion of the optic nerve; B, proximal portion of the optic nerve; C, optic tract; D, lateral geniculate body. In each case the dorsal aspect is above, the medial to the left

however, form a disturbing factor; they enter the nerve on its outer aspect, where they are spread over an area which is triangular in section, with the apex towards the centre of the nerve (Fig. 4.3). These *papillo-macular fibres* soon become more centrally situated, so that in the posterior part of the nerve they are all in the centre. Tracing the nerve fibres still farther backwards, a partial decussation occurs wherein the nasal fibres cross in the chiasma, while the temporal ones enter the optic tract of the same side to reach the dorsal part of the laternal geniculate bodies. The axons of their corresponding neurones of the third order are also widely distributed in the central part of the optic radiations and end at the most posterior part of the visual cortex at the tip of the occipital pole; each half macula (R. and L.) is thus represented in the corresponding occipital pole (Fig. 4.2).

The fibres from peripheral regions of the retina similarly form two distinct groups, corresponding to the temporal and nasal halves of the retina. The distinction is very exact, as if a vertical line divided the retina into two halves at the level of the fovea (Fig. 4.2). The fibres from the temporal half of the retina enter the chiasma and pass into the optic tract of the same side; thence they run to the lateral geniculate body where all the visual fibres end. The fibres from the nasal half of each retina enter the chiasma, decussate, and pass into the optic tract of the opposite side, the arrangement being such that the direct and crossed fibres pass to alternating laminæ in the lateral geniculate body. The corresponding neurones of the third order pass by the optic radi-

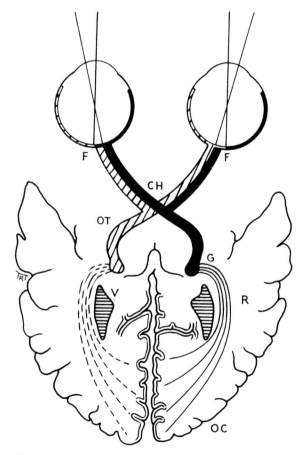

Fig. 4.2 The visual nerve paths showing lines of projection of the fixation area and the blind spot (from Traquair's 'Clinical Perimetry'): F, fovea; CH, chiasma; OT, optic tract; G, lateral geniculate body; R, optic radiations; OC, occipital cortex; V, lateral ventricle

ations to the corresponding occipital lobes. It follows that a lesion of one occipital lobe or optic tract will cause blindness of the temporal half of the retina on the same side and of the nasal half of the retina on the opposite side. Projecting this outwards, such a lesion will cause loss of vision in the opposite half of the binocular field of vision, a condition which is known as *hemianopia*. The afferent pupillo-constrictor fibres have a similar semi-decussation in the chiasma (Fig. 4.7).

The visual fibres in the optic radiations, like other sensory tracts, run behind the motor fibres in the internal capsule. Thereafter they separate considerably, the

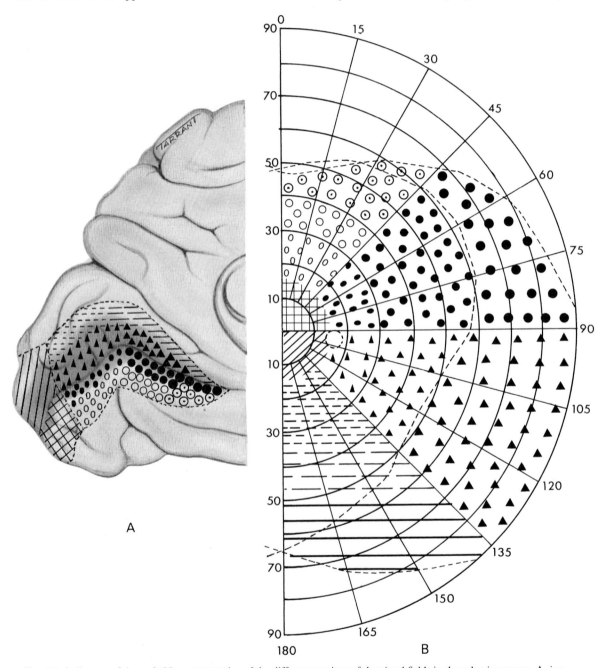

Fig. 4.4 A diagram of the probable representation of the different portions of the visual fields in the calcarine cortex. A, is a drawing of the medial surface of the left occipital lobe with the lips of the calcarine fissure separated so that its walls and floor are visible. The markings of the various portions of the visual cortex which is thus exposed correspond to those shown on the chart B of the right half of the field of vision. (By courtesy of Gordon Homes)

ventral fibres (projecting the lower quadrant of the retina or the upper quadrant of the visual field) running forwards into the temporal lobe before they turn backwards to the lower portion of the visual cortex, the dorsal fibres (projecting the upper retinal quadrant or lower field) running backwards in a more direct course to the upper part of the visual cortex (Fig. 4.2). They pass close to the posterior cornu of the lateral ventricle, so that they are liable to pressure here when the ventricle is distended.

The occipital cortex in and about the calcarine fissure differs from the cortex elsewhere in the possession of a white line, the line of Gennari, interpolated in the grey matter. This area, which is the primary visual or visuosensory area (Fig. 4.4A and B), is the cortical projection of the corresponding halves of both retinas. In this projection the same spatial arrangement is maintained — the part above the calcarine fissure represents the upper corresponding quadrants, the part below represents the lower corresponding quadrants of both retinæ, and the posterior part of the occipital lobe represents the macula.

THE PUPILLARY PATHWAYS AND REACTIONS

The pupils are controlled by two muscles of ectodermal origin — the sphincter and dilatator. The responses of these muscles to stimuli are very rapid and delicate and are easily observed, and the size of the pupil may be looked upon as essentially the resultant of their opposing forces. The constrictor centre possesses 'tone' and is perpetually sending out impulses to the sphincter which keep the pupil slightly contracted. Abnormal enlargement of the pupil is called *mydriasis*, abnormal contractions, *miosis*.

The pupillary pathways

The innervation of these muscles is seen in Figures 4.5 and 4.6.

The sphincter is supplied by cholinergic nerves of the parasympathetic system through the third cranial nerve. The fibres start in the Edinger–Westphal nucleus near the third nucleus in the floor of the aqueduct of Sylvius. This nucleus has connections with the dilatator centre as well as with the frontal and occipital cortex. From it the fibres pass out of the mid-brain and run in the main trunk of the third nerve as far as the orbit. Here the fibres pass into the branch which supplies the inferior oblique muscle, leaving it by the short root of the ciliary ganglion. From the ciliary ganglion they pass by the short ciliary nerves to the eye, piercing the sclera around the optic nerve in company with the short ciliary arter-

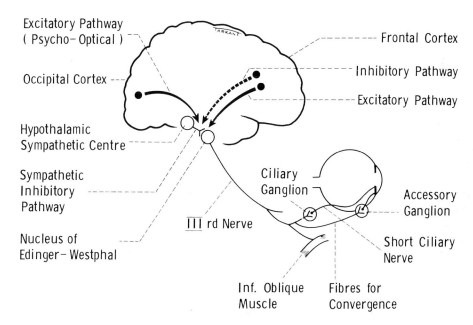

Fig. 4.5 The parasympathetic pupillary system. *Cortical control*: a) excitatory pathways from the frontal and occipital (psycho-optical) cortex; (*b*) inhibitory pathway from the frontal cortex.
Sympathetic control (inhibitory) from hypothalamic centre.
Pathway — Edinger-Westphal nucleus → third nerve → inferior division → branch to inferior oblique →
    (*a*) *Light reflex* — short root of ciliary ganglion → ciliary ganglion → short ciliary nerves → sphincter of iris
    (*b*) *Near reflex* — leaving the third nerve at an unknown point → (?) accessory ganglion → sphincter of iris

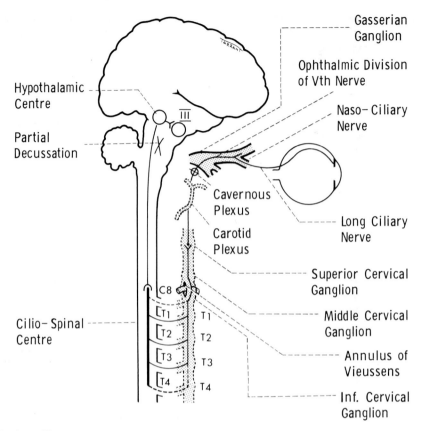

Fig. 4.6 Sympathetic pupillary system.

I. Central. *Centre* in hypothalamic region — inhibitory pathway to Edinger–Westphal group of Nucleus III. *Tract* (hypothalamic–spinal) with a partial decussation in the mid-brain so that each hypothalamic centre supplies each cilio-spinal centre but especially the contralateral: it traverses the reticular *substance of the mid-brain* and the lateral column of the cord.

II. Pre-ganglionic sympathetic. Cilio-spinal centre of Budge in the intermedio-lateral tract of the grey matter of the cord. Leaves by ventral roots of C 8, T 1, 2 and 3 (largely T 1) via the white rami communicantes → cervical sympathetic chain in which the fibres traverse the inferior cervical ganglion and the anterior loop of the ansa of Vieussens and terminate in the superior cervical ganglion.

III. Post-ganglionic sympathetic. Sup. cerv. gang. → enter the skull with the carotid plexus → cavernous plexus → travel over the Gasserian ganglion → along first division of V → naso-ciliary nerve → long ciliary nerves, entering the globe with the long ciliary arteries (some perhaps running without a relay along the long and/or sympathetic root of the ciliary ganglion → short ciliary nerves), traversing the epichoroidal space to reach the iris and terminate in the dilatator muscle.

ies. The nerve fibres pass forwards in the choroid and ciliary body to the iris.

The dilatator pupillæ is supplied by the adrenergic fibres of the cervical sympathetic nerve (Fig. 4.6). The dilatator tract probably commences in the hypothalamus not far from the constrictor centre, and it also has connections with the cerebral cortex.

From the hypothalamic centre the dilatator fibres pass downwards through the medulla oblongata into the lateral columns of the cord. The fibres leave the cord by the ventral roots of the first three dorsal and probably the last two cervical nerves, enter the rami communicantes, and run to the first thoracic or stellate ganglion. From here they pass by the anterior limb of the ansa of Vieussens into the cervical sympathetic. In this nerve

they run up the neck to the superior cervical ganglion, whence they pass with the carotid plexus into the skull. They run over the anterior part of the Gasserian ganglion and pass into the first or ophthalmic division of the fifth nerve, following the nasal branch, which they finally leave to enter the long ciliary nerves, thus avoiding the ciliary ganglion. The long ciliary nerves enter the eye on each side of the optic nerve, accompanying the long ciliary arteries. Like them, they run forwards between the choroid and sclera, enter the ciliary body and thus reach the iris.

The balance of tone between these two antagonistic innervations maintains the pupil at its normal size. The essential factor being the superior tone of the sphincter. The pupils are normally equal on the two sides; it is rare to meet with unequal pupils (*anisocoria*) in a normal person; such cases do occur, but every pathological cause must be eliminated before we rest content that the condition is an idiosyncrasy. On the other hand, the size of the pupils varies much in different people under the same conditions of illumination. In old people it is smaller than in the young, sometimes to so great an extent that the pupils are almost 'pin-point'. They are often smaller in hypermetropes, and larger in myopes than in emmetropes and are commonly smaller in blue eyes than in brown.

The pupillary reflexes

The pupils participate in several reflexes, three of which are of clinical importance:

1. The *light reflexes*, whereby if light enters an eye the pupil of this eye contracts (the *direct light reflex*), an activity shared equally by the pupil of the other eye (the *consensual light reflex*).

2. The *near reflex*, whereby a contraction occurs on looking at a near object, a reflex largely determined by the reaction to convergence, but in which accommodation also plays a part.

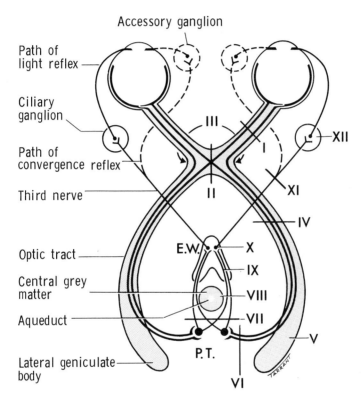

Fig. 4.7 The pupillary pathways for the light reflex. E.W, Edinger–Westphal nucleus; P.T., pretectal nucleus. The numbers denote lesions accompanied by the following symptoms

I. Optic nerve: *unilateral amaurotic paralysis* (abolition of the direct reaction on the ipsilateral side and the consensual on the contralateral side: retention of the consensual on the ipsilateral side and the direct on the contra-lateral side). Retention of the near reflex and the lid reflex.

II. Medial chiasma: *bitemporal hemianopic paralysis*.

III. Lateral chiasma: *binasal hemianopic paralysis*.

IV. Optic tract: *contralateral hemianopic paralysis* (Wernicke's reaction).

V. Lesion of the proximal part of optic tract: (normal pupillary reactions).

VI. Superficially in the region of the brachium and tectum: *contralateral hemianopic paralysis*.

VII. Central decussation: *bilateral reflex paralysis* — inactivity to light (direct and consensual) with retention of the near reflex, the lid reflexes and the psycho-sensory reactions (*bilateral Argyll Robertson pupil*) (according to Behr).

VIII. Between the decussation and the constrictor centre: ipsilateral abolition of direct and consensual reactions with retentions of both contralaterally — *unilateral Argyll Robertson pupil* (according to Behr).

IX. A partial lesion corresponding to VIII: ipsilateral abolition of direct reaction with retention of consensual reaction; retention of both contralaterally.

X. Nuclear or extensive supranuclear lesion: ipsilateral absolute pupillary paralysis.

XI. Lesion of IIIrd nerve: absolute pupillary paralysis.

XII. Lesion of ciliary ganglion: abolition of the light reflex with retention of the near reflex (*Argyll Robertson pupil*).

3. The *psycho-sensory reflex*, whereby a dilatation occurs on psychic and sensory stimuli.

The *light reflex* is initiated from the rods and cones throughout the retina. The fibres run up the optic nerve, partially decussate in the chiasma and enter the optic tracts with exactly the same distribution as the visual fibres (Fig. 4.7). Near the upper end of the tract, however, they part company with these and, instead of running to the lateral geniculate body, they enter the pretectal region. Here they are relayed in a small *pretectal nucleus*, and the new fibres, suffering a partial decussation in the mid-brain, travel to the Edinger-Westphal nucleus on each side. From these nuclei the constrictor fibres travel to each iris as already described.

The decussation is important for it explains the mechanism of the consensual as well as the direct reaction to light and also accounts for several pathological reactions such as the Argyll Robertson pupil (*q.v.*). It is obvious from a study of these paths that a lesion distal to the chiasma will abolish the direct reaction in the eye on the affected side and the consensual reaction on the other (Fig. 4.7); a lesion in the optic tract will produce a hemianopic reaction involving both eyes, while blindness due to a lesion affecting the visual pathways in or above the lateral geniculate body will leave the pupillary reactions unaltered. It is also obvious that if one eye sees and the other is blind, stimulation of the first by light will elicit the consensual reaction in the second, provided the reflex pathways in the mid-brain and third nerve are intact and the iris of this eye functioning.

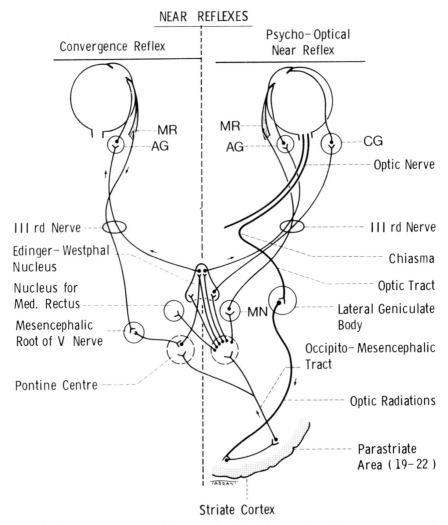

Fig. 4.8 The nerve paths of the two components of the near reflex. The afferent pathway for the convergence reflex is indicated as running up the IIIrd nerve: this is not certain. That for the accommodation reflex follows the visual fibres to the striate area of the calcarine cortex (area 17), is relayed to the parastriate area (19), whence the efferent path travels to the Edinger–Westphal nucleus via the occipito-mesencephalic tract and the pontine centre for convergence. AG, accessory ganglion; CG, ciliary ganglion; MN, nucleus for medial rectus; MR, medial rectus

The *near reflex* is initiated mainly by fibres from the medial rectus muscles which contract on convergence (Fig. 4.8). From these muscles afferent fibres run centrally, probably by the third nerve to the mesencephalic nucleus of the fifth nerve, to a presumptive convergence centre in the tectal or pre-tectal region. From this the pathway is relayed to the Edinger–Westphal nucleus and along the third nerve to the sphincter muscle of the iris, so that the pupil contracts commensurately with convergence. At the same time, accommodation reinforces the reflex by visual impulses relayed from the cortex to the Edinger–Westphal nucleus.

The *sensory reflex*, which is initiated by the stimulation of any sensory nerve to the extent of causing pain or by emotional states and excitement, is more complicated than the light reflex, for both the dilatator and the constrictor centres play a part in its production. Sensory stimulation causes first a rapid dilatation of the pupil due to augmentation of the dilatator tone through the cervical sympathetic, and then a second dilatation, rapid in onset but slow in disappearance, due to inhibition of the constrictor tone.

Minute examination of the pupil when the intensity of the light entering the eye is altered, shows that the pupil contracts and then oscillates rapidly, finally settling down into a condition of contraction which is slightly less than the summit of the first wave. In its sudden response, the pupil as it were oversteps the mark, oversteps it again in the opposite direction, and so on. Two different types of exaggeration of this oscillation are met with in abnormal conditions. One is the condition in which the oscillations are very large and easily seen, and are to a great extent independent of the light falling upon the eye. This is called *hippus*; it depends upon the rhythmic activity of the nervous centres, and is not a peripheral phenomenon. It is found in association with multiple sclerosis. More important is the lack of sustained contraction under the continued influence of light. Here the pupil contracts sluggishly when the intensity of the light is increased, but while the light is still kept constant it slowly dilates, often with superimposed sluggish oscillations. This is a pathological phenomenon dependent upon diminished conductivity in the afferent path of the light reflex, usually in the optic nerve as in optic neuritis.

The action of drugs on the intra-ocular musculature

Pupil-dilating drugs are called *mydriatics*; pupil-constricting, *miotics*; drugs which paralyse the ciliary muscle, *cycloplegics*. All drugs which dilate the pupil also paralyse the accommodation in greater or less degree; similarly, all miotics stimulate the ciliary muscle to contract, so that the eye assumes a condition of partial or complete accommodation.

All these drugs, when instilled into the conjunctival sac, are rapidly absorbed through the cornea and become effective in the inner eye. Constriction of the pupil by the third nerve is due to the liberation of acetylcholine which, almost as soon as it has been formed and has accomplished its immediate purpose, is destroyed by an enzyme, cholinesterase. One type of drug, of which atropine is the prototype, abolishes the action of acetylcholine and thus causes mydriasis by making it impossible for the sphincter to contract (*parasympatholytic drugs*). A second type of drug acts as a parasympathetic stimulant and thus causes miosis (*cholinergic drugs*); this can be done in two ways. (1) The drug may act as a direct stimulant on the myoneural junction, supplementing the normal effect of acetylcholine (the acetylcholine-like drugs, of which pilocarpine is the prototype). (2) The drug may act as an indirect stimulant by abolishing the effect of cholinesterase so that the acetylcholine formed on the activity of the third nerve continues its effect and a sustained miosis results (anticholinesterase drugs, of which eserine is the prototype.)

A further class of drugs acts on the sympathetic which exerts its activity at the post-synaptic receptor sites owing to the liberation of noradrenaline; when it has performed its function, noradrenaline diffuses back across the synaptic cleft and is actively taken up into the presynaptic neurone. As with the parasympathetic mechanism, drugs are available which stimulate the sympathetic apparatus either by stimulating the receptor sites directly or by suppressing the uptake of noradrenaline. The prototype of such *sympathomimetic drugs* is adrenaline which produces a mydriasis. The opposite effect of inducing a miosis by a paralysis of the sympathetic (*sympatholytic drugs*) is less commonly used in ophthalmology in the form of thymoxamine 0.5%.

Finally, a miosis may be induced by direct stimulation of the muscle cells by a drug such as histamine.

Parasympatholytic mydriatic drugs

Atropine is the strongest mydriatic at our disposal; it completely paralyses the sphincter pupillae and ciliary muscle. It takes a considerable time to cause complete paralysis; one drop of 1.0% atropine sulphate solution causes wide dilatation of the pupil in 30 to 40 min, and marked paralysis of accommodation in about 2 h; the effects do not pass off entirely for three to seven days.

Homatropine acts more quickly than atropine, and the effects pass off rapidly; as a 1.0% solution its effect is fully evident in three-quarters of an hour, especially if combined with cocaine (2%) which facilitates absorption and acts synergically by stimulating the dilatator mechanism. The effects pass off completely in 48 h, or much more quickly if a drop of eserine (0.5%) is instilled.

Scopolamine (*hyoscine*) (0.1–1.0%), and *duboisine*

(*hyoscyamine*) *sulphate* (0.5%) have a similar but less powerful action than atropine.

Other useful drugs of this type which have been recently introduced are *cyclopentolate hydrochloride* (Cyclogyl, Mydrilate) (0.5–2%) and *bistropamide* (Mydriacyl) the reactions of which are both rapid and temporary.

Sympathomimetic mydriatic drugs

Adrenaline (*epinephrine*) which acts on the dilatator fibres directly, produces dilatation after the instillation of four drops of a 1 in 1000 solution, the instillation being repeated in 5 min. Other drugs in this class are *phenylephrine* (*neo-synephrine hydrochloride*).

Cocaine, besides its anæsthetic effect upon the endings of the fifth nerve, inhibits the active uptake of noradrenaline into the post ganglionic sympathetic nerves. Thus noradrenaline released from the nerve remains in the synaptic cleft and activates the α receptors of the smooth muscle of the iris. It does not paralyse the sphincter, so that the dilatation of the pupil is only moderate, and the pupil continues to react to light even after prolonged application. Cocaine is therefore ineffective and adrenaline effective when the sympathetic nerve is paralysed.

Ephedrine, paredrine (*hydroxyamphetamine*) and *benzedrine* (*amphetamine*) penetrate the neurone, enter the vesicular store and cause noradrenaline to be released into the synaptic cleft.

Parasympathetic stimulatory miotics

(a) Direct stimulants (acetylcholine-like drugs). *Miochol* consists of acetylcholine chloride 1% and mannitol 5% in powder form. It is made up immediately before use in a diluent and is used to contract the pupil after cataract extraction.

Pilocarpine (0.25–5.0%) causes miosis by directly stimulating the myoneural junctions of the sphincter muscle, and is thus still active after degeneration of the nerve fibres. The action is not prolonged and may be followed by a fatigue-reaction — slight mydriasis.

Other drugs in this class are *metacholine chloride* (*mecholyl chloride*) (10–20%), usually used with neostigmine, and *furmethide* (furfuryl-trimethyl-ammonium-iodide) (10%).

(*b*) Indirect stimulants (anticholinesterase drugs). *Eserine* (*physostigmine*) (0.25–1.0%) is a powerful and useful miotic. It is able to overcome the dilatation produced by 1% atropine only with difficulty. On the other hand, it readily overcomes the dilatation produced by homatropine and cocaine. Owing to its mode of action eserine fails to produce constriction of the pupil after blocking of the third nerve. Normally it begins to contract the pupil and cause spasm of accommodation in about five minutes; its maximum effect is reached in 20 to 45 min. The effect on accommodation lasts only an hour or two, that on the pupil two to three days. When instilled into the conjunctival sac it causes some smarting and an unpleasant 'dragging' sensation; indeed, it may be so irritating as to cause vomiting, but this only occurs in very sensitive persons or when the drug is pushed. Owing to these symptoms it should not be instilled more frequently nor in stronger doses than are necessary to ensure the desired result. A 0.5% solution or one considerably weaker is often adequate.

Other drugs in this class are *neostigmine bromide* (*Prostigmin*) (3–5%), less powerful than eserine, *demecarium bromide* (Humorsol, Tosmilen) (0.5%), and three very powerful organophosphates, *di-isopropylphosphorofluoridate* (*DFP*) (0.1%), *tetra-ethylpyrophosphate* (*TEPP*) (0.1%), and *ecothiopate iodide* (Phospholine) (0.06–0.25%).

Two drugs are sometimes employed which combine the direct and indirect methods of stimulation — *doryl* (*carbachol*) (carbamyl-choline chloride) (1.0%) and *urecholine* (carbaminoyl-β-methyl-choline chloride) (1.0%). Both of these require the assistance of a wetting agent (zephiran chloride) (p. 105) to traverse the cornea with ease.

Sympatholytic miotics are rarely used topically although Thymoxamine in 0.5% solution is a powerful miotic. It is an adrenergic alpha-blocking agent, inhibiting the dilator of the pupil and leaving the sphincter unopposed.

SECTION 2

Ophthalmic optics

5

Elementary optics

It is obvious that sharp images of external objects must be formed upon the retina if these are to be clearly seen. Before considering how this is effected it will be advisable to outline the elementary principles of optics.

If white light, such as sunlight, is passed through a suitable prism or diffraction grating a spectrum is formed, consisting of rays differing from each other in wavelength. Of these certain are visible and appear to the majority of people as pure colours — red, orange, yellow, green, blue and violet in the order named, the red having the longest and the violet the shortest wavelength. The visible spectrum extends from about 723 mμ[*] at the red end to 397 mμ at the violent end, or roughly from 700 mμ to 400 mμ. Beyond the red end are infra-red rays of greater length which, when absorbed, cause a rise in temperature and are commonly known as heat rays. Beyond the violet end are waves of smaller length, the ultra-violet rays, which are capable of causing chemical actions. The longer visible rays also cause a rise in temperature, and the visible rays are also actinic, though less so than the infrared and ultra-violet, respectively. Glass absorbs some of the heat rays and many of the ultra-violet but prisms and lenses made of quartz allow most of the ultra-violet rays to pass unimpeded. The media of the eye are uniformly permeable to the visible rays between 600 mμ and 390 mμ but the cornea absorbs rays shorter than 295 mμ, the lens rays shorter than 350 mμ, and the vitreous has an absorption band with its maximum at 270 mμ. Rays between 400 mμ and 295 mμ can therefore reach the lens, those between 400 mμ and 350 mμ can reach the retina in the normal eye, and those between 40 mμ and 295 mμ can reach the retina in an eye from which the lens has been removed. Whenever absorption occurs there is the possibility of pathological changes resulting. Sunlight at sea-level is poor in ultra-violet rays, which are absorbed in the atmosphere. Ordinary glass used for spectacles absorbs rays beyond 350 mμ. Heat radiation from 1100 mμ to 700 mμ passes into the eye almost unchecked, and a large amount of it reaches the retina. The pigment epithelium on the back of the iris absorbs radiation of all wavelengths, and the same is true of the retinal pigmentary epithelium at the back of the eye.

RAYS OF LIGHT AND IMAGES

It is a familiar fact that a naked light emits light in all directions. This is transmitted in straight lines, so that we may imagine it coming from the source as an immense number of diverging straight lines, each of which is called a *ray*. Every point on such a ray represents, or is the image of, the point of light from which it springs.

This is shown by a simple experiment carried out in a dark room. Make a pinhole in a piece of cardboard (A, Fig. 5.1) and hold the cardboard in front of the candle (C) at a little distance from it. Beyond the cardboard hold up a white screen (B), so that the cardboard is between the screen and the candle. A dim image (D) of the flame will be thrown upon the screen, and it will be noticed that it is upside down so that an inverted image of the flame is formed. This is due to the fact that the cardboard cuts off all the rays of light from the candle except such as can pass through the hole. The only rays from the top of the flame which can pass through the hole are those which are caught upon the lower part of the screen. The image is dim because only a few rays of light can pass through the small hole. Now make another hole a little distance away from the first.

* A mμ is a convenient unit of length equal to 1 millimicromillimeter, or 10^{-6} mm; in the terminology standardized in 1960, the term nanometer (nm) has the same significance.

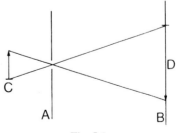

Fig. 5.1

Another inverted image of the flame is seen. If a dozen holes are made, a dozen images appear and if the holes are close together the images will overlap. If a large hole is made, so that many images overlap and all resemblance to the original flame is lost, then part of the screen becomes uniformly illuminated. If we take away the cardboard altogether the whole screen becomes illuminated, and we now know that this is because we have an infinite number of images of the flame all overlapping each other.

The speed of light varies when it traverses different substances. If the velocity is less in one medium than another, the first medium is said to be optically denser than the second.

When light, travelling in one medium, meets another medium it breaks up into two parts: part is *reflected* back into the first medium; part is *refracted* into the second medium. If the second medium is opaque none of the light is refracted.

REFLECTION

Let us now consider what happens to a ray of light when, travelling in one medium, it is reflected from the surface of a denser medium. Before it meets the surface it is called an *incident ray*; after it is reflected from the surface it is called the *reflected ray*. If a line is drawn at right angles to the surface at the point where the incident ray meets it (the *normal*), it is found to be an invariable rule that the incident ray makes the same angle with this line as the reflected ray. Put in formal language, this law of reflection is that *for all surfaces the angle of incidence is equal to the angle of reflection, and is in the same plane with it* (Fig. 5.2).

These principles can now be applied to the types of mirror which interest the ophthalmologist.

Plane mirrors. If P (Fig. 5.3) is a luminous point in front of the mirror AB, the ray PQ will be reflected towards R, and the ray PS towards T; thus the reflected rays QR and ST appear to come from *p*, a point as far behind the mirror as P is in front of it. As the rays QR and ST have to be produced backwards in order that

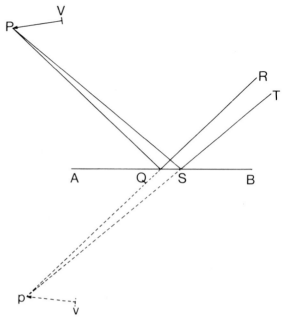

Fig. 5.3

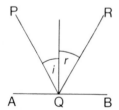

Fig. 5.2 The ray from P which strikes the mirror AB at Q is reflected to R so that PQ and QR are in the same plane, i.e., that of the paper, and the angle of incidence, *i*, is equal to the angle of reflection, *r*

they may meet, no real image is formed, and such an image is called a *virtual image*. Note that the rays reflected from a plane mirror are divergent. The same reasoning holds good for every point on the object PV, its image being *pv*, as far behind the mirror as the object is in front of it: moreover, the size of the image is equal to that of the object.

Concave mirrors. Here the normal to the surface is the radius of the sphere of which the mirror forms a part; around any radius an incident ray must be symmetrically reflected. If AH (Fig. 5.4) is part of the section of a concave mirror and PB is an object, K being the centre of the sphere, then the line HKB is called the *axis* and H the apex of the mirror. The ray PK through the centre of the sphere will obviously be reflected along itself, so that the image of P must be on PK. The ray PA, parallel to the axis and reflected symmetrically around the radius, will meet PK in *p*. Hence *p* is the image of P. Now it is found that all rays parallel to the axis and not very far removed from it cut the axis in the same point, F, and this point bisects the line HK. This point is called the *principal focus* of the mirror. If the object PB were removed a very great distance away from the mirror, all the rays which fell upon a small portion of the mirror near H would diverge so little from each other than they would all be practically parallel to BH, and the image of PB would be extremely small and situated at F. In each of these cases the image is an inverted one of the object.

It is an axiom of optics that the direction of the rays is reversible. Hence, if *pb* were an object, it would have its

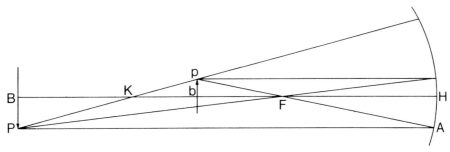

Fig. 5.4

image at PB, and if there were an object at F, all the rays from it reflected by the mirror would be parallel to the axis, and the image would be infinitely large and situated at infinity.

If the object were situated between F and H (Fig. 5.5), the rays would diverge on reflection as if they came from an object behind the mirror, much as they do with a plane mirror. The image would therefore be a virtual one, situated behind the mirror: it would be erect and larger than the object.

The important fact to remember with regard to concave mirrors is that if the object is farther away from the mirror than its focal distance, i.e., than half its radius of curvature, the image is real and inverted, situated also in front of the mirror. This is the condition which is almost always present in the ordinary use of ophthalmic instruments.

Convex mirrors. We are not accustomed to using convex mirrors in ophthalmic instruments, but it is necessary to know what happens with them, since the cornea acts as a convex mirror. By the same construction, as will be seen from Fig. 5.6, the image is always virtual, erect, and smaller than the object. As with the concave mirror, if the object is a long way off, the image will be situated at the principal focus, i.e., at a distance equal to half the radius of curvature behind the mirror.

REFRACTION

We have now to consider what happens to the refracted

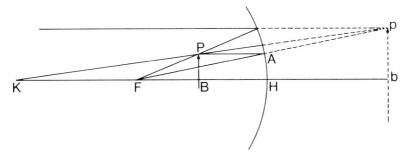

Fig. 5.5 The ray from P parallel to the axis is reflected through F, the principal focus. The ray FP is reflected parallel to the axis. The ray KP is normal to the surface, and is therefore reflected on itself. The meeting point of any two of these rays will give the situation of *p*, the image of P

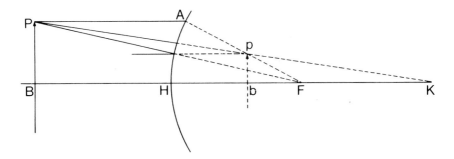

Fig. 5.6 Reflection by a convex mirror. The description of Figure 5.5 applies equally to this figure

ray when the incident ray, travelling in one medium, e.g., air, meets an optically denser medium, e.g., glass. Since the light will now travel more slowly it will be deviated towards the normal to the surface, and it will be more deviated the greater the difference in optical density between the two media. If the density of air is taken as unity, then the ratio of its density to that of the second medium is called the *index of refraction* of the medium.

Plane lamina. When an incident ray, such as LM (Fig. 5.7), meets the surface of a plate of glass with parallel sides it will be deflected towards the normal at M. When the ray passes out of the glass on the other side, it will obviously be deflected away from the new normal at N just as much as LM was deflected towards it. Hence the emergent ray NO will be parallel to the incident ray LM. If the plate of glass is very thin, NO will be practically continuous with LM.

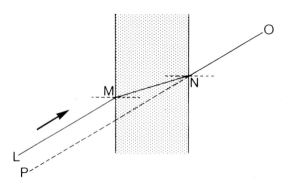

Fig. 5.7 Refraction by a plane lamina

Prisms. If we imagine the two sides of the plane lamina to meet at a point A, a prism will be formed (Fig. 5.8). In this case, being similarly refracted with reference to the normals at these surfaces, the ray will be deflected along DEFG. The ray is thus deviated towards the base of the prism. When the angles of incidence and emergence are equal, the ray is said to pass symmetrically through the prism. In these circumstances, if the prism is made of crown glass, the angle of deviation of

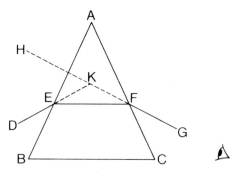

Fig. 5.8 Refraction by a prism

the ray (DKH) is approximately equal to half the refracting angle of the prism.

We are accustomed to project objects along the direction of the rays of light as they enter the eye, and in doing so we ignore the effect of refraction, since it enters relatively little into our everyday experience. If, therefore, we look at a light D through a prism, as in Fig. 5.8, the light will appear to come from H. Objects, then, seen through a prism, appear displaced towards the apex of the prism. Prisms may be categorized according to the apical angle or the angle of deviation, but more usually in *prism dioptres* ($\triangle$), a unit indicating the strength of the prism which will produce a linear apparent displacement of 1 cm of an object situated 1 m away.

Lenses. Ordinary lenses are pieces of glass with spherical surfaces. The line passing through the centres of curvature of the surfaces is called the axis of the lens. Figure 5.9 shows the chief varieties of lenses: (1) biconvex, (2) biconcave, (3) plano-convex, (4) plano-concave, (5) convexo-concave or meniscus: these names require no further explanation.

The effect of a biconvex lens upon rays of light meeting it is very similar to what would occur if it were replaced by two prisms set base to base (Fig. 5.10).

If the incident rays are parallel to the axis they will be refracted in such a manner that they all cross the axis in a single point upon the other side of the lens. This point is called the *principal focus* of the lens, and its distance

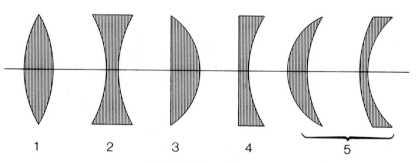

Fig. 5.9 Types of lenses

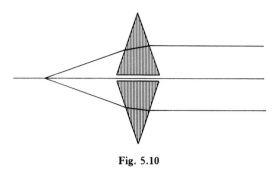

Fig. 5.10

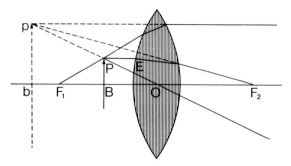

Fig. 5.12 The description of Figure 5.11 applies equally to this figure

from the lens is called the *focal distance* or *length* of the lens. When the lens has the same medium, such as air, on each side of it, the two principal foci, one on each side of the lens, are situated at equal distances from it. For thin glass lenses of low power the focal distance is equal to the radius of curvature of the two surfaces when these are equally curved. If there is an object a very long distance away from the lens, the rays which come from it are practically parallel. Hence in this case an image of the object will be formed by the lens at its principal focus; it will be inverted and very small. If the object is gradually brought nearer and nearer to the lens (Fig. 5.11) the image will recede farther and farther from it; from being very small it will grow larger, until, when the object is at the principal focus, the image will have receded to infinity and it will be infinitely large. All the rays coming from an object at the principal focus are therefore parallel to the axis and to each other after refraction. If the object is brought closer to the lens than its focal distance (Fig. 5.12) it will be found that its image is a virtual one behind the object, and that it is erect and larger than the object. The positions of the object and image bear a constant relationship to each other and are called *conjugate foci*.

There is a point in the middle of a biconvex lens which is called its *optical centre*. With thin lenses any ray which passes through this point suffers little or no de-

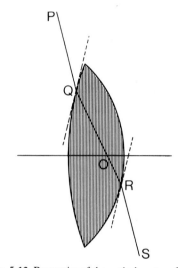

Fig. 5.13 Properties of the optical centre of a lens

viation. It is easy to understand why this is so. If PQRS (Fig. 5.13) is such a ray and tangents are drawn to the two surfaces at the points Q and R, these two tangents will be parallel to each other. Consequently, the lens acts for such a ray as if it were a plate with parallel sides, and we have already seen that in such a case the

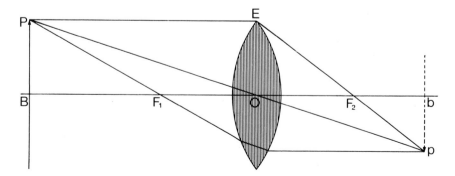

Fig. 5.11 The ray PE, parallel to the axis, is refracted through the second principal focus F_2. The ray PF_1, through the first principal focus, is refracted parallel to the axis. The ray PO, through the optical centre of the lens, is not deflected. The meeting point of any two of these rays gives the situation of p, the image of P

emergent ray is parallel to its original direction. If the lens is very thin the refracted ray will be practically continuous with the incident ray.

If we know these facts — that rays passing through the optical centre are not deviated, and that rays passing through the principal focus are parallel to the axis after refraction — we can easily construct the image of an object in any given position.

Thus, in Figure 5.11, if PB is an object, the ray PO through the optical centre O will not be deviated; the ray PE parallel to the axis will pass through the second principal focus F_2; and the ray PF_1 through the first principal focus will be parallel to the axis after refraction. Hence *pb* must be the image of PB.

The effect of a biconcave lens upon rays of light meeting it is very similar to what would occur if it were replaced by two prisms set apex to apex (Fig. 5.14).

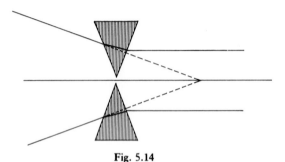

Fig. 5.14

Here, if the incident rays are parallel to the axis they will be divergent after refraction, and the amount of divergence of the individual rays will be such that if they are produced backwards they will all cross the axis in a single point upon the side of the lens from which they came. This and the corresponding point on the other side of the lens are called the principal foci. The biconcave lens also has an optical centre, situated upon the axis within it and having the same properties as in the

case of the convex lens. The image of any object formed by a concave lens can be constructed in exactly the same manner as for a convex lens (Fig. 5.15). It will be found that in every position of the object the image is always virtual, erect and smaller than the object.

Plano-convex and plano-concave lenses act like biconvex and biconcave lenses respectively, but in them the optical centre is on the curved surface at the point where the axis cuts it. Menisci act as convex or concave lenses according to whether the convex or the concave surface has the greater curvature. In them the optical centre is outside the lens.

It will have been noticed that the refractive power of a lens varies inversely as the focal distance, i.e., a lens with a short focal distance will bend the rays more than one with a longer focal distance. It is necessary to have some system of numbering lenses so as to indicate their refractive power. The most convenient system for ophthalmic purposes is that which takes a lens with a focal distance of 1 metre as a standard. Such a lens is said to have a refractive power of 1 *dioptre*.

A lens with a focal length of 0.5 m will be twice as strong as one with a focal length of 1 m: the refractive power of such a lens is therefore 2 dioptres. Similarly, a 3 D (3 dioptre) lens has a focal length of one-third of a metre, or 33 cm; a 4 D lens, 25 cm; and so on. The dioptric power is thus the reciprocal of the focal length (D = 1/F). It is important to remember that in this system the standard is a metre, not a centimetre or a millimetre; otherwise confusion may arise.

Convex lenses are indicated by a plus sign (+), concave by a minus sign (−) before the number.

Cylindrical lenses are also used in ophthalmology; their nature and use will be considered at a later stage.

We often wish to find out whether a lens is convex or concave, and what is its refractive power. There are several ways of doing this, but the simplest is the following. Hold a convex lens up near the eye and look at distant objects through it; then move the lens a little

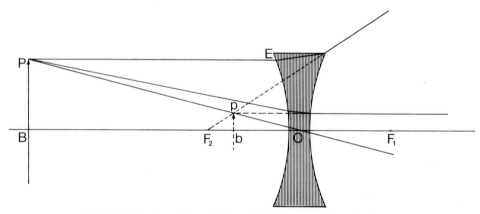

Fig. 5.15 The description of Figure 5.11 applies equally to this figure

from side to side: the distant object will seem to move in the opposite direction to that in which lens is moved. If we repeat the process with a concave lens the objects seem to move in the same direction as the lens. The reason is to be found in the fact that a convex lens forms an inverted, whilst a concave forms an erect image. If we place two lenses of opposite sign but equal curvature in contact with one another the combination will make a plate with parallel sides: such a plate, as we know, causes no practical deflection of the rays of light. Hence we can determine the strength of a lens by exactly neutralizing it with a lens of the opposite sign.

Let us take a concrete example of a particular lens which we wish to determine. We hold it up and find that distant objects seem to move in the opposite direction to the lens. We know that it is a convex lens. We then put a weak concave lens in contact with it and repeat the process. We find that with a -2 D lens objects still seem to move in the opposite direction, though not so much. With a -3 D lens there is only a trace of

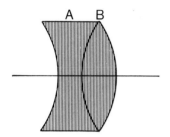

Fig. 5.16

movement, and with a -3.5 D lens there is no movement at all. We conclude that the original lens was $+3.5$ D. In performing this test it is important to have the two lenses as closely in contact as possible, and also to have their centres in contact (Fig. 5.16). If the centre of one lens is higher than that of the other they will obviously not counteract each other exactly. If they are not in contact the result will be either too high or too low.

Systems of lenses. This leads us to consider what happens when more than one lens is used, the combination forming an optical system. We will confine ourselves to cases where the system is *homocentric*, that is when all the component lenses are centred on a common optic axis in which event the principles already discussed are additively applied.

When the lenses are in contact the refractive power of the combination (D) is equal to the algebraical sum of the refractive powers of the two lenses (d_1, d_2): i.e., $D = d_1 + d_2$, or $\dfrac{1}{F} = \dfrac{1}{f_1} + \dfrac{1}{f_2}$ where F, f_1, f_2, are the respective focal distances (Fig. 5.16).

Suppose, however, that two convex lenses are separated by a distance c (Fig. 5.17). The lens A will make parallel rays converge towards a, but after a distance c they meet the lens B: hence the convergence of the rays is not expressed by $\dfrac{1}{f_1}$ but by $\dfrac{1}{f_1 - c}$. Therefore the combined effect of the lenses D, or $\dfrac{1}{F}$, is now equal to

$$\dfrac{1}{f_1 - c} + \dfrac{1}{f_2}$$

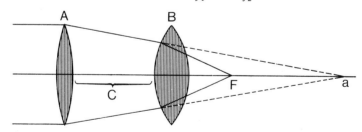

Fig. 5.17

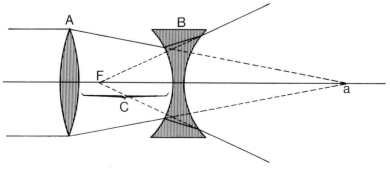

Fig. 5.18

If the second lens (B) is concave (Fig. 5.18) its effect will be one of divergence, so that it must have a negative sign, and D will now be equal to $\dfrac{1}{f_1-} - \dfrac{1}{f_2}$

It is to be noted that in the formula

$$\frac{1}{F} = \frac{1}{f_1 - c} + \frac{1}{f_2}$$

F is now the posterior focal length, the incident light impinging upon the lens the focal length of which is f_1, and being directed towards the lens the focal length of which is f_2. The following formula gives the equivalent focal length (F_e) of the combination, irrespective of the direction of light:

$$F_e = \frac{f_1 f_2}{f_1 + f_2 - c.}$$

6

Elementary physiological optics

THE OPTICAL SYSTEM OF THE NORMAL EYE

In the previous chapter we have shortly outlined the effect of a convex lens in bringing parallel rays of light to a focus (Fig. 5.11). The optical system of the eye can be deduced from this simple analogy. At first sight the matter would seem to be much more difficult, for instead of a simple convex lens with the same medium (air) on either side, the system comprises a curved optical plate (the cornea), the aqueous humour, the crystalline lens, itself optically complex, and the vitreous body. The object of this more complicated arrangement is to shorten the focal distance of the system, so that the eye may be smaller and more compact. Moreover, the medium in front is air, while behind the lens there is the vitreous which has a higher refractive index. Fortunately great simplifications can be made. The cornea has almost the same refractive index as the aqueous, which is also equal to that of the vitreous. The anterior surface of the cornea may be regarded as nearly spherical, the radius of curvature being 8 mm. The centres of curvature of the cornea and the two surfaces of the lens are all on the same straight line, which is called the *optic axis*. Indeed, from the optical point of view, with little loss of accuracy, the entire system can be regarded as one lens with one optical centre (the *nodal point*, N) which lies in the posterior part of the crystalline lens (the *schematic eye*) (Fig. 6.1).

Since the rays enter and leave the refracting system through media of different optical density, the anterior and posterior focal distances are different, the former being about 15 mm in front of the cornea, the latter about 24 mm behind it. It follows that if parallel rays fall upon the cornea they will be brought to a focus 24 mm behind it. Since the small bundles of rays which enter the pupil may be considered parallel, the image formed by the eye of distant objects will be at this point, which in the normal eye lies on the retina. Hence the normal eye in its condition of rest is so constituted that distant objects form their images upon the retina (Fig. 6.2).

The optic axis, produced backwards to meet the retina, cuts it almost exactly at the fovea centralis. Hence, any distant object on the prolongation forwards of the optic axis will have its image at the fovea, which is the best spot for distinct vision. Here, just as with a convex lens, the image is inverted; it is re-inverted psychologically in the brain.

It is easy to find the size of the retinal image which any external object will form, since the nodal point (N) corresponds to the optical centre of a convex lens. As in the case of lenses, any ray which passes through this

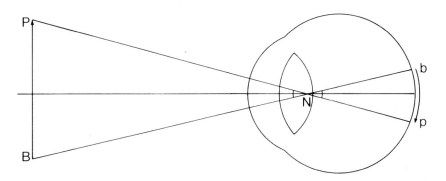

Fig. 6.1 The formation of retinal images in the schematic eye. The image *pb* of an object PB is formed by drawing lines from P and B through the nodal point (N). PNB or *p*N*b* represents the visual angle

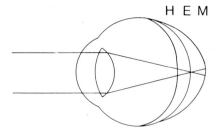

Fig. 6.2 Emmetropia, hypermetropia and myopia. In emmetropia (E), parallel rays of light are focused upon the retina. In hypermetropia (H), the eye is relatively too short; in myopia (M), it is too long

point will not be appreciably deflected. If, therefore, there is an object PB (Fig. 6.1) in front of the eye, the size of its retinal image *pb* is found by joining the extremities of the object and the nodal point and producing these lines until they meet the retina. The lines will enclose an angle, PNB, which is called the *visual angle*, the angle subtended by the object at the nodal point. It is of course equal to the angle *pNb*, which is subtended by the retinal image at the nodal point.

THE OPTICAL SYSTEM OF THE ABNORMAL EYE

In some eyes the retina is not situated in exactly the right place for the images of distant objects to be clearly focused upon it. It may be too far forward, or too far back (Fig. 6.2); in the former case the eye is said to be *hypermetropic*, in the latter *myopic*. If we consider the effect upon parallel rays we shall see that in the hypermetropic eye they have not yet come to a focus, whereas in the myopic eye they have not only come to a focus but have commenced to diverge. In each case a blurred image will be formed upon the retina, and vision will be impaired. Such conditions are called *errors of refraction* or *ametropia* (α, privative, μετρόν, measure; not according to measure). In contradistinction to hypermetropia and myopia the normal condition is called *emmetropia*. The condition of an eye, whether emmetropic, hypermetropic or myopic, is called its refraction, or more accurately its *static refraction*, since the term applies to the eye at rest. When, as commonly happens, the refractions of the two eyes are different, the condition is called *anisometropia* (α, privative; ισός, equal; μετρον, measure).

It has already been stated that in optics the direction of the rays is reversible. If we imagine a minute point on the emmetropic retina to be luminous, it will give out rays which will diverge in all directions. The rays which pass through the pupil out of the eye will have to submit to exactly the same optical deviations as the parallel rays

falling upon the cornea when they passed into the eye and will therefore be parallel to each other when they leave the eye.

Suppose, however, that the eye is hypermetropic because it is too short (Fig. 6.2). The rays coming from a point on the retina will be relatively more divergent than the corresponding rays of the emmetropic eye before they fall upon the back of the lens. (Compare the effect of placing an object closer to a convex lens than its principal focus, Fig. 5.12.) They will therefore still be divergent when they leave the eye, though of course not so divergent as when they were passing through the vitreous. In fact, their direction will be the same as if they came from a point behind the eye. The nearer the retina is to the lens, the more divergent they will be, and the nearer to the back of the eye will be the point from which they seem to come. This virtual point (R) behind the eye is called the *remote* or *far point* of the eye. The point on the retina and this point behind the eye are really *conjugate foci* (Fig. 6.3).

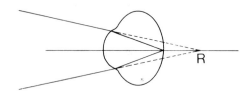

Fig. 6.3 Hypermetropia eye. Rays from a point on the retina are divergent when they emerge from the eye, as if they came from the point, R, behind the eye

Suppose now that the eye is myopic because it is too long (Fig. 6.2). The rays coming from a point on the retina will be relatively less divergent than the corresponding rays in the emmetropic eye before they fall on the back of the lens. (Compare the effect of placing an object farther away from a convex lens than its principal focus, Fig. 5.11.) The refractive media in front will therefore cause them to converge more than in the emmetropic eye. They will thus be convergent when they leave the eye, and will cross at a point (R) somewhere in front of the eye (Fig. 6.4). The farther the retina is from the lens, i.e., the higher the degree of myopia, the more convergent they will be, and the nearer to the front of the eye will be the point where they

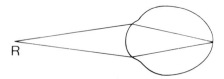

Fig. 6.4 Myopic eye. Rays from a point on the retina are convergent when they emerge from the eye, so that they cross at a real point, R, in front of the eye

cross. This point is again the conjugate focus to the point of the retina, but in this case it is a real point. It is also called the remote or far point of the eye.

We have seen that in the emmetropic eye the emergent rays are parallel to each other. Since parallel rays meet at infinity, the far point of the emmetropic eye is at infinity.

We have seen also that in every case the far point and a point on the retina are conjugate foci. Using the principle of the reversibility of rays, any object situated at the far point of any eye will have a sharp image upon the retina (Fig. 6.4). Thus the emmetrope sees only distant objects clearly with his eyes at rest, since the rays from such objects are nearly parallel; for practical purposes this applies to objects more than six metres away. On the other hand, a patient with myopia can only see things which are near; he is 'short-sighted'. He can see things at a distance better if he screws up his eyes because he thus makes a narrow slit through which to look, and this slit acts in the same way as the hole in the cardboard in the experiment illustrated in Figure 5.1. The term myopia originated in this peculiarity ($\mu\upsilon\epsilon\iota\nu$, to shut; $\omega\psi$, the eye). Again, a patient with hypermetropia can see neither distant nor near objects clearly with his eyes at rest, since the far point is virtual, and it is impossible to place an object at its situation. We shall see later that when young he is better off than the myope since he can alter his refractive power by accommodation.

Errors of refraction may be due to causes other than axial shortening or lengthening of the eye (*axial ametropia*). They may be due to alterations in the refractive indices of the media, or to alterations in the curvatures of the refractive surfaces; ametropia due to these causes is called *index or curvature ametropia*, respectively. Index ametropia is rare, apart from changes in the refractivity of the lens.

Curvature ametropia has a special importance because it is the cause of another very troublesome error of refraction, called *astigmatism*. In most eyes the areas of the refractive surfaces uncovered by the pupil and used in vision are very nearly spherical. Sometimes, however, they are not. In most of these cases it is the cornea which is at fault, and the error is generally of such a nature that its surface is flatter from side to side than it is from above downwards, perhaps because the pressure of the lids on the globe tends to squeeze it above and below.

When the cornea has its direction of greatest and least curvature at right angles to one another, the condition is called *regular astigmatism*. In the commonest form when the vertical meridian is the more curved, the condition is generally called regular astigmatism 'according to the rule'; the reverse is said to be 'against the rule', but not infrequently the axes are oblique. Often, as after ulceration, the surface of the cornea is irregular so that the rays of light are refracted irregularly without any symmetry and different groups form foci in various positions. This is called *irregular astigmatism*: it cannot be corrected, and can only occasionally be improved by lenses.

Although astigmatism is chiefly due to faulty curvature of the cornea, in some cases there is also lenticular astigmatism. This is not generally due to unequal curvature of the surfaces, but to slight tilting of the lens, so that the incident rays fall upon it obliquely. If we look through a tilted glass lens at printed matter we shall see that the letters become distorted and elongated in one direction; this is a form of astigmatism. The astigmatism of the crystalline lens is generally of such a nature that it tends to counteract the corneal astigmatism although sometimes it adds to the effect.

A regularly astigmatic surface is said to have a *toric* curvature. In it the more curved meridian will have more refractive or convergent power than the less curved: hence if parallel rays fall upon such a surface

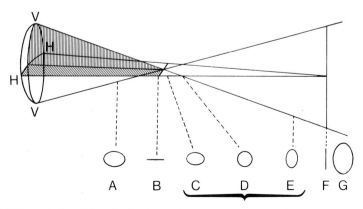

Fig. 6.5 Sturm's conoid. VV, vertical meridian of refracting surface, more curved than H H, the horizontal meridian. A, B, C, D, E, F, G, sections of conoid. From B to F is the focal interval of Sturm. D shows the circle of least diffusion

the vertical rays will come to a focus sooner than the horizontal. The rays after refraction will be perfectly symmetrical when referred to the vertical and horizontal planes but they will have two foci. The whole bundle of rays is called *Sturm's conoid*, and the distance between the two foci is called the *focal interval* of Sturm. It is difficult to represent this conoid on a plane surface (Fig. 6.5), but we can see what sections of the bundle or pencil of rays would look like at different distances from the refractive surface (Fig. 6.5, A–G).

At A the section will be a horizontal oval or oblate ellipse, because the vertical rays are converging more rapidly than the horizontal. At B the vertical rays have come to a focus, while the horizontal are still converging: the section will be a horizontal straight line. At C, D, and E the vertical rays are diverging and the horizontal are still converging. At one place in this focal interval there will be a spot (D) where the vertical rays have diverged from the axis exactly as much as the horizontal rays have converged towards it. Here the section is a circle, which is called the *circle of least diffusion*. At F the horizontal rays come to focus while the vertical are diverging: the section will be a vertical straight line. Beyond this point, as at G, both sets of rays are diverging, and the section will always be a vertical oval or prolate ellipse.

If the retina is situated at any of these points of section, it is obvious that the retinal image will always be blurred; it is because the rays never come to a focus in a single point that the condition is called *astigmatism* (α, privative; $\sigma\tau\iota\gamma\mu\alpha$, a point). If the retina cuts the conoid at A, where none of the rays has come to a focus, every meridian will be in the same condition, though in different degree, as in the axial hypermetropic eye: this condition is therefore called *compound hypermetropic astigmatism*. If the retina is at B the vertical meridian will be in the condition of an emmetropic eye, while the horizontal will still be in the condition of hypermetropia: this condition is called *simple hypermetropic astigmatism*. At C, D and E the vertical meridian will be in the condition of a myopic, and the horizontal still in that of a hypermetropic eye: this is called *mixed astigmatism*. At F the vertical meridian is still myopic, whilst the horizontal is in the same condition as in an emmetropic eye: this is *simple myopic astigmatism*. Beyond F, as at G, both meridians are in the condition of an axial myope, the rays having crossed in the vitreous: this is *compound myopic astigmatism*. All these positions of the retina are met with in actual practice, although there is often a combination of axial and curvature defects.

Distant vision is often found to be surprisingly good with relatively high degrees of mixed astigmatism, probably because the circle of least diffusion falls on or near the neuro-epithelium of the retina.

THE CORRECTION OF AMETROPIA WITH LENSES

It is obvious that, in hypermetropia, if we give the rays the requisite amount of convergence before they enter the eye by placing a convex lens in front of it, they will be brought to a focus upon the retina (Fig. 6.6). This is what is done by means of spectacles. The refractive or convergent power of a convex lens is the reciprocal of its focal distance. Hence in hypermetropia of 1 D, a convex lens of 1 D or 1 m focal distance placed in contact with the cornea, acting in combination with the refractive power of the eye, would bring the rays to a focus on the retina. But lenses are only rarely worn in contact with the cornea. If the lens is placed 20 mm in front of the cornea its focal length will have to be 1020 mm instead of 1000 mm, but this small difference is negligible, and we are accustomed to measure errors of refraction by the strength of the lens which is required when it is placed in the ordinary position of a spectacle lens.

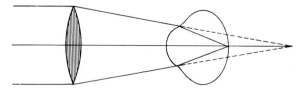

Fig. 6.6 Hypermetropic eye. Parallel incident rays brought to a focus on the retina by means of a suitable convex lens

Similarly in myopia, if we give the rays the requisite amount of divergence before they enter the eye they will be brought to a focus upon the retina. We do this by placing a concave lens in front of the eye (Fig. 6.7). Here we should want a –1 D lens in contact with the cornea to correct a myopia of 1 D, i.e., an eye the far point of which is 1 m in front of the eye. If the glass is worn about 20 mm in front of the eye it will have to be somewhat stronger, i.e., it will have to be a focal distance of 980 mm instead of 1000 mm.

There is an advantage in having the correcting lenses in axial ametropia in the position of the anterior focus of the eye, because in these conditions the size of the retinal image is the same as if the eye were emmetropic (Fig. 6.8A and C). The anterior focus is about 15 mm in front

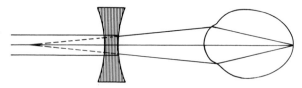

Fig. 6.7 Myopic eye. Parallel incident rays brought to a focus on the retina by means of a suitable concave lens

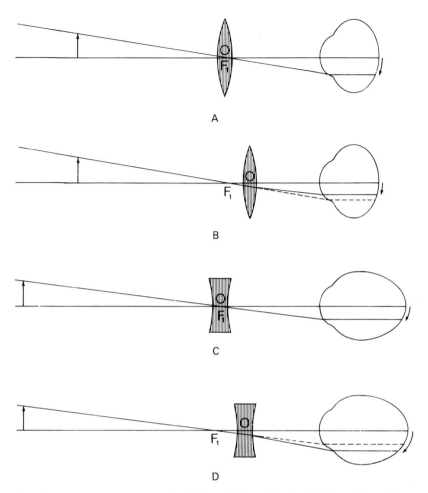

Fig. 6.8A and C Effect of correcting lenses upon the size of the retinal image. In A and C where the optical centre of the lens, O, coincides with the anterior focal point of the eye, F_1, the size of the retinal image is the same as in emmetropia. When the lens is closer to the eye than the anterior focal distance of the eye the size of the retinal image is diminished (convex lens, B) or increased (concave lens, D)

of the eye. The optician aims at placing the optical centre of the spectacle lens 12–13 mm from the cornea. We have already discovered that the farther the lens is from the eye, the convex lens in hypermetropia has to be weaker, and the concave lens in myopia stronger. There is also an effect on the size of the retinal image (see Fig. 6.8B and D). If the lens is more than 15 mm from the cornea the retinal image in hypermetropia is larger, and in myopia smaller than the emmetropic image. The increase in size in hypermetropia is advantageous, but the diminution in myopia is a disadvantage, especially in very high degrees. Consequently, in the latter the spectacles ought to be made to fit as closely to the eyes as possible.

In astigmatism we must obtain some means of affecting one set of rays more than the other. This means is found in cylindrical lenses.

Suppose CDEF is a cylinder of glass (Fig. 6.9): AB is called the axis of the cylinder. If a slice is cut off the cylinder by a plane parallel to the axis, it would form a cylindrical lens. Figure 6.10 gives representations of a convex and a concave cylinder. The direction ab is called the axis of the cylinder, since it is parallel to the axis of the original cylinder from which the slice may be supposed to have been taken. It is important not to confuse the axis of a spherical and the axis of a cylindrical lens, as they are totally different things. The axis of a cylinder has just been described: the axis of a spherical lens is the line joining the centres of curvature of the two surfaces.

Parallel rays falling upon a cylindrical lens will be affected in different ways. In the direction of its axis it is simply a plane lamina with parallel sides, so that it will have no effect upon the rays. In the direction at right angles to its axis it is spherical on one side and plane on

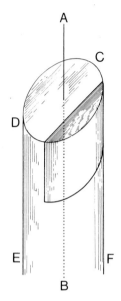

Fig. 6.9

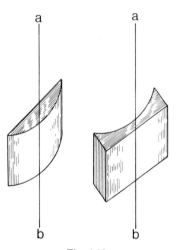

Fig. 6.10

It is to be noted that the line is in the direction of the axis of the cylinder. If another convex cylinder of the same strength were held with its axis at right angles to the first, it would obviously form a focal line perpendicular to the first focal line. If the two cylinders are put in contact with their axes at right angles, all the rays after refraction must pass through both lines. The only place where they can go through both lines is where the lines intersect. Hence we see that two cylindrical lenses of equal strength, placed in contact with their axes at right angles, act exactly like a convex spherical lens of the same strength as either of the cylinders.

Optical aberrations

As in all optical systems in practical use, the eye is by no means optically perfect; the lapses from perfection are called *aberrations*. To a large extent, however, they affect the peripheral rays and are thus eliminated by the iris which acts like the diaphragm of any ordinary optical system, such as a photographic camera or a microscope. In discussing the effects of spherical mirrors in reflecting, and of spherical surfaces in refracting rays of light, we said that in each case they were all brought to a focus in a single point. This is really only an approximation which is sufficiently accurate for rays close to the axis. In a convex spherical lens, for instance, only parallel rays near the axis meet at the principal focus; rays farther away from the axis, however, are refracted too much, so that they cut the axis nearer the lens than the principal focus thus causing a blurring of the edges of the image (*spherical aberration*) (Fig. 6.13). A diaphragm cutting off these peripheral rays would prevent the blurring. In the eye the surfaces are not spherical, especially near the periphery, so that much more aberration is liable to occur, but the iris reduces the effects to a minimum.

There is also another form of aberration due to the imperfect refraction at spherical surfaces. White light is made up of all the colours of the spectrum. The component rays are refracted differently, the short violet rays most, the long red least. Hence there is a tendency for the white light to be split up into its components, in which case the image will have a coloured edge (*chromatic aberration*); this effect in the eye, however, is small.

Several other aberrations occur which are relatively unimportant; their effect, however, may be increased and others introduced, particularly affecting oblique

the other: it will therefore act exactly like a plano-convex or a plano-concave lens, i.e., it will make the rays either converge or diverge (Fig. 6.11). If a convex cylinder is held between a point of light and a screen, a position can be found for the screen such that a sharp bright line is thrown upon it (Fig. 6.12): this is the *focal line* of the cylinder.

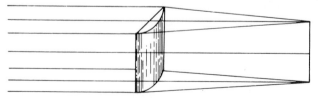

Fig. 6.11 Refraction of parallel rays through a plano-convex cylinder

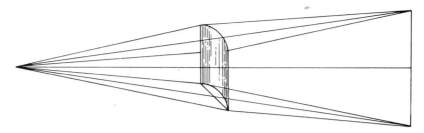

Fig. 6.12 Refraction of divergent rays from a point of light through a plano-convex cylinder

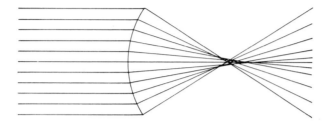

Fig. 6.13 Spherical aberration

and peripheral rays, when the optical system is complicated by spectacles.

ACCOMMODATION

We have to consider now how a person with normal sight can see not only distant objects, but also near ones. If an object is situated near the eye, as at ordinary reading distance (about 30 cm), the divergence of the rays which it emits cannot be neglected. Since the converging power of the refractive media of the emmetropic eye is only strong enough to make parallel rays come to a focus on the retina, it is obvious that divergent rays falling upon the cornea will not have come to a focus (Fig. 6.14). The necessary increase in their convergence is accomplished by augmenting the refractive power of the crystalline lens by increasing the curvature of its surfaces in the act of *accommodation*.

The curvature of the surfaces of the lens at rest in the eye is approximately spherical, the radius of curvature

of the anterior surface being 10 mm, that of the posterior surface 6 mm. In accommodation, the curvature of the posterior surface remains almost the same, but the anterior surface changes so that in strong accommodation its radius of curvature becomes 6 mm. The eye in this condition, which is called its *dynamic refraction*, has a much increased converging effect upon the incident rays.

The mechanism by which this change in the curvature of the lens is brought about has excited much controversy. It would seem that the lens itself has a considerable amount of elasticity which determines its normal non-accommodated form (Fig. 6.15). The capsule, however, is more elastic, and when the ciliary muscle contracts the ciliary body approaches the lens, thus slackening the zonule so that the capsule, relieved of tension, is able to mould the lens into its accommodated form. The peculiar shape assumed by the lens thus deformed may be due to the peculiar configuration of the capsule which is thicker behind the iris than in the central area. The shape of the lens at any one time is thus the

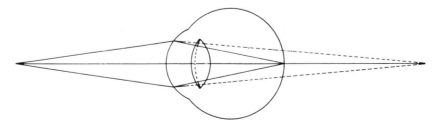

Fig. 6.14 Effect of accommodation. The dotted lines show the curvature of the anterior surface of the lens and the course of rays with the eye at rest (static refraction). The solid lines show the curvature of the anterior surface of the lens and the course of rays with active accommodation (dynamic refraction)

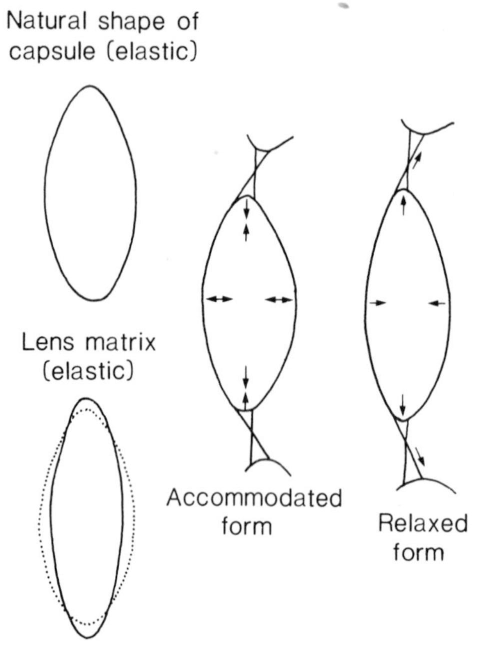

Natural shape of
capsule (elastic)

Lens matrix
(elastic)

Accommodated
form

Relaxed
form

Fig. 6.15 The changes in the lens with accommodation. During accommodation the elastic capsule imposes its natural conoidal shape on the elastic lens substance which resists the former (after Weale)

result of a balance between its own elasticity and that of its capsule.

Our control over the ciliary muscle, though involuntary, is very delicate, so that all distances up to quite close to the eye can be accurately focused. The nearest point at which small objects can be clearly distinguished is called the *near point*, or *punctum proximum*. At this point accommodation is exerted to its maximum, the lens capsule is as slack as it is possible to make it, and an object closer to the eye could only be seen clearly by using a convex lens.

It has been shown that the *far point* or *punctum remotum* of the eye varies according to its static refraction, that is, whether it is emmetropic, hypermetropic, or myopic. The near point also varies with the static refraction, and again with the age of the patient, the reason being that the lens becomes less plastic as age advances. We have stated that the lens is a mass of epithelium of which the central part is the oldest; as it gets older the central cells become tougher and more compressed, thus forming a relatively hard nucleus. The nucleus is less plastic than the younger cortex and, as age advances, more and more of the fibres become converted into nucleus. Consequently the lens tends to respond less and less to changes in tension of the capsule. Thus, a child of 10 is able to see a small object clearly when it is only 7 cm from the eye, while a person of 30 years of age may not see clearly at less than 14 cm.

Normally the ciliary muscle has a considerable amount of tone which cannot be relaxed so that the full degree of hypermetropia is only apparent when this muscle is paralysed by a cycloplegic drug. This portion of the total hypermetropia which can only be revealed under atropine is called the *latent hypermetropia*. The remainder, which is normally uncorrected, is called the *manifest hypermetropia*. The sum of the two gives the *total hypermetropia*. Of the manifest hypermetropia, that part which can be relaxed by accommodation is termed *facultative*; that which cannot be thus relaxed, *absolute*. In extreme youth nearly all the hypermetropia is latent: the lens is so resilient that it is impossible to prevent its responding to the slightest stimulus. As the lens becomes less plastic more and more of the hypermetropia becomes manifest, until finally, when accommodation disappears entirely, all the hypermetropia is manifest. The older the patient, therefore, the more nearly the manifest hypermetropia represents the total amount.

We have pointed out that the refractive power of a lens in dioptres is the reciprocal of its focal distance measured in metres and that the same method is applied to measure the static refractive powers of the eye. Applying the same method to the dynamic refractive power, the child of 10, whose near point is 7 cm from his eye, has a refractive power of $100/7 = 14$ D, and a man of 30, whose near point is 14 cm from his eye, has a refractive power of $100/14 = 7$ D.

By this means we can obtain a general rule for indicating the amount or *amplitude of accommodation*, not only of emmetropic but also of hypermetropic or myopic eyes. This is given by the formula $A = P - R$, which states that the amplitude of accommodation (A) is equal to the refractive power of the eye when fully accommodated (P) (i.e., the reciprocal of the distance of the near point in metres) less the refractive power of the eye at rest (R) (i.e., the reciprocal of the distance of the far point in metres).

Thus, the emmetropic child of 10 has an amplitude of accommodation of $100/7 - 1/\infty = 14 - 0 = 14$ D. Similarly in the case of an emmetrope whose near point is 12.5 cm from his eye, the amplitude of accommodation (A) $= 1000/125 - 1/\infty = 8$ D. Again, a myope of 2 D whose near point is 8 cm in front of his eye will have an amplitude of accommodation (A) $= 100/8 - 2 = 10.5$ D. Again, in the case of a hypermetrope of 3 D whose near point is 12.5 cm from his eye, the far point is behind the eye and distances measured in this direction must have the opposite sign to those measured in front of the eye. Hence A $= 1000/125 - (-3) = 8 + 3 = 11$ D.

The numbers given by these calculations for the amplitude of accommodation give the strength of the convex lens which would have to be placed in contact with the cornea in order that the near point might be brought to the required distance without using the accommodation. Several interesting facts come to light from the calculations. Thus a hypermetrope of 3 D has to exert 11 D of accommodation in order that he may see clearly at 12.5 cm, while an emmetrope has to exert only 8 D of accommodation to bring about the same result. We see, then, that the hypermetrope has to exert an amount of accommodation equivalent to the amount of his hypermetropia in order to focus parallel rays upon his retina and see distant objects clearly. Again, the myope of 2 D, whose far point is 0.5 m or 50 cm, from his eye, can see clearly at that distance without accommodating, but he has to exert 10.5 D of accommodation in order that he may see clearly at 8 cm from his eye. This patient, then, has to exert nearly as much accommodation to alter his points of clear vision from 50 to 8 cm, i.e., through 42 cm, as a hypermetrope of 3 D has to employ in order to move his point of distinct vision from infinity up to 12.5 cm. We see, therefore, that the *range of accommodation*, that is, the distance between the far point and the near point, is not always the same for a given amplitude.

The effect of age upon the static and dynamic refraction is given in Figure 6.16, which is compiled from a large number of statistics. From this graph we see that even the far point alters in advanced age. After about 50 years the eye tends to become hypermetropic, so that at 80 it has about 2.5 D of hypermetropia; this is due to an alteration in the refractive index of the lens so that it has a weaker converging power.

The refractive indices of the successive layers of the lens increase from the periphery towards the nucleus. The effect is two-fold: it tends to correct aberration by increasing the convergence of the central rays, and the total refractive index of the whole lens is increased, becoming greater than the refractive index of the nucleus. The lens may be looked upon as a central biconvex lens encapsulated in two menisci (Fig. 6.17); these act as concave lenses because the curvature of the nucleus is greater than that of the periphery of the lens. Hence they tend to counteract the effect of the central lens, but not so much as if their refractive indices were the same. In old age the index of the peripheral layers usually increases, so that the total refractive index of the lens becomes less, and the eye becomes hypermetropic.

If we turn our attention to the curve of the near point

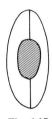

Fig. 6.17

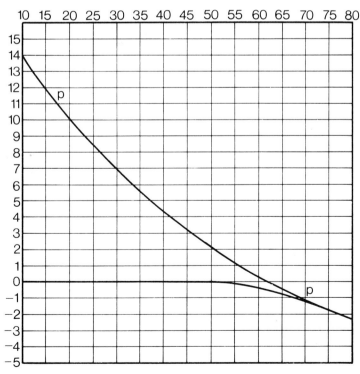

Fig. 6.16 Chart of static (lower curve) and maximum dynamic (upper curve) refraction at various ages (Donders). Abscissa, ages; ordinate, accommodation in dioptres

in Figure 6.16 we see that the amplitude of accommodation gradually diminishes throughout life. Since we are accustomed to hold books for reading at about 25 cm from the eye, in order to see clearly we must exert 100/25 or 4 D of accommodation which is all that an emmetrope has available at a little over 40 years of age; he will still be able to see clearly at 25 cm, but not closer. If he is about 46 he will have only 3 D of accommodation left and will have to hold his book farther off, at 100/3 or 33 cm, a disability which will increase as age advances. This is the condition which is called *presbyopia* (πρεσβυς, old).

It is a common error to think that presbyopia is a condition which commences at about 45 years of age in emmetropes, and earlier in hypermetropes. It is important to remember that the condition has been increasing throughout life and first becomes troublesome when the near point of the eye has receded so far that it is beyond comfortable reading or working distance.

There are two other phenomena which occur with accommodation, one affecting the iris, the other the direction of the eyes. In order that we may see a near object with both eyes they must each turn inwards or *converge*. The amount of convergence, like the amount of accommodation, depends upon the distance of the object so that there is a close relationship between accommodation and convergence. We shall have more to say upon this subject when we consider the various forms of squint.

When we accommodate for a near object the pupil becomes smaller, or contracts. Experiment has shown that this movement of the iris is associated with the accompanying act of convergence rather than with accommodation. This contraction of the pupil during accommodation helps to diminish aberration by cutting out the peripheral parts of the lens, increases the depth of focus and compensates for the relative increase of light entering the eye from near objects. It may be noted that in accommodation the ciliary muscle contracts equally all round the circumference and equally and simultaneously in the two eyes, so that the activity can correct neither astigmatism nor anisometropia.

7

The determination of the refraction

In determining the refraction of the eye the best routine is, first, to estimate the condition objectively, and then to verify and adjust these findings by subjective tests. The objective methods commonly employed are retinoscopy and the use of the refractometer or (for the corneal astigmatism) the keratometer.

RETINOSCOPY

The theory of retinoscopy

Retinoscopy or, more correctly, *skiascopy or the shadow test*, is the most practicable method of estimating the condition of the refraction objectively. It depends upon the fact that when light is reflected from a mirror into the eye the direction in which the light travels across the pupil varies with the refraction of the eye. The light seen in the pupil is the blurred image of the illuminated area of the fundus as seen by the observer when he accommodates for the observed pupil; it is bordered by a shadow representing the image of the edge of the illuminated area. If the light is thrown into a myopic eye from a concave mirror at a distance of 1 metre and the mirror is tilted in any direction the light, or, what is easier to observe, the shadow, moves across the pupil in the same direction (Fig. 7.1). If a plane mirror is used,

the other conditions remaining the same, the shadow will be seen to move in the opposite direction to the movement of the mirror. If the eye is hypermetropic the direction in which the shadow moves is the opposite to that with the myopic eye. If the eye has one dioptre of myopia no shadow will be visible; the pupil will be either completely illuminated or completely dark. The method therefore consists in placing lenses in front of the eye until no shadow is seen; if the surgeon is 1 m away from the patient the combination of the optical system of the patient's eye and the lenses is equal to 1 dioptre of myopia.

A simple optical explanation is as follows. Rays from a point of light in front of the eye illuminate a circular area of the fundus, varying in size according to the refraction of the eye (Fig. 7.2). If the point of light moves upwards, the light on the retina will move downwards.

In the hypermetropic eye the rays reflected from the illuminated area will be divergent, as if they came from a point behind the eye. This far point, corresponding to the illuminated area, will move in the same direction, i.e., downwards. If an observer, placed in front of the eye, looks towards a point of light situated at the position of the far point, but accommodates for the position of the observed pupil, he will see a circle of light with a blurred margin, not a point, because he is not accommo-

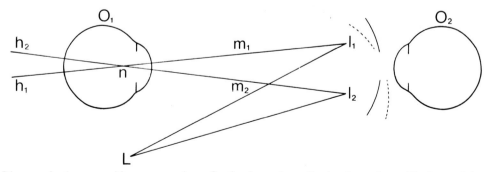

Fig. 7.1 Diagram of retinoscopy with a concave mirror. O_1, the observed eye; O_2, the observer's eye. The image of the source of light (L) is formed at l_1 (the immediate source of light) by the mirror. If O_1 is hypermetropic a virtual image of l_1 is formed on the line $l_1 n$, passing through the nodal point n, as at h_1. If O_1 is myopic a real inverted image is formed as at m_1. If the mirror is tilted downwards, as shown by the dotted line, l_1 *moves to* l_2, h_1 to h_2. and m_1 to m_2. This shows that the shadow moves in the opposite direction in hypermetropia and the same direction in myopia

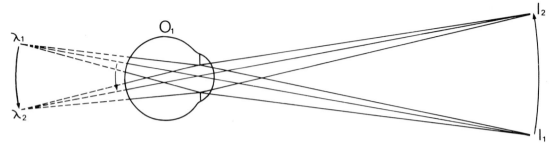

Fig. 7.2 Showing the course of incident rays and field of illumination of the fundus in hypermetropia: l_1 forms a virtual image at λ_1; l_2 at λ_2. The field of illumination is determined by the pupil of O_1

dating accurately for the far point. When the illumination on the retina moves down, the circle of light which the observer sees will appear to move down also (Fig. 7.2).

In a highly myopic eye, on the other hand, the rays of light reflected from the illuminated area on the fundus will be convergent and will cross at a real point in front of the eye. This far point, corresponding to the illuminated area, will move upwards when the illuminated area moves downwards. If an observer placed in front of the eye and farther from it than the far point, looks towards the far point but accommodates for the observed pupil, he will see a circle of light with a blurred margin. When the illumination on the retina moves down, the circle of light which the observer sees will move up, i.e., in the opposite direction to the movement in the case of the hypermetropic eye (Fig. 7.3).

If the observer's eye is one metre in front of the observed eye, and the latter has 1 D of myopia, the far point of the observed eye will be at the situation of the observer's eye (Fig. 7.4). In this case a very slight movement of the light on the observed fundus will throw the image at the far point off the observer's eye altogether; in other words, the observed pupil will appear to be completely bright or completely dark.

If, again, the observed eye is emmetropic, its far point will be at infinity; we may regard it as being infinitely far behind the observed eye. Here, again, there will be scarcely any shadow, although in reality there is a very faint shadow moving in the same direction as for the hypermetropic eye.

The type of mirror used is an entirely subsidiary matter; it merely determines the direction of movement of the immediate source of light, i.e., the point of light in

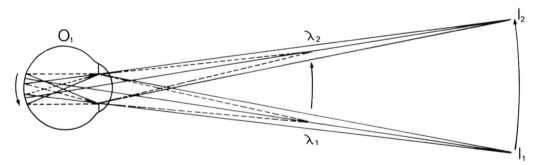

Fig. 7.3 Showing the course of incident rays in myopia

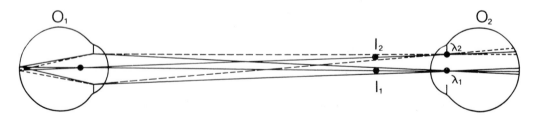

Fig. 7.4 Showing the course of the emergent rays at the point of reversal. So long as λ_1 is in the pupillary area of O_2, the pupil of O_1 appears uniformly illuminated, and there is no shadow. Directly λ_1 passes to λ_2 the whole of the light is cut off, so that the pupil of O_1 becomes completely dark

front of the eye which has been considered above. The image of a real light behind the patient's head, formed by a concave mirror, is situated in front of the mirror. If the mirror is tilted up, the image moves up. The image of a real light behind the patient's head, formed by a plane mirror, is situated as far behind the mirror as the light is in front of it. When the mirror is tilted up, the image moves down.

Hence under the actual conditions of retinoscopy with a *plane mirror*, when the mirror is tilted to the right the immediate source of light moves to the left, and

a. In the hypermetropic eye, the circle of light on the fundus and the shadow seen in the pupil move to the right,

b. In the myopic eye (above −1 D) the circle of light on the fundus moves to the right, and the shadow seen in the pupil moves to the left.

c. In the myopic eye of −1 D there is no shadow,

d. In emmetropia and myopia of less than −1 D there is a very faint shadow moving to the right.

Stated as a mere guide to practice, with the plane mirror the shadow moves in the same direction as the mirror in hypermetropia and in the opposite direction in myopia above one dioptre; in myopia of one dioptre there is no shadow and in emmetropia and myopia of less than one dioptre there is a very faint shadow moving in the same direction as the mirror.

In actual retinoscopy the whole of the image of the illuminated area of fundus cannot be seen at once; the shadow is part of the circumference. In high degrees of ametropia the shadow has a distinctly curved border, it is very dark, and it moves slowly. In low degrees of ametropia the border of the shadow looks straight; it is faint, and it moves rapidly.

The movement of the shadow, being a purely optical phenomenon, is, of course, independent of the cause of the ametropia. Consequently, in astigmatism, if one axis

is hypermetropic and the other myopic (mixed astigmatism) the shadow moves in opposite directions in the two meridians. Often the periphery of the cornea is flatter than the centre; correction of the refraction of the central part, which is the more important, will then differ from that of the peripheral part. These variations produce very puzzling shadows in many cases.

The practice of retinoscopy

Retinoscopy is conducted in a dark room at least six metres long. The surgeon sits at one metre from the patient. The patient wears a trial frame (Fig. 7.5) and fixes a spot of light at the far end of the room. A light may be placed behind and above the patient's head and the surgeon manipulates a plane mirror, perforated with a central hole through which he looks as he reflects light into the patient's eye, or he may use a self-luminous retinoscope with a corresponding optical arrangement.

The light is reflected into the eye, and as the mirror is slowly tilted from one side to the other, the direction in which the shadow moves is noted. The horizontal meridian should be observed first, then the vertical. If the shadow appears to swirl round, not moving in the same meridian as the mirror, the eye is astigmatic, and the mirror is not moving in a direction which corresponds to either axis. A direction of movement can then be found in which the shadow will move either directly with or against the mirror; this is one of the principal axes of the astigmatism. The other axis is at right angles in regular astigmatism.

If the shadow moves with the mirror, progressively stronger convex lenses are put in the trial frame in front of the eye until no shadow can be seen. A still stronger convex glass is placed in the frame when the shadow probably moves against the mirror. We now know that the refraction has been over-corrected. The point at which there is absolutely no shadow — the point of re-

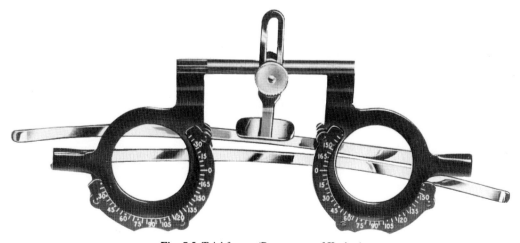

Fig. 7.5 Trial frame. (By courtesy of Keeler.)

versal — is somewhere between the last two lenses, and we know that at that point the refraction of the eye *minus* the lens is equivalent to one dioptre of myopia.

If, for example, the shadow can still be seen to move with the mirror with +4 D lens in the frame, and moves against it with +4.5 D, we shall not be far wrong in considering that the point of reversal is +4.25 D. A lens of +4.25 D would therefore make the eye one dioptre myopic. The actual refraction is therefore +3.25 D.

Similarly, for spherical myopia, if −4 D eliminates the shadow against the mirror and −4.5 D gives a distinct shadow with the mirror, we know that −4.25 D will still leave the eye with − 1 D. Hence the refraction is −5.25 D.

In astigmatism each principal meridian is corrected separately in the same way. When one meridian is approximately corrected the shadow assumes the shape of a band, the edge of the band being parallel to the axis of the corrected meridian. Even if the light is not moved in a direction accurately at right angles to this meridian, the shadow still seems to move in the same direction. This is due to an optical illusion. If, in Figure 7.6, a straight edge, AB, is placed obliquely behind a circular hole in a card and is then moved horizontally in the direction of the arrow C, it will appear to be moving in the direction of the arrow D at right angles to its own edge. The shadow is most sharply defined if the mirror is moved at right angles to its edge, i.e., at right angles to the corrected meridian.

The strength and direction of the axis of the cylinder are then verified by placing the appropriate sphere and cylinder in the trial frame and again studying the shadow effects. If there is any shadow in any direction the appropriate correction should be made. A further accurate test may be made by the surgeon leaning towards and then away from the patient, repeating his observations on each occasion. In the first case a shadow should move in the same direction as the tilt of the mirror, in the second in the opposite direction. If the expected change does not occur in both directions symmetrically, the correction is wrong.

Streak retinoscopy. Wherein, instead of a circular source of light as is obtained by an ordinary plane mirror, a streak of light is used, has some advantages. The streak effect is obtained by using a plano-cylindrical retinoscopy mirror or a similarly adjusted electric retinoscope. The appearances are more dramatic (Fig. 7.7A–C). The band of light in the pupillary aperture moves 'with' or 'against' the band of light outside the pupil, the axis of astigmatisim is more easily determined, and on neutralization the streak disappears and the pupil appears completely light or completely dark.

Cycloplegics in refraction

The use of cycloplegics, whereby the ciliary muscle is paralysed and the pupil dilated, has definite indications and contra-indications. Because of their strong accommodative reserve, very young people should always be given atropine or hyoscine, but less powerful drugs

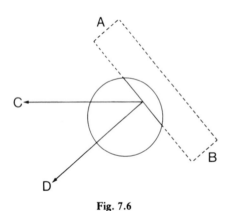

Fig. 7.6

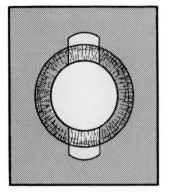
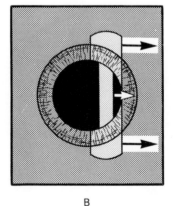
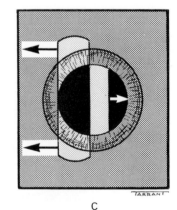

A   B   C

Fig. 7.7 Streak retinoscopy: A, shows the reflex at the point of neutralisation; B, the reflex and streak in a 'with movement in hypermetropia' plane mirror; C, the reflex and streak in an 'against movement in myopia' plane mirror

should be used with most hypermetropes below 16. In older patients the ideal refraction is the one estimated in the absence of cycloplegics. There is no need for cycloplegia as a routine although the pupillary dilatation is helpful for the beginner. They should be used, however, if there is a suspicion that the accommodation is abnormally active, if the objective findings by retinoscopy do not agree with the patient's subjective desires, if definite symptoms of accommodative asthenopia are present which do not seem to be explicable by the error found without a cycloplegic, and if the pupil is small and the refraction presents technical difficulties. A mydriatic may also be indicated for ophthalmoscopic purposes, in order to see the macula or the periphery of the fundus. It is to be remembered, however, that the refraction under cycloplegia is pathological because the shape of the lens has been altered, and after the lens has assumed its normal shape, minute errors cannot reasonably be transposed to the dioptric system in the ordinary conditions of use; a post-cycloplegic test is therefore advisable. Moreover, with a mydriatic the refraction of the peripheral part of the lens is often estimated, not the central part which in practice is used for vision. When the refraction is estimated under cyclopegia a correction must be made to compensate for the normal tone of the ciliary muscle. As an average one dioptre is deducted, somewhat more in young hypermetropes and somewhat less in myopes.

Atropine is the most powerful cycloplegic and for young children should be instilled two or three times a day for three days before examination; in older children a drop of 0.05% hyoscine in oil is effective after an hour or cyclopentolate 1%. For adults a rapid and transient effect is produced by such synthetic drugs as cyclopentolate hydrochloride (1%). If cycloplegia is desired, however, its effect, which varies greatly in different people and even in the two eyes of the same person, should be tested by estimating the residual accommodation which should not exceed one dioptre. Any mydriatic should be used with care in adults in whom the angle of the anterior chamber is narrow, owing to the danger of glaucoma. In older people mydriasis should be counteracted by pilocarpine (1%); and if suspicion of a tendency to closed-angle glaucoma exists and dilatation of the pupil is necessary, cocaine itself may be used.

To avoid ambiguity in ordering glasses the axes of cylinders should be uniformly numbered according to the method recommended by the International Council of Ophthalmology (Fig. 7.8).

Difficulties in retinoscopy

The shadows in regular astigmatism are not always easy to correct, owing chiefly to differences in curvature of different parts of the cornea. Usually the periphery of the cornea is flatter than the centre. The centre of the pupillary area will then be corrected by a different lens from the periphery, especially when the pupil is dilated. Various conflicting shadows may thus be seen, the commonest being the so-called 'scissors' shadows, where two shadows appear to meet each other and cross as the light is moved in a given direction. These difficulties are diminished with the undilated pupil. In irregular astigmatism the shadows move in various directions in different parts of the pupillary area and an accurate correction cannot be made by spherical or cylindrical lenses. In conical cornea a triangular shadow with its apex at the apex of the cone appears to swirl round its apex as the mirror is moved.

In conclusion, a word of warning must be given. The correction of a given refraction by retinoscopy may be easy or difficult. A large number of refractions should have been carefully corrected and confirmed by subjective tests before the beginner should consider himself justified in ordering spectacles without supervision.

Retinoscopy for near vision

The method of retinoscopy just described gives an objective measurement of the static refraction for distant vision. *Dynamic retinoscopy* has been introduced to give a similarly objective basis of the refraction of the eye when focused for near vision. The principle employed is to perform retinoscopy at the working distance with a self-luminous retinoscope on which is set a target for which the patient accommodates. The method gives an indication of the dynamic refraction, but our knowledge of the problems thus raised is insufficient to allow dogmatic conclusions to be drawn from the subtleties of the findings.

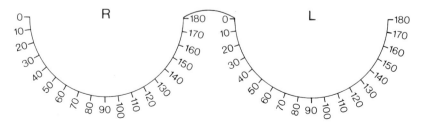

Fig. 7.8 The standard notation of axes of cylinders

REFRACTOMETRY AND KERATOMETRY

Refractometry utilizes the principle of indirect ophthalmoscopy wherein a condensing lens brings rays emergent from the retina to a focus at a convenient distance. The rays from a test-object are collimated to enter the pupil as a parallel beam, and consequently, if the eye is emmetropic, are focused on the retina; emerging from the eye as a parallel beam, they are focused again by the objective lens at the position of the test-object. If the eye is myopic the emergent rays will be convergent and the image will be formed at a nearer point; if hypermetropic, the emergent rays will be divergent and the image will be formed further away by an amount depending on the degree of ametropia. This is estimated by the direct observation of this image, the end-point being the maximum sharpness of focus. A more accurate device is to employ the principle of displacement by parallax which was elaborated by Henker in his parallax refractometer. By displacing the line of view to one side, the optical system is arranged so that if (as in emmetropia) the distances of the object and the image from the objective lens are equal, the image will be superimposed on the object and will not be seen. If (in myopia) the image is nearer the lens than the test-object, it will be displaced to the side next the illuminating tube. If (in hypermetropia) it is further away, it will be displaced to the other side. When the two do not coincide the test-object is moved until coincidence is attained when the refraction can be read from a scale.

A more accurate principle has been utilised by Fincham and Hartinger in their *coincidence optometers*. In these instruments, when the target is not in a position which is conjugate to the subject's retina, the retinal image is displaced from the axis. The image is viewed through a system of prisms which divides the field into two and reverses one half, so that when the image is out of alignment the halves of the line-image move in opposite directions; the setting is correct only when an unbroken line is formed.

The keratometer (ophthalmometer) measures the astigmatism of the anterior surface of the cornea at two points about 1.25 mm on either side of its centre. Since considerable lenticular astigmatism may exist, the technique is untrustworthy except in aphakia. The method is based on the fact that the surface of the cornea acts as a convex mirror so that the size of the image reflected by it varies with the curvature: the greater the curvature of the mirror, the smaller the image. To measure the size of the image a device is employed, originally adopted by Thomas Young, of doubling the images by a double refracting prism. The object consists of two illuminated 'mires' (AB, Fig. 7.9A) disposed on a rotatable circular arc, and the curvature of any diameter of the cornea can be measured by observation through the telescope (T). The mires are shaped as in *ab* (Fig. 7.9B) and are con-

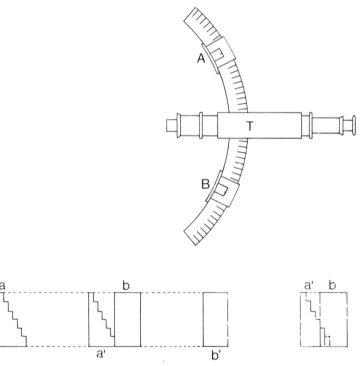

Fig. 7.9A–C The principle of the keratometer of Javal and Schiötz

sidered as the ends of a luminous object which appears in the cornea in duplicate as ab and $a'b'$. A and B are adjusted on the arc so that the two images $a'b$ just touch each other as in Fig. 7.9B. The arc is now rotated through 90° and a similar reading made. If a' and b still touch there is no astigmatism. If the curvature in this meridian is greater, the image is smaller and the mires will overlap as in Fig. 7.9C. The mire a' is so constructed that each step corresponds to a dioptre of refractive power, the number of dioptres of astigmation being thus read off directly.

THE SUBJECTIVE VERIFICATION OF THE REFRACTION

After the refraction has been estimated objectively it should always be verified subjectively by testing the visual acuity (p. 97), and if a cycloplegic has been used, the process should ideally be repeated in a *post-cycloplegic test*. These tests are made with the appropriate lenses, as found by the objective test, inserted in the trial frame (Fig. 7.5). Each eye is tested separately while an opaque disc is placed in the other compartment of the frame, and then the two are finally tested together.

If a cycloplegic has not been used the patient is asked to read the test types, and the effects of slight modifications in the lenses are tried in each eye separately, any small change being made which gives a marked improvement in visual acuity.

These manouvres are greatly facilitated by the use of a *cross-cylinder*, a mixed cylindrical combination of various strengths in which the spherical component is one half the (opposite) power of the cylindrical with the axes at right angles (Fig. 7.10). The most convenient form is a combination of a − 0.25 D sphere with a + 0.5 D cylinder. To check the strength of the cylinder in the optical correction, the cylindrical axis of the cross-cylinder is first placed in the same direction as the axis of the cylinder in the trial frame and then perpendicular to it. In the first position the cylindrical correction is enhanced by 0.5 D, in the second it is diminished by the same amount. If the visual acuity is unimproved in either of these positions, the cylinder in the trial frame is correct. If the visual acuity is improved, a corresponding change should be made in the correction unless it is especially contra-indicated; and the new combination verified by running through the cycle again.

To check the axis of the cylinder the principles of obliquely crossed cylinders are applied. A moderately strong cross-cylinder (± 0.5 or ± 1.0) is held before the eye so that each axis lies alternately 45° to either side of

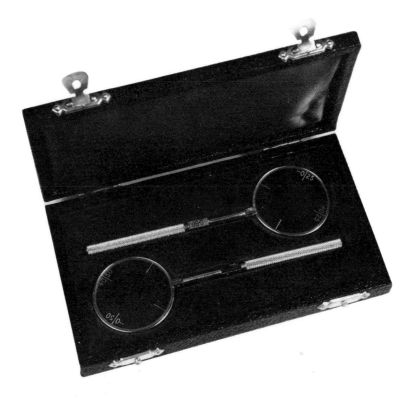

Fig. 7.10 Cross-cylinders. (By courtesy of Keeler.)

the axis of the trial cylinder. If visual improvement is attained by one or other alternative, the correcting cylinder is turned slightly in the direction of the axis of the cylinder of the same denomination in the cross-cylinder. The test is then repeated several times until the position of the trial cylinder is found at which rotation of the cross-cylinder gives no alteration in distinctness in either position.

It is not always easy for the patient to give definite answers with the use of the test types alone, especially in cases of small degress of astigmatism. In these the results may be confirmed by the use of some type of *astigmatic fan* (Fig. 7.11). On looking at such a figure, if any of the lines are seen more clearly than the others, astigmatism must be present; if the vertical lines are clear, the diffusion ellipses on the retina must be vertical, that is, the horizontal meridian must be more nearly emmetropic than the vertical and vice versa. A cylinder placed in front of the eye with its axis horizontal will therefore correct the vertical meridian, and when the correct glass is found all the lines will appear equally distinct.

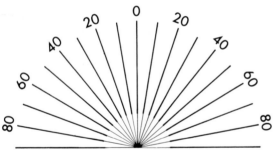

Fig. 7.11 Astigmatic fan

The cylinder which thus renders the outline of the whole fan equally clear is a measure of the amount of astigmatism, and the axis of the cylinder is at right angles to the line which was initially the most clearly defined.

As a clinical routine the test should be carried out with the patient's vision slightly fogged by an amount sufficient to over-correct every meridian by + 0.5 D, and the patient is asked to observe if any of the lines stand out more clearly than the others. If astigmatism is present he will see one or a neighbouring group of lines more sharply defined by a degree depending on the amount of astigmatism; concave cylinders are now added, their axis lying at right angles to this until all the lines — including that at right angles to the first — are equally clear, additional convex spheres being added to maintain the fogging if necessary.

The entire examination must be done slowly and leisurely, and the patient is given the strongest hyper-

metropic or the weakest myopic correction with which he can attain normal vision.

The *correction of near vision* should be preceded by the determination of the near point with the distance correction in place.

For this purpose appropriate test-types should be used. Snellen's reading test-types were constructed on the same principle as his distance types (p. 97) and are therefore theoretically accurate. Ordinary types in common use, however, are more legible and more easily obtained. Jaeger, therefore, introduced a series of test-types in print such as was in common use a century ago corresponding so closely in size to those of Snellen as to be sufficiently accurate for practical purposes. These are still widely used and the sizes of print are numbered J1, J2, etc. Recently a similar card of modern types has been standardised by the Faculty of Ophthalmologists numbered from N5 to N48, corresponding to the modern Times Roman type in various sizes from 5 pt to 48 pt.

The patient is given the reading test types and asked to hold them at the distance at which he is accustomed to work or read. When they are not distinctly seen, appropriate convex lenses should be added to the distance correction so that the near point is brought within the working distance, and the types are easily and confortably read. The position of the *near point* should now be determined. This is most accurately done by approximating to the eye a card on which is drawn a fine line 0.2 mm in breadth, until the line appears blurred (not doubled). For practical purposes it is sufficient to use the smallest test-type and move it towards the eye until it can no longer be easily read. The last position at which it can be read gives the near point. The distance of the near point from the eye is then measured with a tape. This distance is transformed, if necessary, into millimetres (25 mm = 1 inch), and the range of accommodation is deduced from the formula A = P – R. The correction given should be such that some amplitude of accommodation (about one-third) is kept in reserve.

Presbyopic spectacles should never be prescribed mechanically by ordering an approximate addition varying with the age of the patient. Each patient should be tested individually, for the individual variation is large, and those lenses should be ordered in each case which give the most serviceable and comfortable, not necessarily the clearest, vision for the particular work for which the spectacles are intended. In all cases it is better to under-correct than to over-correct since, if the spectacles tend to be too strong, difficulties will be experienced with convergence, and the range of vision will be limited. In any case, lenses which bring the near point closer than 28 cm are rarely well tolerated (that is, a total power of 3.5 D), and if for any reason the demands of fine work require a higher correction, the convergence should be aided with prisms as well as the accommodation with spheres (see Chapter 30).

THE CORRECTION OF ERRORS OF REFRACTION

The correction of errors of refraction has already been briefly sketched. It will be well, however, to outline the method to be adopted in systematically examining for and correcting these errors, and to indicate the requirements which should be satisfied by spectacles.

1. External examination in diffuse light (Chapter 10).

2. Examination of the motility of the eyes (Chapter 29).

3. The cover test to elicit heterophoria and squint (Chapter 30).

This is best done at this stage. The detection of a squint may account for a marked deficiency of vision in the deviating eye, which, if it is not recognised early in the examination, may give rise to some concern.

4. The examination of the eyes by focal illumination, and by the plane mirror, and the ophthalmoscopic examination by the indirect and direct methods (Chapter 10–11).

5. The trial frames are put on and centred.

6. The testing of visual acuity, uniocularly and binocularly (Chapter 13).

6. The testing of visual acuity, uniocularly and binocularly (Chapter 13).

7. The retinoscopy.

8. The subjective verification of the retinoscopy with the test types, astigmatic fan and cross-cylinder.

9. With the full correction in place, the testing of the muscle balance for distant vision.

10. With the full correction in place, the determination of the near point of accommodation and convergence (Chapter 28).

11. The additon of the correction for near work (if necessary), and the testing of the acuity with the near types, uniocularly and binocularly.

12. With the additional correction for near work, the estimation of the muscle balance for near vision (Chapter 30).

If the patient is less than 5 years of age. 1–5 are done on the first visit. Then order ung. atropinæ, 1%, to be inserted three times a day for three days. The ophthalmoscopic examination is repeated and 6, if possible, and 7 are done. The spectacles may then be ordered with the appropriate deduction for cycloplegia.

If the patient is between 5 and 15. The same procedure should be undertaken but the entire examination can be done at one visit using cyclopentolate (1.0%) or 0.05% hyoscine in oil as a cycloplegic.

If the patient is between 15 and 20. The same procedure should be undertaken, but the lowered activity of the ciliary muscle and the economic disability imposed by long cycloplegia allow cyclopentolate or homatropine with cocaine to be employed; a post-cycloplegic test is advisable.

If the patient is between 20 and 40. Cycloplegia followed by a post-cycloplegic test may be used as seems indicated (p. 52) but is usually not required. 1–10 should be performed as a routine.

If the patient is above 40. Cycloplegia is rarely necessary, should only be used with care and should always be neutralised by the instillation of 1.0% pilocarpine. Mydriasis (as with cocaine) may be employed in difficult cases. 1–12 should be performed as a routine.

Spectacles

In children, spectacles with large round or oval lenses should be ordered, otherwise the child may look over them. In adults with astigmatism rigid spectacles must be ordered.

It is very important that all spectacles fit accurately. For distant vision the lenses must be centred so that the optical centres are exactly opposite the centres of the pupils when the visual axes are parallel. For near vision the lenses are decentred slightly inwards and tilted so that the surfaces form an angle of 15° with the plane of the face: they are then approximately at right angles to the visual axes when the eyes are directed downwards in reading.

Various forms of bifocal or trifocal lenses are sometimes used. In the former the upper part contains the distant correction, the lower part the near; in the second a strip for an intermediate distance is interposed between the two; in multifocal lenses a continuous gradation from the near to the far point is incorporated. If any of these are recommended, patients should be warned that they may experience some initial difficulty in moving about, particularly going downstairs, since vision through the reading portion of the lenses will be blurred and prismatic effects cause the apparent displacement of objects.

If tinted glasses are desirable, as in high myopia, albinism or in tropical countries, the correcting lenses may be tinted.

Contact lenses

In cases of irregular corneal astigmatism and high myopia great improvement of vision occurs when a suitably curved glass meniscus is in actual apposition to the cornea or separated from it by a thin fluid meniscus. Contact lenses are made of plastic; if resting on the sclera they must fit with great accuracy, but microlenses resting on the cornea are easier to fit and to wear, although they sometimes may cause epithelial abrasions. As optical instruments they undoubtedly form the theoretically ideal correction for ametropia and are free of many of the disadvantages of spectacles. In all cases the prismatic effects of spectacles are eliminated and the field wherein clear vision is possible greatly increased; they are therefore particularly valuable in high errors of refraction, especially myopia or aphakia. Moreover, their effect in tending to maintain the size of the image approximately that of the emmetropic eye, makes them useful in cases of anisometropia, wherein the refractions of the two eyes are widely different (the most dramatic example of which is unilateral aphakia); while, since these lenses eliminate the corneal curvatures, high errors of astigmatism, as in conical cornea, are optically abolished. They cannot, however, be tolerated in all cases, their fitting must be of extreme accuracy, and perseverance is necessary to acquire facility in their insertion and removal. Even at the best they are not free from the danger of causing corneal injury unless they are used with care.

In cases wherein retinal disease is a cause of visual failure, *telescopic spectacles* may provide sufficient magnification to permit reading. They incorporate the optical principles of a Galilean telescope, but their use is difficult, particularly in view of the small size of the visual field. In such cases an ordinary convex lens held in the hand or on a fixed stand as a reading lens is often found more useful.

8

Errors of refraction

Ametropia

The condition in which incident parallel rays of light do not come to a focus upon the light-sensitive layer of the retina, may be due to one or more of the following conditions:

A. Abnormal length of the globe — too long in myopia, too short in hypermetropia — *axial ametropia*.

B. Abnormal curvature of the refracting surfaces of the cornea or lens — too strong a curvature in myopia, too weak in hypermetropia — *curvature ametropia*.

C. Abnormal refractive indices of the media — *index ametropia*. In index myopia the refractive index, either of the cornea, the aqueous or of the lens (produced whether by a high index in the nucleus or a low in the cortex or both) is too high, and that of the vitreous may be too low. In index hypermetropia the opposite conditions are operative, and the error is high when the lens is absent.

D. Abnormal position of the lens — displacement forwards in myopia, backwards in hypermetropia.

Of all these factors the axial length of the globe is perhaps the most important.

Emmetropic eyes may differ in length by as much as 1–2 mm, and the radius of curvature of the cornea may vary from 7 to 8 mm. Emmetropia therefore results from the integration of all the variables mentioned in the previous paragraph and a deviation in one factor is often compensated by the opposite tendency in another. Statistically one might expect its incidence to resemble the Gaussian frequency curve, but since the full development of emmetropia is never present normally at birth the curve will have a certain 'skew deviation'. Most infants are born hypermetropic; almost inevitably some cases will fail to reach emmetropia and remain hypermetropic, while others will proceed too far and become myopic. Of these the former are by far the more numerous. Most cases of low ametropia (including myopia) are merely biological variants around a mean and cannot be regarded as pathological (Fig. 8.1).

Myopia

Otherwise known as 'short sight' is that dioptric condition of the eye in which, with the accommodation at rest, incident parallel rays come to a focus anterior to the light-sensitive layer of the retina. The majority of cases merely results as variants in the frequency curve of axial length and curvature, the former being the more important although curvature myopia occurs commonly as a factor in astigmatism. Such cases of *simple myopia* are in no sense pathological, there are no degenerative changes in the fundus although peripheral retinal degeneration often becomes evident in later life, and they do not progress after adolescence when a degree of 5 or 6 dioptres may be attained. In severe illness, however, or states of debility, the sclera may stretch and the myopia increase.

Rarely a *developmental myopia* occurs. In this case the child is born with an abnormally long eye, the fundus may lack pigmentation and the choroidal vessels are evident while a myopic crescent (p. 60) may be seen at the disc. The refraction soon after birth may be — 10 D; but in this type of case progression is rare.

Pathological axial myopia is degenerative and progressive. The refractive change appears in childhood, usually between the ages of five and 10, and increases steadily up to 25 or beyond, finally amounting to 15–25 D or more. The degenerative changes in the fundus, on the other hand, do not appear until later in life, becoming marked at about the fifth decade. The condition is strongly hereditary, being commoner in women than in men. It has racial tendencies, being common, for example, among Jews and Japanese, and most cases are of genetic origin. Many other aetiological theories have been advanced — excessive accommodation and convergence in near work, vascular congestion due to a dependent position of the head, and so on — but they have little to recommend them.

The condition is essentially a disturbance of growth on which are imposed the degenerative phenomena; these will be considered at a later stage (p. 165). Endocrine or nutritional disturbances, debility or illness, probably act as incidental factors which may increase the general tendency; but, despite popular belief which still lingers, environmental conditions such as excessive

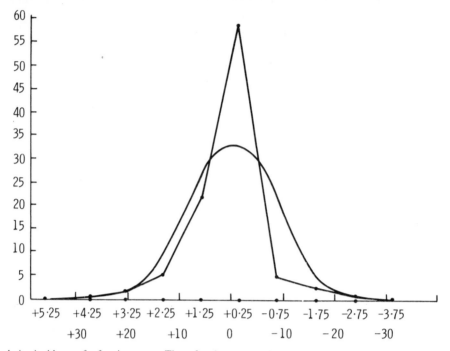

Fig. 8.1 The relative incidence of refractive errors. The refraction curves of Scheerer and Betsch (the higher curve) compared with the theoretically derived binomial variation curve (the lower curve and lower figures). The abscissae are refractions measured without cycloplegia

near work probably have little influence upon the condition which is genetically predetermined, except in so far as they inhibit normal healthy development.

Pathological curvature myopia is seen typically in conical cornea. *Index myopia* accounts for myopia as a premonitory symptom of senile cataract, when it is due to the increased refractive index of the nucleus of the lens; it also accounts for myopia in some cases of diabetes, with or without cataractous changes in the lens.

In degenerative axial myopia the increase in length of the eye affects the posterior pole and the surrounding area; the part of the eye anterior to the equator may be normal (Fig. 8.2). The elongation is probably not due to stretching but to a primary degeneration of the coats of the eye including the posterior half of the sclera. In the high degrees, the sclera may bulge out at the posterior pole to form a *posterior staphyloma*, distinguishable clinically by the optical condition and the associated changes in the fundus. The edges of the bulge may be actually visible by the indirect method of ophthalmoscopy owing to the presence of a crescentic shadow two or three disc-diameters to the temporal side of the disc and concentric with it and to the change in course of the retinal vessels.

Two typical ophthalmoscopic appearances are seen in high myopia — changes at the disc typified in the development of a myopic crescent, and changes in the central area of the fundus described as chorioretinal myopic

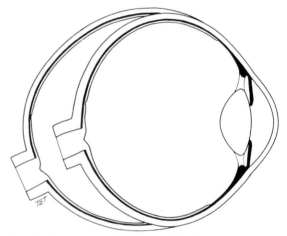

Fig. 8.2 The two eyes of the same indiviudal superimposed: the one emmetropic, the other with −15 D of myopia

degeneration (p. 165). Degenerative changes also occur at the periphery of the retina which may lead to the occurrence of a retinal detachment, and degenerative changes in the vitreous are common, giving rise to dust-like vitreous opacities or large floaters composed of elements of the vitreous framework. These 'floaters' are seen more plainly by myopic than by other eyes because the entoptic image is larger. These degenerative changes may have serious visual consequences; in fact they are among the more common causes of severe visual disability.

The only symptom in low myopia may be indistinct distant vision. In other cases and in high myopia there is often, in addition, discomfort after near work, due largely to disproportion between the efforts of accommodation and convergence (q.v.). The eyes may be sensitive to light. Black spots may be seen floating before them, and sometimes flashes of light are noticed; the latter may occur irrespective of any tendency to detachment of the retina. In very high myopia the eyes are prominent, the pupils are large, and the anterior chamber appears deeper than normal, probably only owing to the dilatation of the pupil. There may be an apparent convergent squint due to a large negative angle γ (q.v.). Vision may be very poor, even with optical correction; scotomata may be present, both central and peripheral.

As regards *prognosis*, low or moderate degrees of simple myopia (up to 5 or 6 D), unless occurring in young children, have a good prognosis. They are not likely to progress, and in some of the conditions of civilized life they may even be an advantage to the individual. The same condition in a child before the age of six or seven should give rise to anxiety if it is not of the congenital type, since the degenerative condition is clinically indistinguishable from the simple at this stage. The former is of grave prognosis, because it is almost certain to progress so that eventually there may be 10 or 15 D of myopia or more, accompanied by serious degenerative changes in the fundus and defects of vision. The likelihood of these developments must be judged by the acuity of vision after correction, the condition of the fundus and the evidence of heredity.

Treatment. Consists in wearing suitable correcting spectacles and attention to the hygiene of the eyes. Each case must be considered on its merits.

With regard to the ordering of spectacles in myopia, every surgeon agrees that *myopia must never be overcorrected*. Opinions differ as to details. In low myopia, up to 5 or 6 D, no harm is done by ordering the full distance correction for constant use, and if this is done the patient must be warned not to hold near work closer than ordinary reading distance. Many surgeons order lenses weaker by 2 or 3 D for near work with a view to diminishing accommodation. As we have seen, this is based on an old and erroneous ætiological view, but many patients are more comfortable for near work with the weaker lenses. Any advantage in comfort in the young, however, tends to be neutralised by the disturbance of the normal relationship between accommodation and convergence.

In practice, in low myopia, the full correction may be ordered for constant use; in the event of any discomfort being experienced, weaker lenses may be ordered for near work, especially if much reading or close work is done. Children should wear their distance correction constantly — not particularly in the interests of their eyes but in the interests of their mental development — for children with even low degrees of uncorrected myopia cannot be expected to take a normal interest in their surroundings since they cannot see distant objects as clearly as their fellows. Their mental horizon is constricted, they tend to become unduly introspective, and they are thrown more and more into finding their interest in reading and near work. Adults need not wear their correction constantly in the absence of symptoms provided they resign themselves, when they do not wear spectacles, to their poor vision and do not impose the strain upon their eyes of attempting to see the difficult or impossible. In low degrees of error, spectacles for near work are rarely required after the presbyopic age.

In high myopia it is wise always slightly to undercorrect even for distance, and the same or still weaker lenses may be ordered for near work. In the highest grades the patient often sees best with lenses which are decidedly weaker than the full correction; he should be allowed to choose those he prefers. One reason is that strong minus lenses considerably diminish the size of the retinal images and make them very bright and clear. The retinal images are diminished because the lenses have to be worn farther from the eye than the anterior focal plane (p. 42); spectacles for high myopia should therefore be made to fit as closely to the eyes as possible; toric lenses may be ordered. The very bright, clear images are uncomfortable because the retina has become accustomed to large and indistinct images. Moreover, much artificial astigmatism and therefore distortion of the image, is produced by looking obliquely through strong lenses. Very short-sighted people thus get into the habit of turning the head rather than the eyes to avoid looking obliquely through the lenses. Indeed, some high myopes can find their way about better without any spectacles. Contact lenses may be of great value in cases of this type when they can be tolerated.

In very high myopia the requisite amount of convergence for near work, if spectacles are not constantly worn, may be impossible. In this case the effort to converge is abandoned so that reading and other near work become uniocular and the disused eye becomes divergent.

As regard hygienic measures in myopia, especially in the young, near work, apart from being held in the proper position and being undertaken in good illumination, need not be restricted if the general health and physical development of the child are not being undermined thereby. Only if the visual acuity of the child is such as to make it difficult for him to keep pace with his fellows at school need special educational methods be adopted wherein most of the teaching is oral and visual instruction is limited to specially printed large types. In all cases the most important factor is the maintenance of the general health, and if the myopia is rapidly progressive, and especially if the child is under stress, the temporary cessation of schooling and a change of air to the country with plenty of healthy exercise may well be desirable from this point of view.

Owing to the gravity of the prognosis in later life, for economic reasons high myopes with degenerative changes in the fundus or a family history thereof should avoid an occupation wherein close work is necessary. Consideration should also be given to the hereditary propagation of the disease; at the least, two high myopes with pronounced degenerative changes in the fundi should not have children.

Operative treatment for high myopia. If an eye has axial myopia of 21 D, its length will be about 31 mm (p. 63). If the crystalline lens of such an eye is removed, parallel rays will be focused upon the retina without the intervention of any correcting lens, and the retinal images of distant objects will be larger than those of the emmetropic eye. Hence extraction of the lens has been advocated in high myopia often with immediately satisfactory results. The operation is, however, attended with considerable danger for such eyes withstand operative measures badly, the vitreous is likely to be fluid and the retina and choroid are probably degenerate so that the tendency to retinal detachment is increased.

Hypermetropia (Hyperopia)

Otherwise known as 'far sight' is that dioptric condition of the eye in which, with the accommodation at rest, incident parallel rays come to a focus posterior to the light-sensitive layer of the retina.

As in myopia, the chief factor in clinical hypermetropia is *axial* — an abnormal shortness in the length of the eye. It must be remembered that a small eye, although too short, is not necessarily hypermetropic since there may be uniform diminution of all the parts. This is, perhaps, most easily understood if a diagram such as Figure 6.2 is considered; if such a diagram is uniformly diminished, as by photography, the parallel rays will still come to a focus on the retina. As a matter of fact, however, highly hypermetropic eyes are almost invariably also smaller than normal.

Curvature hypermetropia occurs commonly as a factor in astigmatism; it is almost unknown as a cause of spherical hypermetropia. *Index hypermetropia* accounts for the hypermetropia of old age (p. 47), and it is to be attributed to the increased refractive index of the cortex of the lens.

Hypermetropia rarely exceeds 6–7 D, which is equivalent to a shortening of the optic axis of 2 mm. Individual cases of much higher degrees without other anomaly have been recorded — up to 24 D.

In the young the condition may cause no symptoms. When symptoms are present or arise, they are chiefly referable to the abnormal amount of accommodation to which these eyes are subjected, and to the lack of balance between accommodation and convergence (*q.v.*). As has been pointed out, the healthy youth has an ample reserve of accommodation, and if he happens to be hypermetropic he accommodates for distant and near objects without being conscious of the act. If he is weakly or does much near work the perpetual overaction of the ciliary muscle is likely to produce symptoms; the condition is often called *accommodative asthenopia* or 'eye-strain'. The symptoms are noticed chiefly after close work, especially in the evening by artificial illumination. The eyes ache and burn; they may feel dry, so that blinking movements are more frequent than usual, or there may be lacrimation. The conjunctiva and edges of the lids become hyperæmic and if near work is persisted in, headaches, usually frontal, develop.

In young children hypermetropia is a predisposing cause of convergent strabismus (*q.v.*). Latent convergence is often found in hypermetropes, although other forms of heterophoria may occur (*q.v.*). The presence of heterophoria increases the tendency to headache and other symptoms of eye-strain.

In older patients no symptoms may be caused until the power of accommodation has diminished to the extent that the near point is beyond the range of comfortable reading distance and work has to be held farther off than usual in order to be seen clearly. The greater the degree of hypermetropia the sooner will this symptom arise; in other words, apparent presbyopia commences at an earlier age than usual.

Ophthalmoscopically the fundus may exhibit no abnormality. A bright reflex, suggesting the appearance of watered silk, is commoner in hypermetropic than in emmetropic or myopic eyes; and in some cases optic neuritis is nearly simulated — pseudopapillitis (*q.v.*).

Anatomically, the smallness of the eye is not confined to the post-equatorial segment as in myopia, nor are abnormalities found in the retina or choroid. The diameter of the cornea is often reduced and regular astigmatism is common while the anterior chamber is shallower than usual, owing partly to the normal size of the lens, a configuration which predisposes to closed-angle glaucoma.

The new-born are almost invariably hypermetropic (average 2.5 D). In the first decades of life the incidence of hypermetropia falls rapidly, remaining at about 50% after the twentieth year. There is no predilection for either sex. It is interesting that primitive races and the higher mammals, especially the carnivora, are generally hypermetropic.

Treatment. Consists in prescribing the correcting

lenses. Unless there are definite symptoms there is no reason for insisting upon the use of spectacles in the young or middle-aged. In elderly people the hypermetropia must be corrected for near work: the ordinary presbyopic addition must be added to the hypermetropic correction, but care should be taken that these cases are rather under- than over-corrected.

Astigmatism

This is that condition of refraction in which a point of light cannot be made to produce a punctate image upon the retina by any spherical correcting lens. The varieties of regular astigmatism have been already enumerated (p. 41).

Regular astigmatism, the only form susceptible to optical correction by lenses, invariably produces some defect in visual acuity. It is particularly liable to cause the worst forms of asthenopia or 'eye-strain'; the asthenopia in these cases is only in part accommodative. It is often worse in the lower degrees of astigmatism than in the higher because of endeavours to accommodate so as to produce a circle of least diffusion upon the retina (p. 41). Aching of the eyes and headaches are common symptoms; the eyes quickly become fatigued with reading and the letters are described as 'running together'.

Regular astigmatism is usually a congenital defect, due in most part to differences in the curvature of the cornea in different meridians. It must be remembered that frequently the cornea is not alone at fault, for corneal astigmatism may be increased or partially corrected by lenticular astigmatism. Regular astigmatism may be traumatic following a wound, frequently surgical, in the corneo-scleral margin since the contraction of the scar causes flattening of the cornea in the meridian at right angles to the wound. The astigmatism due to this cause continues to alter for some weeks after the injury so that final spectacles should not be ordered for at least six weeks thereafter.

The higher degrees of astigmatism cause much lowering of visual acuity: this is usually least in mixed astigmatism, probably because the circle of least diffusion falls upon or near the retina.

Treatment. If the astigmatic error is small and not associated with symptoms, spectacles are unnecessary unless the highest visual acuity is desired; but in all cases in which astigmatism causes asthenopic symptoms the full optical correction should be ordered for constant use, that is, both for distant and near vision.

Aphakia

This is the condition of the eye when the crystalline lens has been removed. The eye is extremely hypermetropic if it had been emmetropic or had only a low grade of ametropia before removal of the lens, and all accommodation is lost. The hypermetropia, as estimated by

the correcting lens required when worn in the usual position, is about 10 or 11 D if the eye were previously emmetropic.

The optical conditions of the aphakic eye are very simple. It consists of a curved surface, the cornea, separating two media of different refractive indices, air and aqueous plus vitreous. Knowing the radius of curvature (8 mm) and the refractive indices (1 and 1.33), it is easy to calculate the focal distances; the anterior focal distance is 23 and the posterior 31 mm, as compared with 15 and 24 mm, respectively for the normal eye. If the aphakic eye were 31 mm long, parallel rays falling on the cornea would be brought to a focus on the retina and no correcting glass would be required for distance. The axial myopia of a phakic eye which is 31 mm long equals — 21 D.

The retinal image of the aphakic eye is about a quarter larger than the emmetropic retinal image. Hence vision of 6/6 with a correcting lens after extraction is not quite so good as it seems; and, owing to the disparity of the images, any attempt to correct unilateral aphakia with spectacles when there is good vision in the other eye leads to an intolerable diplopia. With contact lenses, however, comfortable binocular vision may be attained.

In addition to the hypermetropia, there is always some astigmatism in those cases in which a corneal or corneo-scleral section has been made. If the section is in the upper part of the cornea, the astigmatism is against the rule since the cornea is flattened in the vertical meridian. The astigmatism usually amounts initially to 2 or 3 D but gradually diminishes.

Treatment. The refractive error is determined by retinoscopy and by subjective tests; the ophthalmometer may afford help in determining astigmatism. The optical condition of aphakia with a strong correcting lens and with no accommodation is difficult and great patience is often necessary if the patient is to adapt himself to it. Sometimes these difficulties can be much improved by a contact lens provided the patient can manipulate and tolerate it.

The difficulties of aphakia and its correction by spectacles include:
1. An image magnification of about 30%.
2. Spherical aberration producing a 'pin cushion effect'.
3. Lack of physical co-ordination.
4. A 'Jack-in-the-Box' ring scotoma from prismatic effects at the edge of the lens.
5. Prismatic errors resulting from displaced optical centres of the lenses.
6. Reduced visual fields and poor eccentric acuity.
7. Inaccurate correction because of erroneous vertex distances.
8. Physical inconvenience and cosmetic deficiency of heavy spectacle lenses.

In an attempt to overcome these difficulties aphakic

spectacles may be had in various forms, namely spherical, lenticular, and full field (hyperaspheric). In aspheric lenses the front lens surface has a progressive peripheral flattening starting 12 mm. from the centre with the power ground on the posterior surface. The smaller lenticular lens (40 mm diameter) has a bull's-eye effect with a −3.50 D rear curve, moderate asphericity (1.50 D power drop), a small peripheral field, a smaller more central scotoma, less distortion, greater central magnification and better eccentric acuity. The reduced distortion makes it more suitable for a first aphakic lens. The full-field lenses have a flat rear curve, more asphericity (2−5 D power drop peripherally), variable but usually larger diameter, larger peripheral field, larger but more peripheral scotoma, somewhat more distortion, less central magnification and poorer eccentric acuity. These full-field lenses have increased field, more secure mobility and improvement in eye-hand co-ordination and spatial orientation.

General problems in the use of contact lenses in aphakic persons include:
1. Lack of dexterity in older patients.
2. Intolerance of the feeling of a foreign body.
3. Cleansing of mucus commonly present on the lens and sterilisation.
4. Lens spoilage from dislodgement or loss, breakage or deterioration.

Ocular complications of increasing seriousness include:
1. Oedema of the corneal epithelium with blurring of vision from over-wearing.
2. Corneal epithelial erosions from trauma in removing the lens.
3. Papillary conjunctivitis perhaps related to mucus.
4. Peripheral corneal vascularisation.
5. Corneal ulcers from infection.

The advantages of intra-ocular lens implantation are freedom from patient handling, minimum aniseikonia, rapid return of binocularity and normal peripheral vision.

The operation however carries added risks and the complications which may arise are corneal dystrophy, implant dislocation, pupil block glaucoma, cystoid maculopathy, increased severity of post-operative iridocyclitis and greater post-operative astigmatism.

Intra-ocular lenses are made of monomer-free polymethylmethacrylate (P.M.M.A.). Lenses are biconvex or plano/convex 4−6 mm in diameter. The standard power lens of 19.50 D in aqueous is approximately equivalent to an 11.0 D sphere spectacle lens. Lens power measurements for primary implantation necessitate axial length measurement with ultrasonography, keratometry and the use of standard calculation tables. In children a stronger lens of 22.50 D strength is required.

Lens loops are made from nylon or prolene, the latter being more stable and recently of methylmethacrylate.

Anisometropia

This is the condition in which the refractions of the two eyes show a considerable difference. A slight difference is very common but all varieties and degrees of anisometropia occur. The condition may cause asthenopic symptoms. In the lower grades there is usually binocular vision, although it is imperfect and the effort of fusion may produce symptoms of eye-strain. In the higher grades this is impossible; vision is then uniocular, and there is some danger of the eye which is not used becoming divergent.

Treatment. The correction of anisometropia is often difficult. It has already been mentioned that if correcting lenses are placed at the anterior focal plane of the eye, the retinal images in axial ametropia are the same size as the emmetropic retinal image. In practice the lenses are nearer to the eyes so that with convex lenses the retinal image is diminished, with concave, enlarged. In high grades of anisometropia, therefore, there will be a considerable difference in the size of the retinal images of the two eyes (*aniseikonia*). Patients find it difficult or impossible to fuse these sharp but diverse images. Moreover, on looking obliquely through the lenses the prismatic effect and the distortion are different in the two eyes, enhancing the discomfort. The use of ordinary spectacle lenses thus presents difficulties, and if a full correction cannot be borne a compromise may be adopted wherein each eye is under-corrected. *Iseikonic* or *size-lenses*, which correct such a difference in their optical construction, require specialised methods of manufacture and their clinical results are often disappointing. Contact lenses diminish these optical defects and may be ordered in suitable cases. Alternatively, resort may be had to uniocular vision, one eye being used at a time, a habit which grows more comfortable with practice as is seen in the use of a uniocular microscope or monocle. It is particularly fortunate when one eye is nearly emmetropic and the other myopic for the former can be used for distant, the latter for near vision without the aid of spectacles.

9

Anomalies of accommodation

Insufficiency of accommodation

In this condition the accommodative power is below the lower limit of what might be accepted as normal for the patient's age; in a sense presbyopia (p. 47) is a physiological failure of accommodation due to hardening of the lens. Such an insufficiency is usually due to weakness of the ciliary muscle, the aetiology embracing all the causes of muscular fatigue (general debility, anæmia, toxæmia, etc.) accompanied by excessive use of the eyes particularly for close work. A rapid failure of accommodation also occurs in the prodromal stages of glaucoma, due probably to impairment of the effectivity of the ciliary muscle by the increased pressure.

The symptoms are those of eye-strain with particular difficulty associated with near work. The treatment should be directed essentially to the causal condition, but if close work is difficult reading spectacles may be prescribed, the same procedure being adopted as that recommended for presbyopia. In general the weakest convex lenses which will allow adequate vision should be ordered so that the accomodation may be exercised and stimulated rather than relieved.

Paralysis of accommodation or cycloplegia

This occurs in disease as well as from the direct action of cycloplegic drugs. Unilateral cycloplegia is generally due to drugs (often through rubbing the eyes after using a belladonna liniment), contusion (*q.v.*), or to paralysis of the third nerve. Bilateral paresis, less commonly paralysis, occurs typically after diphtheria, but may appear after debilitating illness, or with syphilis, diabetes, alcoholism and cerebral or meningeal diseases.

In diphtheritic cases the paralysis of accommodation follows the primary attack after an interval of several weeks, and is often associated with paralysis of the palate, loss of knee jerks, etc. The sore throat may have been very slight and its diphtheritic character unrecognized.

In complete paralysis the sphincter pupillae is also generally paralysed so that the pupil is widely dilated. In paresis the pupil may be scarcely affected, especially after diphtheria, but in this disease the reverse of the Argyll Robertson pupil may be met with — loss of reaction to accommodation with retained reaction to light. The symptoms depend upon the condition of the refraction. If the patient is myopic, the defect may pass unnoticed; if he is emmetropic, near vision alone will be affected; if he is hypermetropic, both distant and near vision will be affected, but particularly the latter. In paresis it may be possible to diagnose the condition only by carefully measuring the range of accommodation.

The prognosis is good in cases due to drugs or diphtheria. In traumatic cases the condition may be permanent.

Treatment is that of the cause. Whenever the condition is bilateral, near work can be carried on by using suitable convex lenses, as in the correction of presbyopia. Miotics are sometimes used, but they may do harm and seldom do good.

Spasm of accommodation

It has already been mentioned that the ciliary muscle has physiological tone which is abolished by atropine, and is equivalent to about one dioptre. In spasm of the ciliary muscle, it is found that atropine produces a much greater effect. The condition is found only in young patients and, contrary to what might be expected, particularly in myopes. An actual or relative myopia is produced and in these cases subjective testing without a cycloplegic indicates too high an error. Spasm of accommodation is produced artifically by the instillation of miotics.

In spontaneous spasm of accommodation there is nearly always some error of refraction and the eyes have usually been subjected to too much near work in unfavourable circumstances which may include such factors as bad illumination, a bad position, mental stress and anxiety, and so on. The condition should not be diagnosed unless proved to be present by the use of atropine.

Treatment consists in the use of atropine for several weeks together with assurance and if indicated psychotherapy.

SECTION 3

The examination of the eye: therapeutics

10

External examination

In this section we shall confine ourselves essentially to conditions affecting the globe itself.

When the cornea is inflamed or ulcerated the eye is irritable and resistant to examination in bright light so that the slightest attempt to separate the lids is accompanied by violent blepharospasm, especially in children. In such a case the lids must be separated by retractors, preferably under general anaesthesia.

Examination of the anterior segment of the eye is made by three methods: 1. General inspection in a good diffuse light. 2. Examination in focal (or oblique) illumination using the loupe or slit-lamp. 3. Examination of the recess of the angle of the anterior chamber with the gonioscope.

Focal or oblique illumination using a binocular loupe is carried out with the help of a small electric torch, the beam of which can be focused to a point or converted into a slit (Fig. 10.1).

With a *binocular loupe* a stereoscopic effect is obtained, and the depth of opacities can be determined with great accuracy. The degree of magnification amounts to three or four times; greater accuracy is attained with the slit-lamp.

The *slit-lamp* is essential when minute examination of the eye is required (Fig. 10.2). It employs the same principles of focal illumination wherein a brilliant light is brought to a focus as a slit or a point by an optical system supported on a movable arm, and observations are made through a binocular microscope. Plate 7 (Fig. A) shows a general view of the eye illuminated by a beam of light of moderate width coming from the slit-lamp entering the eye from the left side. Optically homogeneous media appear quite black; structures like the cornea, lens and suspended particles in the aqueous scatter the light. Hence, on the left of the diagram is seen the illuminated portion of the cornea forming a parallelepiped, the brighter areas corresponding to the surfaces, the darker to the section of the cornea. The black space to the right is the anterior chamber. Then follows the 'phantom' of the lens, in which can be distinguished the dim central interval, formed by the embryonic nucleus with its Y-sutures, outside which are the successive 'zones of discontinuity' — the fetal nucleus, the infantile nucleus, the adult nucleus and the cortex. Still farther to the right is the faintly striated vitreous.

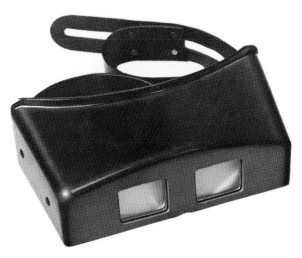

Fig. 10.1 Binocular loupe (by courtesy of Keeler Instruments Ltd)

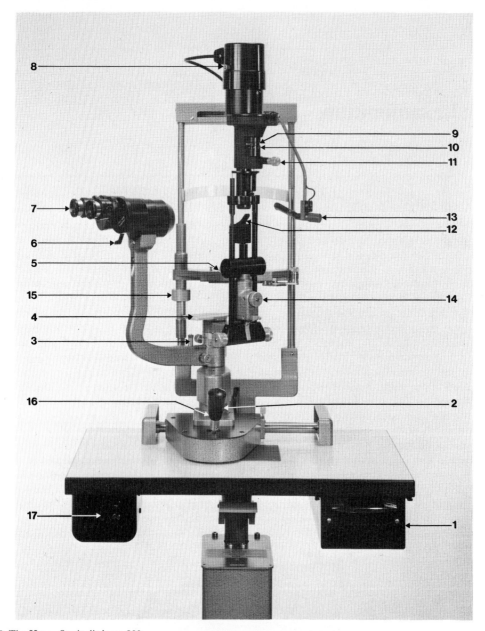

Fig. 10.2 The Haag–Streit slit-lamp 900

1. Accessory box.
2. Joy-stick lever for horizontal coarse and fine adjustments.
3. Roll for setting the angle between microscope and illumination unit.
4. Guide-plate for pre-set lenses and applanation tonometer.
5. Chin support.
6. Lever for changing objectives.
7. Interchangeable eye-pieces.
8. Lamp-casing.
9. Lever for four different light filters.
10 Lever for six different diaphragms.
11. Ball-handle for turning slit-image.
12. Interchangeable illumination mirror.
13. Fixation lamp with annular fixation marker.
14. Centring screw.
15. Level adjustment control for chin support.
16. Height adjustment control of slit-lamp.
17. Transformer with switch.

The conjunctiva

In order to examine the whole conjunctival sac it is necessary to expose the palpebral conjunctiva and the fornices. The lower fornix is easily exposed by drawing down the lower lid while the patient looks towards the ceiling. The upper palpebral conjunctiva is exposed by everting the upper lid.

Eversion of the upper lid requires some practice.

Place a probe or thin pencil along the skin of the upper lid at the level of the upper broader of the tarsus, the patient looking towards his feet. Grasp the eyelashes between the left index and thumb, and draw the lid away from the globe, using the probe as a fixed point. Rotate the lid in a vertical direction round the probe, which is then withdrawn (Fig. 10.3A and B.)

In many cases the upper lid is everted with the examiner standing behind the patient, who may be lying on a couch. In this case the following is the best method: place the left index finger vertically upon the lid while the patient is looking towards his feet. Grasp the lashes with the right index and thumb, and rotate the lid around the tip of the left index.

Having everted the upper lid we can examine the palpebral conjunctiva, but we are still unable to see the upper fornix. This can usually be effected in adults by the use of a retractor following local anaesthesia.

In general, congestion of the conjunctival vessels, leaving a relatively white zone around the cornea and accompanied by mucous or muco-purulent secretion, is indicative of conjunctivitis. If there is much irritation and photophobia with some blepharospasm and weep-ing, we suspect the presence either of a foreign body or misplaced lashes or other irritation of the cornea (abrasion, erosions, ulcer, and forms of keratitis). Careful examination shows that the vessels in the circumcorneal zone are bright red, and that the corneal loops of the limbal plexus are also dilated and visible.

In ciliary congestion, on the other hand, which indicates involvement of the inner eye, particularly inflammation of the iris or the sclera, the pink perilimbal injection is supplemented by the dusky lilac tint of congestion of the anterior ciliary vessels.

These types of congestion, however, are frequently combined so that they then cease to have special diagnostic importance.

Lacrimal apparatus

Conjunctival congestion of one eye only, or signs of irritation such as watering, should lead us to suspect the efficiency of the lacrimal apparatus. Simple *epiphora* or a flow of tears onto the cheek may be due to malposition of the lower punctum, or to blockage of the canaliculi or nasal duct. Displacement of the lower punctum, which is often very slight, may be easily overlooked but it should be remembered that it is not normally visible without slightly everting the lids. The presence of distension and inflammation of the lacrimal sac should also be noted. This structure is situated in the lacrimal fossa between the inner canthus and the nose, and pressure inwards and backwards at this position will fall upon it. If the sac is distended, the contents — lacrimal fluid, mucus or pus — may regurgitate into the conjunctival

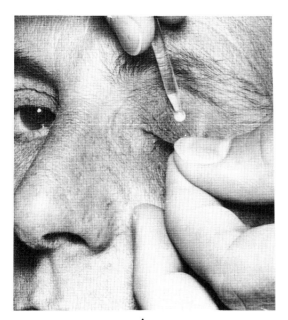

A

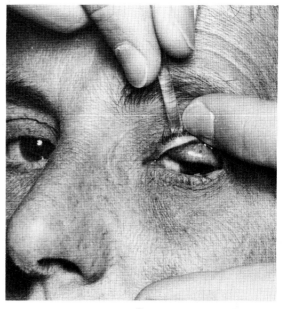

B

Fig. 10.3. Eversion of the upper lid (by courtesy of Hansell)

sac by way of the canaliculi and will be seen pouring from the puncta. The special methods of testing the patency of the lacrimal passages will be described subsequently (Ch. 32).

The sclera

Inspection of the sclera around the cornea may reveal the raised congested nodules of episcleritis, while deep scleritis may be shown by dusky ciliary congestion and opacification of the deeper layers of the cornea at the periphery.

Definite blue coloration of the circumcorneal sclera, except in young children, is pathological. It is most frequently due to a herniation of uveal tissue (a ciliary staphyloma) owing to weakness of the sclera (injury, scleritis, etc.) or to increased intra-ocular pressure (glaucoma). Discoloration may be due to pigmentation. Slight duskiness around the points where the anterior ciliary vessels perforate the sclera is not uncommon in people with dark complexions, but otherwise pigmentation in this neighbourhood, either in the conjunctiva or sclera, should be regarded with suspicion as indicative of melanosis.

The cornea

The corneal surface should be bright, lustrous and transparent. Any loss of substance, such as an abrasion, may easily be overlooked without special methods of examination.

1. An accurate assessment of the corneal surface may be made by *Placido's keratoscopic disc* (Fig. 10.4), on which are painted alternating black and white circles. The observer looks through a hole in the centre at the corneal image as reflected from a light behind the patient; a loss in the sharpness of the outline of the image denotes a loss of the normal polish of the corneal surface, while irregularities in the rings betray irregular-

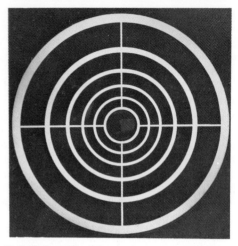

Fig. 10.5 Photograph of the normal corneal reflex; for an abnormal reflex, see Figure 16.13

ities on the corneal surface. The image may be photographed to provide an objective record of the optical and anatomical condition of the cornea (Fig. 10.5). Minor degrees of keratoconus deform the corneal rings.

2. To determine the state of the corneal epithelium, the technique of *corneal staining* with a vital dye should be employed by which lesions often minute and invisible to the naked eye are dramatically accentuated in vivid

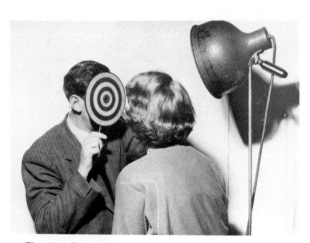

Fig. 10.4 Placido's disc

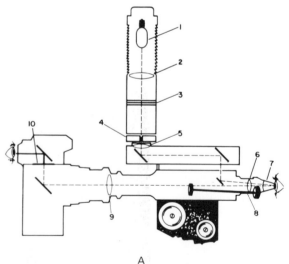

A

Fig. 10.6A Schema of the clinical specular microscope with: 1, viewing lamp; 2, condensing lens; 3; xenon flash tube; 4, slit aperture; 5, condensing lens; 6, objective lens; 7, dipping cone lens; 8, attachment for focusing; 9, eyepiece lens; and 10, viewing screen. (By courtesy of W. M. Bourne and H. E. Kaufman. Published with permission from the Am. J. Oplthalmol. 81 : 319–323, 1976. Copyright by the Ophthalmic Publishing Co. April 24, 1981) B Speciman microscope with camera (by courtesy of Keeler instruments Ltd.) C Normal corneal endothelial cells (by courtesy of Keeler Instruments Ltd)

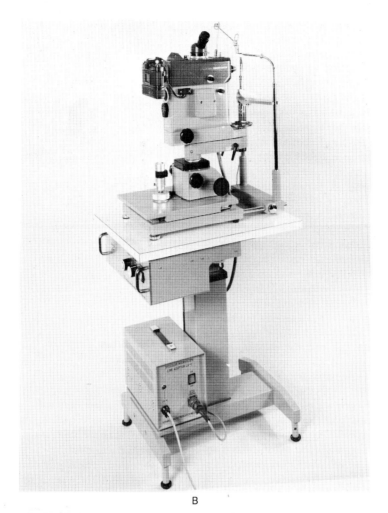

B

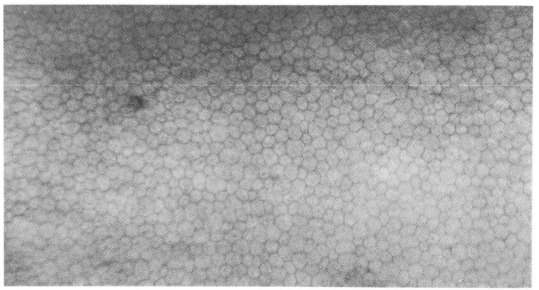

C

colours. Three dyes are usually employed (App. I).
Fluorescein is the most useful to delineate areas denuded of epithelium (abrasions, multiple erosions,
ulcers) which are stained a brilliant green, while Bengal
rose stains diseased and devitalised cells a red colour (as
in superficial punctate keratitis). Alcian blue dye stains
mucus selectively and delineates excess mucus produced
when there is a deficiency in tear formation.

Opacities of the cornea may be so faint that they require minute investigation, and the same is true of the
details and depth of gross opacities. These can best be
studied with the slit-lamp. Of particular importance is
the detection of the minute epithelial or subepithelial
lesions of a *punctate keratitis* as well as of *keratic percipi-
tates* ('k.p.'), small accumulations of cells which adhere
to the endothelium and are derived from the uveal tract.
The importance of their presence is that they form an
indication of inflammation in the uvea, and they are
usually associated with an oedematous condition of the
corneal endothelium itself.

The corneal endothelium is examined by the clinical
specular microscope which makes it possible to observe
a relatively large number of endothelial cells, photograph them and study their morphology (Fig. 10.6B).

With the instrument as described by Bourne and co-
workers (Fig. 10.6A) light passes through a slit aperture
into a system of mirrors which directs the light through
an objective lens and its attached 'dipping cone' and into
the cornea. The dipping cone lens has a flat surface extension on the 20 water immersion objective that ap-
planates the cornea as in applanation tonometry. The
focusing knob adjusts the excursion of the dipping cone
to focus the image of the cornea for different thick-
nesses. The focusing process is used to provide an objective measurement of the corneal thickness. The light is
reflected from the endothelium and back through the
objective lens eye pieces at 200 magnification and may
be observed through an eye piece or directed into a
single-lens reflex camera (Fig. 10.6B). An Xenon flash
cube permits clear photographs despite continuous small
eye movements. Linear magnification of the image on
the film is approximately ×70.

The average cell count is 2800 cells per square millimetre (Fig. 10.6C). There is a significant decrease in
cell density with age. The microscope enables the
surgeon to perform a cell count before using material for
corneal grafting. In cataract extraction, endothelial loss
ranges from 0 to 8%. With intra-ocular lens insertion
cell loss ranges from 24 to 62%. This loss results from
endothelial touch by the implant. Cell loss is greater still
following phako-emulsification.

In many diseases *new vessels* are formed in the cornea.
An exact knowledge of their position, whether superficial or deep, and of their distribution, whether local-

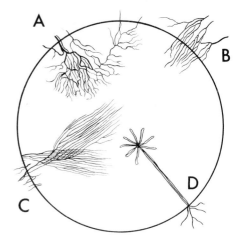

Fig. 10.7 Types of corneal vascularisation: A, arborescent
(superficial) type; B, terminal loop type; C, brush type; D,
umbel type

ised, general, peripheral, above, and so on, is of diagnostic importance.

Superficial vessels in the cornea are distinguished
from deep (Fig. 10.7) by the following features:

1. Superficial vessels can be traced over the limbus
into the conjunctiva, while deep ones seem to come to
an abrupt end at the limbus.

2. Superficial vessels are bright red and well defined,
while deep ones are ill-defined, greyish red, or cause
only a diffuse red blush.

3. Superficial vessels branch in an arborescent
fashion, dichotomously, while deep vessels run more or
less parallel to each other in a general radial direction,
and branch at acute angles; their course is determined
by the lamellar structure of the substantia propria.

4. Superficial vessels may raise the epithelium over
them so that the surface of the cornea is uneven, while
with deep vessels the cornea, though hazy, is smooth.

The *sensibility* of the cornea may be tested by
touching it in various spots with a wisp of cotton-wool
twisted to a fine point and comparing the effect with
that on the opposite side. Normally there is a brisk reflex closure of the lids. The sensibility is often dis-
minished in corneal affections, but the change is of
diagnostic significance in certain cases, particularly
herpes.

The anterior chamber

The anterior chamber is shallow in extreme youth and
in old age: at other periods of life it is normally about
2.5 mm deep. The depth of the anterior chamber is estimated by the position of the iris, and the iris is viewed
through the cornea, which is a strongly refracting convex surface. The effect of this is to magnify the iris and

pupil, and to make them appear farther forwards than they really are.

The anterior chamber is usually shallow in closed-angle glaucoma; abnormally deep in iridocyclitis. It is frequently unequal in depth in different parts. For example, it may be deeper at the periphery than in the centre in iridocyclitis; on the other hand, when the iris is bowed forwards (iris bombé) it is funnel-shaped, the centre being deep, the periphery shallow. Tilting (subluxation) of the lens causes it to be deeper on one side than on the other as does angle-recession following trauma.

After considering the depth, attention must be paid to the contents. In inflammatory conditions of the uveal tract when the permeability of the vessels is increased, the aqueous may contain particles of protein or floating cells. These are of considerable diagnostic importance. In slighter degrees their presence produces an *aqueous flare* which may be visible only with the slit-lamp when its beam is focused to a point (Fig. 10.8); in its more extreme degrees a turbidity exists easily distinguishable by the loupe. The presence of such an opalescence should, of course, lead to a careful examination of the posterior surface of the cornea to detect whether any protein material or cells are deposited thereon (k.p.). In infected wounds and ulcers of the cornea, and occasionally in iridocyclitis, there is pus in the anterior chamber forming a sediment at the bottom, the surface of which is level (*hypopyon*). A similar collection of blood may occur after contusions or spontaneously (*hyphæma*).

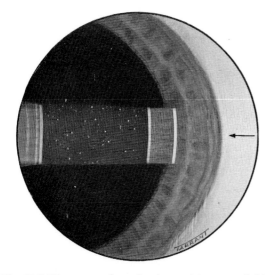

Fig. 10.8 The aqueous flare, showing particles suspended in the anterior chamber as seen by a slit-beam (coming from the right) in a case of cyclitis

The iris

The *colour* of the iris and the clarity of its pattern should first be noted. The two irides or parts of the same iris may be of different colour, conditions which are known respectively as heterochromia iridum or iridis. A grey iris with an ill-defined pattern suggests atrophy from cyclitis and patches of atrophy suggest glaucoma. Darkly pigmented spots in the iris, not raised above the surface, are common as freckles. 'Muddiness of the iris' is the expression used for indistinctness of the pattern, caused by inflammatory exudates; a muddy iris, with small irregular pupil and sluggish reaction to light, is indicative of iritis.

The *position* of the iris must be noted, especially the plane in which it lies. Special attention should be paid to any adhesions (*synechiae*), anterior (to the cornea) or posterior (to the lens capsule). *Tremulousness* of the iris (iridodonesis) is seen when the eyes are moved rapidly if this tissue is not properly supported by the lens; this occurs in absence, shrinkage, or subluxation of the lens. The phenomenon is best seen in a dark room with oblique illumination.

The lens

The lens cannot be thoroughly examined without the assistance of the slit-lamp and the ophthalmoscope. By inspection, aided by focal illumination, we note any opacities in the pupillary area.

When the light is concentrated by focal illumination upon the pupil of a young person's eye the lens substance seems almost perfectly clear; at most we see a faint bluish haze. If we examine the lens of an old person in the same manner the haze is much more pronounced; the lens substance in fact looks slightly milky. We might conclude that the patient has cataract but examination with the ophthalmoscope shows a clear red reflex. The explanation is that the refractive index of the lens substance increases with age, and thus the scattering of light from its surface will be greater; the milkiness is due to rays of light which are reflected from the lens and enter the eye of the observer.

Opacities in the lens itself are seen by oblique illumination as grey, white or yellowish patches; by retro-illumination with the ophthalmoscope they appear black. According to their distribution and nature we diagnose the various forms of cataract, but our observation must always be confirmed and controlled by ophthalmoscopic examination and the opacities localised by examination with the slit-lamp (Plate 7, Fig. A). A spot in the centre of the pupil, looking as if it were on the surface of the lens, may be a pupillary exudate or an anterior polar cataract. Triangular spokes of opacity with their apices towards the centre are indicative of senile cataract. A white appearance over the whole pupillary area suggests a total cataract; if it is yellow and the iris is tremulous we suspect a shrunken calcareous lens. Finally, the pupil may be blocked with uveal exudates (inflammatory pupillary membrane, blocked pupil).

The pupils

The condition of the pupils should be examined at an early stage in every routine examination of the eyes, certainly before any mydriatic is employed. Such an examination requires careful attention to details and is best carried out as follows:

Place the patient facing the light, which should not be too bright, and arrange so that the two pupils are equally illuminated. Note the size, shape and contour of each pupil. To elicit the *direct reaction to light* cover both eyes with the palms of the hands, preferably without touching the face. While the patient looks straight ahead remove one hand and watch the pupil, noting if its constriction to light is well maintained. Replace this hand and remove the other, watching the other pupil.

The *consensual reaction to light* is determined by removing one hand so that this eye is exposed to light (it should be shaded from intense light) and watching the pupils as the hand is removed from the other eye. The process is repeated whilst watching the other pupil.

'*Swinging-flashlight test*'. A bright light is shone onto one pupil and a constriction noted. After two to three seconds, the light is rapidly transferred to the opposite pupil. This swinging to and fro of the light is repeated several times while observing the response of the pupil to which the light is transferred. When the input down both optic nerves to the mid-brain is equal, the pupil to which the light is transferred will remain tightly constricted since the consensual response has the same magnitude as a direct response. Should there be a lesion of one optic nerve the input from that side is less than from the normal side. In that case when the light is transferred to the diseased eye the pupil will dilate, and on swinging back to the normal side the pupil will constrict. Dilatation or 'escape' that occurs is due to removal of the light from the normal side.

This finding is commonly called the *Marcus Gunn pupil* or an afferent pupillary defect and may be the earliest indication of optic nerve disease.

The *reaction to convergence and accommodation* is determined by asking the patient to look to the far end of the room. While he does so the index finger is suddenly held up vertically at about six inches from the patient's nose and he is told to look at it. The movement of the pupils is studied while he converges for the finger.

When the reaction to light is feeble and the pupils are already small, it is difficult to be certain of the results in bright diffuse daylight. In such cases the examination should be made in a dark room and light concentrated upon one pupil by focal illumination so that it shines upon the macula, the most sensitive area from which to elicit the light reflex. By slight lateral movements the focus of light can be moved on or off the pupil, the pupillary movements being watched the while. Still finer observations can be made with the slit-lamp, when the microscope is focused on the pupillary margin and the beam is abruptly switched from the side into the pupillary aperture. If there is no movement in these conditions we may conclude that the reaction to light is absent.

The same method will elicit the *hemianopic pupillary reaction* (Wernicke) in the rare cases (lesion of one optic tract) in which it is present. To test for it, the light is placed in front, but rather to one side of the patient. The light is focused on the opposite side of the retina, and the pupil watched. The light is then moved to the other side and is now focused on the other side of the retina. The best source of illumination for this purpose is the focal beam of the slit-lamp reduced to a spot. If the reaction is present the pupil will react briskly when one half of the retina is illuminated, but very slightly when the other half is illuminated. It usually reacts slightly owing to the impossibility of preventing diffusion of light onto the sensitive half of the retina, and for this reason the test is rarely unequivocal.

If these directions are carried out we shall have reliable information as to the shape and relative size of the pupils and their reactions. A few of the commoner conditions may be enumerated here.

Abnormal size of the pupil

Dilatation of the pupils with retained mobility is found sometimes in myopia and in conditions of impaired tone or nervous excitement. Conversely the pupils are small in babies and in old people.

Very large pupils will suggest that a mydriatic has been used, perhaps inadvertently as when a patient has been using a liniment containing belladonna, and has rubbed (usually) his right eye with soiled fingers. These pupils are usually immobile, and the patient complains of dimness of vision, especially in near work.

The pupil is also large and immobile in lesions affecting the retina and optic nerve causing blindness (Fig. 4.7). The most common are complete optic nerve atrophy and absolute glaucoma. In acute glaucoma it is usually large, immobile and oval, with the long axis vertical. It is to be remembered that the presence of a direct reaction to light does not eliminate the possibility of the patient being blind owing to a central lesion affecting the visual pathways above the level of the lateral geniculate body (post-basal meningitis, hæmorrhage, uræmia, etc.)

Dilated and immobile pupils also result from third

nerve palsies (*absolute paralysis of the pupil*); if the paralysis also affects the third nerve fibres to the ciliary muscle, accommodation is also paralysed (*ophthalmoplegia interna*). This results from cerebral syphilis affecting the third nerve nucleus, meningitis, encephalitis, diphtheria, lead poisoning, orbital disease or trauma affecting the third nerve or ciliary ganglion or the eye itself.

Unilateral dilatation may result from irritation of the cervical sympathetic as by swollen lymph nodes in the neck, apical pneumonia, phthisis, apical pleurisy, cervical rib, thoracic aneurysm, etc.; it may also be due to syringomyelia, acute anterior poliomyelitis and meningitis affecting the lower cervical and upper dorsal part of the spinal cord and to pressure on the sympathetic fibres leaving the cord in the lower cervical and upper dorsal ventral roots. Many of these causes eventually lead to constriction of the corresponding pupil from sympathetic paralysis.

Small immobile pupils suggest the use of drugs, either locally (miotics), or through the general system (morphia). A small sluggish pupil with muddiness of the iris is associated with active iritis. A small immobile pupil suggests old iritis with posterior synechiæ, and should lead to investigation with a mydriatic such as cyclopentolate to see if the pupil dilates regularly.

Bilaterally small pupils may be due to irritation of the third nerves, arousing suspicion of central nervous disease in their vicinity. The condition can also be due to palsy of the sympathetic, as in pontine hæmorrhage. Most of the conditions causing an irritative dilatation lead eventually to constriction. When all the sympathetic function on one side is lost, resulting in miosis, a narrowed palpebral fissure and slight enophthalmos (due to loss of tone of Muller's muscle), sometimes with unilateral absence of sweating, the condition is called *Horner's syndrome*.

Abnormal reactions of the pupil. These are equally important. We have already seen that loss of the light reflexes results from a lesion in the retina or optic nerve causing blindness and that a hemianopic reaction results from lesions in the tract (Fig. 4.7). A lesion in the third nerve abolishes both the light and the convergence reflexes.

More complex lesions may result from damage to the relay paths in the tectum between the afferent and efferent tracts. The most important of these is the *Argyll Robertson pupil*, usually cau d by a lesion, almost invariably syphilitic, in this region. In it the pupils are small (spinal miosis) and do not react to light, but the contraction to convergence is retained.

The *tonic pupil* (of Adie) somewhat resembles the Argyll Robertson pupil; it is of unknown etiology, not associated with syphilis, occurs usually in young women, is often unilateral and associated with absent knee-jerks. The tonic pupil is slightly dilated and always larger than its fellow; the unilateral Argyll Robertson pupil is always smaller. Although in the tonic pupil the reaction to light seems absent at first sight, careful examination shows it to be present although slight. The pupil reaction on convergence is sluggish with a long latent period and it is unduly sustained. The tonic pupil dilates well with atropine; the Argyll Robertson pupil does not; finally, the tonic pupil constricts to weak pilocarpine (0.1%).

An analysis of the pupillary reactions to drugs frequently allows a differential diagnosis to be made of the causal nerve lesion; the rationale of these tests will be understood from the reaction of the various drugs (p. 27).

If an enlargement of the pupil is due to sympathetic irritation (*spastic mydriasis*), light and accommodation will cause constriction, cocaine will not cause further dilatation since the sympathetic is already stimulated, eserine will cause considerable but not maximal constriction (since the tone of the sphincter overcomes that of the dilatator), and atropine will cause maximal dilatation since the dilatator is now completely unopposed.

If the enlargement is due to paralysis of the third nerve (*paralytic mydriasis*), the reactions to light and accommodation are absent, cocaine and atropine cause a further dilatation and pilocarpine causes constriction if the lesion is proximal to the ciliary ganglion.

If the pupil is small due to irritation of the third nerve (*spastic miosis*), light, accommodation and eserine will cause no appreciable increase in constriction, cocaine a slight and atropine a greater dilatation.

If the miosis is due to sympathetic palsy (*paralytic miosis*), light, accommodation and eserine will cause maximal constriction, cocaine will be inactive and atropine relatively inactive since both muscles are now paralysed.

Gonioscopy

With the methods of examination which we have discussed it is impossible to see into the recesses of the angle of the anterior chamber since this region is covered over by the projecting shelf of the sclera at the limbus. In many conditions such as glaucoma, foreign bodies or tumours, a close inspection of this region is important. It can, however, be made accessible by the slit-lamp provided the beam is diverted at an angle. For this purpose several types of *gonioscope* have been developed, the simplest of which is that of Goldmann (Fig. 10. 9) whereby a contact lens is inserted between the lids to lie upon the anæsthetised cornea; the lens is fitted with a mirror in which the image of the recesses of the angle is reflected.

In this way a clear view of the whole of the angle is provided. Figure 10.10 shows the main features of the gonioscopic picture. The landmarks from behind for-

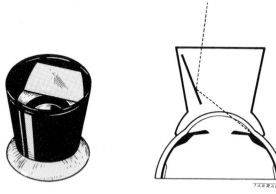

Fig. 10.9 The Goldmann contact lens used for gonioscopy with the slit-lamp microscope. The figure on the right shows the path of the rays through the lens. They are reflected by the mirror in their path into the angle, and again, as they emerge, into the objectives of the corneal microscope

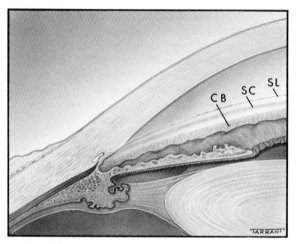

Fig. 10.10 The angle of the anterior chamber seen gonioscopically: SL, Schwalbe's line; SC, Schlemm's canal; CB, ciliary band

wards are: 1. the anterior surface of the iris; 2. the antero-medial surface of the ciliary body; 3. the trabeculae covering the canal of Schlemm; 4. Schwalbe's ring (a glistening white line corresponding to the break-up of Descemet's membrane); and beyond this 5. the posterior surface of the cornea which is seen as a convex dome.

Transillumination

In this method of examination an intense beam of light is thrown through the conjunctiva and sclera whereupon the pupil normally appears red; if, however, a solid mass lies in the path of the light, the beam is obstructed and the pupil remains black. For this purpose, special transilluminators may be employed or, more simply, a cap with an open hole at the end may be

fitted over the bulb of an electric ophthalmoscope.

In this way a solid mass can be delineated and a tumour differentiated from a cyst. An opaque foreign body can be seen in a cataractous lens, while pupillary reactions may be tested in the presence of a cornea so opaque that accurate vision through it is impossible, although light may be transmitted. Only the anterior half of the eye can be transilluminated in this way, but if there is a mass in the posterior segment of the globe, it can be transilluminated at the time of an operation after the capsule of Tenon has been opened and the transilluminator inserted within it. In the latter type of case a somewhat less reliable method is that of *indirect transillumination*, wherein a powerful source of light is placed in the mouth illuminating the eyes from behind; normally the pupils have a strikingly luminous appearance but if a solid mass occupies the fundus, they appear black.

The tension

Last in the external examination, but by no means of least importance, the tension of the sclera should be assessed; depending on its degree of rigidity, which varies between individuals, it is increased when the intra-ocular pressure is raised, though not necessarily *paripassu*. It may be done digitally in the same manner as testing for fluctuation in other parts of the body.

Instruments known as *tonometers* have been devised for measuring the tension of the intact eye and are of two types. The most common *indentation tonometer* in clinical use is that of Schiötz (Fig. 10.11); with it the depth of the indentation of the cornea, anæsthetised

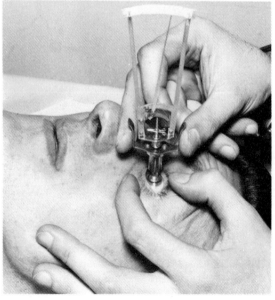

Fig. 10.11 Schiötz tonometer (by courtesy of Hansell)

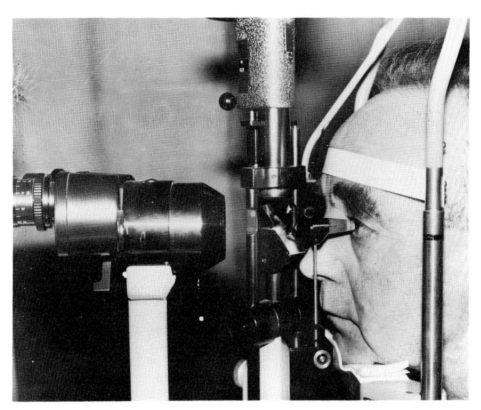

Fig. 10.12 The applanation tonometer (by courtesy of Hansell)

with benoxinate solution, made by a weighted stylet is measured by a lever which travels over a scale. There are four weights (5.5, 7.5, 10 and 15 gm) and the greatest accuracy is attained with the weight which gives a deflection of the lever of 2–4 mm. The instrument is calibrated so that the equivalents of the readings in millimetres of mercury can be read off a chart. The readings are inaccurate when transformed into pressures in millimetres of mercury largely because of wide individual variations in the rigidity of the corneo-sclera, but the tonometer is certainly useful to obtain approximate readings and particularly for comparative measurements, as between the two eyes or between successive measurements on the same eye. To allow for this inaccuracy the type of tonometer should always be cited and the reading expressed in this form –20 mm Hg (Schiötz).

An *applanation tonometer* is more accurate than an indentation tonometer since the factor of ocular rigidity is not involved. When the cornea is flattened by the application to it of a plane surface, the intra-ocular pressure is directly proportional to the pressure applied and inversely to the area flattened. The most popular applanation tonometer was designed by Goldmann for use with the Haag-Streit slit-lamp (Fig. 10.12). In it a flat circular plexiglass plate 7 mm in diameter is applied to the anaesthetised cornea so as to flatten an area 3.06 mm in diameter. The constancy of the area is ensured by an ingenious duplicating optical device; a force of 0.1 gm exerted by a spring-and-lever system corresponds to a pressure of 1 mm Hg. To avoid the necessity of using a slit-lamp, simpler instruments have been devised based on the same principle. With these instruments the average ocular tension is approximately 15 mm. Hg (applanation).

11

Examination of the fundus

In ordinary circumstances the pupil looks black, and no reflex is obtained from the fundus. If, as in Figure 11.1, there is a source of light L, in front of the eye, and the eye is focused upon it or accommodated for it, the light and a spot upon the retina are conjugate foci so that the image of the spot of light is a spot on the retina. Reversing the direction of the rays, all rays from the illuminated spot of the retina are brought to a focus at the source of light. It follows that no rays will enter an observing eye unless it is situated at the source of light. The problem of ophthalmoscopic examination is to make the observing eye at the same time the source of illumination of the observed fundus.

If the eye is not focused for the source of light the conditions are different, and some slight luminosity of the pupil may be seen. This is one cause of luminosity in the pupils of very hypermetropic eyes and in pathological conditions when the retina is displaced forwards as in detachment or by a tumour.

In hypermetropia the conjugate focus of the source of light, L, is a point, l, behind the retina (Fig. 11.2). Hence the emergent rays from the illuminated area of the fundus are divergent, as if coming from l. Therefore an observing eye situated anywhere within the area l_1 l_2 of the cone of emergent rays will catch some of them, and the pupil of the observed eye will appear feebly illuminated. In these circumstances it is not necessary for the observing eye to occupy the exact position of the source of light, but only a spot in its immediate neighbourhood. On the same principle, the extremely hypermetropic retina pushed forwards by a tumour can be seen well by focal illumination.

The luminosity of albinos' eyes is due to light entering the eye, not only through the pupil, but also through the iris and sclera. That this is the true explanation is shown by the fact that the pupil looks black if it is observed through a small hole in an opaque screen. Only a small amount of light passes through the sclera in the normal eye.

OPHTHALMOSCOPY

It will help us to understand the principles of the ophthalmoscope if we say a few words about its historical development. The ophthalmoscope was invented by

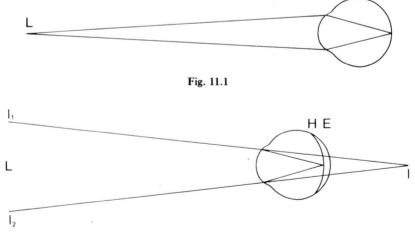

Fig. 11.1

Fig. 11.2

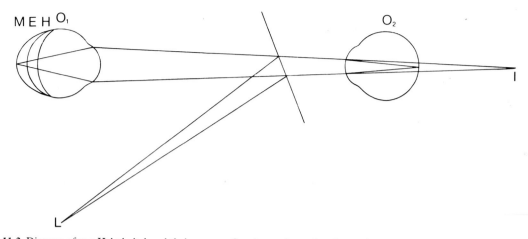

M E H O₁ O₂ l L

Fig. 11.3 Diagram of von Helmholtz's ophthalmoscope: O_1, observed eye; O_2, observer's eye; L, source of light; l, image of L formed by the plane mirror — immediate source of light; M E H, relative positions of retina in myopia, emmetropia, and hypermetropia respectively, showing the relative size of the areas of retina illuminated in each case

Babbage in 1848, but its importance was not recognised, and it was re-invented by von Helmholtz in 1850. The original ophthalmoscope of von Helmholtz was merely a plane plate of glass (Fig. 11.3). A source of light was placed beside the observed eye and the glass plate obliquely in front of it, so that a portion of the light was reflected from the surface of the plate into the eye. On looking through the transparent plate an observer could now receive some of the rays from the fundus into his own eye, and thus obtain an image of the illuminated fundus. Since but a small proportion of the light received upon the plate is reflected at its surface, the illumination is feeble. von Helmholtz next increased the amount of light reflected by superimposing three plane plates. The back of the glass was next converted into a more powerful mirror by silvering it, leaving a small portion unsilvered or a hole in the mirror, through which the observer might look. The illumination was still feeble, since the rays reflected by a plane mirror are divergent. Reute (1852) therefore introduced the perforated concave mirror which is still generally used. The final modification was the addition of a battery of small lenses of various strengths, which might be brought into position behind the aperture. The many forms of ophthalmoscopes are merely various mechanical contrivances for doing this most conveniently.

The *routine of ophthalmoscopic examination* should be as follows:

1. Preliminary examination with the plane mirror alone at a distance of about 1 m from the patient.

2. Examination with the mirror alone at a distance of about 22 cm. from the patient.

3. Ophthalmoscopic examination by the indirect method.

4. Ophthalmoscopic examination by the direct method.

The following facts show the wisdom of this procedure. By (1) we obtained knowledge of the nature of the refraction of the eye under examination; this will prevent many difficulties when we come to closer quarters. By (2) we see any gross changes, especially opacities in the refractive media; these may at once be made evident by this method, whereas they may be very puzzling if first observed by (3) or (4). In addition, we shall see the details of any very hypermetropic part of the fundus, such as a detachment of the retina or a tumour; these also are sometimes by no means difficult to miss by (3) and (4). By (3) we get a general view of the fundus — the largest possible area under moderate magnification; it is comparable to microscopic examination with a low power. By (4) we examine details under a high magnification; it is comparable to microscopic examination with a high power. All these examinations are easier if the pupils are dilated with a mydriatic.

The patient is taken into the darkroom and the eye should be as much as possible in darkness. For *examination with the plane mirror alone* the observer sits facing the patient, about a metre from him. He reflects the light from the plane mirror into the eye, meanwhile looking through the sight-hole. An adjustable electric ophthalmoscope or the retinoscope (p. 50) can provide the same illumination. When the light falls on the eye he notices a red reflex from the pupil. There ought to be no black spots in the pupillary area, but either a uniform red reflex or obscure details of the fundus. By tilting the mirror to and fro in various directions he can obtain an approximate idea of the refraction of the eye.

The observer now approaches the patient until his eye, still with the plane mirror, is about 20 cm from the eye under observation. He can now see the cornea and iris clearly, and can confirm any points which he has made out previously by the external examination.

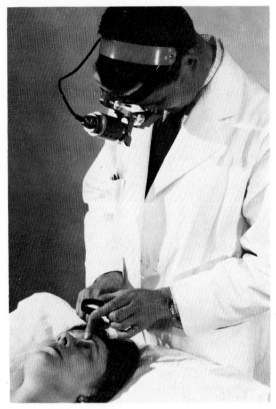

Fig. 11.4 Indirect opthalmoscopy (by courtesy of Hansel)

Examination by indirect ophthalmoscopy. The binocular indirect ophthalmoscope is applicable to all refractive errors and as its beam penetrates most medial opacities and there is a reduced image size, it is possible to obtain a wide view of the retina and its defects (Fig. 11.4).

The lens is held between the thumb and forefinger of the left hand with the curved surface towards the examiner, and with the lens itself in a plane parallel to the iris plane of the observer. The strength of the lens may be + 30 D, + 20 D or + 14 D, the weaker lenses giving images of increasing size. The periphery of the retina may be brought into view by scleral depression and it is best seen with the patient recumbent. Drawings

should be made on a retinal detachment chart with accurate delineation of the vascular structure of the retina and careful assessment of its relationship to retinal holes or areas of degeneration.

Having obtained a good general view of the fundus, the observer again approaches the patient and proceeds to *direct ophthalmoscopy*. Using the self-luminous ophthalmoscope, he looks through the sight-hole and directs the light upon the eye; this is best effected from a short distance away. When the light is on the pupil and the observer can see the red reflex, he slowly approaches until his brow is almost touching the patient's brow. If both the patient and the observer are emmetropic and the latter keeps his accommodation relaxed, he will then probably see the fundus clearly. If either is ametropic, the observer brings into position the appropriate lenses in the ophthalmoscope; and if he cannot relax his accommodation he should use extra concave lenses. The image is erect, the opposite of that by the indirect method. Here again practice is needed, and a knowledge of the optical conditions is essential.

1. Preliminary examination with the mirror at 1 m
We will suppose that the observer is emmetropic or that his refraction has been corrected, and that the accommodation of the observed eye is at rest or paralysed by a cycloplegic.

If the eye is emmetropic or has a low refractive error, the rays issuing from any point on the retina are parallel, and since the bundles of rays from two points on the retina diverge after leaving the eye, the observer cannot receive portions of both bundles simultaneously through his pupil (Fig. 11.5). He cannot therefore see two spots on the retina but can only focus one at a time, and thus sees only a general illumination. In the hypermetropic eye, however, the emerging rays are divergent, and the two bundles of rays from two points on the retina will form two divergent bundles (Fig. 11.6). These will appear to come from two points behind the eye where an imaginary erect image is formed. Since each bundle diverges, some of the peripheral rays of each will be received by the observer's pupil, so that he will obtain a clear image of

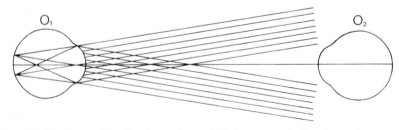

Fig. 11.5 Examination with the mirror at 1 m: O_1, observed eye, which is emmetropic; O_2, observer's eye: none of the rays from the widely distant points on the fundus of O_1 enters O_2. If the points are close together the rays of the two bundles will be nearly parallel, and would form a clear image on the retina of O_2 if the accommodation of O_2 were almost completely in abeyance

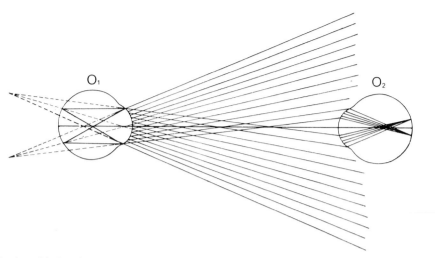

Fig. 11.6 Examination with the mirror at 1 m: O_1, observed eye, which is hypermetropic; O_2, observer's eye, emmetropic, but accommodated for the divergent rays from O_1

each point and thus see the virtual image behind the patient's eye. In myopia, on the other hand, the rays coming from the two points will be convergent and will form a real inverted image in front of the eye (Fig. 11.7). Continuing from this image the rays will diverge in two bundles, the peripheral parts of which will enter the observer's pupil. He will thus see a small inverted image of the fundus. If the observer now moves his head from side to side, the erect image in hypermetropia will appear to move in the same direction, and the inverted image in myopia in the opposite.

It therefore follows that in the preliminary examination with the plane mirror, if the fundus reflex is seen as a uniform red glow (the *red reflex*), the eye is emmetropic or approximately so; but if any details of the retinal structure are seen, a considerable degree of ametropia exists. If the picture thus presented appears to move in the same direction as the observer's head, the refraction is hypermetropic; if it moves in the opposite direction, it is myopic. This may be verified and a more accurate assessment of the refraction gained by retinoscopy.

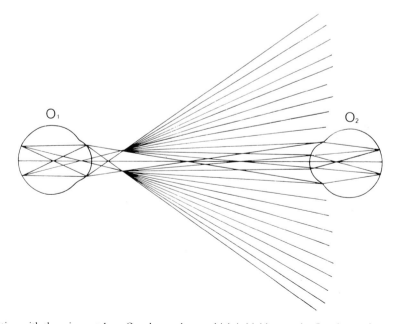

Fig. 11.7 Examination with the mirror at 1 m: O_1, observed eye, which is highly myopic; O_2, observer's eye, emmetropic, but accommodated for the divergent rays from the far point of O_1

2. Preliminary examination with the mirror at the convenient distance for near vision (22 cm)

At this distance the observer will be most suitably situated for distinct unaided vision, and he will be able to examine the superficial parts of the eye more accurately. If he is hypermetropic or presbyopic he will naturally have to use a convex lens. The purposes of a preliminary examination in this manner are (1) the recognition of opacities in the refractive media; (2) the recognition of a detached retina or other structure not far behind the lens; (3) the confirmation of the results found by the external examination.

1. *The diagnosis of opacities in the refractive media.* If there is any opaque body in the course of the rays reflected from the fundus it will stop these rays and will therefore appear black. The whole field may be black, as when the lens is entirely opaque, or when there is blood in the vitreous. If small opacities are seen their motility is determined by telling the patient to turn his eye in different directions; a floating opacity will then continue to move after the eye is brought to rest, in which case it must be either in the aqueous or vitreous which latter in this event must be fluid. The exact position may be determined by observing its *parallactic displacement*.

In Fig. 11.8, if 4 is the centre of rotation of the eye, and if there are opacities at 1, 2, 3, 4, 5, then, when the eye is rotated a small amount, all the opacities except 4 will move, the amount of movement being greater the farther the opacity is from the centre of rotation. Since all the movements will be referred to the edge of the pupil for comparison, to an observer situated at A, all the opacities will appear as a single spot in the centre of the pupillary reflex. If he shifts his position to B, or if the eye is rotated in the opposite direction, the opacity 2 will remain in the centre of the pupil, whilst 1 will appear to move towards one edge of the pupil, and 3, 4 and 5 towards the opposite edge, 5 being lost behind the iris.

Hence we deduce the rule that if the eye is moved slightly in a given direction, opacities in the pupillary plane will appear stationary; those in front of that plane will move in the same direction, and those behind will appear to move in the opposite direction, the amplitude of apparent movement being a rough indication of their distance from the pupillary plane.

The *corneal reflex*, the image of the mirror formed by the cornea, can also be used as a guide. It is a virtual image situated about 4 mm behind the anterior corneal surface, that is, a short distance behind the anterior surface of the lens (behind 2 in Fig. 11.8). The centre of curvature of the cornea is situated 8 mm behind its anterior surface (less than 1 mm behind 3 in Fig. 11.8). By this method of examination the corneal reflex will always cover this latter spot, the centre of curvature of the cornea, no matter what the position of the eye. Hence an opacity situated here will always be covered by the corneal reflex: opacities in front of the corneal reflex move in the same sense with regard to the reflex as the eye moves; and opacities behind it move in the opposite direction to the movement of the eye.

This method of examination affords the surest means of discovering the edge of a *dislocated lens*, or the notch in the edge of the lens in congenital *coloboma of the lens*. When the edge of the lens crosses the pupillary area it is seen as an intensely black crescent, since the whole of the light reflected from the fundus which falls upon the extreme edge of the lens is totally reflected within the lens; none of it leaves the eye, so that none of it can enter the observer's eye.

2. *The recognition of a detached retina or a tumour arising from the fundus.* We have already discussed the optical conditions rendering such lesions visible, the retina being in the position of the fundus of a very hypermetropic eye. When light is thrown in from the mirror a difference of reflex in different directions is noticed, red in some, grey or black in others. More minute investigation will reveal a whitish or greyish uneven surface upon which the retinal vessels are seen as black wavy lines, an important observation since the appearance of a detached retina by ophthalmoscopy may be puzzling to the beginner.

3. *Confirmation of the results found by the external*

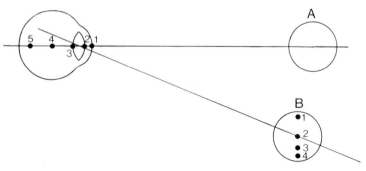

Fig. 11.8 Parallactic displacement

examination. We are able by this method not only to confirm the results peviously arrived at by external examination, but also to supplement some of them by important subsidiary information. Thus we are able to map out the limits of opacities in the lens much more accurately, since they now appear black on a red background. A black spot in the iris may allow a red reflex through it and thus show itself to be a hole. Similarly a black patch at the ciliary margin of the iris may be a melanotic tumour of the ciliary body growing forwards and implicating the iris: or it may be a separation of the iris from its ciliary attachment (irido-dialysis); in the latter case it will be possible to obtain a reflex through it by the mirror, whereas in the former it will be opaque.

By this method, also, superficial opacities, such as those in the cornea and near the anterior surface of the lens, can be seen in their natural colours at high magnification by approaching still nearer to the eye and using stronger convex lenses behind the mirror. Thus if we approach very closely to the eye and place a + 20 D lens behind the mirror the opacities in the cornea are seen highly magnified, while those in the lens may be brought more clearly into focus with a slightly weaker lens.

3. *The indirect method*

The indirect method of examination with the ophthalmoscope consists essentially in making the eye, whatever be its refraction, highly myopic by placing a strong convex lens in front of it so that a real inverted image of the fundus is formed between the observer and the convex lens (Figs 11.9–11.10). In all cases the image is magnified, the amount of magnification depending upon the refraction of the eye, the strength of the lens and its distance from the eye. With a lens of + 13 D the fundus of an emmetropic eye is magnified about five times.

It will be seen that with the same lens the inverted image is formed at different distances beyond it accord-

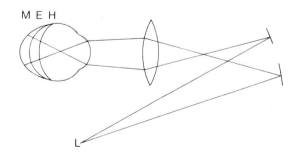

Fig. 11.9 Indirect method. Illumination of the fundus, showing the course of rays from the source of light to the mirror, through the lens, and through the eye; also the area of the field of illumination

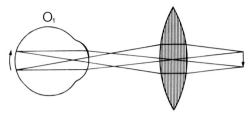

Fig. 11.10 Indirect method. Emergent rays from the fundus, showing the formation of the image. In the figure the lens is situated at the anterior focal plane of the eye; the rays which are parallel inside the eye, therefore, pass through the optical centre of the lens. The rays which pass through the nodal point of the eye are rendered convergent by the lens. The points where these two systems of rays cross give the position of the image, which is seen to be inverted

ing to the refraction of the eye. If the lens is kept at a constant distance from the eye, for example, its own focal distance, the emmetropic image will be formed at the focal distance of the lens beyond it: the myopic will be nearer to the lens, the hypermetropic farther from it (Fig. 11.11). Since in all cases the image is formed in the air between the lens and the observer's eye, the observer must not approach too closely to the patient (a natural impulse in order to see the aerial image clearly with his unaided eye); if he does so he will find it necessary to put up an appropriate convex lens, which, incidentally, will magnify the image.

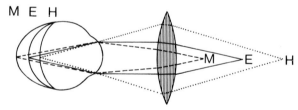

Fig. 11.11 Indirect method. Position of the image according to the refraction of the eye. In this figure the lens is situated at its own focal distance from the cornea. In emmetropia the parallel emergent rays, therefore, cross at the principal focus of the lens at E. In myopia the convergent emergent rays cross nearer to the lens than its principal focus, at M; in hypermetropia the divergent emergent rays cross farther from the lens than its principal focus, at H

One of the difficulties in the indirect method is the reflexes formed by the eye and the surfaces of the lens. The cornea forms a reflex of the mirror which, when seen through the convex lens, is magnified, so that it may cover the pupil and prevent anything behind being seen. The surface of the lens towards the observer acts as another convex mirror and forms another reflex situated behind the lens. Similarly the surface of the lens near the patient acts as a concave mirror and forms a reflex on the observer's side of the lens. These reflexes are troublesome, but they may be got out of the way by tilting the lens so that they move in opposite directions and a view is obtained between them. The tilting should not be overdone since the optical effect of astigmatism is produced and the fundus appears distorted.

Theoretically, to obtain the maximum field, the best place for the lens is its own focal distance from the patient's pupil; but this is the worst place for the corneal reflex. Since the latter is situated near the level of the iris, if the convex lens is at its focal distance from it, the rays from this image will be made parallel by the lens and the reflex will fill the whole area of the lens so that nothing else is seen. The best position of practical purposes is either nearer to or farther from the eye than this, and the convenient distance is where the lens is at its focal distance from the anterior focus of the eye. Here, slight tilting of the lens, besides shifting the lens reflexes out of the way, will also move the corneal reflex and the image of the fundus in opposite directions, allowing an uninterrupted view.

Differences of level of two points near each other on the fundus are made very evident by parallactic displacement with the indirect method. Thus, in Figure

11.12, if there are two points, *a* and *b*, at different levels in the fundus, for example, on the edge of the disc and at the bottom of a glaucomatous cup, when the lens is shifted slightly so that its optical centre moves from o_1 to o_2, the images of *a* and *b* will move from a_1 to a_2 and b_1 to b_2.

4. The direct method.

In the direct method the patient's eye is approached as closely as possible by the observer whose eye thus receives the emergent rays from the fundus directly (Fig. 11.13).

If the patient is emmetropic (E, Fig. 11.14), the issuing rays will be parallel, and will be brought to a focus on the retina of the observer. If he is hypermetropic, the emergent rays will diverge (H, Fig. 11.14), and consequently will only be brought to a focus on the observer's retina if he accommodates, or by the help of a convex lens. If he is myopic, they are convergent (M. Fig. 11.14) and must be made more divergent by the interposition of a concave lens if a similar focus is to be formed. In emmetropia, therefore, the image of the re-

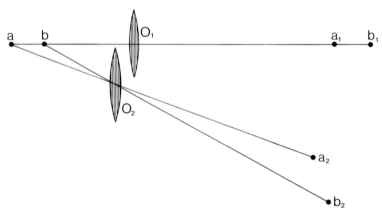

Fig. 11.12 Indirect method. Parallactic displacement

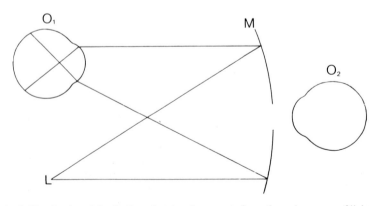

Fig. 11.13 Direct method. Illumination of the fundus, showing the course of rays from the source of light to the mirror and through the eye: also the area of the field of illumination. Compare with Figure 11.8

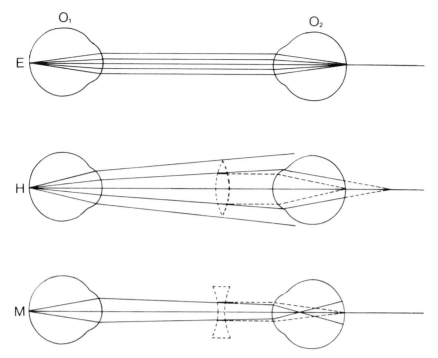

Fig. 11.14 Direct method. Emergent rays from the fundus of the observed eye, O_1, showing the formation of the retinal image on the retina of the observer's eye, O_2. In emmetropia, E, the emergent parallel rays are brought to a focus on the retina of O_2 if the accommodation of this eye is absolutely at rest. In hypermetropia, H, the emergent divergent rays are brought to a focus on the retina of O_2, either by means of accommodation or by placing a convex lens in front of O_2. In myopia, M, the emergent convergent rays can only be brought to a focus on the retina of O_2 by placing a concave lens in front of O_2

tina is seen clearly without any lens in the ophthalmoscope; in ametropia, in order that the image be clearly seen, a lens corresponding to the refractive error must be used. If, however, the eye is very highly myopic its punctum remotum will be situated somewhere in space between the eye itself and the observer's ophthalmoscope so that it may be impossible to obtain a clear image with any correction; in such cases a view of the fundus may be possible if the patient's spectacles are left in place and the examination is made through them.

Much stress is generally laid upon the necessity and the difficulty of relaxing one's accommodation in examination by the direct method. It is difficult to relax the accommodation entirely when the eye is apparently close to the object looked at. The observer should try to think that he is looking at a very distant object, but even then, as soon as he directs his attention to details of the picture, he is almost certain to accommodate. It is best for the beginner not to worry himself about this point: if he cannot see an emmetropic fundus clearly, let him put up minus lenses until he does. When he has acquired facility in seeing anything at all it will be soon enough for him to grapple with this difficulty.

The image by the direct method is always erect and is also more magnified than by the indirect method. In emmetropia the fundus is seen magnified about fifteen times, somewhat less in hypermetropia and more in myopia.

The area of the fundus which can be seen by the direct method varies with the distance of the observer from the eye and with the refraction. It increases as the eye is approached, is greatest in hypermetropia, least in myopia, and intermediate in emmetropia. Thus, we see the largest area, least magnified, in hypermetropia, and the least area, most magnified, in myopia. In astigmatism the magnification is greatest in the more myopic meridian, and least in the more hypermetropic so that there can be no clear image of the whole field. *Only lines perpendicular to the meridian which is corrected are seen clearly.*

If there is a difference in level between two points on the fundus, it is made manifest in the direct method also by parallactic displacement if the observer moves slightly to one side; an object farther forward always moves in the opposite direction to the movement of the observer's head.

The difference in level can be accurately measured. Thus the bottom of a cupped disc will be relatively myopic to the edge so that a more concave lens will be required to see the vessels at the bottom of the cup clearly, while the top of an eminence, such as a swollen disc or a tumour, will require more convex lenses than are needed to see clearly a blood vessel on a normal part of the retina near the disc. It can be proved that *if the correcting lens is at the anterior focus of the emmetropic eye* a difference of 3 D is equivalent to approximately 1 mm difference of level at the fundus. It is important to get as close as possible to the eye when measuring differences of level and to relax the accommodation, because only then are the conditions of accuracy fulfilled. In order to eliminate the effect of the observer's accommodation the lowest minus lens or the highest convex lens which allows clear vision must be chosen for the purposes of measurement.

An opacity in the vitreous provides the same optical conditions as the fundus of a hypermetropic eye. Such an opacity can be examined by putting up convex lenses until it is clearly focused; by using convex lenses from 0 to + 20 D and by withdrawing slightly from the eye, we can thoroughly explore the emmetropic eye from the fundus to the surface of the cornea. The appearance of opacities in the vitreous or lens will vary with their density and with the amount of light reflected from their surfaces; if they are very dense they will appear black against the background of the red reflex, but if they are semi-transparent they will appear red or whitish according to the relative amounts of light transmitted from the fundus and reflected from their surface. A detached retina may therefore look red or white according to its degree of transparency, and if much light is reflected from the surface details may be seen upon it.

EXAMINATION OF THE FUNDUS BY FOCAL ILLUMINATION

The ordinary slit-lamp, as we have seen, cannot be used to explore the eye further back than the anterior parts of the vitreous because the beam of light is ordinarily brought to a focus in this region. If, however, the beam is made more divergent by eliminating the refractive influence of the corneal curvature by using a contact lens with a flat anterior face, or (more simply) by interposing a− 55 D lens in front of the cornea, the posterior part of the vitreous and the central area of the fundus can be examined by the binocular microscope in the focused beam of light. Such an examination requires full mydriasis. By this method fine changes in the posterior part of the vitreous and in the retina and at the optic disc can be readily studied, areas of œdema are clearly outlined in the optical section, and difficult problems in diagnosis such as the difference between a cyst or hole at the macula are clearly demonstrated (Plate V, Figs A and B).

Three types of lenses are available for biomicroscopic examination of the vitreous and fundus.

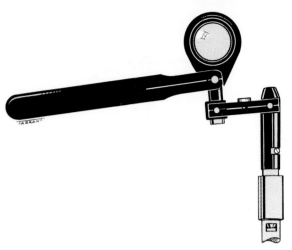

Fig. 11.15 Hruby lens

1. Hruby lens (Fig. 11.15)
The lens has a plano-concave surface mounted on a holder attached to the chin rest of the Haag-Streit slit lamp. It has a dioptric strength of -58.6 D so that images of objects in the fundus are brought to a focus at the distal focal point of the lens which lies in the anterior segment of the eye (Fig. 11.16.1). The concave surface should face the patient and be placed as near to the observed cornea as possible.

This lens provides a small field with low magnification and cannot visualise the fundus beyond the equator (Fig. 11.16.2).

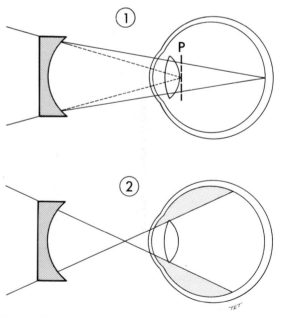

Fig. 11.16 Optics of Hruby lens. 1. fundus image appears in plane P. 2. Area of the fundus seen is limited

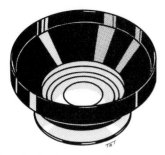

Fig. 11.17 Posterior fundus contact lens

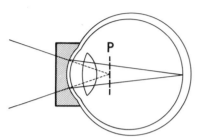

Fig. 11.18 Posterior fundus contact lens with the image appearing in plane P

2. Posterior fundus contact lens (Fig. 11.17)

This is a modified Koeppe lens. The image produced is virtual and erect, situated in the anterior vitreous cavity and is most helpful in exploring the posterior fundus (Fig. 11.18).

3. Goldmann three-mirror contact lens (Fig. 11.19)

Three mirrors are placed in the cone, each with a different angle of inclination (B, C, D). The central part of the contact lens allows a view of the posterior fundus (A). The peripheral fundus can be examined by each mirror, bringing into focus a different area (Fig. 11.19.3).

The basis of biomicroscropy of the vitreous body is the Tyndall effect and this is maximal with a high intensity of projected light, a good contrast between the observed structure and background, a large angle of separation between observer and illumination axes and when viewed by a dark adapted eye. The patient's pupils must be widely dilated, so that the peripheral retina may be explored in combination with scleral depression.

Fluorescein angiography

Fluorescein angiography of the fundus is based on the sensitivity of the recording film to the presence of fluorescent light from the dye. This fluorescence is produced by irradiation of the dye with light of a wavelength within the absorption band of the fluorescein and blood mixture (420–490 nm). The emitted fluorescence (510–530 nm) is passed through a barrier filter to the film with complete exclusion of the irradiating light.

Fluorescein is readily bound to albumen in the blood stream. The blood–retinal barrier by preventing dye leakage in the physiological state facilitates the delin-

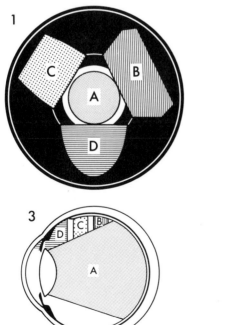

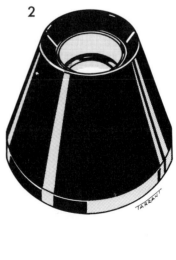

Fig. 11.19 Goldman-three-mirror contact lens and diagram of optical principles

eation of retinal vessels of all calibres. In the choroidal circulation fluorescein passes freely across the endothelium of the capillaries to the extravascular spaces. A physiological barrier to the dye prevents the passage across Bruch's membrane and the intact retinal pigment epithelium.

Fluorograms reveal dissolution of the physiological barriers by the leakage of dye across retinal vessel walls and across Bruch's membrane and having leaked the dye may persist for longer than can be explained on physiological grounds. Fundus pigment and red cells absorb fluorescent light and such tissues may therefore mask fluorescence in deeper structures. On the other hand migration of pigment gives access to deeper fluorescence — a window effect.

When the dye enters the eye there is at first a choroidal blush and then the dye can be followed through the retinal arterioles, the capillary bed and into the veins which are at first laminated. A late phase is usually recorded 5–30 min after injection (Fig. 11.20A–D).

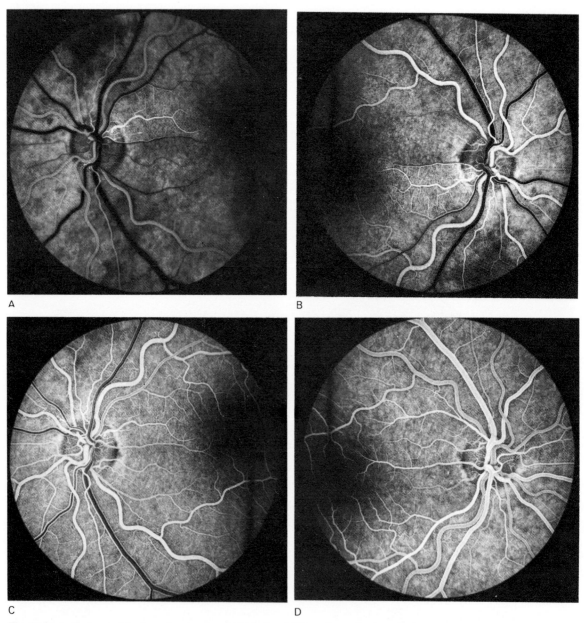

A

B

C

D

Fig. 11.20 A. Early arteriole phase showing choroidal blush and filling of a small cilio-retinal vessel. B. Arterial phase. C. Arterio-venous phase showing laminar flow in the retinal veins. D. Venous phase. (By courtesy of T. J. ffytche.)

Fluorescein angiography is particularly helpful in exposing the depth of pathology in diabetic retinopathy and reveals neovascularisation occurring in any area of the fundus. It gives a clear idea of the integrity of the vascular tree itself, and is also useful in the assessment of fundus disorders including neoplasia and disorders of the optic nerve head such as papilloedema.

Fluorescein angiography is also helpful in the interpretation of neovascularisation of the iris when leakage from the iris vessels may be the first sign of rubeosis. Vitreous fluorophotometry allows measurement of fluorescein concentration in all parts of the vitreous chamber visible through the eyepiece of the slit-lamp. By this technique minimal amounts of fluorescein in the range of $10^{-8}-10^{-9}$ g/ml may be detected in the vitreous. One of the early signs of diabetes in the eye is an alteration in permeability of the blood-aqueous barrier allowing the passage of fluorescein into the vitreous chamber. A similar breakdown in the barrier occurs early in the course of retinitis pigmentosa and also in carriers of this disease.

ULTRASONOGRAPHY

Diagnostic ultrasound is used in the investigation of patients with opacification of the ocular media or with orbital problems. Ultrasonic frequencies in the range of 10 MHz are used for ophthalmic diagnosis. The sound is coupled to the eye by means of a saline bath. Three

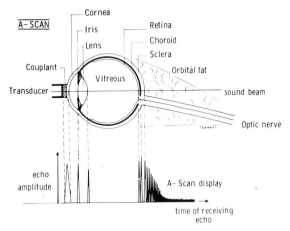

Fig. 11.21 A-scan technique. (By courtesy of Restori.)

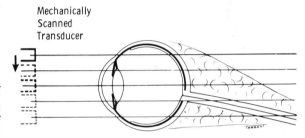

Fig. 11.22 B-scan technique. (By courtesy of Restori.)

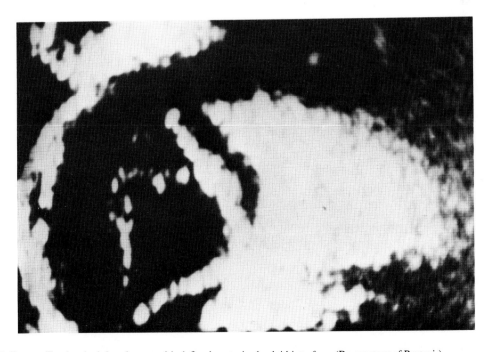

Fig. 11.23 B-scan. Total retinal detachment with defined posterior hyaloid interface. (By courtesy of Restori.)

different 'pulse echo' techniques are A-scan, B-scan and C-scan.

A-scan

The transducer is positioned so that the ultrasonic beam passes through a chosen ocular meridian. Pulses of high frequency sound are transmitted from the transducer into the eye. In the time intervals between pulses, echoes are received by the same transducer and recorded as spikes on a cathode ray tube. The height of the spike indicates the size of the echo, while the position of the spike along the horizontal axis indicates the time of receiving the echo (Fig. 11.21).

B-Scan

Echoes are plotted as dots instead of spikes, and the brightness of the dot indicates the size of the received echo. The transducer is moved to several positions above the eye, and a whole series of intensity registrations are plotted. The resulting B-scan is comparable to a histological section through the eye and orbit. If the transducer is moved in the manner shown in Figure 11.22 a 'linear B' scan' is produced. Such B-scans may be taken in the horizontal, saggital or oblique planes. (Fig. 11.22 and 11.23).

C-scan

The technique is illustrated in Figure 11.24. A strongly focused transducer scans mechanically a 4 cm square aperture in which the eye is centralised. The focal plane of the transducer is arranged to lie at the plane of in-terest and only echoes from this plane are recorded; these echoes are plotted on a cathode ray tube as dots, the brightness of which indicate the size of the echo. The C-scan thus displays soft tissues in the coronal plane of the orbit (Figs. 11.24 and 11.25).

In general, ultrasonic techniques are complementary to computerised axial tomography (CAT), the latter out-lining the bone and orbital apex more fully than ultra-sound. CAT scanning has been less successful in tissue diagnosis than ultrasound.

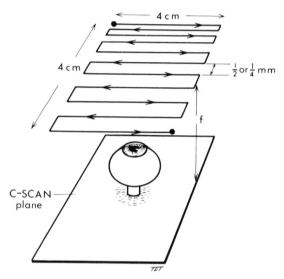

Fig. 11.24 C-scan technique. (By courtesy Restori.)

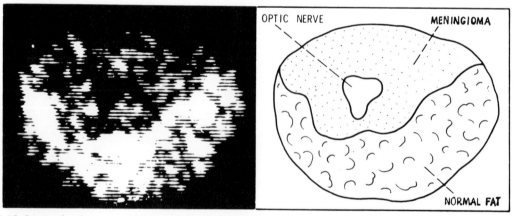

Fig. 11.25 C-scan of optic nerve meningioma giving rise to echoes from psammoma bodies. (By courtesy of Restori.)

12

The fundus oculi

When the fundus is seen it appears a bright red colour: this is due chiefly to the blood circulating in the choroid. In people of dark complexion no choroidal blood vessels are evident on account of the retinal pigmentary epithelium which, while dense enough to blur any details, is not sufficiently so to prevent the colour of the blood manifesting itself.

The optic disc
The first object to be sought is the optic disc (Plate 3, Fig. A). It is pale pink in colour, the tint showing considerable variations within normal limits. It is nearly circular but seldom perfectly so; it is about 1.5 mm in diameter, but, of course, is seen magnified. An oval appearance due to astigmatism must be borne in mind. The edges are usually sharp, but sometimes a little irregular and certain physiological variations without pathological significance should be noted. Not uncommonly, especially in old people, there is a narrow white ring around the pink disc, the *scleral ring*; this is due to the fact that the choroid and the pigmentary epithelium of the retina do not extend quite up to the margin of the disc so that the sclera is seen through the retina. Sometimes there is a ring of black pigment around the margin of the disc due to the heaping up of the retinal pigmentary epithelium. More commonly parts of the circumference have black patches, but they are not continuous.

The disc itself is seldom uniformly pink. The central part is usually paler and may be quite white, and this lighter area may extend nearly but rarely quite to the temporal edge of the disc so that the temporal side is normally paler than the nasal. The central vessels emerge from the middle of this white area, usually from a funnel-shaped depression, the *physiological cup*. This cup varies in different eyes. When it is deep the central part may be seen to be speckled with grey spots representing the meshes of the lamina cribrosa through which the nerve fibres pass. Sometimes there is scarcely any physiological cup, in which case the disc is more uniformly pink and the central vessels may have already divided before they come to the surface. The true nature of the physiological cup is best understood by compar-

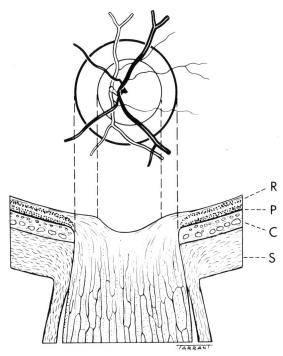

Fig. 12.1 Physiological cup: R, retina; P, pigmentary epithelium; C, choroid; S, sclera

ing the ophthalmoscopic picture with a microscopic section vertically through the nerve-head (Fig. 12.1).

The colour of the disc is due to the white fibres of the lamina cribrosa seen through the vascularised nerve tissue. Where the nerve fibres are thinnest, in the centre, the white lamina shines more brightly through. The grey spots in the lamina, when they are seen, are due to the non-medullated nerve fibres reflecting less light than the white connective tissue fibres.

The retinal vessels
The retinal vessels are derived from the central artery and vein, which usually divide into two branches at or near the surface of the disc to form a superior and an inferior trunk (Plate 1A). Each trunk usually divides into

two, one of which sweeps up (or down) towards the temporal side, the other up (or down) towards the nasal side — the superior and inferior temporal and nasal arteries and veins. These divide dichotomously into innumerable branches the mode of division being subject to great variations, but the nasal branches run more radially than the temporal which make a decided sweep to avoid the macula.

The arteries are distinguished from the veins by being lighter red and narrower. The veins have a purplish tint and are often more convoluted although less frequently the arteries are tortuous. Ophthalmoscopically the blood column is seen, not the vessel wall which is normally transparent. Each, but especially the arteries, may have a bright silvery streak running longitudinally down the centre, due to reflection of light from the convex cylindrical surface.

The macula lutea
This is situated about 3 mm or 2 disc-diameters (2 d.d.) to the temporal side of the edge of the disc, a little below the level of the horizontal meridian (Plate 3, Fig. A). It is difficult to see without a mydriatic unless dim illumination is used, for the bright light on this most sensitive spot causes maximal constriction of the pupil: the corneal reflex then often obliterates all view. It varies in appearance according to illumination, refraction and complexion. In general, it is a small circular area of a deeper red than the surrounding fundus, and in its centre there is nearly always a *foveal reflex*, due to reflection of light from the walls of the foveal depression. This is most frequently seen as a silvery ring of light hiding everything behind it: it may be circular or oval, according to the incidence of the light and the refraction of the eye. Often there is an intensely bright spot at or close to the fovea, also due to reflection.

The macular region is supplied by twigs from the superior and inferior temporal arteries, and by small branches coming straight from the disc. There are no retinal blood vessels at the fovea itself, and none can be seen ophthalmoscopically for a little distance around. Occasionally small arteries (cilio-retinal) derived from the ciliary system start near the edge of the disc, run inwards, and then bend sharply outwards towards the macula.

The general fundus
The appearance of the general fundus varies considerably in health. In people who are neither very dark nor very light in complexion the spaces between the retinal vessels show a uniform redness, occasionally with a very delicate punctate stippling, especially towards the periphery. In albinos the choroidal vessels are seen clearly, the spaces between them being white where the sclera shines through. In partial albinos in whom the hair is very fair in infancy, the macular region usually shows a uniform normal redness, the lack of pigmentation being manifested peripherally. In very dark people the fundus is a darker red, and indications of the choroidal vessels are often seen as indefinite brighter red streaks. Sometimes the pigment between the choroidal vessels is particularly dense, or the pigment is deficient in the retinal pigmentary epithelium, while the choroid is deeply pigmented: the choroidal vessels are then seen to be separated by deeply pigmented polygonal areas (*tigroid* or *tesselated fundus*).

There is no difficulty in distinguishing the choroidal from the retinal vessels when both are visible (Plate 5, Fig. E). The former are broader and ribbon-like, without any central reflex streak: they anastomose freely, whereas the retinal vessels do not anastomose at all. Moreover, in certain parts, their anatomical distribution is characteristic (p. 12).

The order of examination of the details of the fundus should be systematic. Applying the indirect method we obtain a general view. The patient is instructed to fix his gaze in such a direction that the disc is brought into view. The shape and colour of the disc, the arrangement of the vessels, the colour of the choroidal reflex (its uniformity or tesselation), gross abnormalities (white or pigmented spots, etc.), are readily noted. The patient is then directed to look up, to the right, to the left, and down. In this manner the periphery of the fundus is brought into view.

A binocular ophthalmoscope supported on the forehead and carrying its own source of (powerful) illumination for indirect ophthalmoscopy is of great value in the analysis of fine details of the retina, particularly in the periphery. It is especially useful in the search for small retinal holes in cases of detachment.

The macula is next examined. It may be brought into view by telling the patient to look into the light; but it is best to fix the temporal edge of the disc and pass horizontally outwards for a distance of about two disc diameters (a convenient unit in ophthalmoscopic topography), when the macula will be found. Any abnormality at or near the macula is of the utmost importance. Black or white spots are often difficult to distinguish from shadows or reflexes: if either has a sharp contour, and if they do not seem to shift when a minute movement is made with the ophthalmoscope, it may be concluded that they are pathological entities.

Finally, the periphery of the fundus is investigated. With full dilatation of the pupil it is possible to see almost to the ora serrata, and especially if the sclera over the ciliary region is slightly indented with a thimble depressor after the eye has been lightly anæsthetised. The periphery, even in an emmetropic eye, is usually best seen with a low convex lens, owing to the obliquity of the axis of the rays as they pass through the crystalline lens.

Vascular pulsation

In normal conditions no pulsation can be seen in the retinal arteries. In some 10–20% of people, however, retinal *venous pulsation* may be seen at or near the edge of the disc or, indeed, wherever veins take a very sharp bend; we have already noted that this is due to transmission of the intra-ocular pressure. The venous pressure is lowest at the point near the disc, and there is a certain amount of obstruction to the flow of blood as the vessels pass through the narrow neck at the lamina cribrosa. With each arterial pulsation the intra-ocular pressure is suddenly slightly raised so that the increased pressure on the outside of the walls of the veins tends to make them collapse. This causes a sudden increased obstruction to the outflow of blood from the eye during systole, but the venous circulation recovers itself during the arterial diastole. The venous pulsation can be increased or made manifest if absent by increasing the intra-ocular pressure by slight pressure with the finger on the globe. It will be noticed that it is diastolic and therefore has been called the *negative venous pulse*.

Visible *arterial pulsation* is always pathological. Since the pressure in the central retinal artery is far above the intra-ocular pressure, it would not be surprising if the pulse wave were transmitted and could be seen. Normally, however, the intra-ocular pressure damps the pulsation, and the increase in pressure which accompanies each pulsation is spread over the whole volume of the contents of the globe and is transmitted to the plastic sclera; such pulsations as survive this damping effect are too slight to be observed in such small vessels by ordinary ophthalmoscopic examination.

Two types of arterial pulsation occur pathologically: (1) a true pulse wave, accompanied by locomotion of the vessels; (2) an intermittent flow of blood or pressure pulse. The true arterial pulse occurs in such conditions as aortic regurgitation, aneurysm or exophthalmic goitre; it is not confined to the disc. In the pressure pulse the arteries fill only with the heart-beats, being empty between them; it is only visible on the disc, and may be produced in a normal eye by external pressure upon the globe by a finger applied to the lid. This type of pulsation is purely a pressure phenomenon, and is caused by a considerable increase of intra-ocular pressure with normal or lowered blood pressure, as in glaucoma, or by any considerable diminution of blood pressure with normal intra-ocular pressure, as in syncope or orbital tumours.

Capillary pulsation is seen only in aortic regurgitation as a systolic reddening and diastolic paling of the disc.

Ophthalmodynamometry. In view of the fact that the central retinal artery is a branch of the ophthalmic artery, itself a branch of the internal carotid just at its termination, the arterial pulse seen at the optic disc when the intra-ocular pressure is raised can be used to assess the pressure in this important vessel particularly on a comparative basis between the two sides. If the intra-ocular pressure is raised sufficiently to stop the circulation in the artery at the disc, we are measuring the lateral pressure of the ophthalmic artery which is virtually the pressure of the internal carotid. A spring-loaded plunger calibrated in G. of pressure exerted (*dynamometer*) is pressed against the sclera of the anæsthetised eye over the insertion of the lateral rectus, and the disc is observed with the ophthalmoscope. The pressure is increased until the circulation in the central artery is obliterated; as the pressure is lessened the first sign of pulsation to reappear gives the systolic pressure in the ophthalmic artery; and as the pressure is further lessened the pulse disappears to give the diastolic pressure. A unilateral fall of pressure of more than 30% suggests a stenosis or occlusion of the carotid system proximal to the origin of the ophthalmic artery; in cases of aneurysm a low diastolic ophthalmic pressure indicates that carotid ligation might be hazardous; while in glaucoma an approach of the intra-ocular pressure to the diastolic pressure indicates that the margin of safety before retinal damage may occur is small.

Examination of retinal function

The functional examination of the eye consists of testing the acuity of the forms of visual perception which have already been mentioned — the light sense, the colour sense, and the form sense. They are usually tested in the reverse order. Each eye must be tested separately throughout.

The acuity of vision

The acuity of *distant central vision* is now almost invariably tested by means of Snellen's Test Types (Fig. 13.1). These are constructed upon the standard that the average minimum visual angle is 1 min.

The types consist of a series of letters arranged in lines each diminishing in size. The breadth of the lines of which the letters are composed is such that the edges will subtend an angle of 1 min at the nodal point of the eye at a particular distance. Each letter is of such a shape that it can be placed in a square the sides of which are five times the breadth of the constituent lines. Hence the whole letter will subtend an angle of 5 minutes at the nodal point of the eye at the given distance (Fig. 13.2).

To fulfil these conditions a letter used as a test a long distance from the eye must be larger and the constituent lines must be broader than in the case of a letter to be used nearer the eye. In Snellen's types the largest letter will subtend 5 min at the nodal point if it is 60 m from the eye. Those in the subsequent lines will subtend 5 min if they are 36, 24, 18, 12, 9 and 6 m from the eye. Sometimes smaller letters corresponding to 5 and 4 m are used. A person with average acuity of vision ought therefore to be able to read the top letter at 60 m, the second line at 36, the third at 24, and so on.

For convenience the patient is kept at a fixed distance from the types. This distance should never be less than 5 and preferably 6 m. At such a distance the divergence of the rays in the small bundle which enters the pupil is so slight that the rays can be considered parallel and accommodation is thus eliminated.

A normal patient 6 m from the types ought to be able to read every letter from the top to the end of the 6-m line; many people can read more in a good light. If the patient can only read the 18-m line, his distant vision is obviously defective. The numerical convention which is used to record this is a fraction in which the numerator is the distance at which he is from the types, and the denominator is the distance at which a person with normal vision ought to be able to read the last line which he succeeds in reading. The patient under consideration will therefore have his distant vision recorded thus: $V = 6/18$. The normal patient's vision will be $V = 6/6$.

These fractions should not be reduced, because they are conventions giving an accurate numerical estimate under special conditions. In its original form it indicates the actual types used and the distance away from the test-types.

In the United States of America the metric system is not usually employed (6 m $= 20$ f): vision of $6/6$ is therefore $20/20$; of $6/60$, $20/200$; of $1/60$, $3/200$ (approx.), etc. (see Appendix 2).

Other notations than the original suggestion of Snellen are widely used. On the continent of Europe many employ Monoyer's scale in arthmetical progression wherein the relative sizes of the test types are $10/10$, $10/9$, $10/8$ . . . giving a relative visual acuity of 1.0, 0.9, 0.8 . . . 0.1.

The amount of illumination on the test card has a considerable influence on normal visual acuity. It has been found that the acuity rises rapidly as the illumination is increased from zero up to $5-10$ foot candles; and more slowly up to 1000 or more ft. cs. (Chap. 37). The illumination of the test card should never be allowed to fall below 20 ft. cs., and to allow for the deterioration of lamps with use it would be advantageous if a standard of 100 ft. cs. were used.

If the patient cannot read the largest letter he is told to walk slowly towards the types. At a certain distance he may be able to see the top letter. He should then be moved back a little, since he may not have understood exactly where to look. In this manner the farthest point at which he can distinguish the top letter is determined. If this is 3 m, the vision is recorded thus — $V = 3/60$. If he is unable to see the top letter when close to it, he is asked to count the extended fingers of the surgeon's

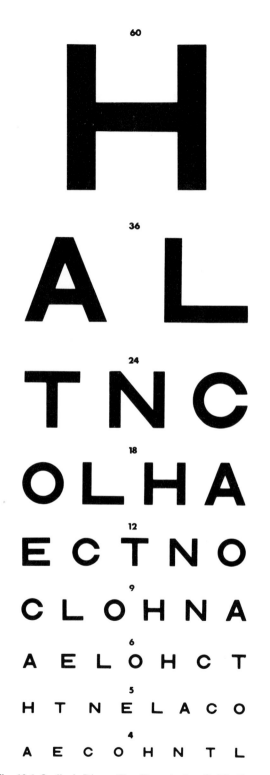

Fig. 13.1 Snellen's Distant Test Types (reduced). The lines, from above downwards, should be read at 60, 36, 24, 18, 12, 9, 6, 5 and 4 m, respectively, i.e., at these distances the letters subtend a visual angle of 5′

hand, held up at about 1 m against a dark background; this is recorded thus — V = fingers at 1 m. If he cannot count fingers the surgeon's hand is moved in front of the eye; if he can distinguish the movements the vision is recorded as V = hand movements. If he is unable to see these he is taken into the dark room and a light is concentrated on his eye and he is asked to say when the light is on the eye and when it is off. If he succeeds in doing this, V = p.1 (perception of light) and he may be able to give some indication of the direction from which the light is coming (projection of light, good or bad). If he fails to see the light the vision is recorded as V = no p.1.

The measurement gives the visual acuity of the eye unaided by lenses. It is necessary in all cases, however, to determine the function of the macula in the best optical conditions, and for this purpose the refraction of the eye, including the manifest hypermetropia must be determined, and the visual acuity taken again in the same way with the correcting glasses in place. If, for example, there are two dioptres of hypermetropia, *corrected visual acuity* is then written: V = 6/12 + 2D = 6/6.

The ordinary test-types cannot be used with young children. Simple pictures constructed on Snellen's principles may be used. A very effective test is the 'E-test' wherein the examiner holds in various positions cards whereon is printed the letter E in various sizes, and the child standing 6 m away, if the matter is treated as a game, will readily respond on request by indicating the direction of the letter with his hand or by holding a similar card in the same positions so long as he sees it. The system of character matching is exploited by the Sheridan Gardiner test when children will identify Snellen letters on a hand-held card.

An objective measure of the visual acuity may be made by utilizing the phenomenon of *optico-kinetic nystagmus.* If a white drum with vertical back stripes is rotated before the eyes, they follow a stripe with a slow motion and then as it disappears, switch suddenly back to pick up a new stripe. This is an automatic reflex persisting so long as the individual stripes are seen, and by varying their breadth or the distance of the patient from the drum, an assessment of the acuity can be made, particularly in unco-operative or malingering patients. It is interesting that in cases of hemianopia the response is absent in lesions of the parietal lobe.

Photo-stress test. One eye is covered and the patient reads the smallest possible line on the near chart. A bright light is shone into the eye for 15 sec following which he is asked to read the same line of print and the recovery time noted. The test is repeated with the other eye. In normal people and those with optic nerve disease there is no significant difference in the time taken for the two eyes to recover from the photostress. In a sub-

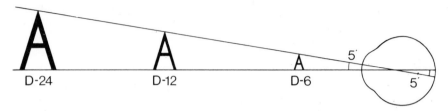

Fig. 13.2

ject with macular disease the recovery time is prolonged; the significant difference is at least one third longer than the recovery time of a normal eye.

When photo-receptors are diseased there is a marked delay in the visual pigment regeneration process so that the after image of the light persists longer on the diseased side. The test is useful in early macular disease, particularly central serous retinopathy, where there may be minimal deterioration in visual acuity and yet an easily detectable decrease in photo-receptor reserve capacity.

The field of vision

There are several methods of testing the field of vision.

1. A rough, but very useful, method is the *confrontation test*, which should be applied in every case, at any rate if there is the slightest suspicion of a defect, as follows:

The surgeon stands facing the patient at a distance of about 2 ft. The patient covers his left eye with the palm of his hand. He is told to look straight into the surgeon's left eye. The surgeon closes his right eye. He then moves his hand in from the periphery towards the common line of vision of the patient's right and his own left eye, keeping his hand in the plane half-way between the patient and himself. Directly he sees it himself the patient ought to say that he also sees it. The movement of the hand is repeated in various parts of the field — above, below, to the right, to the left, and so on.

This method is extremely simple, rapidly applied, and an excellent test. It will be seen that the surgeon tests the range of the patients's field by that of his own, which may be considered normal; moreover, he is continually watching the patient's eye, so that he can at once observe any deflection from the point of fixation. Better results are obtained by face-outline perimetry. The object is brought from behind forwards into the patients' field at a distance of several centimetres from the face. This is repeated in 10–12 meridia. A hemianopic defect can easily be detected if the surgeon extends each hand to either side and asks the patient how many hands he sees.

If any defect is indicated by these methods or is suspected from other features of the case it must be accurately mapped out and recorded with the perimeter.

2. *The perimeter* consists essentially of a half sphere within which a spot of light can be moved, e.g., Goldmann's perimeter (Fig. 13.3), or a rotatable arc, capable of being revolved round a pivot and along which a test-object can be moved (e.g., Lister's perimeter). The former is the more standardized. The chart, which has concentric circles marked upon it corresponding to degrees on the arc, is under the surgeon's control at the back of the perimeter. In self-registering perimeters, which are almost invariably used, the readings are recorded by perforations with a sharp point.

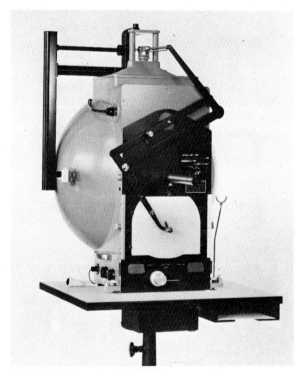

Fig. 13.3 Goldmann perimeter

The details of taking a perimetric chart can only be taught by actual demonstration. It will suffice to emphasize here the chief procedures to be followed in order that accuracy may be attained.

The patient is seated with his chin upon the chin-rest and the face vertical; one eye is covered. The other eye, situated at the centre of the arc, fixes the white dot around which the arc revolves.

The field should first be taken with a white object 5 mm in diameter. At least eight meridians must be investigated, preferably, 16 and the object should be carried up to the fixation point as there may be areas inside the limits of the field which are blind (*absolute scotomata*). These should be mapped out with the same accuracy as the limits of the field, and the plotting should always be from a blind to a seeing area. If the scotomata are small the limits should now be determined with a small object (1 or 3 mm diameter). The size of the test object and its distance from the patient's eye are usually recorded by a convention similar to the mode of recording visual acuity, e.g., 5/330, both measurements being expressed in millimetres. With small objects *relative scotomata* can be found which are not demonstrable with large objects.

Perimetry is a relatively rough test and purely subjective. Every student should have his own field taken: he will then appreciate the difficulties which patients experience. The normal physiological response to an object in the peripheral field is to turn the eyes towards it.

In charting the field of vision this normal response must be suppressed, fixation being rigidly maintained while attention is directed to an object at the periphery. Hence the first fields taken should be regarded with suspicion, especially in the case of dull or neurotic patients. With good illumination an object subtending a visual angle of 0.5° will give the full normal field for white. The 5 mm object used at the ordinary distance of 33 cm (5/330), corresponds to a visual angle of approximately 1°.

The extent of the normal field, with a 5 mm object in good illumination, is shown in the accompanying chart (Fig. 13.4). The peculiar shape is essentially due to the shape of the sensitive area of the retina as projected outwards, modified by interference caused by the nose and the brows; this complication can be eliminated if, when the field of the right eye is being taken, the head is turned somewhat to the left, and vice versa. It is seen that the field for white extends upwards 60°, outwards rather more than 90°, downwards 70°, and inwards 60°. The size varies with the illumination, the size of the test object, the contrast of the test object with the background, and the state of adaptation of the eye.

If the charts of the two eyes are superimposed there

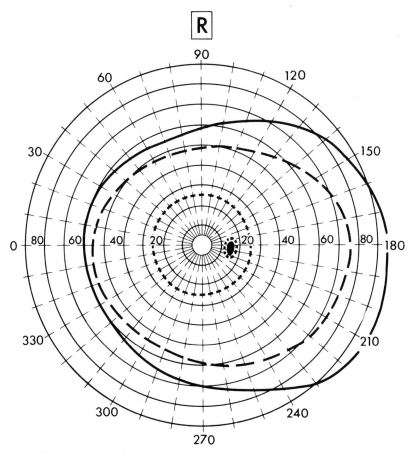

Fig. 13.4 The right visual field for a white object determined on the perimeter. (5/330, 1/330, 1/2,000 in good daylight.)

will be a large central area which is common to both eyes: this is the *field of binocular vision*.

Having mapped out the field for white the process may be repeated with coloured objects of similar size. The limit of the field for a colour is the point at which, passing from the periphery to the centre, the colour first becomes evident; peripheral to this limit the object is perceptible but appears grey in ordinary illumination. The exact limit is difficult to determine, for most colours appear to change in hue and saturation as the object passes from the fixation point towards the periphery. Red or green should be used first, then blue or yellow. In ordinary conditions, the blue field is largest, slightly smaller than the white: then follow the yellow, red and green, in the order named.

The field for blue and yellow is roughly 10° less in each direction than that for white, that for red and green another 10° less. The limits of the colour fields vary not only with the intensity of the light, but also with saturation of the colour, and above all with the size of the object. If these are sufficiently great, colours may be recognized almost, if not quite, at the periphery. Deductions made from variations in the colour fields are particularly unreliable except in compressive lesions when the red field is affected first. This is particularly helpful in the diagnosis of bitemporal hemianopia due to chiasmal compression and in the central scotoma of retrobulbar neuritis.

3. For more accurate investigation of details *campimetry* must be employed, but it is applicable only to the central and paracentral areas. It consists of placing the patient 2 m from the centre of a large black screen, 2 m or more in diameter (Bjerrum's screen). He fixes a spot in the centre of the screen and small white targets in the form of discs, 1–10 mm in diameter, attached to a long black rod are brought in from the periphery on a level with the screen. A grey screen with a spot of light the size of which can be controlled may be used in a similar fashion; this method has the advantage of eliminating the distraction caused by the rod. At this distance a 3 mm object subtends a visual angle of about 5 min. It will be noticed that since the angles are projected onto a flat surface, tangents are recorded, not angles themselves as with the arc (Fig. 13.5). Hence only a small area be investigated, and the distortion must be taken into account. Some points of diagnostic importance which cannot be elicited by the perimeter can be brought out by this method. Various *scotometers* have been devised on the principle of Bjerrum's screen.

Stimuli may be presented perimetrically in three different ways:
1. In threshold static perimetry targets of different intensities are presented at designated points in the visual field until the patient's threshold is determined, as in the Tubingen instrument.

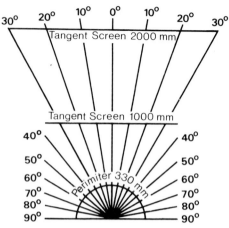

Fig. 13.5 Diagram of the right field, showing the relationship of the retina to the degrees of the perimetric arc, and the relative value of the latter when projected on a tangent scale

2. In supra-threshold static perimetry targets of a given intensity explore designated points in the visual field, as in the Friedmann analyser.
3. In threshold kinetic perimetry a target of given luminance is moved from a blind area until the patient sees it, as in the Bjerrum screen.

Automated instruments may exploit all types of stimuli and the choice of instrument consists of:
1. An inexpensive non-computerized test such as the Friedman analyser.
2. A computer-assisted technique such as the Baylor visual fields programmer designed as an attachment to the standard Goldmann Perimeter and incorporating a computer to guide the perimetrist.
3. A super threshold static device [Fieldmaster, autofield or Ocuplot] which displays targets on a cupola in random sequence at a varying luminance, duration and time interval. Each has an electronic fixation control and an automatic recording of missed points.
4. A static threshold instrument, the Octopus which permits a 3-dimensional representation of the island of vision.

It would seem that automation facilitates screening. If a qualitative assessment of the visual field is required of high order there is no substitute for manual perimetry possibly because rapport is established between the patient and the technician which keeps both parties alert and interested.

The light sense

This should never be measured until the patient has become thoroughly dark-adapted by remaining at least 20 min in a dark room. For this measurement instruments called *photometers* (or *adaptometers*) have been used, but none of them is of easy clinical application. There are individual differences in the rate of development of dark adaptation and facility of behaviour under low illumination which must be considered normal, but the rate of dark adaptation may be prolonged in pathological conditions such as pigmentary dystrophy of the retina, vitamin A deficiency or glaucoma. Such investigations, however, do not lend themselves readily to routine clinical investigation.

Contrast sensitivity

This may be measured by sinusoidal grating patterns. Figures 13.6 A, B, and C show examples of sinusoidal gratings and D shows a square grating together with their diagramatic representation. Of all the gratings in the figures the two main variables are the degree of blackness to whiteness, the *contrast*, and the distance be-

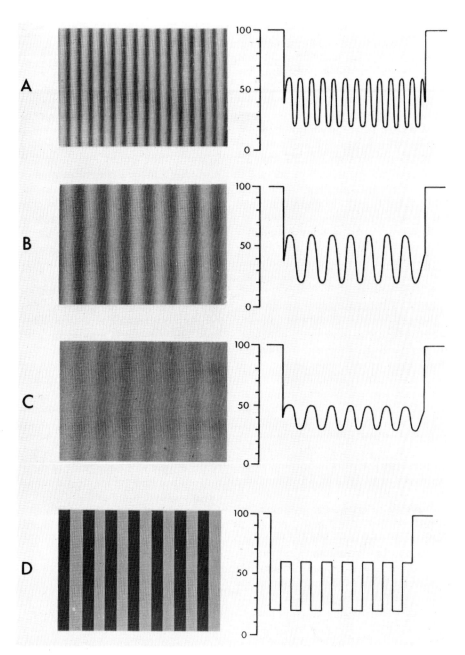

Fig. 13.6 A, B & C Sinusoidal grating patterns. D Square grating pattern. A and B differ in spatial frequency, B and C in contrast, defined as (L max − L min)/(L max + L min) where L is the light intensity recorded by a photocell scanning across the gratings, as indicated in the diagrams to the right of the illustrations. (Figure kindly supplied by Professor G.B. Arden.)

tween the repeats of the pattern. The distance between the repeats varies, in terms of the retinal image, as the observer moves towards or away from the page. It is usually therefore specified in terms of the visual angle i.e., the number of grating periods, or *cycles per degree* of visual angle. Diagrams on the right of the figure show the output of an ideal reflection microdensitometer as it traverses the grating on the left in a horizontal direction.

A book has been produced which consists of six sheets, each containing gratings which when viewed at 57 cm subtend 0.2, 0.4, 0.8, 1.6, 3.2, and 6.4 cycles per degree. The contrast on the plates is not equal, but has been varied to compensate for the alteration in contrast sensitivity with spatial frequency, hence the gratings appear to vanish about two thirds of the way up the plate. The technique of using the plate is to cover all its lower portion with a piece of card of roughly the same albedo as the grating. What remains exposed is the part with the lowest sub–threshold contrast so that what the patient sees is an area of uniform grey. Then the card is withdrawn slowly downwards exposing successively higher and higher contrasts until the grating becomes visible. When the pattern first appears, it certainly extends into regions which a moment before appeared a uniform grey. The position of the card when the grating becomes visible gives the contrast threshold. An arbitrary scale is placed at the side of the plate so that the position of the card can be read off.

Contrast sensitivity is reduced in many ocular diseases, particularly in glaucoma, macular disease and refractive errors. The Arden rating acuity test appears to be adequately sensitive and specific for screening out visual impairment due to refractive errors or ocular disease and to distinguish between them. Inexperienced medical personnel can carry out the tests satisfactorily with a minimum of training. It is of particular value in screening illiterate patients and where there is a language barrier.

The colour sense
This requires elaborate apparatus for its scientific investigation. The methods used will be discussed later (p. 102).

It is frequently advisable, however, to investigate the central part of the field for red and green, since conditions are not uncommon (such as tobacco amblyopia and retrobulbar neuritis) in which these colours are not recognized by central vision (*central relative scotomata*). In such a test it is sufficient to use perimetric targets of the appropriate colour (5 mm in diameter). It will be found that blue and yellow will frequently be recognized as such but not red and green.

The objective examination of retinal function
The visual function can be explored objectively by *electroretinography* (ERG) whereby changes induced by the

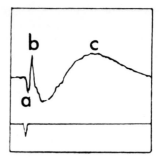

Fig. 13.7 Typical electroretinogram showing *a*, *b* and *c* waves. The dip in the lower line indicates the point of stimulation

stimulation of light in the resting potential of the eye are measured. In the normal dark-adapted eye after a fleeting early receptor potential, three components are seen (Fig. 13.7): a negative *a*-wave, possibly representing the activity of the rods and cones, a positive (composite) *b*-wave arising in the inner retinal layers, and, with strong stimuli, a secondary rise in potential the *c*-wave related not to visual processes but to the retinal metabolism, associated particularly with the pigmentary epithelium. Clinically the simplest technique investigates the dark-adapted eye wherein a minute *a*-wave is followed by the positive *b*-wave (Fig. 13.7). It is measured in dark adaptation with the active electrode incorporated into a contact lens and the reference electrode attached to the forehead so that a monopolar recording is obtained of the electric potentials picked up from the corneal surface. The response is *extinguished* when there is complete failure in the function of the rods and cones (pigmentary retinal dystrophy, complete occlusion of the retinal artery, complete retinal detachment, advanced siderosis, etc.). It is *subnormal* in those conditions wherein a large area of the retina does not function; and *negative* in gross disturbances of the retinal circulation (Fig. 13.8).

The electroretinogram essentially gives an indication of the activity of the periphery of the retina, that is, of the rods and their immediate connections. The photopic electroretinogram makes use of the critical fusion frequency of flicker, but so far has few clinical applications. By using a red filter and sharply focused light,

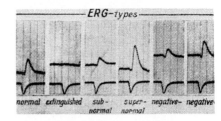

Fig. 13.8 Types of electroretinogram. Upper curve, ERG. Lower curve, photometric record of light-flash

however, an electroretinogram can be obtained from the fovea by the use of averaging techniques; in this way macular degeneration can be diagnosed in cases of cataract.

In the related technique of *electro-oculography* (EOG), changes in the resting current when the eyes are moved laterally are picked up by electrodes placed at the inner and outer canthi. Changes in the potential thus obtained with changes of illumination are indicative of the activity of the pigmentary epithelium and the outer segments of the visual receptors and are diminished or absent in retinal dystrophies and degenerations often before visual symptoms are evident. The technique is thus of value in diagnosing objectively such diseases in their early stages or in cases wherein the fundus cannot be clearly seen.

The electro-encephalogram

The development of the electronic averager has made it possible to detect specific alterations in the electro-encephalogram (EEG) caused by sensory stimuli. The response is known as Visual Evoked Response (VER) The visual stimulus may be unstructured as in flashing light or structured as in some form of pattern to the flash stimulus or the stimulus may be patterned, as in the chequer board. The essential feature is that while the pattern changes the overall illumination remains the same. Black squares go white and white become black, the rate of the lightening of the dark squares being the same as that of the darkening of the light squares.

1. *Flash VER*. This is the crudest of approaches and merely indicates that light has been perceived. It is

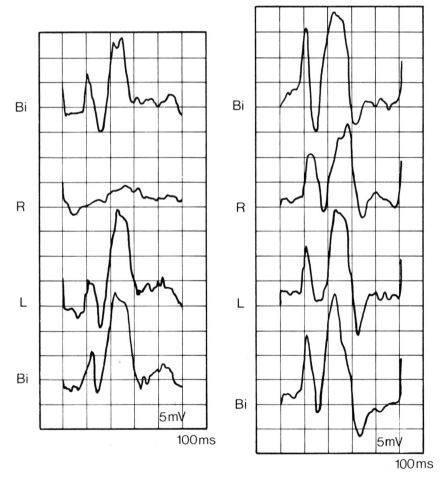

Fig. 13.9 A   Fig. 13.9 B

Fig. 13.9 A. VEP in a patient suffering from an acute attack of retrobulbar neuritis in the right eye. Note the markedly reduced amplitude on the right side. B. VEP in the same patient as in Figure 13.9A after he had recovered from an attack of retrobulbar neuritis in the right eye. Note that the first negative peak in particular is very slightly delayed compared with the left. The difference is small but significant. (By courtesy of Galloway.)

a fovea-dominated response and is relatively unaffected by opacities in the cornea and lens. It is therefore a useful adjunct to retinal tests to assess the integrity of the macula or optic nerve. The test is especially useful when one eye is involved in a disease process.

2. *Pattern reversal VER*. This depends on form sense and may give a very rough estimate of visual acuity.

The timing of the response is more reliable than the amplitude. It has been shown that there is a delay in transmission time in retrobulbar neuritis that persists when vision returns to normal. Delay is therefore an important sign in the diagnosis of a past attack of retrobulbar neuritis (Fig. 13.9.)

14

General therapeutics

Therapeutic substances may be introduced into the eye by five methods — by instillation into the conjunctival sac, by subconjunctival injection, by iontophoresis, by systemic administration and by direct injection into the globe itself.

1. On *instillation* in the form of drops, ocuserts or ointments, drugs enter the eye largely through the cornea and the readiness with which solutes instilled into the conjunctival sac can be detected in the aqueous or (as with atropine) can be evident as acting on the intra-ocular tissues shows the extent of their permeability. The cornea is freely permeable to water, but, largely through the action of the epithelium and to a less extent of the endothelium, it offers considerable resistance to the passage of electrolytes, while the passage of large colloidal molecules is barred. The stroma, like the sclera, is permeable to all water-soluble substances, offering a resistance little greater than an isotonic solution of sodium chloride. In general terms the passage of drugs through the epithelium is determined by the factors controlling the penetration of drugs into other cells, two of the most important of which are fat-solubility and the degree of dissociation of the electrolytes.

Since the epithelium forms the main barrier, permeability is much increased if the epithelium is damaged or abraded or if its vitality is impaired by a local anæsthetic; this is well demonstrated by the staining of the tissue by fluorescein. Theoretically the permeability to water-solube substances is also increased by detergents ('wetting agents') which, possessing a lipophilic grouping, lower surface tension. Such substances, however, are often toxic to the corneal epithelium and should be used, if at all, sparingly, and never in cases of corneal disease.

2. By *subconjunctival injection* a much wider range of substances can be introduced into the eye, for the sclera allows the free and indiscriminate transit of molecules of considerable size. Thus penicillin which does not penetrate the cornea enters the eye freely by this route.

3. By *iontophoresis* an electrolyte is driven into the eye with the passage of a galvanic current. The permeability of the cornea can thus be considerably increased, but in many cases the effect is probably largely due to epithelial damage.

4. The *systemic route*, by which drugs can be given by mouth or injection, has its obvious limitations because of the impermeability of the blood-aqueous barrier. No passage is allowed to large-sized molecules (such as penicillin) and when molecular size is at the border-line, lipoid-solubility is the most important asset. Thus the rate of entry of sulphanilamide (a lipoid-soluble substance) is 16 times that of sucrose although their molecular sizes are comparable; the transformation of urea (non-lipoid-soluble) into the larger-moleculed but lipoid-soluble thiourea increases its ease of passage five times, while among the common antibiotic drugs, the lipoid-soluble chloramphenicol enters the eye the most freely.

5. *Injection into the eye*, either into the anterior chamber or the vitreous, is reserved for desperate cases; it is employed, for example, to flood the ocular tissues with gentisin in acute infective conditions.

CHEMOTHERAPY AND THE ANTIBIOTICS

Antiseptics act by killing both tissues and organisms indiscriminately. Chemotherapeutic and antibiotic drugs, however, are bacteriostatic rather than bactericidal, acting by competing for the raw materials necessary for the existance of the organisms. The result is that since the organisms are inhibited from growing and multiplying, the natural defences of the body can deal with those already present. As soon as the influence of the drug is withdrawn, the remaining organisms can resume growth and multiplication, so that the rationale of treatment is to keep the drug continuously in contact with the infected tissue until the infection is overcome. Since these drugs are rapidly excreted from the body or diffuse from any site of local application, repeated or continuous administration during this crucial period is necessary.

The essential value of all these drugs is in the treatment of acute infections; in chronic infections they are relatively ineffective or relapses follow their use. This applies particularly to the more chronic types of intraocular disease which show little or no response, a circumstance perhaps due to the allergic rather than the directly infective nature of many of these conditions.

The antibiotics

These are a class of substances derived from fungi or other bacteria; their action depends on the inhibitory effect which one organism exerts on another. This 'antibiosis' has long been known, but the discovery of the prototype of such drugs — penicillin — only dates from the work of Fleming in 1929. In the last few years many such drugs have been exploited and used because of their activity against different organisms, the most important of which are penicillin, the cephalosporins, the aminoglycosides and the various tetracyclines. In general, penicillin is effective against Gram-positive organisms and certain spirochaetes; streptomycin against Gram-negative organisms and certain acid-fast species, while the 'broad spectrum' antibiotics — chloramphenicol, tetracycline, chlortetracycline, oxytetracycline, neomycin, soframycin and others — are clinically effective against both Gram-positive and Gram-negative organisms as well as rickettsiæ, the Chlamydia and certain spirochætes and protozoa. With the exception of those due to the *H. aegyptius* and the viruses (epidemic keratoconjunctivitis, herpes, etc.), all the common acute infections of the outer eye are susceptible to one or other of the antibiotics. Many fungi are sensitive to nystatin, amphotericin or trichomycin.

Penicillins

All penicillins have a dicyclic nucleus (6-aminopenicillanic acid) in common. Differences in antibacterial activity, in absorption and in resistance to penicillinase depend on alteration of the side chains attached to the amino group. They are excreted mainly via the kidney and appear in the urine in active forms; a small proportion is excreted via the biliary tract.

In general penicillins act by interfering with cell wall synthesis and they are all bactericidal. Most of them have a rather narrow antibacterial spectrum, being chiefly confined to cocci and Gram-positive organisms. The optimum blood level depends on the sensitivity of the organism. Pencillins diffuse readily into tissue fluids but not into the eye. When given systemically some have to be injected, intramuscularly because they are destroyed in the acid gastric juice; others can be given by mouth. Patients are liable to develop hypersensitivity to penicillin and it is wise to enquire about this matter before starting a course.

Immediate reactions such as urticaria and anaphylactic shock are probably associated with hypersensitivity to the 6-amino-penicillanic acid nucleus. Delayed reactions may be due to hypersensitivity to protein residues occasionally present in penicillin preparations derived from the fermentation process.

Penicillins may be classified into four main groups:

1. Penicillins effective against coccal infections and Gram-positive bacilli. Benzylpenicillin is not acid stable and can, therefore, only be given parenterally.

2. Penicillinase-resistant penicillins. These comprise methicillin sodium (celbenin), cloxacillin sodium (orbenin) and flucloxacillin sodium (floxapen) and their advantage is their activity against penicillin-resistant staphylococci.

3. Ampicillin (penbritin). Ampicillin is absorbed well by mouth and can also be given parenterally. It is a broad spectrum antibiotic and is effective against most cocci other than penicillinase producing staphylococci.

4. Carbenicillin sodium (pyopen). This penicillin is given parenterally and is active against *Pseudomonas aeruginosa*.

Penicillins are in general rapidly absorbed and excreted so that frequent doses are necessary. Prolonged action can be obtained by delaying absorption; thus procaine penicillin will produce blood levels adequate for the treatment of most coccal infections when given parenterally as a single dose of 300 000 international units. By giving probenecid, 1 g twice daily, it is possible to delay the renal excretion of the penicillins and thus maintain higher blood levels.

Penicillins show a synergistic action with antibiotics of the amino-glycoside groups.

In deep-seated inflammations of the orbit or lids, penicillin is administered parenterally; in superficial inflammations of the conjunctiva and cornea it is administered locally as drops or ointment. In intra-ocular infections it is given as injections subconjunctivally.

Benzylpenicillin. A dose of 300 mg, (500 000 units) twice daily is sufficient for sensitive infections and produces high levels in all tissues except the central nervous system and the eye.

Procaine penicillin. This is an intramuscular depot preparation which provides tissue levels for up to 24 h. The fortified injection includes benzypenicillin to give a high initial level, particularly useful in children.

Phenoxymethylpenicillin (penicillin V). This has a similar spectrum to benzylpenicillin but is resistant to gastric acid and is suitable for oral administration.

Methicillin (celbenin), cloxacillin (orbenin) and flucloxacillin (floxapen). These penicillins are not affected by staphylococcal penicillinase and are therefore used for staphyloccal infections which are resistant to other penicillins.

Carbenicillin (pyopen). This is resistant to the penicillinase produced by some strains of proteus, pseudomonas and coliform organisms. The drug is ineffective by mouth.

Ampicillin (penbritin). This is a broad-spectrum penicillinase-sensitive penicillin which is acid resistant and is usually administered orally. It is not as effective as benzylpenicillin and should be used for organisms which are resistant to benzylpenicillin but which do not produce penicillinase.

Flucloxacillin. This has the same activity against penicillin resistant staphylococci as cloxacillin, but blood levels of flucloxacillin after oral administration are approximately twice as high as after an equivalent dose of cloxacillin. This is because flucloxacillin is better absorbed from the gastro-intestinal tract and is also more slowly excreted from the body. Serum levels following intramuscular or intravenous injections of fluclo-xacillin are therefore also greater than with cloxacillin. The dose is 250–500 mg every 6 h.

Amoxycillin (amoxil). This penicillin has an anti-bacterial activity identical to that of ampicillin but its main advantage over ampicillin is that it is well absorbed after oral administration producing serum levels about twice as high as those after an equivalent dose of oral ampicillin. Food in the stomach has little effect on amoxycillin absorption from the small bowel. The adult dose is 250–500 mg every 8 h.

Talampicillin (talpen). This is an ester of ampicillin and has no antibacterial activity until it is hydrolyzed to form free ampicillin. Ampicillin serum levels after oral administration of this drug are approximately twice those attained with an equivalent dose of oral ampicillin. The adult dose is 375 mg (equivalent to 250 mg ampicillin). For practical purposes amoxycillin and talampicillin may be considered pharmacologically improved ampicillins with little or nothing to choose between.

The cephalosporins

These drugs have a similar structure and mode of action to penicillin. Their spectrum is similar to that of ampicillin but they are relatively resistant to staphylococcal pencillinase. Allergy may develop especially in patients already allergic to penicillin. When cephalosporins are used extensively strains of staphylococci emerge which are resistant to Methicillin and cloxacillin as well as the cephalosporins. This limits their use to special situations.

Cephaloridine (ceporin). This must be given by injection but cephalexin (ceporex, keflex) can be given orally only.

All the cephalosporins have a bactericidal action against a wide range of organisms, similar in spectrum to that of ampicillin.

Their clinical use is found in the penicillin-allergic patient. If a penicillin-allergic patient requires a drug with a similar antibacterial spectrum a cephalosporin may be used with caution. If the pathogen is a staphylococcus or a streptococcus, erythromycin may be just as effective.

In some gram-negative infections gentamicin could be considered more appropriate. The main problem in the use of cephalosporins is nephrotoxicity.

Cephradine (velosef, eskacet). This is a cephalosporin porin suitable for either intramsucular or intravenous administration. Its renal clearance is slower than that of cephalordine so that more prolonged blood levels are obtainable and nephrotoxicity is usually not a problem. The usual adult dose is 0.5 g intramuscularly eight hourly.

Cephradine (velosef, eskacet). This is a cephalosporin which can be given by mouth, intramuscularly or intravenously. The dose is 0.5–1.0 g six hourly. Cephra-dine is more stable to the beta-lactamase of *S. aureus* and to the beta-lactamases of some Gram-negative bacilli.

Aminoglycosides

This group includes streptomycin, kanamycin, neomycin, gentamicin and lincomycin. They are bactericidal agents all of which are toxic to the eighth nerve and to the kidney. They all interfere with neuromuscular conduction and cause serious paralysis in patients with myasthenia gravis or those patients who are receiving neuromuscular blocking agents. They provoke allergy and bacterial resistance although they have a broad spectrum of activity.

Streptomycin is bactericidal. It is used in the treatment of mycobacterium tuberculosis, but the organism rapidly becomes resistant so the drug should only be used when the infection has been shown to be sensitive in vitro and in combination with a second drug to prevent resistance developing during treatment. It is more effective when used in combination with PAS.

Gentamicin (gentisin) and kanamycin (kannasym). These may be used parenterally for the treatment of serious infections by Gram-positive and Gram-negative organisms, but as the margin between toxicity and effectivity is narrow they should be reserved for infections resistant to other antibiotics. Gentamicin is effective against an exceptionally wide range of bacteria which includes penicillin-resistant strains of staphylococci and *P. pyocyanea* against which it is one of the most powerful antibiotics known. When administered topically or sub-conjunctivally it penetrates the aqueous well. As it may occasionally cause chemosis, the sub-tenon route is recommended.

Neomycin has similar properties to gentamicin and kanamycin but is too toxic for parenteral use. It can be used topically as eyedrops and sometimes is made up in association with prednisolone (Predsol-N).

Tetracyclines

The tetracyclines are broad-spectrum bacteriostatic agents. Tetracycline (achromycin), chlortetracycline (aureomycin), oxytetracycline (terramycin) and neomycin are broad spectrum antibiotics with a considerable bacterial action against both Gram-positive and Gram-negative organisms as well as some fungi, rickettsiae and the chlamydia; the latter group includes the infective agent of trachoma. Their ability to penetrate the ocular tissues either from the conjunctival sac or after systemic administration is small. They are, therefore essentially employed in the form of drops or ointment for superficial ocular infections; they are too irritative for subconjunctival injection. They may be occasionally used by mouth in chronic staphylococcal infection of the lids and conjunctiva.

The macrolides and the lincomycin group

Erythromycin, linocomycin and clinamycin are relatively narrow-spectrum agents used for treating Gram-positive tissue infections especially when there is a probability of resistance or allergy to penicillin. They may be given orally, (but there is a tendency to cause diarrhoea) or parenterally when liver damage or drug fever is a possible complication. Clindamycin (Dalacin C) is probably the best tolerated drug of the group and should be given six-hourly on an empty stomach, the usual adult dose being 150–450 mg.

Other antibiotics

Chloramphenicol. Originally derived from a streptomyces and now synthesized as chloramphenicol, has a somewhat similar antibacterial spectrum being also effective against the chlamydia. The molecule is relatively small and lipoid soluble so that on systemic administration it enters the eye in therapeutic concentrations. Its effects however on intraocular inflammations are usually not dramatic.

Fusidic acid (fucidin). This is used mainly for penicillinase-producing staphyloccal infections. It reaches all tissues of the body except the brain. It is given orally in a dose of 1.5 g daily in divided doses.

The Polymyxins. Isolated from different strains of the *B. polymyxa*, these are potent antibiotics against Gram-negative bacteria. In view of the fact that most other antibiotics do not affect the organism, they are useful against extra- or intra-ocular infections of *Ps. pyocyanea*, administered as drops in the first case or as subconjunctival injections in the second.

Soframycin. This is highly effective against Gram-positive cocci and Gram-negative bacilli including *P. pyocyanea*. Moreover, being non-irritable, it is suitable for subconjunctival injection which increases its local action many-fold.

Sulphonamides

Sulphonamides are bacteriostatic and act by competing with para-amino benzoic acid which is essential for bacterial cell nutrition. They prevent susceptible microorganisms from synthesizing folic acid.

They find their main use in ophthalmology in their application topically and systemically in the treatment of chlamydial infections — trachoma, inclusion blennorrhoea and lymphogranuloma venereum. They are also helpful as an adjunct of pyrimethamine in the treatment of toxoplasmosis.

Preparations differ in their solubility and in the degree to which they are bound to protein in the body. Sulphonamides are inhibited by the presence of pus. Toxic effects are due to allergic reactions and lead to fever, rashes and occasionally photosensitivity, polyarteritis and the Stevens–Johnson Syndrome. Once an allergic reaction develops the patient is sensitive to all sulphonamides.

The more commonly used are sulphadiazine (185 mg), sulphamerazine (130 mg) and sulphathiazole (185 mg), sulphadimidine and co-trimoxazole (septrin).

Sulphadimidine. This is the best sulphonamide for systemic use. It produces high levels of free drug in all tissues and in the urine. It is given six hourly.

Co-trimoxazole (*septrin*). This is a preparation of trimethoprim and sulphamethoxazole. This combination of a sulphonamide is a blocker of bacterial folic acid metabolism and has a wider spectrum than the sulphonamides alone and is bactericidal. The adult dose is two tablets twice daily for five days, each tablet consisting of trimethoprim 20 mg and sulphamethoxazole 100 mg.

The topical use of sulphonamides for conjunctival or corneal infection has largely been replaced by that of antibiotics; the most effective because of its complete lack of irritability is sodium sulphacetamide (albucid) which may be employed as a solution in drops up to 30% or in an ointment up to 5%.

The sulphones. These were elaborated with a view to attacking the tubercle bacillus but are now widely used with success in the treatment of leprosy. *Dapsone*, a sulphone drug is the most useful antileprotic and is given by mouth. The dose recommended is 25 mg once weekly for one month, 50 mg weekly for the second month and thereafter 100–300 mg weekly for all types of leprosy. It is commonly continued for 2 or 4 years.

Para-amino-salicyclic acid (*PAS*). This is given systemically by mouth in four daily doses of 3 kg each or alternatively, isonicotinic acid hydrazide (isoniazide) in two daily doses of 2.5 mg per kg body weight forms an effective combination with streptomycin against tuberculosis.

The standard treatment of pulmonary tuberculosis now consists of three drugs given together — *Rifampicin, Isoniazide* and *Ethambutol*. Streptomycin is a first reserve. Rifampicin is given in doses of 450–600 mg daily, isoniazid may be given as a single dose of 200–300 mg daily and ethambutol is commonly started at 25 mg per kg of body weight as an initial dose. Treatment is continued with the three drugs for two or three months and then reduced to two drugs for a further 6 or 7 months making a total of 9 months.

Streptomycin is now less commonly used as a first choice but remains the major alternative drug particularly in the not uncommon tuberculous patient with impaired liver function. P.A.S. has been largely abandoned on account of its low efficacy and the high frequency of side effects.

Rifampicin. This is a bactericidal drug which interferes with bacterial nucleic acid metabolism. It is effective by mouth 450–600 mg and is given daily in a single dose before breakfast. It is most effective in combination with ethambutol in the treatment of tuberculosis.

Ethambutol. This is given in a daily dose of 25 mg per kg of body weight daily for the first 2 months and then 15 mg per kg given in a single daily dose. This dose should be reduced in patients with impaired visual function. The chief danger is loss of visual acuity and colour vision due to optic neuropathy which is not always reversible on stopping the drug. Patients on this therapy should be warned to stop the drug and consult their doctor if they notice any visual disturbance.

Diethylcarbamazine (banocide). This is the drug of choice in the treatment of all forms of filariasis. It kills the micro-filariae of all species, and is usually effective against the adult worms.

Antiviral substances

Five-Iodo-2-Deoxyuridine (IDU) inhibits the synthesis of DNA and thus, on topical application prevents the replication of the herpes virus. 85% of initial dendritic ulcers treated with IDU are cured within 2 weeks but some toxicity may be apparent. When corticosteroids are used to suppress the host response responsible for destructive stromal disease along with IDU the antiviral effect of the combination may be insufficient to prevent permanent vascularisation and scarring of the cornea.

Adenine Arabinoside (Ara-A; Vira-A) another antiviral substance has no activity against stromal disease and it produces the same forms of toxicity as IDU. It can only be given clinically in the form of an ointment. This substance blocks the synthesis of the nucleic acids.

Trifluorothimidine (F_3T) given in drop form five times a day results in healing of 90% of herpetic ulcers in a period of two weeks. This drug is more effective than others in the prevention of complications produced by corticosteroids.

Acycloguanosine with Ara-A is an effective combination against herpetic stromal infection. Acycloguanosine is a potent anti-viral drug which appears to have no toxic side effects.

Antifungal agents

Nystatin and *Amphotericin* B are agents used against certain fungal infections, particularly Candida. They are not absorbed by mouth and are usually applied topically. Invasion of the tissues by yeasts and similar organisms is a complication of the use of broad-spectrum antibiotics, cytotoxic agents and corticosteroids. Many of them are normally saprophytic and opportunist: and if they become pathogenic this is an indication for stopping such therapy rather than adding an antifungal agent.

HORMONE THERAPY BY THE CORTICOSTEROIDS

Of recent years much interest has been excited by the therapeutic effect of certain steroids elaborated by the adrenal cortex, the first of which was cortisone. This hormone can be used effectively in ophthalmological conditions; indeed, the eye is a very suitable organ for its exploitation for the undoubted toxic effects resulting from its systemic administration can be eliminated by its topical use in ophthalmological practice. Greater potency for topical application is obtained by the related compound, hydrocortisone; while the newer synthetic drugs such as Prednisone, Prednisolone, Dexamethasone and others, are often preferable for systemic administration since they are less liable to excite the unfortunate side-effects associated with cortisone. They are not, however, without their dangers, among which the possibility of the causation of glaucoma in genetically susceptible persons should be remembered. Clinically the same therapeutic reaction can obtained by the administration of the adrenocorticotrophic hormone of the hypophysis (ACTH); this preparation excites the production of cortisone by the adrenals and is thus only effective on systemic administration.

The general clinical effect in ocular disease of these hormones is a temporary blockage of the exudative phases of inflammation and an inhibition of fibroblastic formation in the process of tissue-repair, whether the cause of the disease is bacterial, anaphylactic, allergic or traumatic. In acute inflammations capillary permeability is decreased and the cellular exudation reduced; while in the stage of healing the formation of granulation tissue, new vessels and fibrosis is reduced. It is, however, of the utmost importance to remember that cortisone does not affect the cause of any disease but merely provides mesenchymal tissues with a temporary protection against an irritant, organismal or otherwise. The tissue-cells become resistant to an injury and are rendered able to function normally in an environment which has become grossly abnormal. The effect is thus limited to the blocking of the pathological evidences of inflammation so long as the administration of the hormone is continued; on its withdrawal the disease forthwith resumes its natural course. It follows that cortisone has its greatest effect in the control of acute disease; it is completely ineffective in the removal of structural damage caused by old or long-standing inflammation, nor is it of any value in the treatment of degenerative conditions.

Cortisone is thus in no sense curative. Its essential function is to hold the acute phases of inflammation in check while cure is obtained by other methods. Thus in infective conditions, cure in the true sense can only be obtained by killing off the invading organisms, as by an antibiotic. In an organ composed of tissues so delicate as the eye, however, this inhibition of the inflammatory reaction is often of the first importance, for damage of a degree which may be tolerated by other tissues may well have a disastrous effect on vision; indeed, if this restraint can be maintained until the organism is dealt with by other means, in the end the eye may escape all permanent damage. On the other hand, if an infection is not otherwise eliminated, the disease resumes its course on the cessation of cortisone treatment and apart from a temporary respite, little good results. In such cases, indeed, the treatment may be a disadvantage, for the tissue-response to injury is essentially protective in its function and its inhibition may not be without danger. The spread of tuberculosis, for example, may be facilitated by the suppression of fibrosis while the organism still lives; while if cortisone is given in an acute infection of the cornea the causal organisms of which are not sensitive to drugs (as in the case of many viruses), since the normal inflammatory response is inhibited, although the eye may seem quiet the infection runs on apace, often with disastrous consequences. The ideal therapeusis is therefore the control of the deleterious aspects of the inflammatory response by cortisone but only if the infective or other cause can be eliminated by other means.

In ophthalmology these steroids may be administered locally or systemically. *Local administration* is by drops, ointment or injection. Drops are used every 2 or 3 h as a 1 in 4 dilution of the standard preparations in saline or a buffered phosphate vehicle. The ointment (25 mg/g) is equally well absorbed into the eye and has a longer action, being particularly useful for administration at night. Subconjunctival injections have a more powerful effect lasting two or three days; 0.2 to 0.4 ml are injected after local analgesia behind the limbus. Retrobulbar injections have been tried with a view to controlling inflammations of the posterior segment of the eye, but they are relatively ineffective. Injections into the anterior chamber may be used in desperate cases.

The steroids may also be administered *systemically*, either by mouth or sub-cutaneous injection, but this requires careful clinical control. The main value of such treatment is in acute inflammatory disease of the posterior segment of the globe which is not readily affected by local therapy. In severe and acute cases the most dramatic effect is attained by the intravenous injection of ACTH. It should be remembered that after the prolonged administration of certain synthetic steroids (prednisone, dexamethasone, triamcinolone) cataractous changes may occur, and (in susceptible patients) steroid glaucoma.

In ophthalmology local therapy by this group of substances has been found beneficial in allergic and certain infective conditions, particularly early deep keratitis (including zoster and other viral diseases), syphilitic interstitial keratitis, phlyctenular and rosacea keratitis, spring catarrh, episcleritis, the acute and subacute phases of iridocyclitis and particularly sympathetic ophthalmitis. Systemic therapy is of value in acute or subacute generalised uveitis or focal choroiditis.

In all chronic inflammations their administration gives temporary or irregular results; in degenerative conditions they are without effect. In no disease are they curative, and if they are relied upon as the only method of therapy, the factor dominating the prognosis in almost every case is the occurrence of the lapses on their cessation unless the malady is eradicable or self-limiting.

SECTION 4

Diseases of the eye

15

Diseases of the conjunctiva

This tissue is frequently the site of disease, for not only is it exposed to all types of exogenous irritants and infections and prone to allergic reactions thereto, but it often becomes involved in endogenous diseases and metabolic disturbances.

Anatomically the conjunctiva is divided into two portions, palpebral and bulbar; the folds uniting these parts are the fornices (Fig. 15.1). The palpebral conjunctiva is said to commence at the anterior margin of the edge of the lid, but from this point to the posterior margin of the edge (the intermarginal strip) and for about 2 mm beyond (to the sulcus subtarsalis) there is a transitional zone covered with stratified epithelium with the characters of both skin and conjunctiva (Chap. 31). There are

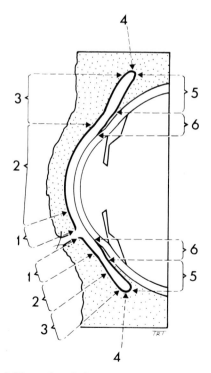

Fig. 15.1 The conjunctival areas: 1, marginal; 2, tarsal; 3, orbital; 4, fornix; 5, bulbar; 6, limbal

two layers of epithelium over the palpebral conjunctiva: from the fornices to the limbus the epithelium becomes gradually thicker, forming once more a stratified epithelium near the corneal margin. Below the epithelium is an adenoid layer, consisting of loose connective tissue containing leucocytes: below this is a fibrous layer, much denser and passing insensibly into the underlying tissues — lid or sclera. The palpebral conjunctiva is firmly adherent to the tarsus, while the bulbar portion is freely movable over the sclera except close to the cornea.

Bacteriology. The conjunctival sac is practically never free from organisms, but owing to its relatively low temperature due to exposure, evaporation of lacrimal fluid and moderate blood supply, bacteria do not readily propagate themselves. Moreover the tears are not a good culture medium, but although they contain a bacteriostatic enzyme, lysozyme, they cannot be regarded as actively bactericidal. Hence they act principally in a mechanical manner, washing away deleterious agents and their products. The bacterial content of the conjunctival sac is increased by bandaging owing to the arrest of movements of the lids and raising the temperature of the sac.

Most of the organisms normally present are non-pathogenic, but some of them are morphologically identical with pathogenic types. Diplococci indistinguishable from pneumococci are sometimes present and in general this organism (as well as *Ps. pyocyanea*) is among the most dangerous in ocular infections. The *Corynebacterium xerosis* is morphologically identical with the *C. diphtheriæ* and is frequently present in the normal conjunctival sac; it can only be distinguished by examination of cultures. Staphylococci are often found; they are relatively innocuous in the absence of other organisms but play an important part in mixed infections. Streptococci, *E. coli*, *B. proteus*, etc., are pathogenic, but rare. Other pathogenic organisms — gonococci, *H. ægyptius*, *Moraxella* — will be discussed later.

Viruses play a large part in conjunctival disease, as also do the Chlamydia. The most common viruses are that of herpes and the adenoviruses.

Hyperæmia of the conjunctiva may be transitory, or recurrent and chronic. The former is caused by temporary irritation, as by a foreign body in the conjunctival sac (which includes the surface of the cornea), concretions in the palpebral conjunctiva or in-growing lashes: in such a case the apparent secretion is almost wholly a reflex secretion of tears. Irritation limited to the lower fornix may be artificial in malingerers and psychopathic patients.

Recurrent or chronic congestion may be caused by conditions such as dusty, ill-ventilated rooms or exposure to heat, but is often due to causes remote from the conjunctiva itself, such as dietary indiscretion or allergic conditions such as hay-fever; in the latter case there may be an excess of eosinophilic cells in the conjunctival secretion.

Simple hyperaemia of the type described causes a sense of discomfort, often described as tightness, grittiness, inability to keep the eyes open and tiredness. Bright light is resented, but there is seldom true photophobia. The conjunctiva often looks normal until the lower fornix is exposed, when it will be seen that the parts in contact are congested and sticky. An increased secretion of a watery nature is the rule and the presence of mucus suggests an infective condition. The discomfort frequently comes on only in the evening or after near work.

Whenever watering of the eyes is complained of, and whenever only one eye is congested or shows signs of conjunctivitis, the lacrimal passages must be investigated. Pressure with the finger backwards and inwards over the lacrimal sac may cause regurgitation of fluid — tears, mucus, or pus — showing that the outflow into the nose is obstructed. If no regurgitation can be detected, the position of the lower punctum must be noted. It ought to be invisible until the lid is slightly everted.

The *treatment* of simple hyperaemia consists primarily in the removal of the cause. Local treatment consists in bathing the eyes with a mild astringent lotion. Transitory relief may be obtained by a drop of adrenaline solution (1 in 10 000) or in allergic cases a preparation such as antistine privine or opticrom.

INFLAMMATION OF THE CONJUNCTIVA

Inflammation of the conjunctiva manifests itself in many grades and many types, but is usually of infective or allergic origin. It is always accompanied by hyperæmia and increased secretion. The hyperæmia varies in degree and in distribution: the secretion varies in nature and amount. The nature of the secretion is of diagnostic importance. It may be watery, due largely to an increased secretion of tears, or mucous, muco-purulent, or purulent, in which case the disease is usually due to a bacterial agency; a serous secretion suggests a viral ætiology. Occasionally the exudation from the abnormally permeable capillaries is retained within the mucous membrane which becomes swollen and gelatinous in appearance particularly in the loosely attached areas of the bulbar conjunctiva and fornices; this phenomenon is called *chemosis* and in severe cases the swollen membrane forms a wall around the cornea. The palpebral conjunctiva is little affected, but the tissues of the lid are often also œdematous, so that the lids are swollen.

In the diagnosis of conjunctivitis, bacteriological investigation should always be supplemented by histological examination of the secretion and of *scrapings of the epithelium* taken by a platinum loop and stained with Giemsa. Apart from the presence of bacteria or inclusion bodies in the cells in specific infections, the cytological picture provides useful information.

Infective types of conjunctivitis

The chief forms of infective conjunctivitis may be divided into two broad clinical groups: acute, and subacute or chronic. Acute conjunctivitis may be classified as serous, catarrhal, muco-purulent, purulent and membranous. Subacute or chronic conjunctivitis includes simple chronic conjunctivitis, angular conjunctivitis and follicular conjunctivitis, while specific clinical pictures are associated with trachoma, tuberculosis, syphilis and tularemia.

Acute catarrhal or muco-purulent conjunctivitis

In its milder forms an infection of the conjunctiva assumes the characteristics of a typical catarrhal inflammation of a mucous membrane. The picture of hyperaemia is associated with a mucous discharge which gums the lids together, particularly in the mornings because of the accumulation during the night.

In the more severe cases the whole conjunctiva is a fiery red ('pink eye'); all the conjunctival vessels are congested, a phenomenon less marked in the circumcorneal zone. Flakes of mucopus and eventually of pus are seen in the fornices and often on the margins of the lids, matting the lashes together with dirty yellow crusts. Flakes of mucus passing across the cornea may give rise to coloured halos, owing to their prismatic action. These 'halos' must be carefully distinguished from those met with in glaucoma (*q.v.*).

The disease reaches its height in three or four days: if untreated it is liable to pass into a less intense, chronic condition. Complications are rare, but abrasions of the cornea are liable to become infected and to give rise to ulcers. Occasionally marginal ulcers form or a superficial keratitis may develop.

Aetiology. Muco-purulent conjunctivitis is caused by a number of organisms and is contagious, being transmitted directly by the discharge.

Among the most common ætiological organisms is the staphylococcus which may also be responsible for other associated conditions such as blepharitis and eczema or impetigo of the skin; it is frequently associated with multiple corneal erosions or other forms of superficial punctate keratitis.

Staphylococci are gram-positive, toxin-producing, nonmotile organisms occurring in grape-like clusters. Strains of *S. aureus* may be recognised by the lysis produced by staphylococcal bacteriophages. Their pathogenicity is proportionate to their coagulase activity. Many strains found in hospitals produce a penicillinase that inactivates benzylpenicillin. The usual source of organisms is the nose. Many other organisms may be responsible for the disease but two deserve special mention.

The *H. aegyptius* of Koch–Weeks is a very slender rod, varying much in length, Gram-negative, staining badly with the ordinary basic dyes. Groups of bacilli found in much degenerated 'skeletonized' pus cells are characteristic. The organism may give rise to widespread epidemics particularly in sandy, semi-tropical countries often associated with severe corneal involvement, but in temperate countries the cases are usually mild and sporadic, although contact transmission is common. An attack confers immunity for some time.

Pneumococcal conjunctivitis is not definitely separable from the other acute forms clinically, but there is usually more œdema (chemosis), small ecchymoses are common, and a membranous film may form — 'pseudo-membranous conjunctivitis'. It ends in a crisis, like pneumococcal infection of the lungs, after which the organism rapidly disappears from the secretion, but may be accompanied by nasal catarrh, which may precede or follow the inflammation. Iritis is rare as a sequel of conjunctivitis, but pneumococcal conjunctivitis is exceptional in this respect and if the cornea is involved a hypopyon ulcer may develop.

Muco-purulent conjunctivitis generally accompanies exanthemata such as measles and scarlet fever.

Treatment. The treatment of muco-purulent conjunctivitis consists of the control of the infection by appropriate drugs. The eyes should not be bandaged, as this prevents the free exit of the secretion, but if there is any photophobia a shade or dark goggles should be worn.

Control of infection is most effectively maintained by the use of bacteriostatic drops. Ideally the appropriate drug should be chosen after tests of bacterial sensitivity have been made. In default of this, one or other of the 'broad-spectrum' antibiotics is the most generally useful (p. 106). An antibiotic ointment is smeared along the lids at bed-time or, in the case of children, as often as they are put to sleep: it prevents the lids from sticking together — a two-fold benefit, that of preventing discharge from being retained, and that of obviating pain on opening them.

For the sake of cleanliness ointments should be prescribed in collapsible tubes from which they are readily applied by expressing a small quantity directly into the lower fornix.

After an attack of muco-purulent conjunctivitis the conjunctiva generally returns to a normal condition. If the case has been neglected and chronic inflammatory signs persist, treatment should be as for chronic conjunctivitis (*q.v.*).

Since the disease is contagious care must be taken to prevent its spread. The patient must keep his hands clean and no one else must be allowed to use his towel, handkerchief, or other fomites.

Purulent conjunctivitis (acute blennorrhœa)

This is a much more serious condition. It occurs in two forms — as ophthalmia neonatorum in babies, and as conjunctivitis in the adult. Many cases are caused by the gonococcus but the same clinical picture may be found with staphylococci, streptococci, *C. diphtheriæ*, and with mixed infections.

Gonorrhœal conjunctivitis. Fortunately, in medically advanced countries gonorrhœal conjunctivitis is now comparatively rare.

The *Neisseria gonorrhœæ* is a bun-shaped diplococcus, staining readily, decolorized by Gram and found within both leucocytes and epithelial cells. The *N. catarrhalis* and the *N. meningitidis*, both Gram-negative, are sometimes found in the conjunctival sac. They may be distinguished from the gonococcus by agglutination tests. The *N. catarrhalis* is rarely found in acute conjunctivitis, but more often in chronic and post-operative forms.

The disease is acute and in adults is due to direct infection from the genitals, occurring usually in males and first in the right eye. There is much swelling of the lids and conjunctiva, a copious purulent discharge, a marked tendency to involvement of the cornea, and constitutional disturbances including a rise of temperature and mental depression.

The incubation period is a few hours to three days. Thereafter the upper lid becomes swollen and tense, overhanging the lower, and edged with pus. Eversion, which is difficult, shows that the palpebral conjunctiva is deep red and velvety; rarely there is a membrane. There is great pain and the pre-auricular lymph node is enlarged and tender and may suppurate. After two or three weeks the purulent discharge diminishes, but subacute conjunctivitis with much papillary thickening of the conjunctiva persists for several weeks longer. The gonococcus is still present — a point of great importance, both as regards contagion and treatment. No immunity is conferred by the attack.

The most important point in diagnosis is the coincidence of urethritis. The most important point in prognosis is the condition of the other eye.

Corneal complications are the rule, and constitute the causes of blindness. There may be diffuse haziness of the whole cornea, with grey or yellow spots near the centre. Ulcers may occur at any part, and are due to necrosis of the epithelium through direct invasion by the organisms. Marginal ulceration, which may extend completely round the cornea, may be due to retention of pus in the angle formed by the chemotic conjunctiva. When ulceration has commenced it progresses rapidly and deeply and perforation is common with all its attendant dangers. Ulceration commencing late is not so dangerous. The greatest care should therefore be taken to prevent injury to the cornea during the manipulation necessary for diagnosis and treatment; abrasions which may ulcerate are easily produced by the finger nails and even by the rough use of wool swabs.

Iritis and iridocyclitis, with attendant complications, may arise independently of perforation of the cornea, and lead to serious diminution of vision. Gonorrhœal arthritis is not uncommon, and endocarditis and septicæmia may arise as complications.

Treatment should be directed first to protection of the other eye. Several drops of a solution of penicillin or other suitable antibiotic are instilled every few minutes for some hours; if these are not immediately available this eye should be given a protective covering.

If the disease is established and there is any purulent discharge, the eye must be irrigated with warm saline and intensive therapy with an aqueous solution of crystalline benzyl penicillin started, using drops in a concentration of 10 000 units per ml every minute, for half an hour. Repeated irrigations are unnecessary since, in the first place, penicillin remains effective in the presence of pus and, in the second, the discharge rapidly disappears. Any pus that does accumulate is wiped away with moist pledgets of cotton-wool. Penicillin drops are continued four hourly for 3 days.

Patients who are allergic to the penicillins should be treated with tetracycline particularly if there is a coexistent infection with Chlamydia trachomatis.

Atropine should be used in all cases in which the cornea is involved since this is always accompanied by some iritis; corneal complications require very active treatment (*q.v.*).

Ophthalmia neonatorum

This is a preventable disease occurring in new-born children due to maternal infection acquired as the result of carelessness at the time of birth; it used to be responsible for 50% of blindness in children, but recently the decline in the incidence of gonorrhœa as well as effective methods of prophylaxis and treatment have almost eliminated its occurrence and the seriousness of the sequelæ in advanced communities. The virtual elimination of this disease has constituted a revolution in ophthalmology within this generation and today the disease is usually mild, due to the *Chlamydia oculogenitalis, Streptococcus pneumoniae* or other organisms. Any discharge, even a watery secretion, from a baby's eyes during the first week should be viewed with suspicion, since tears are not secreted at this early date.

In cases of virulent *gonococcal* infection the discharge rapidly becomes muco-purulent and then purulent. Both eyes are nearly always affected, though one is usually worse than the other. The conjunctiva becomes intensely inflamed, bright red, and swollen, and pours out thick yellow pus. Marked chemosis is a distinguishing feature from severe muco-purulent conjunctivitis, and when the lids are separated by retractors the cornea is seen at the bottom of a crater-like pit. There is dense infiltration of the bulbar conjunctiva, and the lids are swollen and tense. Later the lids become softer and more easily everted, the conjunctiva becomes puckered and velvety, and the blood stasis gives place to intense congestion, with the free discharge of pus, serum and often blood. In some cases a false membrane forms, so that the case resembles a membranous conjunctivitis.

There is great risk of corneal ulceration in untreated gonococcal ophthalmia neonatorum, since this organism has the power of invading intact epithelium. The slightest haziness of the cornea should be viewed with apprehension. Sometimes the cornea is already ulcerated, and not infrequently perforated, when the child comes under observation. Ulceration usually occurs over an oval area just below the centre of the cornea, corresponding to the position of the lid margins when the eyes are closed and consequently rotated somewhat upwards. More rarely oval marginal ulcers are formed as in the gonorrhœal conjunctivitis of adults. The ulcers extend rapidly, both superficially and in depth, and perforation occurs, usually indicated by a black spot or area in the ulcer, caused by a prolapse of the iris. Sometimes perforation is sudden, a large part of the iris prolapses, and the lens may be extruded, while in the worst cases there is a black hole in the cornea filled with clear vitreous.

Metastatic stomatitis and arthritis rarely occur. The arthritic manifestations usually appear in the third or fourth week and affect the knee, wrist, ankle or sometimes elbow. The course is benign, abscesses being rare.

The baby's eyes must be examined with retractors to separate the lids and the surgeon wear protective goggles. A bacteriological examination should be made in every case.

In inadequately treated cases serious sequelæ may occur. If the corneal ulceration heals without perforation there is always much scarring of this tissue, but the nebula clears more in babies than in older people. Perforation may be followed by anterior synechiæ, adherent leucoma, partial or total anterior staphyloma, anterior capsular cataract or panophthalmitis. When vision is not completely destroyed but is seriously impaired by the corneal opacities, the development of macular fixation which takes place during the first six weeks of life is impaired, resulting in the development of nystagmus which persists throughout life; this may not become manifest until a later date.

Inclusion conjunctivitis is a relatively common cause of ophthalmia neonatorum in Western countries. Bacterial examination is negative or inconsequential but the characteristic intracellular inclusion bodies formed by the *Chlamydia oculogenitalis* (a Bedsonian organism) are found (Fig. 15.2). It is a venereal infection derived from the cervix or urethra of the mother. The inflammation is much less severe than the gonococcal type but the conjunctiva may be considerably swollen and œdematous while the discharge may be purulent. In the absence of a subconjunctival adenoid layer at this age there are, however, no follicles as appear in this infection in the adult, but if the disease is allowed to smoulder into a chronic stage these may develop after three months. A complicating superficial keratitis is the rule and occasionally in prolonged cases the corneal periphery may be invaded by pannus.

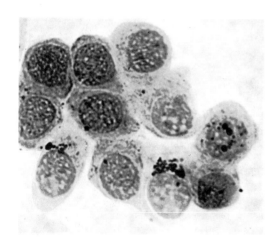

Fig. 15.2 Melanin granules in the cell form a 'cap' over the nucleus suggesting a chlamydial inclusion. (By courtesy of Yoneda.)

Treatment. The disease is preventable; *prophylactic* treatment is therefore of prime importance. Any suspicious vaginal discharge during the antenatal period should be treated, and the most meticulous obstetric asepsis maintained at birth. The new-born baby's closed lids should be thoroughly cleansed and dried. If infection is suspected a drop of silver nitrate solution, 1%, may be instilled into each eye (Credé's method). The eyes must be carefully watched during the first week.

Some considerable controversy still exists over this method of prophylaxis. Many authorities advocate the use of penicillin or other antibiotic drugs but all the organisms which may be present may not be sensitive to the drug employed. If silver nitrate is used the solution should never be stronger than 1%, lest corneal opacities result.

If the disease is established the treatment should be on the lines already indicated for gonorrhœal ophthalmia; fortunately most of the types of infection in ophthalmia neonatorum, including the Chlamydial infection, are amenable to penicillin or tetracycline. The eyes are washed out with saline and if the cornea is involved atropine is instilled. Thereafter intensive treatment with penicillin (or oxytetracycline) is adopted as already described. After about half an hour the clinical picture has altered and although there is some swelling of the lids and conjunctiva, the eye is dry. After a further twenty-four hours' treatment a clinical cure is usually obtained. Topical therapy should be supplemented by parenteral penicillin by intramuscular injection of crystalline benzyl penicillin G 50 000 units to full term, normal weight babies and 20 000 units to premature or low weight babies twice daily for 3 days.

Membranous conjunctivitis (diphtheritic conjunctivitis).
As in inflammation of the throat, the conjunctival surface may become covered by a fibrinous membrane; and similarly, the milder croupous clinical varieties in both can be distinguished from the more severe diphtheritic. It has been placed beyond dispute, however, that mild cases may be diphtheritic, and severe non-diphtheritic; hence it is best to speak simply of membranous conjunctivitis until a bacteriological examination has been done. A variety of organisms other than the diphtheria bacillus, such as the pneumococcus or streptococcus, can produce a membrane, especially in weakly children, particularly after measles and scarlet fever and in association with impetigo; these cases are sometimes called pseudo-membranous but they cannot be distinguished clinically with certainty. The condition occurs chiefly in children who have not been immunised, and shows all degrees of severity.

In mild cases there is some swelling of the lids and a mucopurulent or sanious discharge. On everting the lids the palpebral conjunctiva is seen to be covered with a white membrane which peels off rapidly without much bleeding.

In severe cases the lids are more brawny; the conjunctiva is permeated with semi-solid exudates, which impair mobility, compress the vessels, prevent the formation of a free discharge, and tend to necrosis both of the conjunctiva and cornea. In these cases the membrane separates less readily, the underlying surface bleeding unless it is too infiltrated and solid. The membrane may be patchy or cover the whole palpebral conjunctiva, often beginning at the edge of the lid, but is seldom found on the bulbar conjunctiva. The pre-auricular lymph node may be enlarged and may suppurate.

For six to 10 days there is great peril to the cornea from ulceration usually due to secondary infection. About the same time, also, the sloughs begin to separate and the discharge becomes more profuse. In a few days the conjunctiva assumes a red and succulent appearance and there is danger of adhesions forming between the palpebral and bulbar parts of the conjunctiva (symblepharon).

Post-diphtheritic paralyses, even of accommodation, are rare.

Cases of less severe but more chronic *pseudo-membranous* conjunctivitis are occasionally met with. In *ligneous conjunctivitis* the membrane is cast off, but recurs again and again; the pathology of these cases is not understood. Membrane formation may also occur as a complication of erythema multiforme.

Pathology. There is little or no relationship between the severity of the local condition and the presence or absence of the *C. diphtheriae*. Owing to the difficulty of distinguishing this organism from the *C. xerosis*, with which it is morphologically identical, inoculation tests are the only absolutely reliable diagnostic criterion. It is rare to obtain evidence of primary diphtheria of the throat. Other bacteria which occasionally form membranes are the pneumococcus, streptococcus, *H. ægyptius*, gonococcus, staphylococcus, *E. coli*, etc. Streptococcal conjunctivitis, a very virulent form, occurs chiefly in children, associated with measles, scarlet fever, whooping cough, and influenza.

Streptococci are gram-positive, nonmotile organisms which are spherical and grow in chains. Haemolytic streptococci (beta) are pathogenic; the nonhaemolytic streptococci are saprophytic.

Streptococcal conjunctivitis may be associated with erysipelas which affects the skin of elderly patients usually involving the face and sometimes the skin of the eyelids. It is the result of the haemolytic streptococcal infection of the skin itself.

Other cases may be due to the action of heat, caustics, and other non-bacterial causes.

Treatment. Every case should be treated as diphtherial unless good negative evidence is afforded by films and cultures. This consists of the intensive local and general administration of penicillin together with the prompt injection of anti-diphtheritic serum (4–6–10 000 units repeated in 12 h). Antitoxin given early and in adequate amounts both locally and systemically is curative, but it should be combined with the antibiotic.

In *streptococcal membranous conjunctivitis* the danger of necrosis of the cornea is considerable, so that immediate local and general treatment is necessary. Depending on the sensitivity of the organism this should be carried out with the intensive topical and systemic use of a suitable antibiotic (Chap. 14).

Simple chronic conjunctivitis

This occurs as a continuation of simple acute conjunctivitis, sometimes in spite of orthodox treatment. It is frequent when a cause of irritation is continuous — smoke, dust, heat, bad air, late hours, abuse of alcohol, and so on — or when it is caused by hypersensitivity to an allergen which has not been eliminated. Permanent irritation from concretions (p. 126) in the palpebral conjunctiva, misplaced lashes, dacryocystitis and chronic rhinitis must be remembered and as far as possible eliminated. Unilateral chronic conjunctivitis should suggest the presence of a foreign body retained in the fornix, or inflammation of the lacrimal sac. It is often necessary to make a thorough and systematic investigation of the local and general condition before the cause can be found. It is not infrequently associated with chronic intranasal trouble, and seborrhœa, particularly of the scalp; dandruff is a common accompaniment. The disease is too frequently regarded as trivial, but may be a source of great discomfort.

The essential symptoms are burning and grittiness, especially in the evening when the eyes often become red while the edges of the lids feel hot and dry. Difficulty in keeping the eyes open is a common symptom. The lids may or may not be stuck together on waking for the discharge is slight, but there is frequently an abnormal amount of secretion from the meibomian glands.

Superficially the eyes may look normal but when the lower lid is pulled down the posterior conjunctival vessels are seen to be congested, and the surface of the mucous membrane is sticky. The palpebral conjunctiva, upper and lower, may be congested, with a velvety papilliform roughness; this is due to a hypertrophy of the normal vascularised papillæ in the submucosa. Occasionally it is succulent and fleshy.

Treatment consists in eliminating the cause and restoring the conjunctiva to its normal condition. Chronic nasal catarrh is perhaps most likely to be forgotten. When heat is a prominent aetiological factor (as in cooks or in industry) protective glasses may be ordered. The treatment of the special local conditions mentioned above will be discussed in their proper place. A swab should be taken to eliminate the presence of infective organisms and it is well at the same time to determine the bacteriological flora of the nose and upper respiratory passages; any conjunctival or nasal infection should receive the proper treatment.

Local treatment consists firstly in eliminating any infection by a *short* course of a suitable antibiotic and then in diminishing congestion and restoring the conjunctiva to its normal suppleness and secretory activity. When there is an abnormal amount of secretion from the tarsal glands (*conjunctivitis meibomiana*), this should be squeezed out of the glands by repeated massage of the lid.

Angular conjunctivitis (diplobacillary conjunctivitis)

In this condition the reddening of the conjunctiva is limited almost exclusively to the inter-marginal strip, especially at the inner and outer canthi, and to the bulbar conjunctiva in the same neighbourhood; there is also excoriation of the skin at the inner and outer palpebral angles, which may be very slight — a mere scrufiness — but is nearly always present. There is discomfort, with slight mucopurulent discharge and frequent blinking. If untreated the condition becomes chronic and may give rise to blepharitis. Clear, shallow, corneal ulcers may occur, but are rare; they are usually marginal, but may be central and associated with hypopyon (*q.v.*). A single attack does not confer immunity, and relapses are not uncommon.

Pathology. Such a condition may be caused by the staphylococcus but is typically due to the *Moraxella*, a diplobacillus consisting of pairs of large, thick rods, placed end to end which stain well with basic stains, are decolorised by Gram, and are easily recognised in films. They produce a proteolytic ferment which acts by macerating the epithelium. There is an incubation period of four days. The diplobacilli are strongly resistant to drying. They have been found in the nasal tract of healthy persons, and are often present in the nasal discharge in cases of angular conjunctivitis.

Treatment. Diplobacillary conjunctivitis responds to oxytetracycline applied as ointment. Although less rapidly effective a zine lotion is of great value; this acts by inhibiting the proteolytic ferment. Zinc oxide ointment may be applied to the lids at night.

Follicular conjunctivitis

The occurrence of follicles in the conjunctiva either as an acute, subacute or chronic manifestation of disease is relatively common; they do not occur in the normal conjunctiva. Such follicles appear as rounded swellings, 1–2 mm in diameter, and are due to localised aggregations of lymphocytes in the subepithelial adenoid layer, and unless an acute inflammation is present, the conjunctiva over them remains normal (Fig. 15.3). In all types of follicular conjunctivitis the histological nature of the follicles is identical, but in trachoma degenerative changes and eventually scarring distinguish the condition from non-trachomatous types.

It is important to differentiate follicles from papillae — a hyperplasia of the normal system of vascularisation with glomerulus-like bunches of capillaries of new formation growing into the epithelium in inflammatory conditions. Both give rise to a roughened appearance of the conjunctiva and the slit-lamp may be necessary for

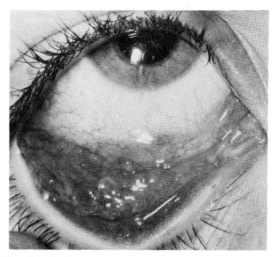

Fig. 15.3 Follicular conjunctivitis

their clinical differentiation. It is interesting that the conjunctiva of the newborn is unable to produce follicles before 2 or 3 months of age, so that an infection very early in life may appear initially as a papillary conjunctivitis and may develop into follicular conjunctivitis if it remains active for longer than 3 months.

Follicular hypertrophy may be due to certain chemicals and toxins, the most notable of which is eserine after prolonged use; a milder manifestation may follow the use of pilocarpine and other drugs such as DFP. This conjunctival reaction is most commonly caused by viruses, particularly those of herpes and the adenoviruses. Isolated follicles, however, may occur particularly in the lower conjunctiva in any conjunctivitis of long standing.

Acute Follicular Conjunctivitis. Several types of acute follicular conjunctivitis occur.

Inclusion conjunctivitis is characterised by a relatively acute onset, the incubation period varying from 5 to 10 days. The follicular hypertrophy is always more prominent in the lower lid than the upper, although in acute cases the follicles may be partially obscured by papillary hypertrophy. The exudate, composed principally of neutrophils, may be moderately abundant, and the cornea is involved in a superficial punctate keratitis occasionally with some pannus-like peripheral vascularisation.

The disease is caused by Chlamydial infection and produces inclusion bodies morphologically identical with those occurring in trachoma (Fig. 15.2). The primary source of infection is a benign subclinical venereal disease producing a mild urethritis in the male and a cervicitis in the female; it is commonly transmitted to the newborn from the mother (p. 115) when follicle formation is less evident. In adults the organism may be transferred from the genitals by the fingers, but a common mode of infection is through the water of swimming pools so that the disease may occur in local epidemics (*swimming-bath conjunctivitis*).

The disease runs a relatively benign course, healing spontaneously when untreated in from 3 to 12 months; the organism, however, is very responsive to treatment with the broad-spectrum antibiotics or systemic treatment by tetracycline 250 mg at 6 hourly intervals for 14 days.

Epidemic kerato-conjunctivitis. This disease is characterised by a rapidly developing follicular conjunctivitis with marked inflammatory symptoms and scanty exudate, associated with a preauricular adenopathy. Occasionally it takes on a membranous form. Seven to ten days after the infection, corneal complications appear — initially punctate epithelial infiltrates followed by the development of discrete subepithelial opacities associated with photophobia. The conjunctival manifestations gradually diminish and finally disappear but the corneal opacities may persist for many months or even years. The condition is markedly contagious and occurs in widespread epidemics, unfortunately often disseminated in clinics by contaminated solutions, fingers or tonometers. It has been associated with several types (3, 7 and particularly 8 and 19) of the adenoviruses. An immunofluorescent test detects the adenoviral group antigen in conjunctival secretions. Diagnosis is based on the demonstration of rising immunoglobulin titres in the blood. Treatment by adenine arabinoside (Ara-A) is promising.

Pharyngo-conjunctival fever is characterised by an acute follicular conjunctivitis in association with pharyngitis and fever and occasionally with pre-auricular adenopathy, appearing chiefly in children in epidemic form. Corneal involvement as a superficial punctate keratitis is rare. The disease is acute and transient and antibiotics have little effect. It is caused by one or other of the group of adenoviruses.

Newcastle conjunctivitis is clinically indistinguishable from the conjunctivitis of pharyngo-conjunctival fever; it is caused by the Newcastle virus derived from contact with diseased fowls.

Acute herpetic conjunctivitis occurs as a primary manifestation of herpes; it is thus usually seen in young children who are as a rule infected by contagion from carriers of the virus. It is comparable with the more common acute stomatitis which results from an initial herpetic infection and may be associated with the usual vesicular lesions on the face. A pre-auricular adenopathy is present and the corneal vesicles which may merge to form dendritic figures (*q.v.*) are frequent. The condition is acute, the follicles are usually large, and corneal sensation is reduced.

Herpes simplex conjunctivitis may occur not uncommonly in atypical form as an acute follicular conjunctivitis without lesions of the face, eyelid or cornea and the condition then resembles epidemic keratoconjunctivitis. Mucosal involvement may be limited to tiny ulcers on the intermarginal portion of the eyelid and they can be demonstrated with fluorescein. Minute microdendrites may be mistaken for the lesions of a coarse punctate epithelial keratitis. Reduced corneal sensation is strongly suggestive of herpetic infection. Herpetic involvement often stimulates the formation of a pannus and this may be a helpful sign.

Where the clinical evidence cannot differentiate herpetic simplex conjunctivitis from epidemic keratoconjunctivitis the viral antigen in epithelial cells may be detected by the fluorescent-antibody (F.A.) technique, or by the demonstration of a rising serum antibody titre during the first one or two weeks of illness or by the isolation of the virus.

Haemorrhagic conjunctivitis is due to the picornavirus. It occurs in pandemic form producing a violent inflammatory conjunctivitis with lacrimation and photophobia. Subconjunctival haemorrhages and enlarged preauricular lymph nodes are common. The cornea is unaffected.

Trachoma

Once known as Egyptian ophthalmia and endemic in the Middle East since pre-historic times, it was spread far and wide in Europe by the French armies during the Napoleonic wars. It is now endemic in many parts of the world, particularly Eastern and Central Europe, the Middle East, Central and Eastern Asia (Iran, India, China and Japan), Indonesia, the Pacific Islands, North and Central Africa, Central, and large areas of South America. It is not a racial disease and no race is exempt; in Western countries infection of the eye or genital tract by *C. trachomatis* is generally spread by sexual transmission from a genital reservoir of infection. It has been estimated that about one-fifth of the inhabitants of the world are affected, and trachoma together with the complicating infections with which it is associated is the cause of more blindness than any other condition.

The disease flourishes among people whose surroundings are unhygienic and who are crowded together in an unhealthy environment wherein dirt abounds. In endemic areas children are infected often in the first few years of life. It is contagious in its acute stages, being spread by the transference of conjunctival secretion by such means as fingers or towels and, above all, by flies, a liability increased by the presence of much discharge. On the other hand, scrupulous cleanliness will prevent extension of the disease to healthy subjects.

The disease usually starts subacutely, but on massive infection, experimental, accidental or clinical, an acute onset may be observed. Its course is determined largely by the presence or absence of a complicating infection and by repeated re-infections from flies and infected relatives. In the absence of such complications a 'pure' trachoma may be a relatively mild disease, so mild and symptomless, indeed, as to excite little or no attention until perhaps cicatrisation manifests itself in later life; in such cases the discovery of follicles or other cicatricial remnants on the upper tarsal conjunctiva when the lid is everted may come as a surprise to the patient and his relatives. On the other hand, in many countries wherein the disease is endemic, particularly in North Africa and the Middle East, secondary infections (as by *H. ægyptius*, the gonococcus or other organisms) result in an acute and incapacitating condition liable to relapses as a result of re-infection and leading to gross cicatricial sequelae which often end in blindness.

The primary infection is epithelial and involves both the conjunctiva and the cornea. The typical *conjunctival signs* are the appearance of a diffuse inflammation characterised by congestion, papillary enlargement and the development of follicles. The conjunctiva covering the upper tarsus is usually most affected and appears red and velvety, a condition which may pass into a uniform jelly-like thickening. The essential lesion is the trachoma follicle. When small, these cannot be distinguished from those of follicular conjunctivitis but they often assume a size (up to 5 mm in diameter) an appearance never seen in non-trachomatous conditions. Their distribution is characteristic. They may commence in the lower fornix but in most cases they quickly appear in the upper fornix also where they are usually most accentuated, often forming a row along the upper margin of the tarsus. They are not, however, limited to these regions but may appear on the caruncle and the plica as well as over the palpebral conjunctiva generally. They are rare on the bulbar conjunctiva but when seen here are pathognomonic of trachoma. Invasion of the lacrimal passages is not common. Trachomatous infiltration may spread deeply into the subepithelial tissues of the palpebral conjunctiva and even invade the tarsal plate. An important diagnostic feature is the appearance at a relatively early stage of signs of cicatrisation of the follicles, often appearing as minute star-shaped scars visible with the slit-lamp.

Trachomatous *implication of the cornea* manifests itself initially as a superficial keratitis, usually of so slight a degree as to be evident only by slit-lamp examination after staining with fluorescein. It occurs typically in the upper part of the cornea where there are numerous epithelial erosions which later become associated with infiltrated areas in the substantia propria.

At a later stage *trachomatous pannus* develops as a lymphoid infiltration with vascularisation of the margin of the cornea, usually limited to the upper half (Fig. 15.4) but tending to spread towards the centre and to involve the whole cornea. The upper part of the margin of the cornea becomes cloudy, and minute superficial vessels,

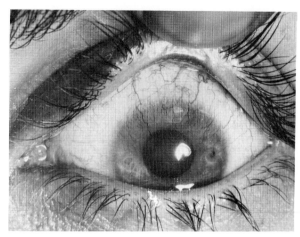

Fig. 15.4 Trachomatous pannus

springing from the corneal loops, grow inwards towards the centre. The haziness and vascularisation increase until the upper half of the cornea is affected. At the same time follicle-like infiltrations may appear near the limbus (Herbert's pits). The vessels are all superficial (p. 74), and microscopic examination has shown that they lie at first between Bowman's membrane and the epithelium, carrying in with them a small amount of granulation tissue. In the later stages Bowman's membrane disappears and the superficial layers of the substantia propria become involved. In more severe cases the vascularisation is not limited to the upper part, but superficial vessels grow in from all sides and the whole cornea becomes vascularised and opaque.

In progressive pannus the vessels are mostly parallel to each other and directed vertically downwards, anastomosing little. They extend to a level which forms a horizontal line, and beyond this line there is a narrow strip of infiltration and haze. In regressive pannus, on the other hand, the vessels extend a short distance beyond the area which is infiltrated and hazy: this difference is useful in estimating the results of treatment. *Corneal ulcers* which may be chronic and indolent may occur anywhere but are commonest at the advancing edge of the pannus. They are shallow, little infiltrated and very irritable, causing much lacrimation and photophobia.

Pannus may resolve completely, leaving the cornea quite clear apart from the obliterated vessels, but only in cases treated early when the pannus has not destroyed Bowman's membrane. In other cases a permanent opacity results.

Pathology. Trachoma is caused by a Bedsonian organism belonging to the psittacosis–lymphogranuloma group — the *Chlamydia trachomatis*; such organisms lie between bacteria and viruses, sharing some of the properties of both. It is seen typically in conjunctival scrapings in colony form in the epithelial cells as Hal-

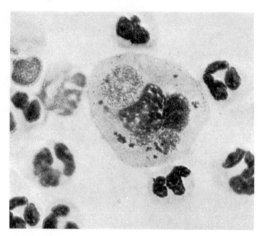

Fig. 15.5 An epithelial cell with multiple inclusions. Above and to the left of the nucleus an elementary body inclusion is deforming the nucleus. A dense probably less mature elementary body inclusion lies adjacent and to the right of the nucleus. (By courtesy of Yoneda.)

berstædter–Prowazek inclusion bodies (Fig. 15.5). The inclusion is first composed of numerous initial bodies. These divide until eventually the cell becomes filled with innumerable elementary bodies embedded in a carbohydrate matrix to form the inclusion body; the nucleus of the cell is displaced to one side and degenerates until eventually the cell bursts and the elementary bodies are set free to attack fresh cells in the cytoplasm of which they increase in size to form initial bodies. Morphologically identical inclusions are found in inclusion conjunctivities so that although they are not histologically pathognomonic of trachoma, the finding of such bodies in scrapings from the conjunctival epithelium is of considerable diagnostic importance. An infection confers little immunity since re-infection is relatively common; its occurrence has been proved experimentally and subsequent re-infections are progressively more acute.

Histologically there is lymphocytic infiltration involving the whole adenoid layer of the parts of the conjunctiva affected. Special aggregations of lymphocytes, without a definite capsule, form follicles which are generally indistinguishable from those of follicular conjunctivitis except that they tend to show necrosis and contain large multinucleated cells (*Leber's* cells). In the late stages hyaline and other types of degeneration occur; and in all long-standing cases fibrous tissue forms around the follicles, giving rise to cicatricial bands such as are never formed in follicular conjunctivitis, and are characteristic. The grosser forms of cicatrisation, however, are found only in cases which have been complicated by a superimposed infection.

Sequelae. Apart from the results of pannus and corneal ulceration the most malign effects of trachoma are

caused by distortions of the lids. A peculiar drooping of the upper lids owing to dense infiltration is very characteristic giving a sleepy appearance to the patient (*trachomatous ptosis*). There is always some scarring and when this is extensive the shape of the lids, especially the upper, is altered, a change aided by the infiltration of the tarsus, causing softening and absorption of its dense fibrous tissue; by the later contraction of the new-formed scar tissue the lids may be turned inwards (entropion), causing the lashes to rub against the cornea often with disastrous effects (trichiasis). These gross changes, however, rarely occur unless complicating infections have played a major part in the illness. (*See* Chap. 31.)

Symptoms. We have already seen that in an uncomplicated trachomatous infection the symptoms may be minimal; when other infections confuse the picture the initial symptomatology depends on these. During the chronic stages there is usually considerable irritation and when the cornea is involved much photophobia and lacrimation, all of which is intensified in the presence of trichiasis. In such cases the disability may be considerable and recurrent irritative phases may result in almost complete incapacity. In endemic areas where trachoma is rife the economic loss thereby entailed may reach enormous dimensions.

Diagnosis. Culture of *C. trachomatis* in irradiated McCoy cells is an expensive test. A simplified micro-immunofluorescence (micro-I.F.) test using pooled antigens rather than individual trachoma inclusion conjunctivitis (TRIC) serotypes has been developed which is practicable for routine diagnostic use. From the clinical point of view, the diagnostic features of trachoma depend on the following characteristics: the presence of follicles, of epithelial keratitis in the early stages most marked in the upper part of the cornea, of pannus in the upper part of the cornea and, in the later stages, of typical trachomatous scarring in the conjunctiva. Depending on the stage of the disease at least two of these signs should be present to establish the diagnosis. It is confirmed by the histological demonstration of the inclusion bodies if inclusion conjunctivitis can be excluded or by the cultivation of the organism.

The disease is frequently designated as occurring in four stages which were initially suggested by MacCallan, an English ophthalmologist who studied trachoma extensively in Egypt. Trachoma I designates the earliest stages of the disease before clinical diagnosis is possible. Trachoma II includes the period between the appearance of typical trachomatous lesions and the development of scar tissue. Trachoma III is the stage when scarring is obvious. Trachoma IV designates the stage when a cure appears to have been effected or the disease has become quiet but when cicatrisation gives rise to symptoms.

Treatment. The ideal antimicrobial treatment has not been developed. Tetracycline, erythromycin, rifampicin and the sulphonamides are effective when administered systemically. Unfortunately, each has some risk of side reactions. Sulphonamides have a high risk of allergic reactions such as erythema multiforme and Stevens–Johnson's syndrome. Tetracycline cannot be given to young children, pregnant women or nursing mothers. Topical treatment with erythromycin ointment, tetracycline or rifampicin is far more effective than with sulphonamides. Such treatment must be persistent in programmes of five consecutive days a month for 12 months. Oral doxycycline 5 mg per kg of body weight once per month is easy to administer and is as efficacious as topical tetracycline. Much of the dramatic effect which results is due to the elimination of secondary infections which almost invariably flourish in trachomatous eyes, but there is no doubt that the organism disappears and that the histological examination of scrapings from the conjunctiva demonstrates the disintegration of the inclusion bodies after the use of these drugs. It is to be remembered, of course, that well-formed follicles take a considerable time to resolve and dense infiltrative tissue does not disappear so that the full effects of a course of such treatment cannot be assessed for some months. It would seem, however, that some cases are resistant to this treatment and it may be that different strains of the organism exist which have different sensitivities to antibiotic drugs, a variation which occurs in many organismal infections. It is desirable that antibiotic drugs should be instilled several times a day until such time as the disease appears to be inactive.

If the follicles in the upper fornix are very large and closely packed it is well to commence treatment by *excising the fornix.* There is always a redundance of tissue here, and no evil results ensue. The upper lid is doubly everted (p. 71) so as to expose completely the retrotarsal fold. A silk suture is then passed through the fold at each end. By dragging on the sutures the whole fold is drawn out; it is then excised with scissors. If the tarsal plate is much diseased or distorted it also may be excised in the operation of *tarsectomy* which frequently gives much relief in chronic cases.

Pannus requires no special treatment for it quietens with the recession of the conjunctival activity. Corneal ulcers must be treated on general principles (*q.v.*).

Tuberculosis of the conjunctiva

This occurs typically in young people who are often free of clinical signs of tuberculosis elsewhere in the body, in which case it is a primary infection of exogenous origin. The disease is rare: it nearly always produces ulceration. Conjunctival ulceration should always suggest either the presence of an embedded foreign body or a tuberculous or syphilitic lesion.

Mycobacterium tuberculosis is a non-motile, encapsulated, rodlike organism which stains with difficulty, but resists decolorisation with strong mineral acids and is therefore referred to as acid fast. Human and bovine varieties produce lesions in man.

The initial or primary lesion is an acute process, healing in a short time, and producing an inconspicuous parenchymal lesion and caseation of the draining lymph nodes. The post-primary lesion or reinfection occurs in an individual who has developed a hypersensitivity to the bacteria and this lesion is chronic and associated with severe parenchymal involvement with a minor effect on the regional lymph nodes.

The disease is chronic, and the ulcers are indolent. The pre-auricular lymph node is often enlarged and may suppurate, but there is little pain or irritation unless the ulceration is extensive.

Pathology. Scrapings may show tubercle bacilli and sections typical giant-cell systems, while inoculation experiments may be made by the intraperitoneal inoculation of guinea-pigs.

Treatment. If the disease is a primary focus, it should preferably be eradicated by excision of the affected conjunctiva; if this is not feasible it should be thoroughly scraped and cauterised by diathermy. In all cases antibiotic treatment topically and systemically is administered. (Chap. 14). Cases of lupus frequently respond to calciferol.

Sarcoid

Patients affected with sarcoidosis not infrequently show lesions in the conjunctiva. These typically take a nodular form, translucent and orange in appearance, located usually in the folds of the lower fornix. Sometimes they are large and confluent. Diagnosis is by biopsy, and treatment is directed to the general condition.

Syphilis

This manifests itself rarely in the conjunctiva in the form of a primary chancre which is less indurated than the ordinary genital chancre and is usually conveyed by an infected mouth. A chronic ulcer or gummatous ulceration of the palpebral or still more of the bulbar conjunctiva is suggestive of the condition particularly when the regional lymph nodes are enlarged. Scrapings should be taken and examined for spirochaetes. Treponema may be demonstrated by dark-ground microscopic examination. A primary chancre of the palpebral conjunctiva may be wrongly diagnosed and treated as a chalazion (*q.v.*).

Tularemia

Tularemia is a disease with a widespread distribution in

America, Europe and Asia caused by an organism (the *Brucella tularensis*) derived from animals, particularly squirrels and rabbits. In the oculo-glandular form ulcers and nodules appear on the tarsal conjunctiva associated with swelling of the pre-auricular lymph node and accompanied by general constitutional symptoms of fever and debility. The diagnosis is made by an agglutination test and treatment, locally and systemically, is by streptomycin.

Ophthalmia nodosa

This is a nodular conjunctivitis which may be mistaken for tuberculosis due to the irritation of the hairs of certain caterpillars, and therefore always commences in the summer months. Small semi-translucent, reddish, or yellowish grey nodules are formed in the conjunctiva, the cornea, and sometimes in the iris. On microscopic examination hairs surrounded by giant cells and lymphocytes are found. The nodules in the conjunctiva should be excised; otherwise the condition is treated on general principles.

Parinaud's oculo-glandular syndrome

This is a generic name which used to be applied to conjunctivitis, usually of the follicular type, associated with pre-auricular (or sub-maxillary) lymphadenopathy.

It is due to lymphogranuloma venereum which is a contagious venereal disease manifested by an initial vesicle which bursts, leaving a grayish ulcer followed by regional lymphadenitis that is frequently suppurative.

The eyelids may be infected venereally or through accidental contamination in laboratory workers.

A number of syndromes related to *erythema multiforme* affect the conjunctiva in association with other mucous membranes such as those of the mouth, the nose, the urethra and vulva, as well as eruptions on the skin associated with general toxic symptoms sometimes of considerable severity. The conjunctivitis may be mild but sometimes is severe when the condition is often known as the Stevens–Johnson syndrome; it may be of a pseudo-membranous or vesicular type and blindness may result from corneal complications. The disease is an immune vasculitis precipitated by deposition of circulating antigen complexed with complement-fixing antibody. In Reiter's disease an acute conjunctivitis, catarrhal or purulent, is associated with urethritis and polyarthritis; a keratitis and a uveitis, sometimes with hypopyon, occasionally occur. The conjunctivitis associated with Behçet's disease (*q.v.*) is usually mild. Treatment of all these conditions is unsatisfactory. Corticosteroids and broad-spectrum antibiotics do not give consistent results.

Benign mucous membrane pemphigoid

This is a rare but very serious disease of unknown origin affecting both eyes. There is a loss of hemidesmosomal attachment of the epithelium to the basement membrane. Vesicles occur on the conjunctiva, but more commonly greyish white membranous patches are seen. Progressive cicatrisation follows, leading eventually to *essential shrinkage of the conjunctiva*, with consequent opacification of the cornea. Similar lesions may be found in the nose, mouth, palate, pharynx, anus and vagina, and more rarely on the skin. Local treatment, such as transplantation of mucous membrane, is unavailing, as also, indeed, is general treatment. Hydrophylic contact lenses together with artificial tears may be helpful.

Somewhat similar lesions may complicate other aphthous affections of the mucous membranes such as *erythema nodosum, dermatitis herpetiformis, epidermolysis bullosa,* and *hydroa vacciniforme*.

Allergic types of conjunctivitis

The allergic reactions of the conjunctiva may assume three forms — an ordinary acute or subacute conjunctivitis of the catarrhal type, phlyctenular conjunctivitis, a characteristic reaction to endogenous allergens, and vernal catarrh, a characteristic reaction to those of exogenous origin.

Acute or subacute allergic catarrhal conjunctivitis

This type of reaction shows few distinguishing characteristics from the corresponding types of inflammation due to organismal infection except that the hyperaemia is usually marked, the secretion is watery and not purulent but often contains eosinophil cells, and the condition has a chronic habit with a marked tendency to subacute remissions on renewed contact with the allergen.

Sometimes the allergen is a bacterial protein of endogenous nature, the most common being a staphylococcus in the nasal cavity or upper respiratory tract. A more characteristic picture is due to exogenous proteins, in which case the conjunctivitis may form part of a typical hay fever and elevated IgE levels are demonstrable in the plasma and tears. Contact with animals (horses, cats), pollens or certain flowers (primula, etc.) is a frequent cause. Some chemicals, cosmetics and eyelash dyes cause severe conjunctivitis and dermatitis.

Drugs applied locally to the conjunctiva often cause a typical reaction of this type in susceptible persons; it may be violent, almost erysipelatous, in type, spreading widely over the lids and face. The most typical picture of such an acute reaction is that of *atropine irritation*, while eserine and other drugs tend to produce a more chronic response characterised by follicular formation (*q.v.*).

Treatment is logically by removal of the allergen from the environment; if this cannot be done desensitisation may be attempted by a long course of injections. Temporary relief may be obtained by astringent lotions or, more effectively, by the instillation of adrenaline solution (1 in 10 000) or antihistamine drugs (antistine privine, 1.0%). Corticosteroid drops also frequently bring relief in severe cases which do not respond to the topical use of 2% sodium cromoglycate (Opticrom).

In atropine irritation the drug should be avoided. If a mydriatic is imperative, some other should be substituted such as phenylephrine 10% (p. 27), but frequently in susceptible persons an allergy also develops to these drugs. Subconjunctival injections of mydricaine (p. 368) may be used with impunity in these cases.

Phlyctenular conjunctivitis (eczematous conjunctivitis).
In phlyctenular conjunctivitis one or more small, round, grey or yellow nodules, slightly raised above the surface, are seen on the bulbar conjunctiva, generally at or near the limbus; they rarely occur on the palpebral conjunctiva. The disease is frequently complicated by mucopurulent conjunctivitis, in which case the whole conjunctiva is intensely reddened. In pure phlyctenular conjunctivitis the congestion of the vessels is limited to the area around the phlyctens.

The evidence is considerable that phlyctenular conjunctivitis is an allergic condition caused by endogenous bacterial proteins which in most cases are tuberculous, but may in other cases be derived from mild infections of long standing as in tonsils or adenoids. The condition used to be common in Britain and America but is rare today, a change which may in some degree be due to improved hygiene and the control over infection of milk by bovine tuberculosis.

Phlyctens resemble blebs, and there is a true vesicular stage. They may be so small as to be seen only with difficulty, but they usually measure about 1 mm in diameter. In the later stages the epithelium over the surface becomes necrotic and small ulcers are formed; on the conjunctiva this is of little moment since healing takes place rapidly without the formation of a scar, but when it occurs on the cornea, as is very frequently the case, it is much more serious (p. 140).

Simple phlyctenular conjunctivitis is attended with few symptoms. There is some discomfort and irritation associated with reflex lacrimation. If there is no mucopurulent complication and if the cornea is not involved there is little or no photophobia. Corneal spread, however, is the rule if the condition persists and in this case there is a marked intensification of the symptoms particularly from phlyctens lying astride the limbus.

Treatment. Simple phlyctenular conjunctivitis is usually readily amenable to treatment, which must be both local and general. Steroids given as drops or ointment usually have a most dramatic effect (Chap. 14). If there is any corneal complication, or evidence of its imminence, atropine is added. The eyes should not be bandaged but dark glasses or a shade, covering both eyes and extending well over the temples, may be ordered.

Spring catarrh (vernal conjunctivitis)
This is a recurrent bilateral conjunctivitis occurring with the onset of hot weather, and therefore rather a summer than a spring complaint, found in young people, usually boys. Burning, itching, some photophobia and lacrimation are the chief symptoms accompanied by a characteristic white, ropy secretion. In the cooler months the condition subsides and gives no trouble although the lesions persist, but the symptoms recur with the return of heat. The disease is met with among all classes, is sporadic, and non-contagious. It is a hypersensitive reaction to exogenous allergens and is mediated by IgE as indicated by the accompanying eosinophilia.

Two typical forms are seen: (1) the palpebral form; (2) the bulbar form. Both may be combined, but this is relatively rare.

The *palpebral form* is easily recognised. On everting the upper lid the palpebral conjunctiva is seen to be hypertrophied and mapped out into polygonal raised areas, not unlike cobble stones (Fig. 15.6). The colour is bluish white, like milk, and this appearance may be seen also over the lower palpebral conjunctiva. The flat-topped nodules are hard, and consist chiefly of dense fibrous tissue, but the epithelium over them is thickened, giving rise to the milky hue. Histologically they are hypertrophied papillae — not follicles. Eosinophilic leucocytes are present in them in great numbers and are found in the secretion. The palpebral form cannot be mistaken if typical, but it may resemble trachoma. The type of patient, the milky hue, the freedom of the fornix from implication and the characteristic recurrence in hot weather will usually prevent mistakes.

The *bulbar form* is less characteristic (Fig. 15.7). In it

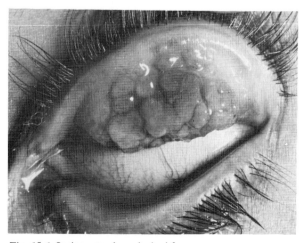

Fig. 15.6 Spring catarrh : palpebral form

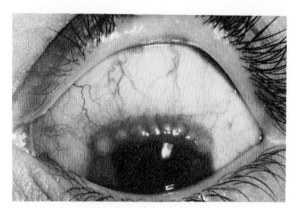

Fig. 15.7 Spring catarrh : bulbar form

nodules or a wall of gelatinous thickening appears at the limbus. Both types are complicated by a fine diffuse superficial punctate keratitis.

Serious complications never supervene and the ultimate prognosis is good, and although recurrences may persist for several years the disease eventually subsides. Occasionally some thickening and discoloration of the conjunctiva may remain.

Treatment is purely symptomatic. The irritation is best relieved by the frequent instillation of steroid drops or ointment; after some days the acute irritation usually subsides and thereafter a maintenance dose three or four times a day during the seasonal period of activity generally keeps the symptoms in check. Antibiotics are likely to set up an allergic reaction and so there is no place for a steroid antibiotic mixture. The production of sticky mucus is characteristic. Acetyl cysteine used as 10% or 20% drops is useful in controlling excess mucus. Tinted glasses are often a considerable comfort. In proliferative cases applications of β-radiation at monthly intervals during February, March and April, are sometimes of value in preventing an attack, but do not cure the disease. Cryotherapy of the nodules is sometimes useful. Disodium cromoglycate 2% (Intal) as drops four times daily may act as an adjuvant to steroid topically.

Traumatic conjunctivitis will be considered with ocular injuries when the action of caustics and vesicant gases will be discussed (Chap. 26). Malingerers sometimes induce conjunctivitis by the insertion of a multitude of irritants into the eyes. The irritation is most marked in the lower fornix, and usually the right eye is affected in right-handed people.

DEGENERATIVE CHANGES IN THE CONJUNCTIVA

Concretions ('lithiasis')

These occur as minute hard yellow spots in the palpebral conjunctiva. They are due to the accumulation of epithelial cells and inspissated mucus in depressions called Henle's glands. They never become calcareous, so the term is a misnomer, but they are so hard that when they project from the surface they scratch the cornea and give the sensation of a foreign body in the eye. They are common in elderly people and they should be removed with a sharp needle in those who have suffered from trachoma.

Pinguecula

This is a triangular patch on the conjunctiva, found usually in elderly people, especially those exposed to strong sunlight, dust, wind and so on. It occurs near the limbus in the palpebral aperture, the apex of the triangle being away from the cornea and affects the nasal side first, then the temporal. It is yellow in colour and looks like fat, whence the name (*pinguis*, fat), but is due to hyaline infiltration and elastotic degeneration of the submucous tissue. Since the pinguecula remains relatively free from congestion it is particularly conspicuous when the eye is inflamed: mistakes in diagnosis may then occur. It requires no treatment.

Pterygium

This is a degenerative condition of the subconjunctival tissues which proliferate as vascularised granulation tissue to invade the cornea, destroying as it does so the superficial layers of the stroma and Bowman's membrane, the whole being covered by conjunctival epithelium (Fig. 15.8). The lesion thus appears as a triangular encroachment of the conjunctiva upon the cornea with, in front of its blunt apex, numerous small opacities lying deeply in the neighbouring part of the cornea. The thick vascularised conjunctiva appears to be drawn onto the cornea from the canthus and is loosely adherent in its whole length to the sclera, the area of adherence being always smaller than its breadth so that there are folds at the upper and lower borders.

A pterygium frequently follows a pinguecula and

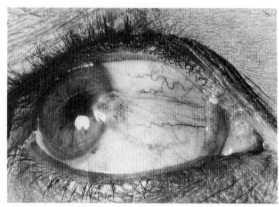

Fig. 15.8 Pterygium

when single is usually on the nasal side; when double the temporal lesion develops later. In the early stages it is thick and vascular; when it ceases to grow it becomes thin and pale, but never disappears. When it ceases to progress, consolidation occurs with the formation of dense fibrous tissue and the development of considerable corneal astigmatism. Ordinarily the condition is symptomless, but vision becomes impaired if it progress into the pupillary area of the cornea.

The condition is common in dry sunny climates with sandy soils as in parts of Australia, South Africa, Texas, or the Middle East. Ultra-violet light is probably an etiological factor.

Treatment. A pterygium is best left alone unless it is progressing towards the pupillary area, or is disfiguring. It cannot be removed without leaving a scar unless it is replaced by a lamellar corneal graft.

Removal is effected by seizing the neck near the corneal margin with fixation forceps, raising it, and shaving or dissecting it from the cornea, starting from the apex. Care must be taken not to go too deeply. The pterygium is then freed from the sclera for about half the distance towards the canthus. Two parallel incisions are then made with scissors to excise as much of the pterygium as possible. The head of the pterygium is then excised and a bare area of sclera remains at the edge of the cornea.

A pterygium sometimes recurs after removal. If it actually re-forms and extends towards the pupillary area, the apex should be freed and a lamellar graft inserted over the affected area. Contact radiation by β-rays may be carefully applied to the limbus. The dose should not exceed 2500 rad given during the first week following surgery. Alternatively thio-TEPA 1 : 2000 solution may be given four times daily for 6 weeks.

SYMPTOMATIC CONDITIONS

Subconjunctival ecchymosis

This is due to the rupture of small vessels and may be the result of minor injury, or more commonly occurs spontaneously. The condition, though unsightly, is trivial. Very minute ecchymoses, or possibly thromboses, are seen in severe conjunctivitis; larger extravasations accompany severe straining, especially in old people as on lifting heavy weights or vomiting. They are not infrequently seen in children with whooping cough and may occur in scurvy, such blood diseases as purpura, or in malaria; as a rule they need arouse no anxiety.

More serious are the large subconjunctival ecchymoses which seep forwards from the fornix which sometimes follow injuries when they are due to an extravasation of blood along the floor of the orbit, the result of a fracture of the base of the skull. In fractures of the sphenoid the blood appears later on the tem-

poral side than elsewhere. Hæmorrhages also result from severe or prolonged pressure on the thorax and abdomen, as in persons squeezed in a crowd or by machinery.

Treatment. The blood becomes absorbed in from one to three weeks without treatment.

Chemosis

Otherwise known as œdema of the conjunctiva, may occur in: (1) acute inflammations; (2) in cases of obstruction to the circulation; (3) in abnormal blood conditions.

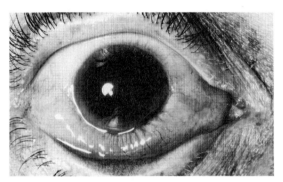

Fig. 15.9 Chemosis

In the first group of cases the inflammation may be in the conjunctiva, as in gonorrhœal conjunctivitis, or within the eyeball, as in panophthalmitis or hypopyon ulcer; it is also occasionally found in acute glaucoma. The inflammation may be in the accessory structures of the eye, as a stye or an insect bite on the lid, dacryocystitis, periostitis, orbital cellulitis or cerebro-spinal meningitis.

In the second group the pressure of an orbital tumour may so interfere with the lymph and blood streams as to produce chemosis; it is also found in pulsating exophthalmos or exophthalmic ophthalmoplegia.

To the third group belong nephritis and the anæmias, urticaria, angioneurotic œdema and occasionally lymphomatous infiltration.

Xerosis (xerophthalmia)

This is a dry, lustreless condition of the conjunctiva which occurs in two groups of cases: (1) as a sequel of a local ocular affection; (2) associated with general disease.

The first type is a cicatricial degeneration of the conjunctiva — (a) following trachoma, burns, pemphigoid, diphtheria, etc., commencing in isolated spots, ultimately involving the whole conjunctiva and cornea; (b) following exposure, due to ectropion or proptosis wherein the eye is not properly covered by the lids.

The chief changes are in the epithelium which becomes epidermoid like that of skin with granular and horny layers and ceases to secrete mucus. A certain amount of vicarious activity is set up in the meibomian glands (Chap. 31) which cover the dry surface with their fatty secretion so that the watery tears then fail to moisten the conjunctiva. The *C. xerosis* grows profusely in these conditions, but this organism has no causal relationship and is of no importance.

It is to be noted that xerosis has nothing to do with any failure of function on the part of the lacrimal apparatus. The conjunctiva can be quite efficiently moistened by its own secretions alone and if the lacrimal gland is extirpated xerosis does not follow. If, on the other hand, the secretory activity of the membrane itself is impaired, xerosis may follow in spite of normal or increased lacrimal secretion.

In the second group of cases xerosis is due to a deficiency of the fatsoluble vitamin A in the diet and occurs usually in a mild form, particularly in children, especially boys, accompanied by night blindness (Chap. 24). It is characterised by small triangular white patches on the outer and inner sides of the cornea, covered by a material resembling dried foam, which is not wetted by the tears (*Bitôt's spots*). The foamy spots are due to horny epithelium which is cast off into the conjunctival sac and accumulates in the lower fornix. The cases usually occur during the summer months, and the children are often not conspicuously ill-nourished. A similar mild form, also associated with night blindness, (xerophthalmia) is found in marasmic children, associated with keratomalacia and necrosis of the cornea (p. 136).

Treatment. Xerosis is a symptom and its treatment must therefore be purely symptomatic. Local treatment consists in relieving the dryness with hypromellose, parolein or weak alkaline solutions; dark glasses should be worn. In the deficiency variety restoration of normal nutrition by the administration of vitamin A is all-important.

Kerato-conjunctivitis sicca, a condition due to deficiency of the lacrimal secretion, is described elsewhere (p. 324).

Argyrosis

This is the staining of the conjunctiva a deep brown from prolonged application of silver salts (nitrate, proteinate, etc.) for the treatment of chronic conjunctivitis and especially trachoma. The staining, which is most marked in the lower fornix, is due to the impregnation of the elastic fibres in the membrane and vessel walls with reduced metallic silver.

CYSTS AND TUMOURS

The only common cysts found in the conjunctiva are due to dilatation of lymph spaces. When small these often form rows of little cysts on the bulbar conjunctiva (*lymphangiectasis*). Occasionally, single though multilocular cysts occur (*lymphangiomata*). Larger retention cysts of Krause's accessory lacrimal glands occur in the upper fornix (Chap. 32). Subconjunctival cysticercus and hydatid cysts are rare. Non-parasitic cysts require simple removal of the anterior walls. *Epithelial implantation cysts* occur rarely after injuries or operations for strabismus.

Tumours

In the conjunctiva these have a tendency to be polypoid owing to the perpetual movements of the globe and lids.

Congenital tumours include dermoids and dermolipomata:

1. *Dermoids* are lenticular yellow tumours, usually astride the corneal margin, most commonly at the outer side (Fig. 15.10). They consist of epidermoid epithelium with sebaceous glands and hairs which may cause irritation. They tend to grow at puberty, and should be dissected off the globe if troublesome, although after removal the site of attachment to the cornea remains densely opaque. This area can be disguised by suitable tatooing or replaced by a lamellar graft.

2. *Dermo-lipomata* or *fibro-fatty tumours* are congenital tumours found at the outer canthus sometimes associated with accessory auricles and other congenital defects in babies. They consist of fibrous tissue and fat, sometimes with dermoid tissue on the surface, and are not encapsulated. The main mass should be removed, but it will be found that the fat is continuous with that of the orbit.

Papillomata occur at the inner canthus, in the fornices or at the limbus. They may become malignant and should be removed.

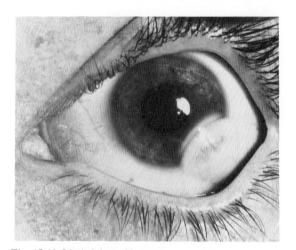
Fig. 15.10 Limbal dermoid

Simple Granulomata, consisting of exuberant granulation tissue, generally polypoid in form, often grow from tenotomy wounds or the sites of foreign bodies. They are common in empty sockets after excision, and at the site of chalazia which have been insufficiently scraped (p. 310). They should be removed by scissors.

Epithelioma (Squamous-celled Carcinoma) usually occurs where one kind of epithelium passes into another; in the conjunctiva it therefore occurs chiefly at the limbus. Papillomata in old people often take on malignant proliferation. *Bowen's intra-epithelial epithelioma* is a rarity. Epitheliomata spread over the surface and into the fornices, rarely penetrating the globe. They have the structural characteristic of such growth elsewhere. They must be removed as freely as possible, the base being cauterised by diathermy; the diagnosis should be microscopically confirmed. On the slightest sign of recurrence the eye must be excised and if recurrence again takes place the orbit must be exenterated and X-ray therapy adopted.

Pigmented tumours

These constitute an important type of neoplasia which introduces difficult clinical decisions: some are simple (nævus), some potentially pre-cancerous (junctional nævus, pre-cancerous melanosis, lentigo malignum) and some frankly malignant (malignant melanoma).

Nævi or *congenital moles* are not uncommon (Fig. 15.11). They are grey gelatinous or pigmented nodules situated by preference at the limbus or near the plica semilunaris. They have the same structure as in the skin — groups, often alveolar, of 'naevus cells' in close connection with the epithelium. They are congenital and tend to grow at puberty rarely becoming malignant. In view of this they should be excised before puberty, but lest malignant changes follow the operative disturbance, they should always be excised completely. It is to be noted that pigmentation at the limbus occurs normally in dark races, and patches in this situation are not uncommon in people with dark complexions.

Pre-cancerous melanosis is a diffusely spreading pigmentation of the conjunctiva occurring rarely in elderly people, which may also involve the skin of the lids and cheek. It is liable to spread slowly and may eventually assume malignant characteristics, giving rise to metastases. The condition should therefore always be viewed as pre-cancerous and at this stage it is radio-sensitive; if allowed to progress to the malignant phase some

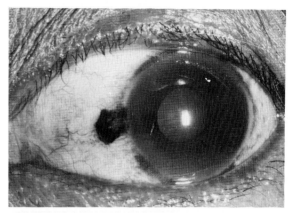

Fig. 15.11 Nævus of the conjunctiva

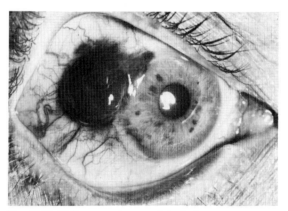

Fig. 15.12 Malignant melanoma of the limbus

cases tend to become radio-resistant in which case the only effective treatment is wide excision with exenteration of the orbit and extensive reconstitution by skin grafting. Beta-irradiation either primary or after tumour excision is the treatment of choice for conjunctival melanomas.

Malignant melanoma is rare (Fig. 15.12). It occurs typically at the limbus, is usually pigmented, and most of the patients are old. It spreads over the surface of the globe but rarely penetrates it; recurrences and metastases occur as elsewhere in the body. The neoplasms may be alveolar — derived from nævi — or round or spindle-celled. The treatment is by excision of the globe or exenteration of the orbit.

Rodent ulcer (Basal-celled Carcinoma) may invade the conjunctiva from the lids (p. 320).

16

Diseases of the cornea

The special importance of diseases of the cornea depends upon the fact that they often leave permanent opacities which seriously lower the visual acuity, while the complications which not infrequently attend them may lead to the loss of the eye.

INFLAMMATION OF THE CORNEA (KERATITIS)

Inflammation of the cornea may arise from three sources.

1. *Exogenous infections.* In these cases the cornea is primarily affected, virulent organisms frequently already present in the conjunctival sac gaining access to the corneal tissues.

2. *From the ocular tissues.* As we have already noted (p. 5), owing to direct anatomical continuity, diseases of the conjunctiva readily spread to the corneal epithelium, those of the sclera to the stroma, and of the uveal tract to the endothelium.

3. *Endogenous infections.* These are of rare occurrence and, owing to the avascularity of the cornea which allows immunological changes to persist for an unusually long time, they are typically allergic in nature.

From the clinical point of view, corneal inflammations are best divided into two categories, superficial and deep. The former may be purulent (corneal ulcers) or non-purulent.

Superficial types of keratitis

Purulent keratitis, ulceration of the cornea
Purulent keratitis is nearly always exogenous, due to pyogenic organisms which invade the cornea from without. It has been pointed out that the only organisms which are known to be able to invade normal epithelium are those of gonorrhœa and diphtheria; but many other bacteria are capable of producing ulceration, notably the pneumococcus, when the epithelium is damaged. Organisms such as the staphylococcus may cause superficial punctate erosions (*q.v.*).

Although minute abrasions of the cornea are probably of everyday occurrence, pathogenic organisms of high virulence are not always present in the conjunctival sac, and if they are, the resistance of the normal tissues may suffice to deal with them. Apart from actual abrasions a diminished resistance of the epithelium will allow the ready intrusion of organisms and lead to rapid and widespread ulceration into the corneal tissues — drying, as in xerosis, necrosis due to deficient nutrition, as in keratomalacia, desquamation as the result of œdema, neuroparalytic keratitis or general malnutrition.

In the commonest form of suppurative keratitis — the corneal ulcer — there is localised necrosis in the most anterior layers of the cornea. The sequestrum is partly disintegrated and cast off into the conjunctival sac, and partly adheres to the surface of the ulcer. Usually the epithelium is desquamated over an area considerably larger than the ulcer itself, and the same applies to Bowman's membrane. The epithelium, however, rapidly advances towards the ulcer, grows over its edge, and even over the slough or purulent infiltration which forms the floor.

The ulcer is usually saucer-shaped, and the walls project above the normal surface of the cornea owing to swelling caused by the imbibition of fluid by the corneal lamellae. The surrounding area is packed with leucocytes, appearing as a grey zone of infiltration. This is the progressive stage.

A line of demarcation forms as in necrosis elsewhere in the body. Here a wall of polymorphonuclear leucocytes forms a second line of defence while the leucocytes exert their digestive functions, macerating and dissolving the necrotic tissues. When the dead material has been thrown off the ulcer is somewhat larger, but the cloudiness has disappeared, the floor and edges are smooth and transparent, and the regressive stage is reached.

Meanwhile vascularisation has been developing. Minute superficial vessels grow in from the limbus near the ulcer supplying the pabulum to restore the loss of substance; they also supply antibodies and therefore play an important role in combating bacterial infection. Sometimes they are so exuberant as to overstep the limits of utility, as in fascicular ulcer (*q.v.*).

While these events occur in the cornea irritative signs are always found within the eye. Some of the toxins elaborated by the bacteria diffuse through the cornea into the anterior chamber, just as atropine does when instilled into the conjunctival sac. Here they exert an irritative effect upon the vessels of the iris and ciliary body, so that hyperæmia of the iris occurs with or without ciliary injection. The irritation may be so great that leucocytosis takes place, and polymorphonuclear cells, poured out by the vessels, pass into the aqueous and gravitate to the bottom of the anterior chamber where they form a *hypopyon* (p. 75).

The *symptoms* of a corneal ulcer are marked. During the progressive stage there is lacrimation, photophobia, blepharospasm, and pain, owing to the exposure of the terminal fibrils of the ophthalmic division of the fifth nerve.

The term photophobia is a misnomer. It is the term applied to the blepharospasm set up by corneal irritation, which becomes greatly increased on the slightest attempt to separate the lids, especially if the attempt is made in bright light. This blepharospasm is not abolished in the dark, but is abolished by thorough cocainisation. It is thus a reflex involving the fifth nerve, not the optic nerve. Serious photophobia only accompanies denudation of the epithelium; but spasm of the sphincter of the iris probably increases the discomfort.

The healing of a corneal ulcer. When the ulcer has become vascularised, everything is prepared for cicatrisation, which is carried out by the formation of fibrous tissue. The new fibres are not arranged regularly as in the normal lamellae, so that they refract the light irregularly; the scar is, therefore, more or less opaque. If it is large and dense some of the larger vessels persist; the smaller ones disappear. Bowman's membrane is never regenerated, and if it has been destroyed, as is the case in all but very superficial abrasions some degree of permanent opacity remains.

The scar tissue which replaces the destroyed portions of the cornea usually fills in the gap exactly, so that the surface is level. It is quite common, however, for some deficiency to remain so that although the resultant cicatrix may be almost transparent, the surface is flattened or even indented. Such *corneal facets* can only be seen by careful examination of the corneal reflex (p. 72) but they may cause considerable diminution of the visual acuity.

If the corneal scar is thin the resulting opacity is slight and is called a *nebula*; if rather more dense it is sometimes called a *macula*; if very dense and white it is called a *leucoma*. Old central leucomata sometimes show a horizontal pigmented line in the palpebral aperture, the

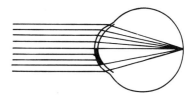

Fig. 16.1 The optical effect of a complete leucoma. Light falling upon it is not irregularly refracted and does not distort the retinal image

nature of which is obscure. A thin, diffuse nebula covering the pupillary area interferes more with vision than a strictly localised dense leucoma, so long as the latter does not block the whole pupillary area.

The reason is that the leucoma stops all the light which falls upon it (Fig. 16.1), whereas the nebula refracts it irregularly, allowing many of the rays to fall upon the retina where they blur the image formed by the regularly refracted rays. An opacity does not necessarily prevent the light from being focused upon the retina immediately behind it. Thus, a central opacity will not prevent the focusing of an object upon the macular region, for the rays passing through the clear peripheral parts of the cornea will be refracted towards the macula; only those rays which are incident to the corneal suface at the opaque region are cut off. There is thus a loss of brightness rather than of definition, although this is impaired by the superimposition of a diffuse entoptic image of the opacity upon the clear image of the external object.

Although some opacity always remains when Bowman's membrane has been destroyed, there is usually a considerable degree of clearing eventually, a process more marked in younger patients. In this vascularisation plays a considerable part, as is shown by the fact that the opacities clear first in the immediate vicinity of the vessels.

Complications. This simple progress of superficial ulceration and subsequent healing is not unfortunately of universal occurrence. If the ulcer has been deep the loss of tissue may lead to a marked thinning of the entire cornea at the site of the ulcer so that it bulges under the influence of the normal intra-ocular pressure. As the cicatrix becomes consolidated the bulging may disappear, or it may remain permanently as an *ectatic cicatrix* (keratectasia from ulcer).

Some ulcers, especially those due to the pneumococcus and septic organisms, extend rapidly in depth so that the whole thickness of the cornea except Descemet's membrane and a few corneal lamellæ may be destroyed. Descemet's membrane, like other elastic membranes, offers great resistance to inflammatory processes. It is, however, unable alone to support the intra-ocular pressure: it therefore herniates through the ulcer as a transparent vesicle, called a *keratocele* or *de-*

scemetocele. This may persist, surrounded by a white cicatricial ring, or it may eventually rupture.

Perforation and its effects. The perforation of an ulcer is usually caused by some sudden exertion on the part of the patient, such as coughing, sneezing, straining at stool, or spasm of the orbicularis. Any such sudden exertion causes a rise in general blood pressure, which at once manifests itself by a rise in intra-ocular pressure and the weak floor of the ulcer, unable to support the sudden strain, gives way. When an ulcer perforates the aqueous suddenly escapes and the intra-ocular pressure sinks to the atmospheric level, the iris and lens being driven forwards into contact with the back of the cornea. The effect upon the nutrition of the cornea is good: owing to the diminution of intra-ocular pressure the diffusion of fluid through the cornea is facilitated, extension of the ulceration usually ceases, pain is alleviated, and cicatrisation proceeds rapidly. The complications which attend perforation are, however, of extreme danger to sight and even to the preservation of the eye. These complications vary according to the position and size of the perforation.

Usually the perforation takes place opposite some part of the iris which is washed into the aperture when the aqueous escapes. If the perforation is small the iris becomes gummed down to the opening, the adhesion organizes and an *anterior synechia* is formed. The blocking of the perforation with iris allows the anterior chamber to be re-formed, fresh aqueous being rapidly secreted. If the perforation is large, a portion of the iris is carried not only into the opening but through it, and a *prolapse of iris* is produced. If this does not include the pupillary margin, the prolapse is hemispherical; if it does, a tag of iris lies free upon the cornea. In either case the colour of the iris soon becomes obscured by the deposition of grey or yellow exudate upon the surface, but eventually the stroma becomes thinned and the black retinal pigmentary epithelium is thrown into relief (Figs 16.2 and 16.3).

Sometimes the whole cornea sloughs with the exception of a narrow rim at the margin, and *total prolapse of iris* occurs. The pupil usually becomes blocked with exudate, and a false cornea is formed consisting of iris covered by exudate. If, however, the perforation takes place suddenly the suspensory ligament of the lens is stretched or ruptured, causing subluxation of the lens, or even dislocation and expulsion through the perforation.

If prolapse of the iris has occurred cicatrisation may still progress. The exudate which covers the prolapse becomes organised and forms a thin layer of connective tissue over which the conjunctival or corneal epithelium rapidly grows. The contraction of the bands of fibrous tissue tends to flatten the protruding prolapse or *pseudo-cornea*. It rarely, however, becomes quite flat; more

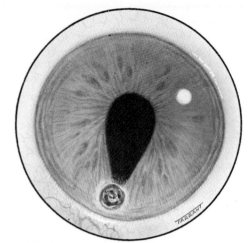

Fig. 16.2 Perforated corneal ulcer with a prolapse of the iris

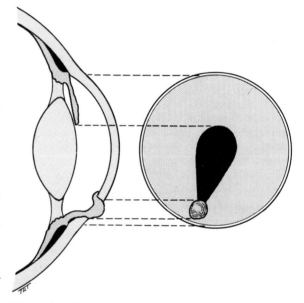

Fig. 16.3 A diagrammatic view of the topography of the lesion

commonly the iris and cicatricial tissue are too weak to support the restored intra-ocular pressure, which is often increased owing to the development of a secondary glaucoma (p. 187). The cicatrix therefore tends to become ectatic; such an ectatic cicatrix in which the iris is incarcerated is called an *anterior staphyloma* which, depending on its extent, may be either partial or total. The bands of scar tissue on the staphyloma vary in breadth and thickness, producing a lobulated surface often blackened with pigment; hence the name.

If the perforation happens to be opposite the pupil, the pupillary margin of the iris often becomes adherent to the edges and the aperture becomes filled with exudate. The anterior chamber is then re-formed very slowly; the lens remains long in contact with the ulcer, and a permanent opacity may occur in it — *anterior capsular cataract*. As the anterior chamber re-forms, the exudate filling the opening is submitted to strain and frequently ruptures, especially if the patient is restless. This process may be repeated so that the opening may become permanent — *corneal fistula*.

The sudden reduction of intra-ocular pressure when the perforation occurs removes support from all the intra-ocular blood vessels which become dilated and may rupture, causing an *intra-ocular haemorrhage*. Rupture of the retinal vessels gives rise to a vitreous hæmorrhage; of the choroidal, to a sub-retinal or sub-choroidal hæmorrhage. It may indeed be so profuse that the contents of the globe are extruded with the out-flowing blood.

Finally, the organisms which have caused the ulceration of the cornea may gain access to the interior of the eye as the result of perforation. *Purulent iridocyclitis* or even *panophthalmitis* may thus be set up, a result especially prone to occur in gonorrhœal ophthalmia and in hypopyon ulcer (*q.v.*).

Treatment of uncomplicated ulcers. Control of infection, cleanliness, heat, rest, and protection are the fundamental principles of the treatment of corneal ulcers. Control of infection is attained by the use of bacteriostatic drugs: surgical cleanliness is the principle which should regulate the use of lotions; heat is employed to prevent stasis and encourage repair; local rest is attained by the use of atropine; rest and protection from deletrious external agencies are attained by the use of a pad and bandage.

The ordinary treatment of a simple uncomplicated ulcer is as follows.

The infection is controlled by the intensive local use of antibiotic drugs as already indicated (Chap. 14). Atropine either as drops or ointment (1 %) should be introduced between the lids two or three times a day; this drug gives comfort by preventing ciliary spasm and forestalling most of the dangerous results of the iritis which always complicate corneal ulceration. Much comfort can frequently be obtained by local heat and in the intervals between treatment a protective pad and bandage may be applied unless there is much conjunctival discharge; in this event any benefit is more than counteracted by the retention of secretion and the pad should be replaced by a shield.

If the reaction is severe, steroids administered either as drops or an ointment may control the symptoms dramatically, but should only be used when it is apparent that antibiotics are controlling the infection, and once the inflammation ceases to progress they should be discontinued since they may retard epithelialisation and inhibit repair by fibrosis.

If the ulcer progresses despite these therapeutic measures, the removal of necrotic material may be hastened by scraping the floor with a spatula, or the ulcer may be cauterised.

Cauterisation may be performed with pure carbolic acid or trichloracetic acid (10–20 %). Carbolic acid has the advantage of penetrating a little more deeply than it is actually applied, thus extending its antiseptic properties more widely; it acts both as a caustic and an antiseptic. Although the parts touched immediately become white, the normal epithelium rapidly recovers. The acid must not, however, touch the conjunctiva lest adhesions form between the lids and globe.

If despite these measures ulceration progresses, pain continues and perforation seems imminent, the latter event may sometimes be anticipated with advantage by *paracentesis*. By this procedure the aqueous is evacuated slowly and the more dangerous results of spontaneous perforation may be avoided while, as has already been pointed out, the nutrition of the diseased cornea is considerably improved.

When cicatrisation is complete and all irritative signs have passed off, attempts to render the scar more transparent are usually disappointing. Cicatrices clear considerably in young patients, and in many others a gratifying improvement may be noticed in the course of some months.

Some improvement in appearance may be obtained by *tattooing* dense leucomata. It is only suitable for firm scars in quiet, blind eyes, and even then is not without danger.

Tattooing with Indian ink has been replaced by impregnation with gold (brown) or platinum (black): of these the latter is preferable. The affected area is denuded of epithelium and a piece of blotting-paper of the same size, soaked in a fresh 2 % solution of platinum chloride, is applied. On removal a few drops of fresh hydrazine hydrate (2 %) solution are allowed to flow over the area, which becomes black. The eye is irrigated with saline, a drop of parolein instilled, and a pad and bandage applied. The epithelium grows over the black deposit of platinum; but at a later stage it may break down.

Lamellar keratoplasty may be advised for superficial scars (Chap. 27) whereby the defect is filled by a correspondingly shaped graft from a human (cadaver) eye. When the scar traverses the greater part or the whole of the corneal thickness, a *full-thickness (penetrating) graft* is similarly used (Chap. 27).

The treatment of a perforated ulcer. If perforation has occurred the treatment depends upon its size and situation. If it is small and in the pupillary area prolapse of iris is not to be feared. Rest in bed, the continued use of antibiotics, atropine, and a firmly applied bandage suffice: all forced expiration — blowing the nose, coughing, etc. — must be avoided. If a small perforation is over the iris, adhesion to the cornea usually occurs to form an *adherent leucoma*. This may become detached when the anterior chamber re-forms, or may be drawn out into a fine thread in which case no special treatment is required.

Hypopyon ulcer

We have already seen that every corneal ulcer is associated with some iritis owing to the diffusion into the inner eye of the toxins elaborated by the bacteria; the resultant iridocyclitis may be so severe and the outpouring of leucocytes from the vessels so great that these cells gravitate to the bottom of the anterior chamber to form a *hypopyon*. Such a hypopyon consists of polymorphonuclear leucocytes which accumulate in the lower angle of the anterior chamber and eventually become enmeshed in a network of fibrin. The hypopyon may be so small that it is scarcely visible, being hidden behind the rim of sclera which overlaps the cornea. It may reach half-way up the iris, having a flat upper surface determined by gravity, or it may fill the anterior chamber, wholly obscuring the iris. The larger hypopyons are usually less fluid owing to the fibrinous network which imprisons the leucocytes in its meshes; these are much less readily absorbed and it may be necessary or advisable to evacuate them.

It is important to remember that the hypopyon is sterile since the leucocytosis is due to toxins, not to actual invasion by bacteria which, indeed, are as incapable of passing through the intact Descemet's membrane as are leucocytes. This accounts for the ease and rapidity with which hypopyon is often absorbed: it may develop in an hour or two, rapidly disappear, and as readily reappear. Such hypopyons are fluid, always moving to the lowest part of the anterior chamber if the position of the patient's head is changed. The fact that the hypopyon is sterile has great practical importance — it is unnecessary to remove the pus, as is the rule in other parts of the body; if the ulcerative process is controlled the hypopyon will be absorbed.

The development of a hypopyon depends on two factors — the virulence of the infecting organism and the resistance of the tissues. Many pyogenic organisms (staphylococci, streptococci, gonococci, *Moraxella*) may produce this result, but by far the most dangerous are *Ps. pyocyanea* and the pneumococcus which is not infrequently present in the normal conjunctival sac and is particularly likely to be present if there is any inflammation of the lacrimal sac (dacryocystitis). The presence of dacryocystitis is therefore a constant menace to the eye. On the other hand, the agent which produces the injury may carry the infection. The commonest causes are scratches with the finger nail and rubbing of the eyes with infected hands following minute foreign bodies, especially of stone or coal in quarries or mines.

Unless the organism be very virulent some lack of resistance on the part of the tissues must be predicted. Hence hypopyon ulcers are much more common in old, debilitated or alcoholic subjects. These ulcers also occur during or after acute infectious diseases, such as measles, scarlet fever or smallpox.

Hypopyon ulcers vary in type according to the infective agent and the age of the patient. In adults the commonest cause is the pneumococcus and the ulcer formed by it is of a characteristic type, called *ulcus serpens* from its tendency to creep over the cornea in a serpiginous fashion.

The typical ulcus serpens is a greyish-white or yellowish disc near the centre of the cornea. The opacity is greater at the edges than at the centre and is particularly well marked in one special direction. A cloudy grey area, made up of fine lines, surrounds the disc, but is also more marked in the same direction. The whole of the cornea may be lustreless or hazy. There is a violent iritis, and the aqueous is cloudy, or there may be a definite hypopyon. The lids are slightly œdematous, and there is conjunctival and ciliary congestion. The subjective symptoms at the early stage are pain in the eye and brow and a variable amount of photophobia. There is remarkably little pain after the initial stage; hence treatment is often unduly delayed, with disastrous results.

The ulcer increases in size and depth. On the side of the densest infiltration, which often looks like a yellow crescent, the tissues break down and the ulcer spreads (Fig. 16.4); on the other side it may be undergoing simultaneous cicatrisation and the edges may be covered by fresh epithelium. In this manner it travels forwards. Often there is infiltration just anterior to Descemet's membrane at a spot exactly opposite the floor of the ulcer, while the intervening lamellæ are normal. This fact accounts to some extent for the great tendency to perforation, since the inflammatory process is going on as it were from both surfaces of the cornea. Meanwhile the hypopyon has become more evident, but it may vary in size from hour to hour. As might be expected, the intra-ocular pressure is often raised.

If left to pursue its natural course the hypopyon will increase and become fibrinous, the ulcer will perforate, usually forming a large opening through which the iris prolapses. The whole cornea, except the narrow rim nourished by the limbal vascular loops, may necrose, and panophthalmitis destroy the eye. In other cases an extremely dense cicatrix in which the iris is incarcerated (*adherent leucoma*) destroys sight. This may be flat or ectatic (anterior staphyloma). Sometimes the iris is bound down to the lens before perforation occurs. In such cases there are posterior synechiæ, which may be annular or total (p. 152), and the pupil may be occluded by exudates which organize into fibrous tissue.

Treatment. In all cases of hypopyon ulcer the treat-

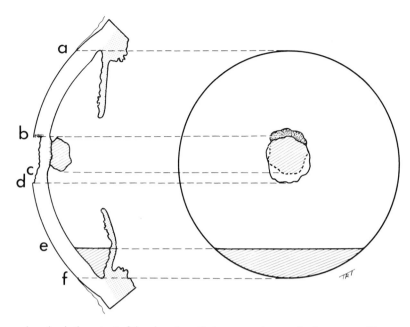

Fig. 16.4 Hypopyon ulcer. b–d, the extent of the ulcer; b, actively progressive margin; b–c, mass of leucocytes and fibrin adherent to the endothelial surface; e–f, hypopyon

ment already indicated for corneal ulcers must be initiated at once and must be energetic. After the overhanging edge and the underlying infiltrated tissue have been curetted with a small spud, intensive antibiotic treatment should be instigated at once and when a bacteriological examination has been made and the sensitivities of the organisms determined, it may have to be reassessed. One of the wide-spectrum antibiotics should be instilled every few minutes for the first hour and thereafter at half hourly intervals; if there is a suspicion of the presence of *Ps. pyocyanea*, gentamicin should be used. Surface application should be supplemented by the subconjunctival injection of this latter drug (p. 369). Atropine is instilled even if the tension is raised (*vide infra*). In many cases the progress of the ulcer and the violence of its clinical symptoms may be controlled by the topical application of steroids (p. 367).

Coincidentally with this treatment the ulcer may be cauterised (p. 133). If this is performed skilfully it does no harm and may save the eye. It is seldom necessary in children.

If these means fail, and especially if the tension of the eye is raised, further measures must be adopted. Of these the most important is *paracentesis*.

The commonest cause of failure in treatment is the development of secondary glaucoma, a complication which usually occurs in elderly people. If the tension rises the effect on the cornea is bad for it diminishes the flow of nutrient fluid and therewith its resistance. The rise of tension is not a contra-indication for the exhibition of

atropine but is an indication for diamox or intravenous mannitol.

If there is a mucocele the lacrimal sac should be drained into the nasal cavities by dacryo-cysto-rhinostomy.

Mycotic hypopyon ulcer. A rare form of ulcer is due to fungus infection such as *Aspergillus fumigatus* or *Candida albicans*. In it the slough is dry in appearance and is surrounded by a yellow line of demarcation which gradually deepens into a gutter and there may be a hypopyon. There is marked ciliary and conjunctival congestion but neovascularisation of the cornea does not occur. Treatment is by means of local nystatin and amphotericin B, but medical therapy is often not effective and the cornea has to be covered with a conjunctival flap.

Marginal ulcer (catarrhal ulcer)

Ulcers not infrequently occur near the limbus, especially in old people; they also occur in association with a chronic conjunctivitis and may be caused by the *Moraxella* or the *H. aegyptius*. They are shallow, slightly infiltrated and often multiple, and may be accompanied by neuralgic pains in the face and head. Sometimes they heal rapidly but as rapidly recur, so that the process tends to drag on indefinitely. Frequently the ulcers become vascularised and the vessels persist. More serious rare forms of deep marginal ulceration also occur in patients with polyarteritis nodosa, systemic lupus erythematosis or Wegeners' granulomatosis caused by deposition or formation of antigen-antibody complexes at the limbus and constituting a *ring ulcer*, sometimes leading to necrosis of the whole cornea.

Treatment. The infection should be treated by an appropriate antibiotic. Mild recurrent marginal ulcers may clear on painting with weak silver nitrate solution, 1%. Steroid drops or ointment may be of benefit, and in severe cases systemic steroids and cytotoxic drugs may be indicated.

Chronic serpiginous ulcer (rodent ulcer, Mooren's ulcer)

This is a rare superficial ulcer of a degenerative type, usually occurring in elderly people, starting at the corneal margin and spreading over the whole of this tissue (Fig. 16.5). Erosion is initiated by autoimmune lysis of the epithelium with consequent release of collagenolytic enzymes. It is accompanied by severe and persistent neuralgic pain and lacrimation. It commences as one or more grey infiltrates; these break down, forming small ulcers which spread and sooner or later coalesce. The ulcer undermines the epithelium and superficial lamellæ at the advancing border, forming a whitish overhanging edge which is characteristic, while the base becomes quickly vascularised. It rarely perforates, but progresses with intermissions for months until eventually a thin nebula is formed over the whole cornea and sight is much diminished. In about a quarter of the cases both corneæ are affected, but not always simultaneously. The cause is unknown.

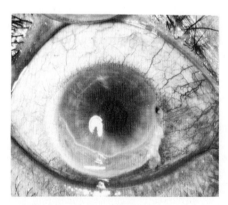

Fig. 16.5 Mooren's ulcer

Treatment is extraordinarily difficult because ischaemia is the underlying etiology. Excision of a 4–7 mm strip of adjacent conjunctiva may prove successful by eliminating conjunctival sources of collagenase and proteoglycanase. Topical antibiotics and steroids are ineffective. If perforation occurs ulcer debridement, cyanoacrylate adhesive and soft contact lenses may be tried. Lamellar keratoplasty with intravenous methotrexate therapy may halt the process.

Keratomalacia

This is common in countries such as India or in the Far East, affects badly nourished children who are lacking vitamin A, often early in the first year of life; the condition is usually bilateral. In the rare cases in which the children are old enough to exhibit this symptom the disease commences with night blindness. The conjunctiva becomes dry and shows xerotic spots (p. 128), while the cornea becomes dull and insensitive; the haze increases and yellow infiltrates form until finally the whole tissue necroses and may seem to melt away within a few hours. A characteristic feature is the absence of inflammatory reaction. The children are usually extremely ill and very frequently die. Owing to their apathetic condition they do not close the lids, so that the cornea is continually exposed.

Treatment must be directed to the general health. Vitamin A should be given in quantity as cod-liver oil, halibut-liver oil or carotene in oil, or in an emergency as an injection.

Keratitis e lagophthalmo

This occurs in eyes insufficiently covered by the lids. The epithelium of the exposed cornea becomes desiccated and the substantia propria hazy. Owing to the drying, the epithelium is cast off and the cornea falls a prey to infective organisms.

The condition is due to any cause which may produce exposure of the cornea (lagophthalmos), such as extreme proptosis as in exopthalmic ophthalmoplegia or orbital tumour, paralysis of the orbicularis, and so on. The absence of reflex blinking is an important factor, as well as defective closure of the lids during sleep, so that patients extremely ill from any disease are liable to this form of keratitis.

Treatment consists in keeping the cornea well covered. In mild cases it is sufficient to bandage the eyes at night. If possible the cause of the exposure must be removed, but in the meantime it may be necessary to sew the lids together (p. 257).

Neuroparalytic keratitis

This occurs in some cases in which the fifth nerve is paralysed, most typically as a result of the radical treatment of trigeminal neuralgia. Nor does it occur in all cases of peripheral lesions of the fifth nerve; thus, if the Gasserian ganglion is removed or the fifth nerve injected with alcohol for trigeminal neuralgia, with proper precautions only a proportion of the cases develops neuroparalytic keratitis, the tendency being decreased if there is an adequate tear film.

The characteristic feature of neuroparalytic keratitis is the desquamation of the corneal epithelium. The surface of the cornea becomes dull and the epithelium is thrown off, first at the centre, then over the whole surface except a narrow rim at the periphery; the whole of the epithelium may thus peel off intact. The substantia propria then becomes cloudy and finally yellow, breaking down into a large ulcer which is usually accompanied by a hypopyon. There is no pain, owing to the anæsthesia, but ciliary injection is marked. Relapses are the rule, the healed scar quickly breaking down again and the whole process being repeated.

Treatment. The ordinary treatment of corneal ulcer should be tried as a preliminary, special care being devoted to the protection of the eye with a shield. Improvement is often marked, but directly the shield is relinquished the ulceration starts anew in some cases. Closure of the lacrimal puncta to conserve moisture by abolishing the drainage of tears is sometimes of great value. If, however, relapses occur, it is best to suture the lids together (*tarsorrhaphy*) (p. 257) and to keep them sutured for a long period up to at least one year. In the operation of lateral tarsorrhaphy after removal or blockage of the Gasserian ganglion, no anæsthetic is necessary since sensation is lost in the conjunctiva and lids. The beneficial effect of this procedure is very striking, for it will invariably succeed in stopping the process.

Non-suppurative superficial keratitis

Superficial nonpurulent keratitis includes a number of conditions of varied etiology. Many of them are viral infections while others such as phlyctenular and rosacea keratitis have a constitutional origin.

Infective (non-suppurative) superficial keratitis. Superficial keratitis may result from a number of infections, most of them of the viral type. Of these the most common are herpes zoster, the adenoviruses and the Chlamydia of trachoma and inclusion conjunctivitis: the last two conditions have already been discussed. More rarely the viruses associated with measles, vaccinia, infectious mononucleosis and mumps, as well as the presumptive viruses responsible for Behçet's syndrome and Reiter's syndrome, may affect the cornea, while a secondary keratitis may follow a lid infection with the viruses of molluscum contagiosum and warts (varrucae). These viral infections give rise to several types of clinical picture, but it is to be remembered that the same appearances may be associated with infection by several types of virus, while one virus may give rise to more than one type of lesion.

Punctate epithelial erosions (multiple superficial erosions) are the most common manifestation of viral infections. In this condition the cornea shows multiple minute defects in the epithelium which stain with fluorescein, frequently associated with an acute onset combined with conjunctivitis; there is considerable pain, photophobia and lacrimation. As a rule the infection is characterised by recurrences when fresh erosions appear in successive crops after the initial lesions have quietened or the orig-

inal erosions have healed; if these recurrences persist for a considerable time, superficial vessels may invade the cornea. A completely non-specific lesion of this type, for example, may be caused by the toxin of the staphylococcus, the organism also giving rise to a blepharitis or conjunctivitis. Some chemical irritants produce the same picture. Associated with a general febrile disturbance this is a well established manifestation of an infection by one or other of the adenoviruses and, as we have seen, constitutes the characteristic picture of early trachomatous keratitis.

Punctate epithelial keratitis (superficial punctate keratitis) is usually a viral infection of both eyes which runs a course of months or sometimes years. It attacks the deeper layers of the corneal epithelium and is sometimes associated with opacities extending into Bowman's membrane and the superficial layers of the stroma (*punctate subepithelial keratitis*). The epithelial opacities appear as superficial slightly raised grey dots scattered over the central area of the cornea which do not stain readily with fluorescein but turn a deep red with rose bengal. A combination of epithelial and subepithelial punctate lesions is also a common occurrence in viral infections (*epidemic keratoconjunctivitis, pharyngoconjunctival fever, herpes, vaccinia* and others (*q.v.*)), but may occur without known cause (*Thygeson's superficial punctate keratitis*).

Treatment of most of these conditions is symptomatic. Topical steroids have a marked suppressive effect.

Herpes (simplex)

The virus of herpes has a widespread distribution; it can be grown in tissue-culture and the elementary bodies can be found by suitable staining methods in the vesicular fluid. The infection is transferable to the corneae of rabbits in which animals a herpetic encephalitis may

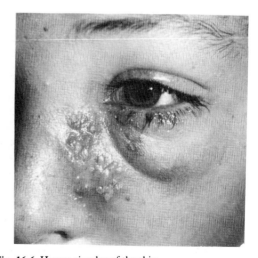

Fig. 16.6 Herpes simplex of the skin

subsequently develop. There is some evidence that the virus has antigenic properties but in practice immunity does not develop after an attack; indeed, a person once infected frequently becomes a carrier, and periodic attacks tend to break out on the lips, nose and genitals as well as on the cornea, the recurrences taking place particularly in association with such intercurrent diseases as a febrile cold, pneumonia or a malarial relapse or exposure to sunlight.

In a primary lesion (usually in children) herpes may manifest itself as a severe follicular kerato-conjunctivitis (*q.v.*); but in the usual recurrent forms the conjunctiva is spared apart from the occurrence of a nondescript conjunctivitis. The cornea essentially is involved, the initial lesion being a *superficial punctate keratitis*. In this condition numerous whitish plaques of epithelial cells appear on the cornea; they are minute, less than the size of a pin's head, and are often arranged in rows or groups. They quickly desquamate, forming erosions which may heal rapidly, leaving no opacity but are accompanied by great irritation, lacrimation, and blepharospasm. Usually, however, fresh crops appear, and the condition may prove very obstinate. After the plaques have desquamated, leaving minute shallow clear facets, the shape of the lesions and the total absence of vascularisation are distinguishing features as well as their grouping, the crenated edges where several have coalesced, and the persisting filamentary shreds of diseased epithelium. In all cases the cornea is relatively insensitive.

In severe forms *dendritic ulcers* develop. The infiltrates, spreading in all directions, coalesce with each other and form a large shallow ulcer with crenated edges. More often grey striæ extend in one or more directions, increase in length, and send out lateral branches which are generally knobbed at the ends so that a dendritic figure, not unlike a liverwort, is formed which resembles no other condition and is pathognomonic (Fig. 16.7). The surface over the infiltrates breaks down and an extremely irritating and chronic type of ulcer is produced, persisting with exacerbations for weeks or months, sending out fresh branches but never extending in depth. Generally only one or two of the infiltrates stain with fluorescein at any given time, but fresh spots are continually being formed and the disease not infrequently recurs; alternatively, a large confluent ulcer may be formed (Fig. 16.7). Meantime the stroma may be implicated and a *disciform keratitis* (*q.v.*), sometimes of considerable extent, may develop (an Arthus reaction). An iritis is invariably associated with a severe herpetic keratitis; sometimes it is of considerable severity and occasionally a hypopyon occurs. The herpetic virus has been isolated from the aqueous in such cases. Immunological tests in diagnosis are limited to immunofluorescence of epithelial scrapings or tissue biopsies.

Treatment. Specific treatment by the topical administration of antiviral substances is encouraging in early cases (p. 108).

Eighty-five per cent of initial dendritic ulcers treated with IDU are cured within 2 weeks. IDU is given along with corticosteroids to suppress the host response. It is not sufficiently active as an antiviral agent to prevent destructive stromal disease in some cases.

Ara-A (Adenine Arabinoside) has similar effects although less toxic. It has little activity against stromal disease and it can only be given in ointment form.

Trifluorothymidine (F_3T) is given in drop form five times a day and is an effective antiviral agent. Of epithelial ulcers 95% are cured within 2 weeks. F_3T is more

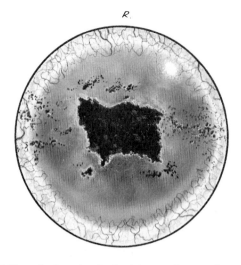
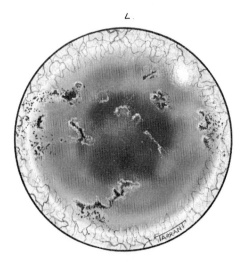

Fig. 16.7 Herpetic ulceration: in the right eye a large confluent ulcer with outlying areas of staining; in the left eye, multiple dendritic ulcers. (By courtesy of Barrie Jones.)

effective than other available drugs in the prevention of complications caused by corticosteroids and the problem of superficial herpes is almost solved. The chemotherapy of stromal disease and iritis remains a problem and is best treated with Acycloguanosine given topically in association with Ara-A. This combination has a significant effect on stromal disease.

Zoster

(Herpes) Zoster is caused by a virus identical with that causing chicken-pox (Varicella–Zoster virus); the two diseases may be associated in epidemics and it may be that after an infection with chicken-pox in youth the virus lies dormant to appear later, particularly in elderly people with depressed cellular immunity causing the clinical picture of zoster. In zoster opthalmicus the chief focus of infection is the Gasserian ganglion whence the virus travels down one or more of the branches of the ophthalmic division of the fifth nerve, so that its area of distribution is marked out by rows of vesicles or the scars left by them, exactly as in zoster in other parts of the body (Fig. 16.8). The supra-orbital, supra- and infratrochlear branches are nearly always involved; frequently the nasal branch; only rarely the infra-orbital branch. It is very rarely bilateral. There may be fever and malaise at the onset, and the eruption is preceded by severe neuralgic pains along the course of the nerves which are so characteristic of zoster that they should arouse suspicion of the nature of the disease before the vesicles appear. The pain sometimes ceases after the outbreak of the eruption, but it may continue for months or even years. The skin of the lids and other areas affected become red and œdematous, so that the

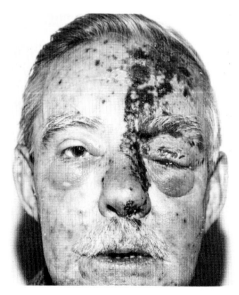

Fig. 16.8 Left-sided zoster affecting the ophthalmic division of the Vth nerve with the naso-ciliary branch

disease may be mistaken for erysipelas, but the characteristic distribution and especially the strict limitation to one side of the middle line of the head should obviate this error. The vesicles often suppurate, bleed and cause small, permanent, pitted scars. The active eruptive stage lasts about three weeks and is followed by some anæsthesia of the skin. Ocular complications arise during the subsidence of the eruption, but may be overlooked during the acute stage owing to the difficulty in examining the eye; they are generally associated with involvement of the naso-ciliary branch of the trigeminal (Plate 7, Fig. B).

With the slit-lamp, numerous rounded spots composed of minute white dots are seen in the epithelium, which soon involve the stroma to form a coarse subepithelial punctate keratitis. Sometimes the infiltration spreads deeply and becomes diffuse in the stroma, associated with iridocyclitis (q.v.). The cornea is usually insensitive. This is tested by touching it with a wisp of cotton-wool, and comparing the reaction with that in the opposite eye; the slightest touch is followed by reflex closure of the lids if the cornea is sensitive. Similar nodules leaving grey scarred areas may appear on the sclera and patches of atrophy may develop on the iris. The intra-ocular pressure is sometimes diminished in the early stage, but subsequently a secondary glaucoma is not unusual. The ocular lesions and the corneal anæsthesia are very obdurate and often persist long after the disease has otherwise passed away. In some cases there is associated paralysis of motor cranial nerves, especially the third, sixth and seventh, which usually passes off within six weeks. Facial palsy adds seriously to the danger to the eye owing to exposure of the cornea.

Treatment. Pain during the first 2 weeks of an attack of herpes zoster is usually severe and is treated with Distalgesic. If this proves ineffective then Fortral or DF 118 may be tried or in very severe cases Pethidine may be necessary.

The accompanying depression in the acute phase should be relieved by the use of Amitriptyline.

Topical Neocortef is required in the treatment of the skin and lids as a spray. In the eye itself an antibiotic-steroid combination of Predsol-N is useful in the acute stage of the disease when lid vesicles are discharging and forming crusts. For chronically scarred lids Chloramphenicol ointment is useful to keep down secondary infection by staphylococci.

When the herpetic infection gives rise to scleritis, scleral keratitis or iritis, Dexamethasone alcohol 0.1% drops four-hourly are used with Betnesol ointment at night. This tends to cut down the ischaemic and fibrotic scarring which may develop. Systemic steroids are recommended in cases of progressive proptosis with total third nerve palsy and at the onset of optic neuritis. These conditions are probably due to occlusive vasculitis. The initial dose is 60 mg. per day and is rapidly reduced to a maintenance dose. Systemic Oxyphenbuta- zone (Tanderil) is useful in severe cases of scleritis which have not responded to steroids.

Artificial tears are required following an attack of herpes zoster if there is any dryness of the eyes or rapid formation of dry spots on the cornea.

Neuroparalytic ulcers of herpes zoster are best treated by tarsorrhaphy of the lateral half of the lids.

Neglected disciform keratitis and scleral keratitis often give rise to dense scarring and lipoid deposits in the central corneal. Such patients may require perforat- ing corneal grafting if the cornea is not too vascularised.

Vaccinia

This affects the eye, usually as an accidental inoculation from a recently vaccinated child. The lids are usually affected (p. 309) but if the conjunctiva and cornea are involved an alarming clinical picture results, with swell- ing of the lids so intense that examination may be dif- ficult. The pre- and post-auricular nodes are always involved. In the conjunctiva the typical lesion is exten- sive ulceration; in the cornea a punctate subepithelial keratitis which may progress to map-like ulceration and stromal abscesses. A disciform keratitis may develop at a later date. *Treatment* is by gamma-globulin from a recently vaccinated person used topically (250 mg in 25 ml distilled water every half-hour) and by intra- muscular injections. IDU (p. 108) has been successfully employed.

Constitutional affections

Phlyctenular keratitis. It has already been pointed out that phlyctens are commonly found at the limbus; they may also occur within the corneal margin. The fact must be emphasised that the disease is essentially conjunctival, and when the cornea is affected it is the conjunctival element of the cornea — the epithelium and the super- ficial layers underlying it — which suffers. As has already been noted it is an allergic reaction to an en- dogenous allergen, notably tuberculo-protein (p. 125).

Corneal phlyctens are localised infiltrations of exactly the same nature as conjunctival phlyctens but cause much pain and reflex blepharospasm (photophobia). They may become absorbed without destruction of the superficial layers of the stroma, in which case they cause no permanent opacity. The epithelium, however, is readily destroyed and the denuded surface easily be- comes infected, usually by staphylococci (p. 115); in this manner a small superficial ulcer is formed. The corneal phlycten is a grey nodule, slightly raised above the sur- face and if the epithelium breaks down, a yellowish ulcer is formed.

Treatment of phlyctenular keratitis is the same as that of phlyctenular conjunctivitis (*q.v.*) until ulceration has occurred when atropine combined with corticosteroids should be intensively administered as drops or oint- ment.

Acne rosacea. This is generally seen in elderly women where, keratitis associated with much irritability and lacrimation may occur. In addition to slight muco- purulent conjunctivitis, yellowish white infiltrates and small ulcers appear in the cornea which always becomes heavily vascularised. They are very intractable and fre- quently recur. In severe cases there is also iritis (Fig. 16.9).

Local treatment is disappointing but should be simi- lar to that for phlyctenular keratitis; the greatest relief usually follows the instillation of corticosteroids as drops or ointment. The essential treatment, however, is that of the skin condition. A course of Tetracyline systemically is often helpful. Patients receive 250 mg orally four times daily for 3 weeks of each month. The dosage is then reduced to three times daily for three weeks and stopped for a week. The dosage is then slowly reduced each month and the drug is stopped if improvement is maintained. For an advancing infiltrate into the cornea due to rosacea, beta radiation may be effective with a dose of 1500 rep. given three times at weekly intervals with the 90 S.R. applicator.

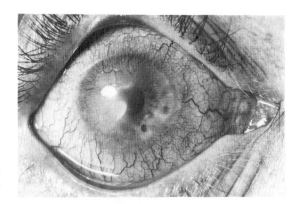

Fig. 16.9 Rosacea keratitis

Superior limbic keratoconjunctivitis. This is character- ised by inflammation of the superior tarsal and bulbar conjunctiva and oedema of the corneoscleral limbal con- junctiva; corneal filaments are frequently present. Fine punctate fluorescein and rose bengal staining of the superior cornea are commonly found. The condition is usually bilateral, occurs frequently in females and fol- lows a chronic course with remissions and exacerba- tions. The prognosis is excellent in that eventual resolution usually occurs.

There is an association with thyroid disease. Treatment is unsatisfactory but removal of a block of conjunctiva extending from the 10.30 to the 1.30 position at the corneo-scleral limbus and 3–4 mm. posteriorly may be helpful. The conjunctival tissue shows varying degrees of keratinisation with areas of acanthosis.

Photophthalmia. Caused by ultra-violet rays, especially from 311 to 290 mμ, it is characterised by extreme burning pain, lacrimation, photophobia, blepharospasm, and swelling of the palpebral conjunctiva and retrotarsal folds. It is due to desquamation of the epithelium to form multiple erosions. There is a latent period of 4 or 5 h between the exposure and the onset of symptoms. The condition is generally caused by the bright flash of a short circuit or exposure to a naked arc light, as in industrial welding or cinema studios. It is rarely due to exposure to enclosed arc lights since the glass globe absorbs the most deleterious rays. In *snow blindness* the cause and symptoms are similar, for the ultra-violet rays are reflected from snow surfaces.

Prophylaxis consists in the wearing of dark glasses when such exposure is to be anticipated, particularly made of such materials as Crookes's glass which cuts off practically all the infra-red and ultra-violet rays. The *treatment* for both types of photophthalmia is by cold compresses and astringent lotions. Comfort will be obtained by bandaging both eyes for twenty-four hours until the epithelium has regenerated. Cocaine, which hinders epithelial healing, should be avoided, but atropine brings some relief.

Deep forms of keratitis

The deep forms of keratitis comprise that due to congenital syphilis, tuberculosis or virus infections (disciform keratitis) as well as lesions of indefinite origin or due to the spread of scleral inflammations (sclerosing keratitis, p. 148).

Interstitial keratitis (parenchymatous keratitis)
This is an inflammation affecting chiefly the stroma of the cornea. It is of infective or more often of allergic origin. Interstitial keratitis and deafness (Cogan's Syndrome) is a rare disease affecting young adults. The keratitis is associated with vertigo, tinnitus and deafness.

Interstitial keratitis due to inherited syphilis affects most commonly children between the ages of five and 15. Delayed interstitial keratitis occasionally occurs in patients over thirty and is more liable to be unilateral but is often severe; the inflammation usually follows an injury to the eye, such as a blow or an operation, the injury acting as an exciting cause in a subject naturally prone to the disease, usually a congenital syphilitic. After slight irritative symptoms with some ciliary congestion, one or more hazy patches appear in deep layers of the cornea near the margin or towards the centre. If they start near the margin they migrate towards the centre; if at the

centre, others appear and fuse, until finally the whole cornea looks lustreless and dull. In two to four weeks the whole cornea is hazy with a steamy surface, giving a general appearance resembling ground glass in which denser spots can always be seen. As a rule the iris can be seen dimly, but in the severest cases the whole cornea becomes opaque, so that this tissue is hidden (Fig. 16.10).

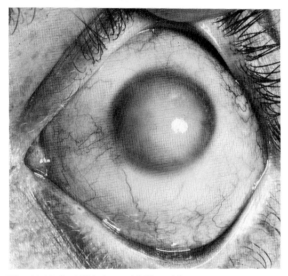

Fig. 16.10 Syphilitic interstitial keratitis

Meanwhile vascularisation has occurred. It is of the deep type (Fig. 10.7, p. 74), consisting of radial bundles of brush-like vessels, and since they are covered by a layer of hazy cornea, their bright scarlet is toned down to a dull reddish pink ('salmon patches') wherein separate vessels can be seen only with difficulty. The opacity extends a little beyond the vessels, which seem to push the opacity in front of them and at the height of the condition the vessels run in radial bundles almost, but seldom quite, to the centre of the cornea. There is often a moderate degree of superficial vascularisation, greater in some cases than in others, but never extending far over the cornea, and at the limbus the conjunctiva may be heaped up like an epaulette. In the absence of treatment this florid stage usually lasts for two to four months when subjective symptoms are very marked — pain, intense photophobia, lacrimation and blepharospasm are so severe that to open the eyes may be difficult or impossible. Vision may be reduced to the appreciation of hand-movements.

After the disease has reached its height the cornea clears slowly from the margin towards the centre, which may long remain hazy, but finally improves except in the worst cases. As the cloudiness disappears the vessels become obliterated, but although they cease to carry blood they remain permanently as fine opaque lines the characteristic radial course of which indicates the previous occurrence of the disease.

Since the infiltration of the cornea is almost entirely limited to the deeper layers lying immediately anterior to Descemet's membrane the corneal surface rarely becomes ulcerated. It is frequently stippled, steamy, and slightly uneven, and this condition may persist. In the worst cases the cornea may be enormously thickened and gelatinous in appearance giving the impression that it is ectatic and that the eye is in a hopeless condition, but it usually improves with some useful vision.

In interstitial keratitis the uveal tract is always profoundly affected and a considerable degree of iritis is invariably present. Sometimes there is severe cyclitis, as shown by the presence of keratic precipitates on the back of the cornea and not infrequently a choroiditis, particularly around the periphery. Indeed, the disease is fundamentally a uveitis, and the keratitis, which clinically masks the uveitis, is secondary. It is important to realize the true pathology, since treatment must be directed to avoiding the deleterious results of iridocyclitis rather than those of keratitis.

Interstitial keratitis is almost invariably bilateral, although an interval of three or more weeks usually intervenes before the onset in the second eye; rarely the interval is several months. The acute stage lasts at least six weeks and may extend to several months. The clearing of the cornea takes many weeks or months, but little improvement can be expected after eighteen months.

Diagnosis A diagnosis depends on other evidences of congenital syphilis and positive serological reactions to this disease. Congenital syphilis is an infectious disease acquired in utero. There is systemic involvement without the occurrence of a primary lesion. Symptoms occur shortly after birth and consist of a rhinitis followed by a maculo-papular eruption. The child is weedy and makes poor headway. The characteristic signs of late congenital syphilis are prominence of the frontal eminences, flatness of the bridge of the nose, Hutchinson's teeth (notching of the two upper central incisors in the permanent dentition), rhagades at the angles of the mouth, shotty cervical nodes and periosteal nodules particularly on the tibiæ.

Treatment. It is usual to order antisyphilitic remedies, but it is doubtful if they have any influence over the course of the keratitis, partly because the cornea is non-vascular and partly because the reaction is probably largely allergic. It is possible however, that intensive systemic treatment with penicillin may shorten the course of the disease.

Local treatment consists primarily in guarding against the evil effect of the uveitis which is an invariable accompaniment of the disease. Atropine is ordered as a routine measure, with the double purpose of keeping the ciliary body and iris at rest and preventing the formation of posterior synechiæ. Radiant heat should be used frequently in the acute stage. The most effective measure, however, is the topical administration of corticosteroids by drops or ointment (p. 109). With intensive treatment the response to this hormone may be dramatic in the early stages and in a few days the symptoms subside, the injection disappears and the eye becomes white. If the treatment is started at a very early stage the attack may thus be aborted, but if it is delayed until necrosis of the stroma has occurred, permanent opacities remain. Particularly in cases wherein the treatment has been instituted at an early stage, however, relapses are common as soon as the treatment is stopped; these should therefore be anticipated and, indeed, it is wise in all cases to continue maintenance doses of steroids (as drops twice a day or as ointment at night) for at least a year until the natural period of the disease has elapsed.

In cases wherein pain and blepharospasm are severe, relief for a week or so may be obtained by the retro-ocular injection of 1.5 ml of procaine (4%) into the region of the ciliary ganglion, followed 7 min later by 1 ml of alcohol (40 %). The pain and blepharospasm are relieved, vascular congestion much reduced, and the child is able to tolerate light.

In the later stages the best results are obtained by corneal grafting, which must be of the penetrating type. In this disease the prognosis for grafting is generally good.

Keratitis disciformis

This is not uncommon: it occurs generally in adults and is unilateral. It is probably, in most cases, associated with a virus infection and has long been known to result from vaccinia affecting the lid margins, or from herpes, and not infrequently develops from a superficial punctate keratitis. The condition is probably not due to a direct infection of the corneal stroma by the virus from the epithelium but seems to be the expression of a tissue-response, sometimes involving necrosis, due to the reaction between antigens liberated by the virus in the epithelium and antibodies produced in the stroma or carried thither by the bloodstream. The pathology may thus be analogous to that of syphilitic interstitial keratitis. The importance of early destruction of the infected epithelium in herpetic cases is thus obvious.

The disease is characterised by the gradual appearance of a central grey disc lying in the middle layers of the stroma usually with a denser central opacity. The slit-lamp shows thickening of the cornea and often folds of Descemet's membrane and an immune ring of the Wesseley type. It is accompanied by moderate irritation which, however, persists for weeks or many months, leaving a permanent opacity. The cornea may become anæsthetic but ulceration does not occur. Owing to the central situation vision is considerably impaired. It is little amenable to treatment, but the symptoms and probably the depth of the permanent opacity may be ameliorated by the local administration of corticosteroids. In the worst cases, particularly when the cornea is anæsthetic, tarsorrhaphy may be indicated (*q.v.*).

DEGENERATIVE CHANGES IN THE CORNEA

A variety of degenerative conditions occurs in the cornea, many of which are of serious clinical import. These are conveniently divided into three categories: primary degenerations, secondary degenerations depending on long-standing changes in the eye itself, and infiltrations associated with metabolic disturbances.

Arcus senilis

This is a lipoid infiltration of the cornea met with in old people. It commences as a crescentic grey line concentric with the upper and lower margins of the cornea, the extremities of which finally meet so that an opaque line, thicker above and below, is formed completely round the cornea. It is characterised by being separated from the margin by a narrow line of comparatively clear cornea, being sharply defined on the peripheral side, fading off on the central. It is never more than about 1 mm broad and is of no importance either from the point of view of vision or of the vitality of the cornea (Fig. 16.11) and is unrelated to secondary forms of hypercholesterolaemia.

Arcus juvenilis

This is exactly similar to arcus senilis but is a rare con-

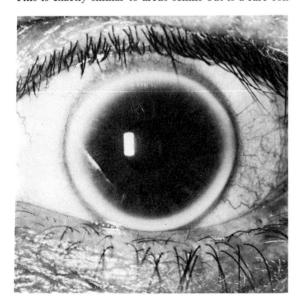

Fig. 16.11 Arcus senilis

dition. If it appears under the age of 40 a serum lipid profile is indicated to eliminate a heritable anomaly with a serious prognosis for life. The characteristic diagnostic feature of both these opacities is the presence of a line of clear cornea between them and the limbus. This is occasionally found in old sclerosing keratitis, but in this case the opacity is usually localised to one part of the cornea and extends farther towards the centre.

Hereditary corneal dystrophies

Occur mainly in males about puberty as bilateral affections of obscure origin involving the central area of the cornea; they rarely affect the corneal margin. The lesions are characterised by the development of discrete areas of opacification mainly in the superficial layers of the stroma due essentially to hyaline deposits between the corneal lamellæ. They tend to increase in number and density until Bowman's membrane becomes eroded and the epithelium desquamates. Relatively symptomless and without inflammatory reaction, they progress slowly until the vision becomes seriously impaired usually over the age of 40. When this occurs treatment is best by keratoplasty.

Four main forms have been differentiated. In the *nodular corneal dystrophy of Groenouw*, which has a dominant heredity, the opacities assume a granular form and subsequently coalesce into various irregular shapes. A *lattice form*, also with a dominant heredity, is characterised by bifurcating criss-cross lines associated with punctate opacities. It is a localised form of amyloidosis. A *macular form* has a recessive heredity and in it the visual acuity tends to be affected at an early age.

Reis-Bucklers' corneal dystrophy (Plate 6, Fig. B)

This dystrophy is an autosomal dominant condition and arises in the region of Bowman's membrane, which eventually is extensively replaced by a cellular connective tissue containing collagen as well as a fibrillar or granular material. The epithelium over this connective tissue shows derangement of the cell layers, œdema and degeneration. The cornea shows irregular dense grey sub-epithelial opacities arranged in a fish net pattern. The opacities lie at the level of Bowman's membrane and are usually more dense in the central portion. The overlying epithelium is irregular and varies in thickness. The material deposited beneath the epithelium may be removed by blunt dissection and this can be repeated if necessary should the condition recur.

Endothelial corneal dystrophies (Plate 6, Fig. A)

Occur rarely, the most common of which is the *endothelial dystrophy of Fuchs*. This is seen in elderly people, particularly females, commencing with fine changes in the endothelium distinguishable by the slit-lamp; these are followed by the formation of hyaline nodules on Descemet's membrane and the eventual atrophy of the underlying endothelial cells (*cornea guttata*). These deep changes are followed by a diffuse dystrophy of the epithelium associated with oedema and the formation of vesicles and a grey opacification as well as punctate opacities in the stroma. Characteristically patients complain of seeing halos in the morning which disappear later in the day as the massaging effect of reflex blinking leads to subsidence of corneal epithelial oedema. Ultimately the entire cornea turns opaque and insensitive. Fortunately the course of the disease is slow so that blindness is usually forestalled by death. Treatment is difficult; corneal grafting is sometimes effective.

Senile marginal degeneration

This is also a rarity occurring in one or both eyes of old people. Bowman's membrane and the stroma suffer fibrillar degeneration and are eventually replaced by vascularised granular tissue. In the process a gutter forms slowly in the periphery of the cornea, starting in the situation of an arcus senilis and eventually becomes ectatic. Treatment is disappointing but reinforcement by a conjunctival flap or a lamellar keratoplasty may be tried.

Band-shaped keratopathy

This is a common condition in old, blind, shrunken eyes and in Still's disease of children. Occasionally it is associated with hyperparathyroidism, Vit. D poisoning or sarcoidosis. It lies in the interpalpebral area, commencing at the inner and outer sides and progressing until it forms a continuous band across the cornea interspersed with round holes in the band itself. Close to the limbus, however, the cornea is generally relatively clear, as in so many degenerative conditions — probably owing to the better nutrition close to the blood-vessels. The condition is due to hyaline infiltration of the superficial parts of the stroma, followed by the deposition of calcareous salts.

It is rarely found, usually bilaterally, in otherwise healthy eyes as a horizontally oval area in the palpebral fissure.

Treatment. In the rare form last mentioned, improvement of vision may be obtained by scraping off the opacity, which is usually calcareous and quite superficial, or dissolving it with the sodium salt of ethylenediamine tetra-acetic acid (p. 369).

Other degenerative changes

These are frequently met with in old leucomata or anterior staphylomata consisting of hyaline infiltration and calcification. Such scars are liable to undergo a serious form of ulceration.

A distinctive form is known as *Salzmann's nodular dystrophy*, a degenerative condition characterised by bluish-white nodules appearing in the superficial layers of the stroma and Bowman's membrane, occurring in persons who have suffered previous corneal disease. The condition tends to be slowly progressive and may be treated by lamellar keratoplasty.

Infiltrations of the cornea

These are rare. A primary *lipid infiltration of obscure origin may occur;* it is a characteristic of gargoylism. Equally rare are primary *calcareous degeneration* and *dystrophia urica* wherein urate crystals form yellow opacities in the cornea. Similarly, deposits of *cystine* may be associated with a generalised cystinosis, renal dwarfism and osteoporosis (*Fanconi's syndrome*).

ECTATIC CONDITIONS

It has already been stated that ectatic conditions of the cornea may result from inflammation, as in keratectasia (p. 131) and anterior staphyloma (p. 132). Two forms of ectasia of non-inflammatory origin are known — keratoconus and keratoglobus.

Keratoconus (Conical cornea)

This is frequently due to a congenital weakness of the cornea, though often it only manifests itself after puberty. The cornea is thin near the centre and progressively bulges forwards, the apex of the cone being always slightly below the centre of the cornea. The cornea is at first transparent, and vision is impaired through the protrusion and alteration in curvature. If the condition is marked the conical shape is easily recognised in profile, particularly by the acute bulge given to the lower lid when the patient looks down. In the less advanced cases distortion of the corneal reflex over the centre is the chief guide, a change best seen with Placido's disc or keratoscope (Fig. 16.12; p. 72) or when the cornea is examined with the ophthalmometer. With the ophthalmoscope mirror at a distance of 1 metre a ring of shadow concentric with the margin is seen in the red reflex, altering its position on moving the mirror. It is due to a zone through which few rays pass into the observer's eye owing to the fact that the emergent rays on the central side are convergent whilst those on the peripheral side are divergent.

The patient becomes myopic, but the error of refraction cannot be satisfactorily corrected with ordinary glasses owing to the parabolic nature of the curvature. The condition is almost invariably bilateral, though frequently more advanced on one side than the other. It may be slight and very slowly progressive, or the reverse. In the later stages the apex shows fine more or less parallel striæ, anastomosing at acute angles, best seen with the slitlamp, and also discrete opacities which become confluent. A brownish ring, probably due to

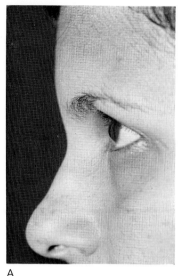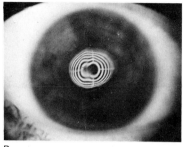

A   B

Fig. 16.12 A Keratoconus B Keratoscopic appearance of the corneal reflex in an advanced case of keratoconus

hæmosiderin, may form in the epithelium encircling the cone (Fleischer's ring). Sometimes ruptures develop in Descemet's membrane in which case the stroma becomes suddenly œdematous and opaque.

Treatment. In the early stage vision may be improved with spectacles, but contact lenses (p. 57) are more beneficial; in this condition they are usually well borne, they eliminate the irregular corneal curvature, and are said to have a supporting effect. If, however, the disease progresses and the cone becomes hydrated, the most satisfactory treatment is the removal of a large whole-thickness disc from the central area of the cornea and its replacement by a corneal graft. Corneal transplants are particularly successful in this condition and should be considered in progressive cases and whenever visual loss has become considerable.

Keratoglobus

This is a hemispherical protrusion of the whole cornea, occurring bilaterally as a congenital anomaly: it is familial and hereditary. It differs from buphthalmos (*q.v*) in that the intra-ocular pressure is normal, the cornea clear, the angle of the anterior chamber normal, and there is no cupping of the optic disc.

SYMPTOMATIC CONDITIONS

There are many pathological conditions of the cornea which are merely evidence of disease in other parts of the eye or of extension of disease. Some are often described as true diseases of the cornea, notably as forms of 'keratitis'; this involves a wrong principle and a misuse of terms which can only lead to confusion. Since it is of great importance to distinguish these conditions from primary affections of the cornea from the points of view of both diagnosis and treatment, it will be well to review the more common here.

Corneal oedema

This is a relatively common condition. It manifests itself first in the epithelium which becomes steamy, an appearance due to the accumulation of fluid between the cells, especially the basal cells. At the same time the accumulation of fluid between the lamellae and around the nerve-fibres of the stroma produces a haziness throughout the entire cornea due to alterations in the refractive condition. If the œdema lasts for a long period the epithelium tends to be raised into large vesicles or bullae (*vesicular or bullous keratopathy*) (Fig. 16.13) This is a peculiarly intractable condition which frequently gives rise to intensely irritating symptoms as the bullæ periodically burst.

Such a corneal oedema may occur in many conditions of an inflammatory or degenerative type of long standing. It is common in long-standing glaucoma when the tension is high; it also tends to occur whenever the endothelium has suffered damage so that the aqueous can percolate through the stroma. After trauma or operation such an œdema is characteristic of endothelial damage, particularly when strands of vitreous remain adherent to the posterior surface of the cornea. Treatment is difficult unless the primary cause of the oedema can be eliminated. Some comfort may be obtained by the application of a bandage contact lens and the frequent instillation of a concentrated saline solution or an ointment containing 15% sodium chloride. An alternative which is frequently effective is to strip off the entire epithelium and to replace it by a thin flap of the con-

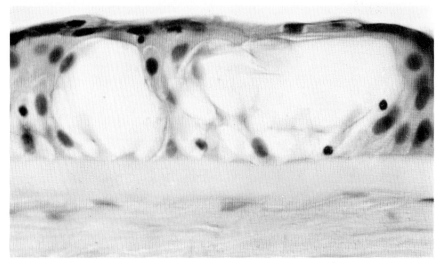

Fig. 16.13 Corneal oedema: vesicle formation

junctiva. Visual improvement depends on full-thickness keratoplasty.

Filamentary keratopathy. Closely allied to bullous keratopathy is the formation of epithelial threads which adhere to the cornea by one end while the other, which is often club-shaped, moves about freely. Such filaments occur in degenerative conditions or in long-standing corneal oedema; they may be seen in cases of viral keratitis, particularly of the herpetic type, in the collagenous diseases and in keratitis sicca (p. 324).

Keratic precipitates

Initially badly termed 'keratitis punctata' or 'k.p.', these are depositions of leucocytes and other cells on the back of the cornea in cyclitis and iridocyclitis and occasionally in choroiditis. The greatest care must be taken not to overlook them, since they may be almost the only objective sign of serious disease. They may be on the back of a clear cornea or the deeper layers may be infiltrated as a result of the intra-ocular inflammation. Their appearance and nature will be described in discussing their cause (pp. 155).

Opacities of the cornea

These are usually secondary to inflammation but some others types may occur.

Congenital opacities of various kinds are sometimes encountered as developmental anomalies; others are due to injury received at birth. The latter are often temporary and diffuse due to oedema caused by ruptures of Descemet's membrane.

Striate opacity occurs in various forms. The commonest form is that seen after operations upon the globe in which a peripheral corneal section has been made, as in cataract extraction. Here, delicate grey lines run from the wound and may pass completely across the cornea;

they disappear spontaneously as the wound heals and are due to slight folding of the cornea whereby Descemet's membrane and the adjacent lamellae become wrinkled. Radial striae are seen around wounds or ulcers; they are partly referable to the same cause, partly to distension of the interlamellar spaces by oedema. The fine hatching which is seen around ulcers and sometimes after tight bandaging is to be referred to similar causes.

White ring opacities (Coats). Occasionally rings or oval formations composed of very dense white spots, about 0.5 mm in diameter, occur beneath Bowman's membrane. The cause is disputed but they frequently follow minor trauma such as results from the impaction of foreign bodies; they do not interfere with vision.

Pigmentation of the cornea

May occur from the prolonged topical use of silver nitrate (*argyrosis*, p. 128). As in the conjunctiva it is due to the permanent impregnation of the elastic fibres and particularly Descemet's membrane with metallic silver.

A similar deposit of copper forms a pigmented ring of a grey-green or golden-brown colour round the periphery of the cornea in the region of Descemet's membrane and the deeper layers of the stroma when a copper foreign body is retained within the eye (*chalcosis* (p. 250)) and in hepato-lenticular degeneration (Wilson's disease) (the *Kayser-Fleischer ring*).

Blood in the cornea is rare. It may occur as a bright red spot or streak superficially at the margin, or as a greenish or rusty stain throughout the whole tissue (blood staining). In the latter case it is derived from blood in the anterior chamber, usually associated with high tension and endothelial damage — a relatively infrequent complication following contusions (p. 244).

Tumours of the cornea have been considered with those of the conjunctiva.

17

Diseases of the sclera

The avascularity of the sclera and the lack of reaction of its dense fibrous tissues to insult whether traumatic or infective, make diseases of this tissue relatively rare; for the same reason, when they do occur they tend to be chronic and sluggish.

INFLAMMATION OF THE SCLERA

Two forms of inflammation of the sclera are described: superficial or episcleritis, and deep or scleritis. They might equally well be considered mild and severe forms of the same disease, but the distinction is convenient since they differ in their evolution.

Episcleritis
This is a benign inflammatory affection of the deep subconjunctival connective tissues, including the superficial scleral lamellae and frequently affecting both eyes. A circumscribed nodule of dense leucocytic infiltration, which may be as large as a lentil, appears usually two or three millimetres from the limbus (Fig. 17.1). It is hard,

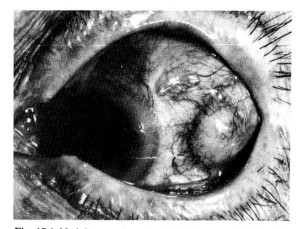

Fig. 17.1 Nodular anterior scleritis. A discrete scleral nodule displacement of deep vessels over the nodule and surrounding inflammation overlying unaffected sclera are characteristic. (By courtesy of P. Watson)

immovable and tender, the conjunctiva moving freely over it, and is traversed by the deeper episcleral vessels so that it looks purple, not bright red. It is usually transient lasting several days or some weeks but has a strong tendency to recur; in this manner the disease may drag on for months. Occasionally the attacks are fleeting but frequently repeated (*episcleritis periodica fugax*). On the other hand, the disease may be extremely chronic, in which case it never ulcerates and may be entirely absorbed, but more frequently leaves a slate-coloured scar behind to which the conjunctiva is adherent. The cornea and uveal tract rarely participate in the inflammation. There may be little or no pain, but usually there is a feeling of discomfort and tenderness on pressure, and often severe neuralgia. In the worst cases the disease extends into the deeper parts of the sclera and thus passes almost imperceptibly into scleritis.

Anatomically dense lymphocytic infiltration of the subconjunctival and episcleral tissues is found.

It is now regarded as an allergic reaction to an endogenous toxin; a history of rheumatoid arthritis is commonly obtained. The condition is sometimes considered to lie within the vague category of collagenous diseases. It is commonest in women.

Treatment is difficult and often unrewarding. Corticosteroids administered topically or Tanderil drops or ointment are sometimes of temporary benefit. Even in cases in which no history of rheumatism can be elicited, salicylates may prove helpful, and should be tried. Prolonged remissions may be induced by Tanderil 600 mg, daily for four days and then reduced to 400 mg, in divided doses.

Scleritis
Scleritis is usually a bilateral disease occurring most frequently in women and more rare than episcleritis. It is associated with connective tissue disease in 50% of cases and thorough investigation is required to eliminate active systemic disease such as polyarteritis nodosa, systemic lupus erythematosus, non-specific arteritis, Wegener's granulomatosis, dermatomyositis and polychondritis. One or more nodules may appear but

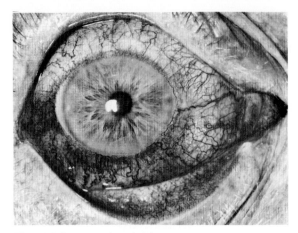

Fig. 17.2 Deep anterior scleritis

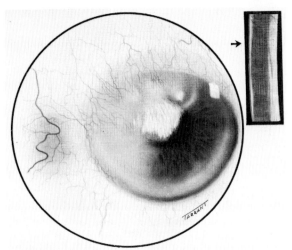

Fig. 17.3 Corneal involvement in episcleritis and scleritis. (By courtesy of P. Watson.)

the area affected is less circumscribed than in episcleritis. The swelling is at first dark red or bluish, later it becomes purple and semi-transparent like porcelain (Fig. 17.2). It may extend entirely round the cornea, forming a very serious condition known as *annular scleritis*. In the diffuse type hard whitish nodules, the size of a pin's head, may develop in the inflamed zone; they disappear without disintegrating. Scleritis differs from episcleritis in that the cornea and uveal tract are involved, some iritis but more usually cyclitis and anterior choroiditis being present. There is no ulceration, but much absorption so that the sclera is thinned, a dark purple cicatrix being formed which occasionally becomes too weak to withstand the intra-ocular pressure, so that ectasia follows (*ciliary staphyloma*). Secondary glaucoma is a common sequel.

Pathologically scleritis resembles episcleritis, but extends more deeply, the essential change being a dense lymphocytic infiltration.

Apart from the intra-ocular complications scleritis may sometimes extend to the cornea causing *sclerosing keratitis* (Fig. 17.3). An opacity develops at the margin of the cornea near the affected scleral area; it is approximately triangular or tongue-shaped, the rounded apex being towards the centre of the cornea. There is little or no corneal vascularisation and ulceration never occurs. Some clearing occurs from the centre towards the periphery as well as near the corneal limbus, but the densest parts usually persist as bluish clouds. The whole margin of the cornea may become opaque like the sclera and occasionally guttered but the pupillary area almost invariably escapes. The most serious corneal complication is keratolysis wherein the stroma melts away.

The patient who presents with episcleritis or scleritis should have the following routine studies carried out — full blood count, rheumatoid arthritis latex agglutina-

tion test, serum uric acid estimation, the Treponema pallidum immobilisation (TPI) test for syphilis, X-rays of the chest and sacro-iliac joints and in certain patients a full immunological survey for tissue antibodies. Soluble immune complexes, complement, lupus erythematosus cells and antinuclear factor (ANF) should be undertaken with a Mantoux test.

Treatment. Systemic steroid therapy is necessary starting with 40 mg Prednisolone daily as a minimum and increasing by 10 mg daily till suppression of inflammation is achieved. Once achieved the dose may be reduced to a maintenance level. In severe and recurrent attacks Tanderil 400 mg daily may be added to the Prednisilone and if vasculitis appears Penicillamine 100 mg should be administered in addition. Local steroids tend to be ineffective and subconjunctival injections of steroids should never be given for fear of rupture of the globe. Likewise biopsy is dangerous as well as uninformative. Cytotoxic immunosuppressive alkylating agents have a place in the therapy of very severe cases administered by physicians familiar with the dangers of this group of drugs.

Gumma of the sclera
This is uncommon.

Tuberculosis of the sclera
In the form of a scleritis, this may be an extension from the conjunctiva, iris, ciliary body, or choroid, or may be primary, forming a localized nodule which caseates and ulcerates. It should be excised or scraped and the tissue examined for the organism. Treatment consists of the local and systemic use of anti-tuberculous drugs.

Collagen diseases

Among these scleral implication is common, particularly in rheumatoid arthritis.

The serological feature of rheumatoid arthritis is the presence of circulating antibodies to immunoglobulin molecules which are known as rheumatoid factors. Between 70 and 90% of rheumatoid patients are seropositive for classical rheumatoid factor.

The lesions of rheumatoid arthritis may be due to the deposition of globulin-antiglobulin complex whereby complexes of modified IgG and locally formed rheumatoid factor in the synovium result in the activation of complement, thereby provoking the release of hydrolytic enzymes and subsequent erosion of adjacent articular surfaces. It would seem likely that the scleral nodules in rheumatoid arthritis represent a granulomatous response to focal deposits of antigen-antibody complexes. The primary event of rheumatoid arthritis is possibly cryptogenic bacterial or viral infection in susceptible individuals provoking an inappropriate immunological response.

Histologically the typical scleral lesion assumes the characteristic combination of a proliferative infiltration by chronic inflammatory cells surrounding a central area of fibrinoid necrosis, as occurs in rheumatoid nodules generally. In the sclera the clinical manifestations take several forms. *Episcleral rheumatoid nodules* may appear and disappear, waxing and waning with the vagaries of the systemic disease. A more serious condition is *necrotising nodular scleritis* wherein a violent and painful anterior scleritis, often circumferential in its extent, characterised by much swelling and the appearance of one or more yellow nodules, usually proceeds to necrosis leading eventually to disintegration of the sclera and exposure of the underlying uvea (Fig. 17.4). In *scleromalacia perforans* the same necrosis of the sclera occurs with exposure of the uvea but without painful symptoms (Fig. 17.5). Finally, in *massive granuloma of the sclera*, proliferative changes are predominant. In the anterior segment of the eye a 'brawny scleritis' results; in the posterior segment the sclera may become so thickened as to simulate an intra-ocular or orbital tumour. In all these cases serious and often destructive extension occurs into the uveal tract, and the general prognosis is poor. Systemic treatment by corticosteroids affords the only known method of amelioration.

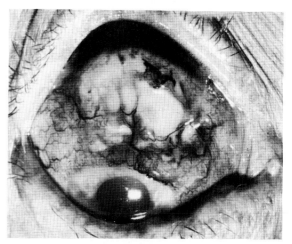

Fig. 17.4 Necrotising nodular scleritis

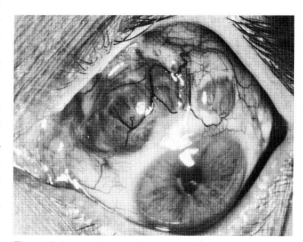

Fig. 17.5 Scleromalacia perforans

Blue sclerotics

The sclera is bluish in babies, but a much more pronounced blue coloration is sometimes seen in several members of the same family as a hereditary condition which persists throughout life; it is frequently associated with fragilitas ossium and deafness. The sexes are about equally involved; only those affected can transmit the disease. Histologically the sclera and cornea are thin so that the uveal pigment shines through to produce the blue colour.

18

Diseases of the uveal tract

Although topographically apparently separate, the iris, the ciliary body and the choroid are so closely related as to form a continuous whole; the diseases affecting the whole uveal tract will therefore be considered together.

VASCULAR DISTURBANCES

While the blood supply of the uveal tract is almost entirely derived from the posterior ciliary arteries, the peculiar distribution resulting in the formation of the major arterial circle of the iris causes involvement of both the iris and the ciliary body in pathological vascular conditions, whereas the blood supply to the choroid, being essentially segmental, results in the formation of lesions restricted to isolated areas. The richness of anastomoses in the anterior part of the uveal tract precludes isolated vascular lesions. Massive hæmorrhages in the choroid occur in expulsive hæmorrhage.

Rubeosis Iridis is a curious and serious condition which occurs in diabetes of long standing and in thrombosis of the retinal vein. It is characterized by the development of new and enlarged vessels in the iris, the neovascularization being frequently accentuated towards its root and in the angle of the anterior chamber. It may be associated with signs of iritis, and a rise in tension often occurs leading to a very intractable neovascular glaucoma. Treatment is difficult; Panretinal photocoagulation of an ischaemic retina prevents the development of neovascular glaucoma. Once it has developed destruction of the neovascular tissue is sometimes achieved by laser application.

INFLAMMATIONS OF THE UVEAL TRACT

The term *uveitis* emphasizes the close relationship between the anatomically distinct parts of the uveal tract, for inflammatory processes tend to involve the uvea as a whole and are not limited to a single part. This feature is particularly well exemplified in inflammation of the iris and ciliary body; iritis never occurs without some cyclitis, nor cyclitis without some iritis and the terms *iritis* and *cyclitis* are used according to whether the iris or ciliary body appears clinically to be the more affected. The same disposition is also seen with regard to the choroid, although in less degree, for the ciliary body is often involved in many cases of choroiditis. A more correct terminology is *anterior* and *posterior uveitis*, while *general uveitis* is commonest in chronic types of inflammation.

The aetiology of uveitis

The determination of the ætiology of inflammations of the uveal tract is one of the most difficult problems in ophthalmology; In some cases the aetiology is obvious and several infections have distinguishing clinical features; but in most cases which present a nondescript clinical picture, our ignorance is profound. It would seem probable that most of these are not due to direct infection but are allergic in origin. The foreign antigen is usually an infectious agent and the uveitis occurs late in the course of the predisposing disease when hypersensitivity mechanisms have been established.

The following classification may prove useful:

1. *Exogenous infections.* Are due to the introduction into the eye of organisms through a perforating wound or ulcer. This results usually in an acute iridocyclitis often of a suppurative type, and sometimes in a panophthalmitis wherein the whole interior of the eye is involved.

2. *Secondary infections*, wherein the inflammation of the uveal tract is due to spread from one or other of the ocular tissues — the cornea, sclera, or retina.

3. *Endogenous infections*, wherein organisms primarily lodged in some other organ of the body reach the eye through the bloodstream. These comprise bacterial infections as tuberculosis, syphilis, gonorrhœa, or brucellosis, viral infections as in mumps, smallpox or influenza wherein an iridocyclitis occurs, and protozoal infections such as toxoplasmosis. The same mechanism causes the violent panophthalmitis seen in septicæmia due to such organisms as the streptococcus, staphylococcus, meningococcus or pneumococcus: in these the inflammation is suppurative in type.

4. *Allergic inflammations* are generally considered to be common. Therein a primary source of infection exists somewhere in the body; at one time the infection was generalized by the escape of organisms into the blood-stream when the ocular tissues had become sensitized to them; and at a later date a renewal of activity in the original focus leads to a further dissemination of the organisms or their proteins which, meeting the sensitized ocular tissues, excite therein an allergic response and lead to the deposition of immune complexes.

Acute iridocyclitis may be comparable to the simple act of antibody formation in a lymph node but it is possible that immunological thymus dependent 'memory cells' may be implanted in the eye without direct local exposure to the antigen. These cells proliferate on contact with the antigen should it reappear in the blood-stream and differentiate to become cytotoxic lymphocytes. This could explain the non-specific focal reaction that may occur in eyes with chronic inflammatory disease after the injection of Tuberculin, foreign protein used therapeutically or following the removal of infected teeth or areas of focal infection.

5. Uveitis can represent hypersensitivity to autologous tissue components. Uveitis is found in association with rheumatoid arthritis, Still's disease in children, systemic lupus erythematosis, Wegener's granulomatosis, sarcoidosis, ankylosing spondylitis, Reiter's disease, relapsing poly-chondritis and Behçet's Syndrome, all of which have an auto-immune component in their aetiology.

Uveitis can also represent a response to antigenic stimuli in other parts of the eye. The uvea may retain sensitised lymphocytes after the initial reaction which provide an immediate response should the cause of the inflammation recur. Thus iridocyclitis is a common accompaniment of severe corneal infection and choroiditis of retinal inflammation.

A number of diseases associated with uveitis occur much more frequently in those persons with certain specific HLA antigens. Thus, in Caucasian patients with ankylosing spondylitis 90% belong to the HLA-B27 antigenic group in contrast to approximately 8% of the normal population. There is also a disproportionately high percentage of patients of the B-27 antigenic group in adult patients with acute anterior uveitis. Patients with acute anterior uveitis and juvenile rheumatoid arthritis are usually negative for the rheumatoid factor and for antinuclear antibodies but belong to the B-27 antigenic group whereas those with chronic anterior uveitis and juvenile rheumatoid arthritis although negative for the rheumatoid factor have a high incidence of antinuclear antibody and a relatively low incidence of B-27 antigens. Other diseases which are associated with specific HLA antigens are the Vogt-Koyanagi-Harada's disease and Behçet's disease.

The general course of (non-purulent) anterior uveitis

Iritis

In order that iritis and the special dangers which attend it may be thoroughly understood, it is necessary to remember the anatomical arrangements of the iris and the pathological changes which occur in it. The iris is practically a diaphragm of blood vessels and unstriped muscle fibres held together by a loose, spongy stroma. In its perpetual movements the pupillary margin slides to and fro upon the lens capsule. The more the pupil is constricted the more of the posterior surface of the iris is in contact with the lens capsule; when fully dilated the iris may not touch the lens.

Inflammation of the iris has fundamentally the same characteristics as in other connective tissues: dilatation of the blood vessels occurs with impairment of the capillary walls and exudation of a protein-rich fluid into the tissue spaces with leuco- or lymphocytosis. Owing to the extreme vascularity of the iris, the peculiar distribution of the vessels and the looseness of the stroma, these generic features of inflammation produce special results. Thus hyperaemia tends to cause the pupil to contract mechanically on account of the radial disposition of the vessels. The extreme vascularity and the looseness of the tissues allow an unusually large amount of exudation on the one hand and swelling on the other. The iris virtually becomes a water-logged sponge full of sticky fluid so that its freedom of movement is impaired, and the normal pupillary reactions become sluggish or abolished. The fluid also contains toxic substances which act as irritants causing the muscle fibres to contract, and since the sphincter overcomes the dilatator muscle, constriction of the pupil results. It follows that in iritis the pupil is constricted, its reactions are sluggish, and the delicate pattern of the iris instead of being clear and sharply defined, becomes blurred and indistinct ('muddy' iris). The colour undergoes considerable change; in fair people the blue iris becomes bluish or yellowish green; brown irides show less difference, but become greyish or yellowish brown. In any case, comparison of the colour of the two irides will usually reveal some difference, for iritis is generally unilateral during the acute attack.

The hyperaemia manifests itself in circumcorneal ciliary congestion, most marked if the ciliary body is seriously involved (p. 71). The conjunctival vessels are also frequently engorged so that care is necessary in distinguishing the condition from conjunctivitis, but the secondary nature of the conjunctival congestion is shown by the relatively slight discharge: any discharge is lacrimal, never mucopurulent.

Since the iris is richly supplied with sensory nerves from the ophthalmic division of the fifth nerve, pain, typically worst at night, is a prominent symptom of acute iritis. It is not confined to the eye, although severe neuralgic pain is felt here, but is also referred to other branches of the nerve, especially to the forehead and scalp, to the cheeks and malar bone, and sometimes to the nose and teeth.

The albuminous exudates escape into the anterior chamber and, particularly if the ciliary body is involved, the aqueous becomes plasmoid (p. 14) containing leucocytes and minute flakes of coagulated protein, or even fibrinous networks in severe cases. It therefore becomes hazy, forming a milky 'flare' in the beam of the slit-lamp which, as it traverses the anterior chamber, should be invisible (Fig. 10.8); this turbidity interferes with a clear view of the iris and is easily mistaken for haziness of the cornea. In very intense cases polymorphonuclear leucocytes are poured out and sink to the bottom of the anterior chamber to form a hypopyon. Hyphaema, or blood in the anterior chamber, rarely occurs.

At the same time the nutrition of the corneal endothelium becomes affected so that the cells become sticky and may desquamate in places. There the exudates tend to stick, forming *keratic precipitates* ('keratitis punctata'). These are seldom present in simple iritis, but form an important feature of cyclitis.

The exudates poured out by the iris and ciliary body also cover the surface of the iris as a thin film and spread into, and sometimes completely over, the pupillary area. When these are profuse the iritis is termed *plastic*. In this manner the pupil may become 'blocked', a condition which seriously impairs the sight. Moreover, the exudates tend to stick the iris to the lens capsule so that it becomes fixed. If atropine is instilled at an early stage the iris may be freed and the pupil again becomes dilated and circular. In such cases spots of exudate or pigment derived from the posterior layer of the iris may be left permanently upon the anterior capsule of the lens, forming valuable evidence of previous iritis (Plate 6, Fig. C); these are easily distinguished from the congenital spots due to persistence of the pupillary membrane (p. 169). If, however, the adhesions are allowed to become organised they are converted into fibrous bands which atropine is unable to rupture; such firm adhesions of the pupillary margin to the lens capsule are called *posterior synechiæ*; they show some predilection for the lower part of the pupil in the early stages, probably owing to gravitation of the plastic exudates. When they are localised and a mydriatic causes the intervening portions of the circle of the pupil to dilate, the pupil assumes a festooned appearance (Plate 6, Fig. C). Such an irregular pupil, intensified by the instillation of a mydriatic, is a sign of present or past iritis. Owing to the contraction of organising exudates upon the iris the pigment epithelium on its posterior surface may be pulled around the pupillary margin so that patches of pigment may be seen on the anterior surface of the iris (*ectropion of the uveal pigment*).

In severe cases of plastic iritis or after recurrent attacks, the whole circle of the pupillary margin may become tied down in this way to the lens capsule. The condition is called *annular* or *ring synechia* or *seclusio pupillae*; it is one of great danger to the eye, since, if unrelieved, it inevitably leads to secondary glaucoma. The aqueous, unable to pass forwards into the anterior chamber, collects behind the iris, which becomes bowed forwards like a sail, a condition which is called *iris bombé*. Regarded from in front, the anterior chamber is seen to be funnel-shaped, deepest in the centre and shallowest at the periphery. The filtration angle is thus obliterated by the apposition of the iris to the cornea at the periphery where eventually adhesions may form (*peripheral anterior synechiae*). The circulation of the aqueous is therefore obstructed and the ocular tension rises (p. 188).

When the exudate has been more extensive it may organize across the entire pupillary area which becomes ultimately filled by a film of opaque fibrous tissue; this condition is called blocked pupil, or *occlusio pupillæ*. If there has been much cyclitis the posterior chamber also becomes filled with exudates which may organize, tying down the iris to the lens capsule; this condition of *total posterior synechia* leads to retraction of the peripheral part of the iris, so that the anterior chamber becomes abnormally deep at the periphery, sometimes deeper than in the centre.

In the worst cases of *plastic iridocyclitis* a cyclitic membrane may form behind the lens where it may be seen with the ophthalmoscope or even by oblique illumination. In young children the condition forms one type of *pseudo-glioma* (p. 241). In the later stages the degenerative changes in the ciliary body prevent it from fulfilling its functions of supplying the eye with intra-ocular fluid and nutriment. The vitreous suffers first, becoming fluid, and later the lens, which becomes opaque. Finally the eye shrinks (*phthisis bulbi*).

During the course of any type of the disease the *ocular tension may be affected*. Most frequently in the active stages this involves a rise determined, in the first place, by the height of the pressure in the widely dilated capillaries and, in the second, by the difficulty experienced by the sticky albuminous aqueous in escaping through the filtration channels at the angle of the anterior chamber (*hypertensive iridocyclitis*). In the later stages when the pupil has been bound down blocking the flow of aqueous from the posterior to the anterior chamber, a secondary glaucoma may also follow. Finally, if the ciliary region becomes atrophic, interference with the secretion of aqueous may lead to lowering of the ocular tension and the development of a soft eye — an ominous sign.

The diagnosis of acute iridocyclitis. Iritis is most frequently mistaken either for conjunctivitis or acute glaucoma. The error of mistaking iritis for acute glaucoma is the most serious which can be made, particularly because the treatment of the two conditions is diametrically opposed. Dilatation of the pupil with atropine, which is urgently necessary in iritis, is the worst possible treatment of closed-angle glaucoma. At the cost of some repetition, therefore, the distinguishing features will be given here.

1. *Injection*. Superficial in conjunctivitis, deep ciliary in iritis and glaucoma.

2. *Secretion*. Muco-purulent in conjunctivitis; watery in iritis and glaucoma.

3. *Pupil*. Normal in conjunctivitis; small and irregular in iritis; large and oval in glaucoma.

4. *Media*. Clear in conjunctivitis; sometimes opacities in the pupil in iritis; corneal oedema in glaucoma.

5. *Tension*. Normal in conjunctivitis; usually normal in iritis; raised glaucoma.

6. *Pain*. Mild discomfort in conjunctivitis; moderate in eye and first division of trigeminal in iritis; severe pain in eye and the entire trigeminal area in glaucoma.

7. *Tenderness*. Absent in conjunctivitis; marked in iritis and glaucoma.

8. *Vision*. Good in conjunctivitis; fair in iritis; poor in glaucoma.

9. *Onset*. Gradual in conjunctivitis; usually gradual in iritis; sudden in glaucoma.

10. *Systemic complications*. Absent in conjunctivitis; little in iritis; prostration and sometimes vomiting in glaucoma.

Cyclitis

This has already been referred to incidentally. In the severe *plastic* form the exudates from the ciliary body pass into the anterior chamber directly from that part which forms a boundary of the chamber (Fig. 1.3), and indirectly by passing forwards through the pupil. The deposition of keratic precipitates on the back of the cornea is a prominent feature, while clouds of dust-like opacities appear in the vitreous. When the exudates organize they not only cause a total posterior synechia, but also surround the lens and extend throughout the vitreous. Behind the lens they form a transverse membrane or *cyclitic membrane*. Strands of fibrous tissue are formed in the vitreous which become anchored to the retina in various places, and by their subsequent contraction may lead to detachment of this tissue. The exudates which organize upon the surface of the ciliary body cause the destruction of the ciliary processes, which results in diminishing or abolishing the secretion of aqueous. Hence the ocular tension becomes lowered (*hypotony*) and the eye may even become shrunken and quadrilateral in shape owing to pressure by the rectus muscles — *phthisis bulbi*; thereafter degenerative changes supervene.

Chronic iridocyclitis (*simple cyclitis*) deserves special mention because of its insidiousness and the difficulty in its diagnosis. It is an extremely chronic disease characterised by diminution of vision with few physical signs. In severe cases there is some ciliary congestion, tenderness on pressure over the ciliary region, a deep anterior chamber, keratic precipitates on the back of the cornea and dust-like opacities in the vitreous. The keratic precipitates indeed, may be the only obvious evidence of the disease, sometimes scattered over a triangular area of the lower part of the cornea, an arrangement due to convection currents in the aqueous and gravitation of the particles towards the bottom of the anterior chamber (Plate 7, Fig. B), but more commonly scattered irregularly over the lower part of the cornea as a few isolated spots. They require great care in examination for their discovery (p. 74) and their importance cannot be overestimated. The smaller spots sometimes coalesce forming small plaques which gradually become translucent ('mutton-fat k.p.').

The vitreous opacities are of the same nature; they are mainly wandering leucocytes but many are coagulated fibrin and particles of albuminous exudate. Their mobility in the vitreous shows that this gel has become fluid.

In the most insidious cases the symptoms and physical signs are minimal. Considerable diminution of vision without obvious cause should always excite apprehension, and the cornea should be most carefully explored with the slit-lamp. A few spots of 'k.p.' are decisive proof of cyclitis and may be the sole physical sign. A change in the colour of the iris due to atrophy is an important sign since it may at once attract attention, especially if the normal eye has a brown iris; it indicates, however, a late stage of the disease.

The disease is generally very chronic and liable to exacerbations with the gradual and insidious formation of posterior synechiae. Vision is diminished during the more acute phases and recovers considerably in the intervals, but each recurrent attack leaves a more permanent defect. The eye may finally become soft and tender and enter into the condition of phthisis bulbi, but this occurs only after many years.

An important and not uncommon complication is a rise of tension in the course of the disease to constitute the clinical syndrome of *hypertensive iridocyclitic crises* (of Posner and Schlossman). In this condition the eye may appear normal but periodically acute or subacute attacks of raised tension occur associated with the presence of an aqueous flare and keratic precipitates, often so few and unobtrusive as only to be seen by examination with the slit-lamp and often of relatively short duration. These attacks, accompanied by the diminution of vision and the appearance of halos around lights with headaches, resemble so closely attacks of closed-angle glaucoma that a mistake in diagnosis is often made. The diagnosis may depend solely on the detection of one or two keratic precipitates, but its establishment is of the utmost importance since in this condition treatment by atropine with topical corticosteroids rapidly resolves the attack, a method of therapy which, of course, would be disastrous in a case of closed-angle glaucoma. These recurrent attacks although controlled by atropine, tend to recur until the cause of the inflammation is eliminated.

Chronic posterior cyclitis, or *Pars Planitis* affecting essentially the pars plana of the ciliary body and the periphery of the choroid, occurs particularly in children and young adults. The condition involves retinal phlebitis with leakage into the vitreous and the late development of collagen in the vitreous. Fluorescein injected intravenously rapidly enters the vitreous chamber. The onset is insidious without dramatic evidences of inflammation and the first symptom is a deterioration of vision due to opacities in the anterior vitreous. The inflammation is non-specific, the cause is usually unknown, and after a long course the results may be serious. Most cases however (80%) do not need any treatment. Therapy is disappointing though cortico-steroids have a place. Immuno-suppressents should only be used in severe cases in which steroids have failed.

Varieties of Anterior Uveitis

While the general description of the course of acute and chronic non-purulent anterior uveitis applies to the majority of cases the aetiology of which is undetermined, a large number of different types are met with clinically. In the most general sense these may be divided into two main varieties — those due to direct organismal infection and those which are an expression of an allergic reaction. The clinical pictures presented by infections with specific organisms will be discussed at a later stage.

Infective (granulomatous) iridocyclitis is due essentially to the invasion of the eye by living organisms. In the absence of allergic sensitivity of the tissues, the inflammation tends to be insidious in onset and chronic in course with a minimum of inflammatory reaction. Such chronic inflammations due to direct organismal infection are typically characterised by dense nodular infiltrations of the tissues rather than by diffuse exudative phenomena (Fig. 18.1). In the absence of immunity these lesions show a slow and gradual extension; if immunity is present they tend to become circumscribed and relapse if the resistance falls. If hyper-sensitivity develops a further organismal invasion leads to necrosis and caseation. Clinically such an inflammation is characterised by the formation of dense synechiæ and large greasy 'mutton-fat' keratic precipitates composed of endothelial cells and lymphocytes (Fig. 18.2). The clinical picture varies considerably with the type of organism concerned; the more important manifestations will be considered presently.

The allergic (exudative) type of reaction, on the other hand, tends to be of acute onset and short duration, diffuse in extension and without focal lesions in the iris. There is a considerable flare in the anterior chamber and the keratic precipitates, if present, are few and composed of lymphoid cells (Fig. 18.3).

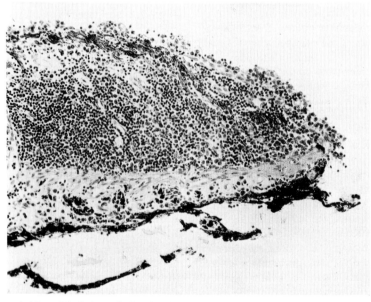

Fig. 18.1 Granulomatous irridocyclitis (in brucellosis). A nodule of lymphoid cells near the sphincter of the iris. (By courtesy of A. C. Woods.)

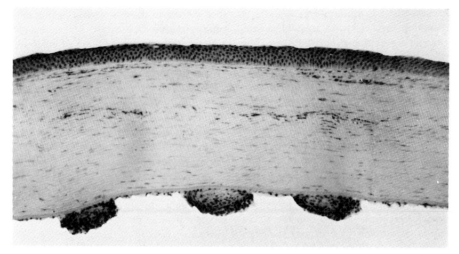

Fig. 18.2 Mutton-fat keratic precipitates

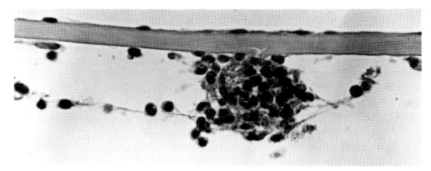

Fig. 18.3 Keratic precipitates in herpes

The course of the disease varies. Milder cases take three or more weeks before the inflammation subsides; improvement is shown by good dilatation of the pupil with atropine, diminution of injection and pain. In the chronic cases the ciliary body is always seriously involved and the inflammatory signs are less. Complete resolution may occur in mild cases treated early and suitably, particularly if early dilatation of the pupil has forestalled the development of posterior synechiæ. In all cases, however, a characteristic feature is the tendency to relapse. Each fresh attack runs a similar course, although usually less severe, often leaving further traces and increased impairment of vision. Repeated attacks of iritis lead to atrophy of the iris, which assumes a dirty grey colour like felt or blotting paper. Red streaks often mark the site of permanently dilated vessels, usually of new formation and therefore not necessarily radial in direction. The pupillary margin is thin and frayed; the reactions are diminished.

The general course of (non-purulent) posterior uveitis

Inflammations of the choroid conform in their general characteristics with those affecting the anterior part of the uveal tract; they may either appear in the form of isolated foci of inflammation or they may be diffuse; in the latter case the anterior uvea is always involved. It is to be remembered that the outer layers of the retina are dependent for their nutrition upon the choroid so that an inflammation of the latter always involves the former secondarily.

Non-suppurative choroiditis

This may occur in two forms. As with iridocyclitis, a *granulomatous* form is associated with direct organismal infection, the essential feature of which is the occurrence of localised accumulations of chronic inflammatory cells (lymphocytes, plasma cells, etc.). This form of choroiditis will be discussed at a later stage.

Exudative choroiditis, on the other hand, is a non-specific plastic inflammatory response characterized initially by more acute cellular infiltration (leucocytes) and much exudation, the aetiology of which is exactly comparable with the similar type of iridocyclitis.

The course of exudative choroiditis. A recent focus is seen ophthalmoscopically as a yellowish area; when near a retinal vessel it lies at a level deeper than the vessel. It is due to infiltration of the choroid, the exudates hiding the choroidal vessels which cause the normal red reflex. In the early stages the membrane of Bruch is intact; in these circumstances only fluid can pass through it, but this suffices to make the overlying retina cloudy and grey so that the edges are hazy and ill-defined. The exudates not only pass into, but also through the retina, so that punctate or diffuse opacities are seen in the vitreous. In the later stages the membrane of Bruch may be destroyed, although like all elastic membranes it offers considerable resistance; when this has occurred leucocytes are enabled to pass through into the retina and vitreous. A marked vitreous haze usually indicates that the ciliary body is also involved; while the presence of keratic precipitates on the back of the cornea and inconspicuous posterior synechiæ proves that in many cases of apparently localized choroiditis the whole uveal tract is implicated (general uveitis).

Owing to the fibroblastic activity of the choroidal stroma the exudates become organized, so that fibrous tissue is formed which destroys the normal structures and fuses the choroid and retina firmly together. The colour of the spots therefore gradually changes to white, partly due to the fibrous tissue deposited, partly to thinning and atrophy whereby the white reflex from the sclera is permitted to shine through (Fig. 18.4).

The pigment of the retinal pigmentary epithelium is extremely resistant, even although the cells which contain it are destroyed. It tends to become heaped up into masses, partly intra-, partly extracellular: moreover, the pigment cells are stimulated to proliferate. Isolated masses of black pigment are thus formed in the white areas, especially at the edges, so that in the atrophic stage the white areas are surrounded by a black zone of pigment (Fig. 18.4). The process has then reached its natural termination, and these sharply defined areas remain permanently unaltered.

The symptoms in the early stages are principally the defects of vision due to the retinal lesions and to cloudiness of the vitreous; they are thus marked when the lesion is in the central area and usually escape observation when in the periphery. The inflamed area is slightly raised, so that the contour of the retina is altered. This causes distortion of the images, giving rise to a similar appearance of distortion of the objects seen — *metamorphopsia*: thus straight lines appear to be wavy. Frequently objects appear smaller than they are — *micropsia*; sometimes larger — *macropsia*: these effects are due to separation or crowding together respectively of the rods and cones. Subjective flashes of light due to retinal irritability (*phtopsiæ*) are seen. These subjective symptoms are often accompanied by the perception of a black

spot in front of the eye, corresponding to the lesion — a *positive scotoma.*

In the later stages the affected areas are incapable of giving rise to visual impulses so that *negative scotomata* exist in the field of vision, wherein there is a hiatus in the field of vision of the same nature as the normal blind spot. Their importance depends upon their situation. Peripheral scotomata may pass unnoticed, a central scotoma destroys direct vision; in the latter case peripheral vision still permits the patient to get about, but all fine work is impossible.

The disease is chronic, organization of the exudates taking several weeks. The occurrence of fresh spots may extend the acute stage over a period of months, and the ultimate defects are permanent. The condition is often bilateral

Non-suppurative choroiditis is usually classified according to the number and location of the areas involved.

Disseminated choroiditis. In this type, small areas of inflammation are scattered over the greater part of the fundus behind the equator. In the milder cases only a few spots are formed and the exudates in the vitreous become absorbed. In the more severe the spots are very numerous, fresh foci arising and passing through the same stages, until finally the whole fundus may be covered with atrophic areas passing through the stages of evolution just described. The vitreous opacities increase, and finally the nutrition of the lens suffers and a complicated cataract results. Owing to the transience of the acute stage the atrophic stage naturally comes much more frequently under observation. Such a condition may be due to syphilis, but in many the cause is obscure.

Anterior choroiditis. This is often syphilitic, and manifests itself in the same form as disseminated choroiditis, but is confined to the peripheral parts of the fundus. On this account it is frequently symptomless and is discovered only on routine examination. It should be clearly distinguished from the similar changes found in high myopia and in old people as a senile degeneration.

Central choroiditis. Occurs in disseminated choroiditis, and occasionally alone.

Juxtapapillary choroiditis (Jensen). Occurs in young persons as an exudation close to the disc, usually oval in shape and about the same size as the disc. The exudates may cover the retinal vessels, and there are vitreous opacities and sometimes 'k.p.' There is generally a sector-shaped defect in the field of vision. The cause is usually obscure. The inflammation slowly subsides, leaving a patch of atrophy, but recurrence may take place.

The general treatment of uveitis

In *anterior uveitis*, dilatation of the pupil with atropine, hot applications, and the control of the acute phases of the inflammation, with steroids, are the essentials of local treatment.

Atropine acts in three ways: (1) by keeping the iris and ciliary body at rest; (2) by diminishing hyperæmia; (3) preventing the formation of posterior synechiæ and breaking down any already formed. It may be used in the form of drops or ointment (1%) which should be pushed in the early stages, better by frequency of application rather than by increased strength; every four hours is usually sufficient. When the pupil is well dilated, twice a day suffices. If atropine irritation ensues one or other of the substitutes for this drug (p. 27) may be used. A very powerful mydriatic effect is also obtained by the subconjunctival injection of 0.3 ml of mydricaine (p. 368), a mixture of atropine, procaine, and adrenaline.

Hot applications are extremely soothing to the patient by diminishing the pain, and are of therapeutic service in increasing the circulation.

Corticosteroids (p. 109) administered as drops, ointment, or — more effectively — as subconjunctival injections are of great value in controlling the inflammation in the acute phase. Occasionally the results are dramatic and the eye becomes white with great rapidity.

Aspirin is very useful in relieving pain, but if it is intense stronger preparations such as distalgesic or DF 118 may be indicated. In the convalescent stage dark glasses are ordered — for both eyes, on account of the consensual reaction to light. Atropine, or its equivalent, should be continued for at least ten days to a fortnight after the eye appears to be quiet, otherwise a relapse is likely to occur.

The treatment of *choroiditis* is unsatisfactory since gross damage is usually done to the retina before the condition can be controlled. The essentials of local treatment are the adminstration of atropine and heat, either by diathermy or an electric pad (p. 371). The systemic administration of corticosteroids or ACTH cuts short an attack and hastens healing (Chap. 14).

Treatment of sequelœ and complications

Secondary glaucoma forms one of the most serious complications of iridocyclitis. If the condition of *hypertensive iridocyclitis* develops in the early stages of the disease before the formation of anatomical hindrances to the circulation of the aqueous humour (posterior or peripheral synechiæ), the most effective treatment is to intensify atropinisation in order to allay the inflammatory congestion. Corticosteroids administered topically and acetazolamide given systemically are frequently very useful in such cases.

Annular synechiæ demand an iridectomy in all cases in order to restore communication between the posterior and anterior chambers, and thus avoid the supervention of secondary glaucoma. No operative procedure of this kind must be undertaken during an acute attack of iritis if it can be avoided, since the traumatic iritis set up will frustrate the object of the operation by filling the opening with exudates. It is best, if possible, to forestall a ring synechia by performing the iridectomy before the adhesion extends round the whole circle. This can often be done because a ring synechia is frequently the result of recurrent attacks and can therefore be performed during a quiescent interval. It is often difficult to get a good gap owing to the atrophy and friability of the iris and the firmness of the adhesions; haemorrhage is common. Iridectomy sometimes has a beneficial effect on recurrent iritis, but should not be done without special indications until all other non-operative measures have failed. The presence of 'k.p.' should generally be regarded as a contra-indication to surgery in the absence of dangerously high intra-ocular pressure.

Purulent uveitis and panophthalmitis

Purulent uveitis is generally caused by infected wounds, whether accidental or the result of operations or ulcers. In the case of ulcers and when the penetrating wound is corneal, the inflammation may remain as an anterior uveitis if the infection is not virulent or if is controlled by treatment; but the usual tendency is for the whole eye to be involved in a *panophthalmitis*. In deeper injuries the vitreous is usually first affected; organisms grow readily in it as in a culture medium, and purulent cyclitis, retinitis and choroiditis develop. The pneumococcus is responsible for many cases, so also are the staphylococcus, the streptococcus, *E. coli*, *Ps. pyocyanea*, *B. cereus* (*subtilis*), and *Cl. welchii* (gas gangrene). Fungal endophthalmitis may occur after intraocular surgery.

Fungal endophthalmitis has an incubation period of several weeks affecting the anterior vitreous and anterior uvea predominantly with the production of a hypopyon. The vitreous becomes a granuloma and the pupils become occluded with inflammatory material.

The endogenous form of purulent uveitis is metastatic in origin. Such cases are now seldom seen as complications of the exanthemata but they may occur as fungal choroiditis in patients receiving cortico-steroids, azothioprine and other drugs given to suppress graft rejection. Mucomycosis extends directly from the nasopharynx in debilitated individuals with ketosis.

In both forms there is rise of temperature, headache, and sometimes vomiting. In the exogenous forms the edges of the wound become yellow and necrotic, a hypopyon appears, there is great chemosis with intense ciliary and conjunctival congestion, and the lids are swollen and red. There is severe pain in the eye, due at first to iritis, later to increased tension. The vitreous becomes purulent, as shown by a yellow reflex with oblique illumination. The anterior chamber soon becomes full of pus, and the cornea cloudy and yellow; ring infiltration may occur (p. 136). There may be proptosis and limitation of movement of the globe due to extension of the inflammation to Tenon's capsule.

In metastatic cases, ophthalmoscopic examination shows that the media are hazy so that the yellow œdematous retina is only dimly seen; there is a yellow reflex, the formation of a hypopyon and rapid failure of vision.

In severe cases the inflammation gives rise to the widespread formation of cyclitic membranes, destruction of the ciliary processes and a fall in ocular tension resulting in shrinkage of the globe. In the most severe cases and when the infection is allowed to take its course, the pus bursts through the walls of the globe, usually just behind the limbus; thereupon the pain subsides and after prolonged suppuration the eyeball shrinks. The prognosis is bad, for vision is almost invariably lost. The condition is not likely to set up sympathetic ophthalmitis.

Treatment. In order to achieve the best results it is essential to treat all cases with a combination of antibiotics and cortico-steroids from the start. The rationale for corticosteroid therapy derives from its anti-inflammatory affects, especially control of the polymorpho-nuclear action leading to preservation of ocular structure. In the majority of cases exact bacteriological and diagnosis is not possible and treatment must be empirical. The cardinal pre-requisite to successful therapy is a selection of antibiotics which are capable of covering all eventualities. Every possible root of administration should be used to maintain a high intraocular concentration of antibiotics throughout treatment. The systemically administered antibiotic should differ from those injected sub-conjunctively so as to allow a greater opportunity for the pathogens to be susceptible to at least one of them. Three antibiotics are recommended, Methicillin a semi-synthetic penicillin with a powerful anti-staphylococcal action penetrates well after sub-conjunctival injection. Sodium fusidate (Fucidin) is a powerful anti-staphylococcal antibiotic which acts synergistically with Methicillin in penicillin resistent strains. Gentamicin has a wide range of effectivity.

Therapeutic Regimen

1. *Subconjunctival therapy*
   a. Immediate:
   The conjunctival sac should be anaesthetised with 4% cocaine and adrenaline drops. Two separate injections are then given.
   (i) One injection, into the upper fornix, consists of methyl-prednisolone acetate (Depomedrone) 40 mg. This ensures an adequate concentration of cortico-steroid in the anterior chamber for up to four weeks.

   (ii) The other injection into the lower fornix consists of the following:
   gentamicin 20 mg (0.5 ml);
   methicillin, 150 mg which is prepared by dissolving 1 g in 1.5 ml of saline solution and using 0.2 ml.;
   mydricaine (atropine, adrenaline, and procaine), 0.3 ml.
   The total volume of the 'cocktail' is 1.0 ml.
   b. Subsequent injections consist of a mixture of:
   gentamicin 20 mg;
   methicillin, 150 mg;
   betamethasone (Betnesol) 4 mg (1.0 ml).
   They should be given at 24- or 48-hourly intervals, depending on the state of the conjunctiva and response to treatment. It is usually unnecessary to give more than four injections over eight days.

2. *Systemic therapy*
   sodium fusidate 400 mg three times a day orally for at least a week.
   prednisolone 10 mg four times a day orally for a week and then gradually reduced.

3. *Topical therapy*
   gentamicin drops hourly for two weeks and then reduced to four times a day for a further two weeks.
   dexamethasone or predsol drops hourly for two weeks and then four times a day until the anterior chamber shows no sign of activity.
   1% atropine drops four times a day.

In centres where vitrectomy is possible recovery from bacterial and fungal endophthalmitis is hastened by removal of the infected vitreous and the introduction of intra-vitreal antibiotics. The main factors influencing the visual outcome in such circumstances are the duration between the onset of infection and institution of therapy and the nature of the infecting organism.

Anterior chamber and vitreous tapping should be performed at once and samples inoculated into blood and chocolate agar plates and also into Saboudaud's media for fungi and thioglycolate for anaerobes. After a vitreous tap a single injection of 400 μg. of Gentamicin and 360 μg. of Dexamethasone is placed in the vitreous cavity. Systemic (intravenous) Gentamicin and topical antibiotics are given for three days. The optimum time for vitrectomy is 24 h after intravitreal injection of antibiotics if the culture proves positive. If a vitreous abscess, however, has formed when first seen an immediate vitrectomy should be undertaken and the same applies to suspected fungal infections. Vitrectomy infusion fluid contains 8 μg per ml of Gentamicin when the vitrophage is in action. In cases of fungal endophthalmitis an intravitreal injection of 5 μg of Amphotericin B is given after completion of vitrectomy.

As soon as it is evident that the eye cannot be saved it should be *excised* or, if there is any danger of the escape of pus during the operation, *eviscerated* (*q.v.*). In most cases a very satisfactory operation which allows more rapid healing than an evisceration and at the same time prevents a spread of the infection up the optic nerve sheath which might give rise to a meningitis, is a *frill excision* (*q.v.*) whereby a collar of sclera is left around the optic nerve.

Specific Types of Uveitis

The more important types of uveitis associated with specific infections will now be discussed.

Syphilis

This accounts for 1% cases in London and may attack any part of the uveal tract. The clinical manifestations of the infection are protean.

Syphilitic iritis. This manifests itself in two forms. A *simple plastic iritis* occurs typically in the secondary stage of the disease, soon after the skin eruptions, usually within the first year after infection, but not before the third month. Posterior synechiae occur between the stromal layer of the iris and the lens; the iritis lasts from two to eight weeks and does not usually recur. In the absence of early anti-syphilitic treatment it is seen in at least 3 to 4% of syphilitics, usually in males, and is generally unilateral, but the second eye may become affected later. The Wassermann reaction is of great value in settling the diagnosis; the *Treponema pallidum* has been found in the aqueous.

A plastic iritis also occurs in congenital syphilis, usually as an accompaniment of interstitial keratitis (*q.v.*). It also occurs in very young babies with congenital syphilis without any corneal complication, but usually with large nodules or gummata on the iris.

Finally, an acute plastic iritis may occur as a *Herxheimer reaction* twenty-four to forty-eight hours after the first therapeutic dose of penicillin, due probably to the flooding of the system with treponemal toxins.

Gummatous iritis. Occurs late in the secondary or rarely during the tertiary stage. These cases are characterized by the formation of yellowish-red, heavily vascularized nodules near the pupillary and ciliary borders of the iris, but not in the intermediate region; they are usually multiple and vary in size from that of a pin's head upwards and are generally associated with much exudation and broad synechiae.

Syphilitic choroiditis. May occur as disseminated choroiditis, peripheral choroiditis or as a diffuse lesion.

The patient is treated by systemic penicillin.

Gonorrhoea

Usually limits itself to the anterior uveal tract.

Gonorrhœal iritis. A very characteristic form may occur during the acute attack of the disease when the anterior chamber contains exudates which have a peculiar gelatinous appearance and a greenish-grey colour which is characteristic. It is a metastatic infection. Extension to the ciliary body may be indicated by fine vitreous opacities. The patients are almost always men, and as a rule both eyes are affected, although not at the same time. A less characteristic plastic form of iritis occurs especially in those cases which have gonorrhoeal 'rheumatism' and seldom supervenes until after an attack of arthritis, usually in the knees or hands. The iritis tends to recur persistently, sometimes associated with arthritis, and often many years after the first attack so that extensive synechiæ result.

Treatment. An intensive course of sulphonamides in full doses should be started at once and may well be supplemented by the local administration of penicillin or other antibiotic (Chap. 14).

Tuberculosis

Tuberculosis may affect any part of the uveal tract. It probably accounts for 1% of uveitis cases in developed countries.

T-cell activity is of significance in tuberculous infection. The ingestion of bacilli by macrophages is a major factor in limiting the spread of infection. In patients, however, who have had previous tuberculous infection, the cell-mediated response is also associated with tissue damage due to the direct effect of sensitized T-lymphocytes on cells containing ingested bacilli.

Tuberculous iritis. The metastatic granulomatous type occurs in a miliary and a conglomerate or solitary form. In the *miliary type* there is a yellowish-white nodule surrounded by numerous smaller satellites, usually situated near the pupillary or ciliary margin. This syndrome develops in severely debilitated patients with impaired immunological responsiveness and massive dissemination of bacilli.

Conglomerate tubercle. In this there is a yellowish-white tumour, although smaller satellites may be present; the nodules contain giant-cell systems.

Exudative type of iritis. This maybe tuberculous in origin, probably allergic in nature. Clinically there is little to distinguish it from other types of the disease. It is usually of a recurrent or very chronic nature with large 'mutton-fat' keratic precipitates (Fig. 18.2). Occasionally minute, translucent nodules appear on the surface of the iris, especially at the pupillary border (*Koeppe's nodules*). These used to be considered of some diagnostic significance.

Tuberculous choroiditis. Occurs in acute or miliary and chronic forms. Miliary tubercles are found in acute miliary tuberculosis, and especially in tuberculous meningitis, usually as a late event. Ophthalmoscopically they appear as round, pale yellow spots, usually near the disc, although any part of the choroid may be attacked Generally only three or four spots ar seen. They afford most important diagnostic evidence of tuberculosis in cases of meningitis and obscure general disease. Microscopically they consist of typical giant-cell systems, containing a variable number of tubercle bacilli. Until the introduction of chemotherapy in the disease, miliary tuberculosis of the choroid was usually a prelude to death, whereas now recovery is common.

The Mantoux dermal reaction is generally used for diagnostic purposes. A positive result is of little value except in children but, of course, does not prove that the ocular condition is tuberculous; but a negative result makes the diagnosis of allergic tuberculosis unlikely. Anergy to tuberculoprotein occurs in patients suffering from sarcoidosis. Hodgkin's disease and other immune deficiency states.

Treatment. Rifampicin with Isoniazid or Ethambutol (p. 109) is of great value.

Onchocerciasis

Onchocerciasis is due to infection with onchocerca volvulus a filarial nematode worm. Micro-filaria are mobile and may reach the eyes and when alive cause little or no reaction. Their death however, produces focal inflammation with reactive destruction of tissues. The vector is the blood sucking black fly Simulium.

The ocular features are microfilaria in the anterior chamber. In the choroid the vessels become attenuated and there is perivascular sheathing. Punctate or sclerosing keratitis is common in the cornea with anterior uveitis and optic atrophy.

Excision of the worm containing subcutaneous nodules may help to reduce the infection particularly if the nodules are close to the eye. Treatment is by Diethylcarbamazine which is effective against microfilariae and Suramin which is active against the adult worm. Patients however may suffer a severe adverse reaction if heavily infected and the treatment must last 2–5 months. Continuous non-pulsed delivery of Diethylcarbamazine at a critical low dosage may succeed in killing the microfilariae without exciting inflammatory reactions dangerous to the host. Transmission of O volvulus may be reduced by efficient larviciding to control the insect vector and is now being carried out in the Volta river basin.

Leprosy

Leprosy (Hansen disease) is caused by an acid-fast rod Mycobacterium leprae, similar to the agent that causes tuberculosis. There are about eleven million cases throughout the world, and about one third have eye complications. The infection involves predominantly the skin, superficial nerves, the nose and throat. It occurs as two principal types: (1) the lepromatous (cutaneous), with depressed cellular immunity and frequent ocular involvement, and (2) the tuberculoid (neural), with systemic resistance and ocular complications caused by neuroparalytic keratopathy (p. 136).

The eyes are usually involved late in the course of the lepromatous type of disease. There may be an initial superficial infection with conjunctivitis, episcleritis, or keratitis. Visual loss arises because of corneal and lens opacities associated with small non-reacting pupils and iris atrophy.

Patients with lepromatous leprosy have impaired cellular immunity and the tissues are laden with leprosy bacilli. Skin papules containing antigen-antibody complex to which the term erythema nodosum leprosum has been given are formed and it may be that the iridocyclitis is another manifestation of immune complex deposition.

In contrast to the lepromatous form uveitis is rare in tuberculoid leprosy and when it occurs it may represent an extension of the more frequent corneal involvement or be caused by the spread of infection along the ciliary nerves. Bacilli are scanty, antibody formation inconspicuous and the tissue lesions are characterised by multiple granulomata which may develop around peripheral nerves producing lagophthalmos and severe exposure keratitis in a cornea which has lost its protective mechanisms through involvement of the trigeminal nerve.

In the treatment of leprosy Dapsone is the drug of choice and the usual daily adult dose is 50–100 mg. Dapsone is a member of the Sulfone group.

Brucellosis (Undulant Fever; Malta Fever; Melitensis)

Infection by *Brucella* (*abortus*, *suis* or *melitensis*) is widespread throughout the world and among the many sites of its manifestations the eye may be affected. Initially there is an acute phase of generalized systemic infection; this is followed by a chronic phase characterized by intermittent bouts of low fever, late in which the ocular manifestations occur. Keratitis and optic neuritis are rare; a uveitis of a chronic granulomatous nature is more common (Fig. 18.1) The disease is prone to relapse and diagnosis can only be suggested from other forms of chronic iridocyclitis or choroiditis by an agglutination test, a cutaneous test, or an opsonocytophagic test. Treatment, apart from the usual measures, is by the sulphonamides or chlortetracycline.

Toxoplasmosis

This is a protozoan infection derived mainly from cats in the form of oocysts which affects both the retina and choroid to form a chorioretinitis; it is probable that in infants the primary seat is most commonly the retina which is involved in association with the brain. As a cause of uveitis toxoplasmosis probably accounts for 25% of all cases in the U.K.

In infants, in whom the infection frequently occurs in fetal life transmitted via the placenta, the ocular lesion is usually associated with an encephalitis, but although almost every tissue of the body may be affected, the retinal picture is so common and often so characteristic as to suggest the diagnosis. In the fundus there are bilateral and frequently multiple chorioretinal lesions, the macular area being particularly involved. The whole thickness of the retina and choroid is destroyed in a necrotizing inflammation so that a punched out, heavily pigmented scar remains; it is probable that many cases labelled congenital 'colobomata' due to intra-uterine inflammation have this ætiology. This lesion is frequently associated with well-marked meningeal changes of the same type. Such infants are usually acutely ill with a history of convulsions and, if they survive, may show hydrocephalus, areas of calcification in the brain, and mental retardation.

In adults toxoplasmic infection probably constitutes one of the more common causes of choroiditis (in Europe). The lesion is usually widespread and is characterised by severe recurrent attacks often at the edge of a previous scar associated with exudation into the vitreous (Fig. 18.4). Encysted trophozoites are insulated from the activities of the lymphoid system but periodic rupture of the cysts releases protozoa which then provoke a secondary immunological response. Possibly all cases of ocular toxoplasmosis are examples of congenital infection.

Pathologically the characteristic feature is a wide area of necrosis of the retina wherein the parasites may be found, either free or encysted. Apart from the demonstration of the parasite, diagnosis depends on sero-

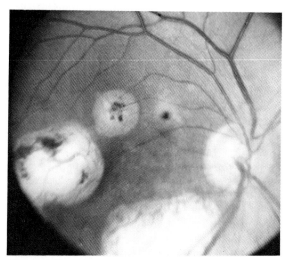

Fig. 18.4 Toxoplasmosis. Recurrent lesion alongside old scars (Perkins)

logical tests (the Sabin–Feldman test with a titre greater than 1 : 16 and the complement-fixation test). Corticosteroids are employed with sulphatriad (sulphadiazine, sulphathiazole and sulphamerazine) in a dosage of three 500 mg tablets every 6 h with 100 mg of pyrimethamine twice the first day and 25 mg daily thereafter. Added to this is 3 mg of citrovorum factor or folinic acid once weekly.

If medical measures fail photocoagulation may protect a threatened macula. An alternative medical attack consists of administrating clindomycin with sulphadiazine each of which operates on unrelated metabolic pathways of Toxoplasma and thus may act synergistically. Clindomycin is given in doses of one 200 mg tablet daily by mouth plus 4 gm of sulphadiazine for 4 weeks.

Sarcoidosis (benign lymphogranuloma)

Boeck's sarcoid is a systemic disease manifested by infiltration of the affected tissue by non-caseating tuberculoid granulomata which either resolve or are replaced by hyalinized scar tissue. It is frequently complicated by a granulomatous iridocyclitis. Uveitis may present as one of the following:

1. *Acute iridocyclitis*. This is often a presenting sign of sarcoidosis in association with hilar lymphadenopathy and erythema nodosum.

2. *Chronic iridocyclitis*. Multiple discrete granulomata develop in the iris in older individuals.

3. *Posterior uveitis*. Choroidal involvement may be associated with granulomata in the retina.

4. *Uveal parotid fever* or *Heerfordt's syndrome*.

Other features are conjunctival nodules in the lower fornix which are sarcoid granulomata; calcification of the cornea associated with hypercalcaemia and keratoconjunctivitis sicca.

The diagnosis is made from the presence of other systemic manifestations of the disease such as pulmonary changes and areas of rarefaction in the bones. Patients with sarcoidosis often fail to react to an intradermal injection of tuberculin indicating a disturbance of immune function. In the Kveim test the skin of patients with sarcoidosis responds to an injection of a suspension of sarcoid tissue by developing a localized granuloma. The course of the iridocyclitis is chronic and the prognosis poor.

Uveoparotitis (Heerfordt's disease)

This is a bilateral affection characterized by a simultaneous involvement of the entire uveal tract, the parotid gland and frequently of the cranial nerves. It appears in young people between ten and thirty years of age, commencing with malaise and fever, sometimes accompanied by a skin rash resembling erythema nodosum. Approximately half the cases commence with a granulomatous iridocyclitis and half with a painful swelling of the parotid resembling that due to mumps; subsequently diplopia due to palsy of the ocular motor nerves or facial paralysis is prone to occur. The disease is self-limiting although the iridocyclitis may cause permanent visual damage; the parotid swellings last for six weeks to two years but also ultimately subside.

Cytomegalo-virus retinitis is characterized by grayish patches or scattered white dots with irregular sheathing of adjacent blood vessels and vitreous clouding. There are superimposed haemorrhages followed by healing along with retinal atrophy. Cytomegalic viraemia is common in renal transplant patients but ocular infection is rare. When it does occur it may produce an acute cytomegalic necrotizing retinitis with irreversible damage and loss of vision. The retina may already be compromised by vascular hypertension. Although the inflammation is self-limiting effective therapy is not available.

In children, infantile cytomegalovirus disease may produce severe brain damage with mental deficiency. The ocular lesion varies from an isolated central retinal lesion to a chorio-retinitis with much disorganization of the globe.

Recurrent iridocyclitis with hypopyon (Behçet's syndrome)
This is a serious condition wherein a severe iridocyclitis usually characterized by a hypopyon is associated with evidence of an obliterative vasculitis with an immunological basis. It is accompanied by ulcerative lesions in the conjunctival, oral and genital mucosae, together with neurological and articular manifestations. It is seen particularly in young adults, and recurs periodically and persistently in attacks of extreme severity so that eventually vision is usually seriously impaired or lost. The syndrome is regarded as belonging to the broad category of connective tissue disorders but it is conceivable that there are two types: the first associated with herpetiform ulcers in the mouth and the second with aphthous ulcers without evidence of an infective basis. Alternatively the syndrome may be initiated by a viral infection and be perpetuated by autoimmune phenomena. There is a significant association with HLA-B5. No specific treatment is known so that non-specific measures only are available such as systemic steroids or preferably oral administration of Chlorambucil 6–8 mg daily for at least a year.

Ankylosing spondylitis and uveitis
Ankylosing spondylitis is a chronic progressive disorder involving the sacro-iliac and the posterior inter-vertebral joints. The onset is insidious with intermittent attacks of pain. Males in the third decade are more frequently affected than females. There is a strong association with HLA-B27.

Acute recurrent irido-cyclitis is part of the syndrome and these attacks may recur. The disease lasts 10–20 years and usually burns itself out. Twenty-five percent of patients suffer from irido-cyclitis so that young males presenting with this ocular disorder should be X-rayed for evidence of axial skeletal involvement.

Reiter's disease and uveitis
This syndrome is also associated with a high incidence of HLA-B27 antigen and affects young males. It tends to affect patients who present with non-specific urethritis, post-gonococcal urethritis or dysentry. Chlamydia has been isolated from urethral discharge in some 50% of cases. There is an association with dysentry due to Shigella Flexneri and it is possible that the Shigella antigen may produce an auto-hypersensitivity in patients who have B27 antigens.

The urethritis associated with Reiter's disease demands administration of Tetracycline orally in a dosage of 500 mg four times a day and it is essential that all sexual partners should be examined for genital infection.

Erythema multiforme (Stevens–Johnson syndrome)
Erythema multiforme is an acute inflammatory polymorphic skin disease which may follow infections such as herpes simplex or other virus diseases in children and the young or the use of drugs in adults. The onset is abrupt with fever followed by a maculopapular rash with vesicles and bullae on the skin and an ulcerative stomatitis and conjunctivits may ensue. The eyes are affected by bilateral catarrhal or pseudomembranous conjunctivitis and in severe cases there may be corneal ulcers and uveitis.

Uveitis associated with vitiligo, poliosis and deafness (the Vogt – Koyanagi syndrome)
This is a rare condition occurring in young adults. The iridocyclitis is chronic and is associated with an exudative choroiditis which often leads to an exudative detachment of the retina. The ocular inflammation is accompanied by a patchy depigmentation of the skin and the hair, the eyebrows and lashes also whitening (poliosis). *Harada's disease* is a closely related condition affecting mainly the choroid and complicated by an exudative detachment of the retina. The cause is unknown but may be viral associated with a secondary immune response.

Heterochromic Iridocyclitis of Fuchs
This is a low-grade chronic cyclitis the only apparent features of which are a lightening of the colour of the affected iris and the presence of a few keratic precipitates on the cornea: the latter distinguish the condition from congenital heterochromia (p. 169). This iris becomes atrophic, loses its markings and readily transilluminates in circumscribed areas, and a cataract frequently develops. The condition is usually said to be associated with some disturbance of the sympathetic

nerve supply; this nerve controls the chromatophores accounting for the depigmentation, as well as the tone of the blood-vessels, so that, in their dilated condition, white cells escape and become deposited on the cornea as precipitates. The cataract has a good operative prognosis, but secondary glaucoma may develop.

Fungal uveitis
Fungal uveitis due to candida albicans is an example of the opportunistic fungi which normally reside on mucous membranes and are not pathogenic. Chorioretinitis with infiltration into the vitreous may be produced by haematogenous spread from the alimentary tract although involvement of the external eye is the predominant manifestation.

Ocular histoplasma syndrome
Disciform lesions at the macula (Fig. 18.5A and B) accompanied by well circumscribed peripheral chorioretinal scars, in the absence of inflammatory signs in the aqueous and vitreous and associated with peri-papillary pigment epithelial atrophy form a characteristic picture occurring in the young and carrying the risk of bilateral central visual loss.

Epidemiologically this syndrome has been related to *H. capsulatum* infection. High incidence of a positive skin reactivity to histoplasma in young patients with disciform macular disease was found in certain areas of North America, particularly the Ohio and Mississippi river basins. Presumed ocular histoplasmosis occurs in the United Kingdom suggesting that other ætiological agents are capable of producing this pattern of ocular fundus disease. When the second macula is threatened it may be possible to halt the progress of the disciform degenerative process by the use of the argon laser.

Measles
This is caused by a paramyxovirus and during the acute phase of the infection visual impairment may be noted and recovery may be followed by residual pigmentary retinal disturbance.

Rarely children who have recovered develop subacute sclerosising panencephalitis. There is permanent loss of vision and pigmentary changes in the retina especially at the macular area. It is possible that SSPE is a slow virus infection wherein the acute phase of measles is followed by persistence of the virus in the brain and retina causing gradual destruction of the non-replicating neuronal cells.

Sympathetic Ophthalmitis, see p. 252.

Routine investigation of uveitis
A limited number of known aetiological factors account for a considerable proportion of cases of uveitis and the problem frequently arises as to which initial investigations, in conjunction with the clinical findings are justifiable and likely to help in a diagnosis.

Anterior uveitis
About 50% of patients with acute anterior uveitis possess HLA-B27. Uveitis is associated with ankylosing spondylitis or Reiter's syndrome in a high proportion of men but overt systemic symptoms are rare in women. The relevant investigations are examination of the urine for WBCs, and X-rays of sacro-iliac joints and lumbar spine. If the urine is abnormal, further urogenital inves-

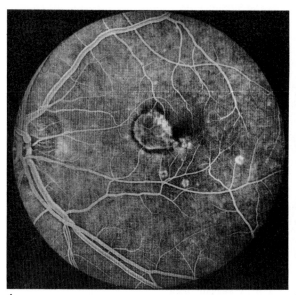 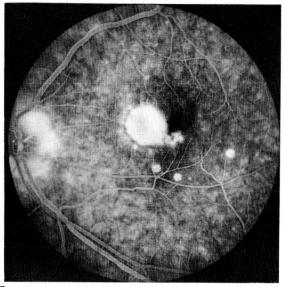

A B
Fig. 18.5 Histoplasmosis of the macula: A. Early fluorescein angiogram; B. Late fluorescein angiogram

tigation is indicated. The ESR and C-reactive protein may be raised.

Sarcoidosis and secondary syphilis may cause an acute anterior uveitis, and if a rheumatic cause has been excluded a chest X-ray and serological tests are indicated.

Chronic anterior uveitis

Heterochromic uveitis should be recognised by the clinical features. Translucent keratic precipitates, posterior polar lens changes and vitreous disturbance should suggest this diagnosis. There are no known pathological investigations of value.

Chronic anterior uveitis in children suggests Still's disease, although the joint changes may be minimal. Anti-nuclear antibody is present in approximately 70% of cases.

A chronic anterior uveitis with nodules on the iris is suggestive of sarcoidosis and these signs are usually accompanied by exudates in the vitreous and perivasculitis. The relevant investigations are a chest X-ray for enlarged hilar glands and a Mantoux test which will be negative or only positive in a low dilution.

Toxoplasmosis never causes a pure anterior uveitis but a severe recurrence of choroiditis, particularly if the lesion is in the periphery of the fundus, may be accompanied by keratic precipitates and posterior synechiae.

Acute posterior uveitis

A focal choroiditis adjacent to a pigmented scar is diagnostic of toxoplasmosis and serological tests are only indicated if the clinical picture is atypical.

Chronic posterior uveitis

Pars planitis is a condition of unknown aetiology and there are no diagnostic investigations likely to indicate the cause. Toxocariasis causes a granulomatous lesion at the posterior pole or in the periphery of the retina of one eye. The patient is usually a child with a history of contact with domestic animals. A blood count may show a low degree of eosinophilia and the toxocaral skin test will be positive. The serum 1gE may be raised.

These initial investigations are summarized in Table 18.1.

DEGENERATIVE CHANGES IN THE UVEAL TRACT

Degenerative changes in the iris

Depigmentation of the iris with atrophy of the stroma is seen in old people and, indeed, is a constant senile phenomenon. Depigmentation of the pupillary margin is common and may occur in the form of small triangular patches or radial fissures. Irregular lacunæ in the pigmentary epithelium may often be seen with transillumination, either with the slit-lamp or by contact illumination.

Essential (progressive) atrophy of the iris is a disease of unknown ætiology characterized by a slowly progressive atrophic change in the tissues of the iris which leads to the complete disappearance of large portions of this tissue. The disease usually starts insidiously in early adult life by the development of large areas of atrophy which coalesce and progress to the formation of lacunæ. Vision is eventually lost by the gradual onset of glaucoma due to down-growth of an endothelial membrane over the tissues at the angle of the anterior chamber. Contraction of the membrane produces synechiae, corectopia, iris atrophy from ischaemia, ectropion uveae and iris nodules. The prognosis is poor; but fortunately the disease is usually unilateral (Fig. 18.6).

Iridoschisis is a rare condition which occurs most commonly as a degenerative senile phenomenon although it may follow as a late result of severe trauma. Large dehiscences appear on the anterior mesodermal layer of the iris and strands of this tissue may float into the anterior chamber as if teased out by a needle; occasionally extensive areas of this layer may become detached. Treatment is unsatisfactory, although the secondary glaucoma induced responds to surgical decompression.

Degenerative changes in the choroid

Degenerative conditions are more frequent and more

Type of uveitis	Possible aetiology	Investigations
Acute anterior	'Rheumatism'	Urine for WBCs. X-ray S.I. Joints. ESR. C-reactive Protein.
	Sarcoidosis	Chest X-ray. Mantoux.
	Secondary syphilis	Serological tests.
Chronic anterior	Heterochromic uveitis	Gonioscopy
	Still's disease	Antinuclear antibody
	Sarcoidosis	Chest X-ray. Mantoux.
Acute posterior	Toxoplasmosis	Serology if appearance equivocal.
Chronic posterior	Pars planitis	None of value
	Toxocariasis	Eosinophil count. Skin test. Serum 1 gE.

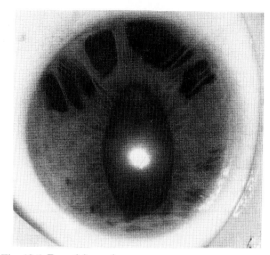

Fig. 18.6 Essential atrophy

important in the posterior than the anterior part of the uveal tract. They may be post-inflammatory or primary.

Secondary degenerations following inflammatory lesions culminating in localized spots of complete atrophy have already been considered. The loss of nourishment to the retina causes atrophy of the outer layers and migration of pigment from the pigment epithelium into the more superficial parts of the retina. The pigment tends to become deposited in the perivascular spaces of the veins, so that the retinal veins may be mapped out here and there by pigment. More noticeable ophthalmoscopically are jet-black branched spots of pigment resembling bone corpuscles, and standing out in sharp relief, an appearance seen in its most typical form in pigmentary

retinal dystrophy (*q.v*). An almost identical picture, although usually without the characteristic distribution of the pigmented spots, may result from choroidal atrophy due to other causes such as syphilis.

Primary choroidal degenerations may be localized or general the localized forms are usually central although circumpapillary changes around the disc are not in frequent in myopia (*q.v.*) or the late stages of glaucoma.

Central choroidal atrophy is most commonly the result of myopia or obliterative vasosclerosis, essentially an age change.

Myopic choroido-retinal degeneration. We have already seen that in pathological axial myopia degenerative changes are common, particularly marked around the optic disc and in the central area of the fundus involving the choroid and retina. These changes are not due to the mechanical effects of stretching but are primary in nature and in their incidence genetic factors play a prominent part. They have been erroneously described as 'myopic choroiditis' but the condition is not inflammatory. They do not run parallel to the degree of myopia and tend to occur after mid-adult life whereas the elongation of the eye is a phenomenon characteristic of the latter part of the first and the second decades. They probably involve both the ectodermal (retinal) and mesodermal (choroidal and scleral) tissues; but since from the clinical point of view the atrophic changes in the retina are secondary to those in the choroid, the entire clinical picture will be considered here. This includes atrophic changes in the sclera, around the disc, in the choroid and retina in the central area and in the peripheral parts of the retina.

In the majority of cases of moderate myopia there is a

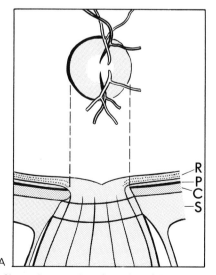
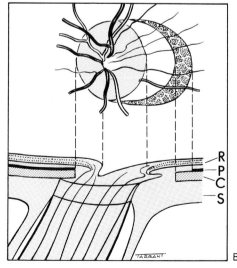

Fig. 18.7 A Shows the normal configuration of the optic disc. B The myopic disc. R, retina; P, pigmentary epithelium; C, choroid; S, sclera. On the temporal side the choroidal and scleral crescents are delineated. Note the oblique temporal direction of the optic nerve fibres and the overlapping on the nasal side resulting in supertraction

myopic crescent (Plate 5, Fig. D). This is a white crescent at the temporal border of the disc; very rarely it is nasal. In higher degrees of myopia it may extend to the upper and lower borders, or a complete ring may be formed around the disc.

The cause of the myopic crescent has given rise to much discussion; it may be absent in high myopia and is often present in low, and is essentially atrophic and not merely due to stretching. It is probably congenital in origin, allied to other congenital crescents (p. 230). Anatomically there is considerable distortion of the disc; on the temporal side the pigment epithelium stops short at a variable distance from the disc and here the choroid is atrophic (Fig. 18.7A and B). In well marked cases the retina, including the pigment epithelium, encroaches over the nasal edge of the disc (supertraction crescent).

The atrophic thinning of the sclera is confined to its posterior half in which region this structure may be very attenuated.

Atrophic changes in the choroid (*myopic choroido-retinal atrophy*) occur mainly in the central area of the fundus (Plate 5, Fig. E). There is a gradual disappearance of the small vessels of the choroid with the development of lacunæ making irregular areas of atrophy which may extend to the region of the disc where they may eventually fuse with each other and with the myopic crescent so as to form an irregular circumpapillary ring. Small hæmorrhages are not uncommon in the macular area and occasionally choroidal thromboses; the latter may give rise to the sudden formation of a circular claret-coloured or black spot at the fovea which may persist (*Fuchs's fleck*). These changes are associated with an atrophy of the overlying retina and involve considerable loss of visual acuity; this tends to be progressive and a central scotoma may result. At the same time the retinal pigmentary epithelium becomes depigmented over most of the fundus so that the choroidal vessels are well seen.

Degenerative changes at the periphery of the retina are also common, typically those of cystoid degeneration (*q.v.*). These may lead to the formation of retinal holes resulting in a detachment of this tissue. Degenerative changes also occur in the vitreous which turns fluid with a breakdown of its colloid structure so that dusty opacities or large membrane-like 'floaters' are formed.

These atrophic changes are one of the commonest causes of grave visual disability; treatment is ineffective.

Senile central choroidal atrophy.

This assumes two chief forms. In central guttate choroidal atrophy (Tay's 'choroiditis') there are numerous minute yellowish white spots in the macular region They are usually round, but the larger spots may have crenated edges, thus showing signs of fusion. There may be indefinite signs of greyish pigmentation of their edges due to the fact that the pigmentary epithelium is stretch-

ed over them. The spots are due to peculiar hyaline excrescences on the surface of the choroid, commonly known as *colloid bodies* or *drusen* (Plate 3, Fig. A); they are of the same nature as Bruch's membrane, and like it are secreted by the pigmented epithelial cells. They are a precurser of disciform macular degeneration in some eyes. The condition is bilateral but causes little impairment of vision.

Central areolar choroidal atrophy (*sclerosis*). Appears as a large circular or oval patch of degeneration in the macular region in which the choroidal vessels are visible owing to atrophy of the retinal pigment epithelium (Plate 5, Fig. A). As a result of the atrophy of the choroid the sclera shines through and the patch appears white, although traversed by choroidal vessels. Only the larger choroidal vessels are seen, the smaller ones having disappeared, and even the large ones may appear smaller than usual owing to degeneration of their walls when they may appear densely white and sclerotic. There is an absolute central scotoma. Occasionally the degeneration progresses slowly to involve most of the fundus. This form of central atrophy is genetically determined.

Geographical choroidopathy

This is a distinct clinical entity in which there are acute, well defined lesions affecting the pigment epithelium. During the evolution of the lesion, which occurs over several months, there is no change in its shape or size. The disease progresses over several years and is characterised by the occurrence of further acute lesions. The earliest changes consist of yellowish-grey areas at the level of the pigment epithelium associated with some swelling of the overlying retina but no inflammatory cells in the vitreous. Fluorescein angiography reveals relative hypofluorescence corresponding with the grey lesion. Over the next three months pigment epithelial and retinal swellings subside and the centre of the lesion takes on a grey appearance and the margin a lighter colour. Fluorescein angiography at this stage shows a relative hyper-fluorescence at the margin of the lesion, whilst the centre of the lesion remains hypo-fluorescent. After a further three months fluorescein studies show uniform hyper-fluorescence of the lesion lasting throughout the angiogram. Old lesions show atrophy of the pigment epithelium and chorio-capillaris leaving the larger choroidal vessels. The margin of the lesion is clearly defined with regular hyper-pigmentation. The ætiology is unknown. The differential diagnosis is from total choroidal sclerosis, placoid pigment epitheliopathy, pigment epitheliitis and serpiginous choroidopathy.

Serpiginous choroiditis. This is a descriptive name for insidious disseminated choroiditis characterized by multiple, confluent foci of exudate and scar formation affecting especially the superficial portion of the choroid. Fluorescein angiographic and histological studies reveal disappearance of the chorio-capillaris and of the pigment epithelium. Ophthalmoscopy shows small greyish disc-like or circular confluent lesions and choroidal scars with slight pigment dispersion leading to depigmentation in a serpiginous configuration. The macula is frequently involved.

There is some evidence of an immunological ætiology. Therapy consists of tuberculo-static drugs alone or in combination with Prednisone. Antimetabolites may be indicated in cases where the macula is threatened such as Cytosine Arabinoside and Azathioprine.

Acute retinal pigment epitheliitis. The condition is characterised by an acute onset with fairly rapid resolution in six to 12 weeks and ultimate recovery to normal vision. The typical lesion is a dark greyish spot which in the acute stage and sometimes afterwards is well defined. It is surrounded by a pale halo-like area. They form in two or four clusters in the macular area and may be unilateral or bilateral. The intervening retina is normal. Fluorescein findings are minimal in the acute stage but hyper-fluorescence corresponding to the initial halo-like zone can eventually be seen.

Acute posterior multi-focal placoid pigment epitheliopathy
This disease affects both eyes in healthy subjects of either sex between the age of 20 and 30 years of age. Spontaneous resolution with good visual recovery is usual.

The primary site of the lesion is at the level of the chorio-capillaris resulting in focal swelling of the retinal pigment epithelial cells and giving rise to the characteristic ophthalmoscopic appearance of cream coloured placoid lesions over the posterior pole within the equatorial region. Fluorescein angiography shows patchy irregular choroidal filling, gradually outlining these lesions which mask the background fluorescence. Each area is stained with fluorescein during the later stages without significant leakage of dye. Upper respiratory symptoms, altered sensitivity to drugs and increased gamma globulin favours a viral or an immune complex mechanism. The differential diagnosis is between multi-focal choroiditis, primary retinal pigment epithelial detachment and acute epitheliitis. Rapid loss of central vision is common followed by prompt resolution of the lesions with significant visual improvement continuing several weeks after the apparent ophthalmoscopic improvement. There is permanent alteration in the retinal pigment epithelium and minimal changes in the chorio-capillaris.

Senile macular degeneration. Much more commonly, minute changes limited to the area at and immediately around the fovea occur in old people and lead to grave disturbance or abolition of central vision. It is generally necessary to dilate the pupil in order that they may be seen. In the early stage the fovea is surrounded by a ring of very fine pigment spots. The stippling is more sharply defined on the foveal side, which usually has a circular or crenated edge, and diminishes rapidly peripherally, where the fundus becomes normal. The fovea gradually becomes paler in colour and the stippling denser, the change being associated with gradually increasing failure of vision, until eventually the small central scotoma becomes absolute. Both eyes are affected, but one is usually attacked before the other which may not be involved for many months. In the majority of cases the atrophy is due to an obliterative sclerosis of the small vessels in the subjacent chorio-capillaris.

Disciform degeneration at the macular (Junius–Kuhnt's disease). In early disciform degeneration the pigment epithelium becomes separated from Bruch's membrane, and blood vessels grow into this space from the chorio-capillaries through breaks in the membrane. Both the detachment of the pigment epithelium and the abnormal blood vessels can be identified by fluorescein angiography. Commonly the abnormal capillaries bleed and the overlying neuroretina may show cystic macular œdema and serous detachment. Eventually the vascular complex fibroses and gives rise to the classical picture of senile disciform macular degeneration (Fig. 18.8).

The patient usually presents with visual loss in one eye due to an advanced stage of this disease. The other eye may be only slightly affected visually at the stage of pigment epithelial detachment or at the stage of development of new vessels provided the latter have remained intact and have not given rise to hæmorrhage. Treatment is often effective by the argon laser by destroying the delicate neovascularisation before hæmorrhage ensues. This method allows exact localisation and treatment by a beam of light with a diameter as small as 50 μm.

Essential (gyrate) atrophy of the choroid. This is a condition due to defective activity of the enzyme ornithine ketoacid aminotransferase and is an inborn error of amino-acid metabolism characterised by hyperornithinæmia and progressive atrophy of the choroid, the pigment epithelium and the retina, starting usually with patchy distribution in early adult life, at first in irregular areas which coalesce so that in the final stages practically all the fundus has disappeared, with preservation only of the macula.

Choroideremia. This resembles the terminal stage of gyrate atrophy although it lacks the fine, dense, velvet-like pigmentation so typical of gyrate atrophy in the late stages. The condition is a hereditary degeneration and the most prominent symptoms are night-blindness and extreme concentric contraction of the visual fields.

Treatment. The treatment of these degenerative diseases which involve a dry scattering of pigment is unsatisfactory. In the types of degeneration, however,

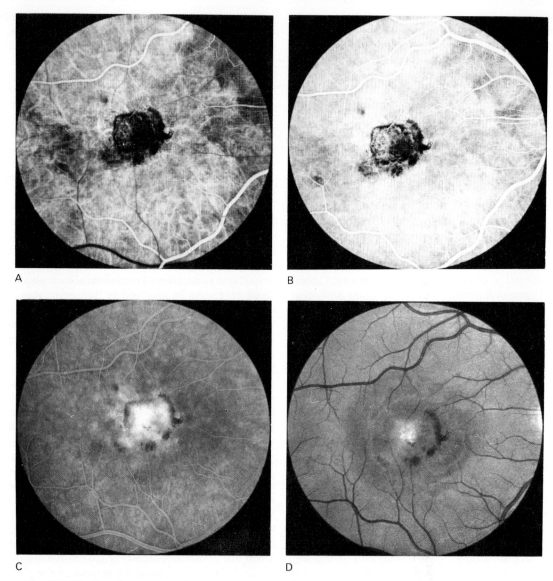

Fig. 18.8 Disciform Degeneration of the Macula. A, B and C are fluorescein angiograms; D is a fundus photograph

involving a separation of the pigment epithelium and neovascularisation the argon laser may prove useful. The patient should be assured that peripheral vision will not become affected, so that, although unable to read or do fine work, he will always be able to see sufficiently well to get about freely. In the early stages reading is facilitated by the use of a magnifying reading aid (p. 58).

Detachment of the choroid

The choroid is often apparently detached from the sclera in eyes which have been lost by plastic iridocyclitis or glaucoma, and this may also result from severe hæmor-

rhage or a new growth. These cases cannot be diagnosed clinically. The condition also not uncommonly occurs during the first days following intra-ocular operations owing to the great vasodilatation and exudation into the outer lamellæ of the choroid which follow the sudden lowering of the intra-ocular pressure. The anterior chamber is shallow and on ophthalmoscopic examination the detached choroid is seen through the pupil as a dark mass; it may also be visible as a dark brown mass by oblique illumination. The prognosis is usually good, the choroid becoming replaced and the anterior chamber reestablished. Occasionally, however, the tension of the eye remains low, and if the iris remains long in contact with the cornea at the angle of the anterior chamber, peripheral synechiae may form so that an obstructive glaucoma may eventually develop. In such circumstances it is well to ensure that the wound or the conjunctival flap is not leaking; if it is it should be reconstituted, if necessary by a conjuctival flap from above. In recalcitrant cases in which the choroidal detachment shows no evidence of subsiding, drainage of the subchoroidal fluid through a diathermy puncture at the most prominent region of the detachment has been suggested while the administration of acetazolamide has sometimes proved useful.

CONGENITAL ABNORMALITIES OF THE UVEAL TRACT

One iris may have a different colour from the other (*heterochromia iridum*), or parts of the same iris, usually a sector, may differ in colour from the remainder (*heterochromia iridis*). The blue iris is due to the absence of pigment in the iris stroma, the pigment in the retinal epithelium being seen through the translucent stroma.

The iris often shows patches of brown pigmentation; these *benign melanomata* are due to abnormal groups of pigmented cells lying in the posterior layers of the stroma

The pupil is normally slightly to the inner side of the centre of the cornea. In some cases it is considerably displaced, usually also to the nasal side — *corectopia* (κόρη, pupil, ἐκ, out of, τόπος, place). Rarely there are other holes in the iris besides the pupil — *polycoria*.

The iris may be apparently absent — *aniridia* or *irideremia* — a condition which is usually bilateral; there is, however, a narrow rim persistent at the ciliary border, but it is hidden from view during life by the sclera. On examination the ciliary processes and the suspensory ligament of the lens can be seen. There is a tendency for secondary glaucoma to develop due to the abnormal structure of the angle of the anterior chamber.

Persistent pupillary membrane
This is due to the continued existence of part of the anterior vascular sheath of the lens, a fetal structure which normally disappears shortly before birth. Fine threads stretch across the pupil, or may be anchored down to the lens capsule. They are distinguished from post-inflammatory synechiæ in always coming from the anterior surface on the iris just outside the pupillary margin, from the position of the circulus iridis minor. Such tags are of frequent occurrence and are of no pathological importance. They are commonest in babies and probably undergo some absorption as age advances, but many persist permanently. Examination with the slit-lamp shows that minute remnants of the pupillary membrane are very common even in adults.

The fetal pupillary membrane consists of a network of small blood vessels supported by a very delicate stroma which contains pigment cells. Sometimes the pigment is left on the lens surface and persists. It forms a stippling of very fine brown dots scattered over a circular area of 5 or 6 mm in diameter in the centre of the pupil. These spots are distinguished from the pigment spots left by posterior synechiæ which have broken down (p. 152) in being much smaller, stellate in shape when magnified under the slit-lamp, much more numerous and regularly arranged, and also by the absence of any concomitant signs of iritis. They do not usually interfere with vision.

Colobomata
Colobomata form one of the commonest congenital malformations of the eye (but are nevertheless rare) in which the tissues of the uvea and the associated retinal tissues or their prolongation onto the back of the iris are badly developed, or deficient. As a rule they are due to defective closure of the embryonic cleft (p. 1) in which case they occur in the lower part of the eye (*typical colobomata*). A *coloboma of the iris* may involve this tissue only, when it is usually pear-shaped, the deficiency extending from the pupil towards, but not always as far as, the ciliary body, usually running downwards and slightly inwards. Colobomata of the iris found in other directions are called *atypical*. (Fig. 18.9) A coloboma of the iris may be associated with a similar *coloboma of the choroid and retina*, or the latter condition may occur alone.

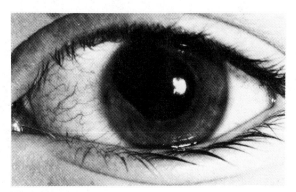

Fig 18.9 Atypical colomboma of the iris

A typical coloboma of the fundus appears as an oval or comet-shaped defect with the rounded apex towards the disc, which may or may not be included. A few vessels are seen over the surface, some retinal, others derived from the choroid at the edges. The surface is often depressed irregularly (ectatic coloboma). The central vision is generally bad, and there is a scotoma in the field corresponding more or less accurately to the coloboma, although this usually contains some retinal elements near the edges.

Albinism

This is a hereditary condition in which there is a defective development of pigment throughout the body. It is divided into ocular, oculo-cutaneous and cutaneous forms, the first being subdivided further on the basis of the tyrosinase test. Owing to absence of pigment in the eye the iris looks pink and the patients suffer from dazzling. Nystagmus, photophobia, and defective vision are usually present and occasionally strabismus. With the ophthalmoscope the retinal and choroidal vessels are seen with great clarity, separated by glistening white spaces where the sclera shines through (Plate 4, Fig. A). Microscopic examination has shown that total albinism is extremely rare, as traces of pigment have always been found in the retinal epithelium.

Partial albinism is commoner, wherein the absence of pigment is limited to the choroid and retina, the irides being blue. The macular regions are pigmented and may therefore look normal. People with dark hair sometimes have relatively slight pigmentation in the periphery of the fundus so that the choroidal vessels are seen: these patients will be found to have had fair hair as children.

Treatment consists in the use of tinted glasses as a protection from glare.

Cysts of the iris

Serous cysts of the iris sometimes occur and are due to closure of iris crypts with the retention of fluid. *Cysts of the posterior epithelium* occur, due to accumulation of fluid between the two layers of retinal epithelium. They look like an iris bombé limited to parts of the circumference — a limitation which is impossible in the case of true iris bombé (*q.v.*). In these cases the posterior layer of epithelium is often adherent to the lens. *Implantation of epithelium* into the iris sometimes occurs after perforating wounds or operations, giving rise to pearl cysts. When such wounds heal badly the corneal epithelium may occasionally spread over the iris and line the whole anterior chamber, causing glaucoma. Such cases are not true implantation cysts. Eyelashes are sometimes carried into the anterior chamber in perforating wounds and, lodging upon the iris, may be associated with cysts formed by the proliferation of the epithelium of their root-sheaths.

Tumours of the uveal tract
See Chapter 25.

19

The lens

Being composed entirely of epithelium surrounded by a capsule, the lens is incapable of becoming inflamed. Some of its fibres, however, are frequently poorly developed and degenerative changes occurring during life are common. Either of these conditions leads to a loss of transparency in the parts affected. As a general rule, developmental opacities are partial and stationary, acquired opacities progressive until the entire lens is involved. Any opacity in the lens or its capsule whether developmental or acquired, is called *cataract*.

Care, however, should be taken in using this term clinically since it often excites anxiety which may be entirely unjustified. This applies particularly to the stationary types of opacity; and it is to be remembered that even in senile cataract the opacities may remain localised for years without causing serious disability, or sometimes without being suspected. It is often wise (and kind), therefore, to tell such patients that they have 'lens opacities' and, if pressed, to suggest that the development of cataract may be long delayed and can be dealt with adequately should the need ever arise.

DEVELOPMENT CATARACT

Developmental cataract assumes the most variegated forms and is common in its minor manifestations; indeed, the lenses of most people show minute points of opacity of this type when examined with the beam of the slit-lamp under full mydriasis. We have seen (p. 11) that the lens is formed in layers, the central nucleus being the earliest formation, around which concentric zones are subsequently laid down, the process continuing until late adolescence (Fig. 1.9). Developmental cataract has therefore a tendency to affect the particular zone which was being formed when this process was disturbed; the fibres laid down previously and subsequently are often normally formed and remain clear. As time goes on, such an opacity is thus usually deeply buried in the substance of the lens by the subsequent formation of normal fibres. Developmental cataract thus tends to follow the architectural pattern of the lens and from its location

an estimate can be made of the stage of development at which the anomaly occurred.

What the deleterious influences may be which may cause such developmental anomalies are yet largely unknown. Maternal (and infantile) malnutrition is certainly one, as in zonular cataract; maternal infections by viruses another, as in rubella: deficient oxygenation owing to placental hæmorrhages possibly a third. Such cataracts tend to be stationary, although progressive opacification of a senile type may occur earlier than is usual. From the functional point of view, most of them are of little or no significance unless they are considerable in size and central in position.

Among the many morphological types the following are the most common.

Punctate cataract

This is the most common manifestation and in minute degree is almost universal in occurrence. When the small opaque spots are multiple and scattered all over the lens, appearing as tiny blue dots by oblique illumination with the slit-lamp, they are known as *cataracta cœrulea*, or *blue-dot cataract*; when crowded in the Y-sutures, the terms *sutural cataract* and *anterior axial embryonic cataract* have been applied. None of these is of significance.

Fusiform cataract, also called *spindle-shaped, axial,* or *coralliform,* is an antero-posterior spindle-shaped opacity, sometimes with offshoots giving an appearance much resembling coral: it is genetically determined and shows a tendency to occur in families. *Discoid cataract* is also a familial form, showing a somewhat ill-defined disc of opacity just behind the nucleus in the posterior cortex.

When the development of the lens has been inhibited at a very early stage, the central nucleus remains opaque — (*embryonal*) *nuclear cataract*. Ordinarily this is of little significance.

A progressive type of congenital cataract, originally nuclear, is associated with the occurrence of *rubella* (German measles) in the mother if the infection is contracted in the second and sometimes in the third month of pregnancy. The virus reaches the fetus before it has developed an immunological defence mechanism so that extensive cellular parasitism occurs.

Rubella is a mild contagious disease with skin eruptions beginning on the face and neck, spreading to the trunk and extremities, and fading in 3 days. There may be pharyngitis and post-auricular adenopathy, with slight fever.

The virus interferes with the translation of DNA to RNA. Pathologically the nucleus is found to be necrotic and the whole lens becomes opaque. Aspiration of the cataract may be followed by a chronic endophthalmitis associated with residual lens matter. There may be an accompanying retinitis which appears as a fine pigmentary deposit at the posterior pole. Other congenital anomalies occur in association with the cataract, particularly congenital heart disease (patent ductus arteriosus), microphthalmos, micrencephaly, mental retardation, deafness and dental anomalies. The frequency of this combination with maternal rubella contracted about the second month of pregnancy raises the question of the advisability of exposing to infection intending mothers who have not had the disease, or the more serious question of abortion if such an illness develops at this crucial stage in pregnancy. The possibility of other viruses traversing the placental barrier is still a matter of conjecture.

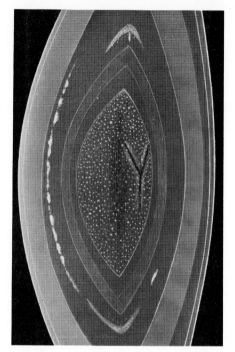

Fig. 19.1 Central pulverulent cataract with zonular opacities in post-adult nucleus

Zonular cataract

Here, development has been interfered with at a later stage and an area around the embryonic nucleus becomes opacified, its extent depending on the duration of the inhibiting factor. The opacity is usually sharply demarcated and the area of the lens within and around the opaque zone is clear, although linear opacities like spokes of a wheel (called *riders*) may run out-wards towards the equator. Occasionally two such rings of opacity are seen. Such cataracts are usually bilateral and if, as is frequently the case, they are formed just before or shortly after birth they may be of sufficient diameter to fill the pupillary aperture when the pupil is undilated; they may thus affect vision (Fig. 19.1).

Such zonular cataracts may have a genetic origin with a strong hereditary tendency of the dominant type. On the other hand, they may be due to a period of malnutrition at some stage of late intrauterine or early infantile life. Lack of vitamin D is apparently a potent factor and evidence of rickets may be found in affected children. This deficiency inhibits the development of other epithelial structures, particularly the enamel of the permanent teeth which is being formed at the time; the permanent incisors and canines particularly have an eroded appearance with transverse lines across them.

Coronary cataract

This represents the same type of developmental cataract

occurring about puberty; it is therefore situated in the deep layers of the cortex and the most superficial layers of the nucleus. It appears as a corona of club-shaped opacities near the periphery of the lens, usually hidden by the iris, while the axial region and the extreme periphery of the lens remain free (Fig. 19.2 A and B). The opacities are not progressive and do not lead to complete opacification of the lens: their importance lies in their recognition as a developmental anomaly, for if they are seen when the pupil is dilated and their character is not recognized, the examiner may be led to diagnose a progressive cataract in a young adult.

Anterior capsular (polar) cataract

This may be developmental owing to delayed formation of the anterior chamber; in this case the opacity is congenital. More commonly the condition is acquired, and follows contact of the lens capsule with the cornea, usually after the perforation of an ulcer in ophthalmia neonatorum (*q.v.*). Fortunately such a reaction is seen only in early infancy. Where contact has occurred, usually in the central pupillary area, a white plaque forms in the lens capsule; sometimes it projects forwards into the anterior chamber like a pyramid (*anterior pyramidal cataract*). Occasionally the underlying layers of cortex are opaque forming an *anterior cortical cataract*. When this occurs it may well be that the subcapsular epithelium grows in between the capsular and cortical

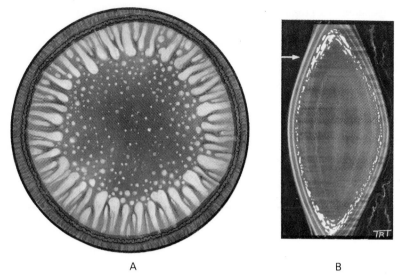

A   B

Fig. 19.2 A, Coronary cataract by oblique illumination; B, in optical section with the beam of the slit-lamp

opacities so that the clear lens fibres subsequently growing therefrom lay down a transparent zone between the two opacities. The buried opacity is called an *'imprint'* and the two together constitute a *reduplicated cataract.* Such opacities are not progressive and rarely interfere with vision.

Posterior capsular cataract
This is due to persistence of the posterior part of the vascular sheath of the lens. In minimal degrees it is common and usually insignificant. Sometimes, however, particularly in cases of persistent hyaloid artery, the lens is deeply invaded by fibrous tissue and a *total cataract* is formed.

Treatment is not required in developmental cataract unless vision is considerably impaired. If the cataract is central and reasonably good vision can be obtained through clear cortex around it, the child should be kept under mydriasis with atropine at least until puberty. An optical iridectomy is an alternative measure if the opacity is stationary. If the opacity is large, the operation of *discission* (*needling*) and irrigation (Chap. 27) may be undertaken. The operation, however, should not be performed unless the vision is seriously impaired. A decision on this question depends upon whether vision with corrected refraction and retained accommodation is to be preferred to probably improved vision after operation without accommodation. Vision of 6/12 or even 6/18, with retained accommodation is probably more valuable than a problematic 6/9 without accommodation, to which must be added the disability of constantly wearing very strong convex glasses for distance and still stronger ones for near work. Contact lenses, however, can often be worn by relatively young children or can be

made available in later life. In such eyes, however, the vision is frequently subnormal.

It is not advisable to operate on lamellar cataracts until the child is one or preferably three years old, but when the lens is completely opaque, or the pupil will not dilate, and when squint or nystagmus is developing, it is wise to operate at an earlier age. Moreover, in unilateral cataracts in children the results of surgery are universally poor unless the operation is carried out early in life and is followed immediately by the fitting of a contact lens. The critical period for developing the fixation reflex in both unilateral and bilateral visual deprivation disorders is between 2 and 4 months of age. The use of a contact lens requires the expert co-operation of interested parents and even with their co-operation binocular vision may be difficult to establish and amblyopia difficult to avoid.

Discission, however, may be difficult or impossible in total or shrunken cataract, and it may be necessary to remove a lens of this type with a modern vitrectomy instrument through a small corneal or pars plana incision.

ACQUIRED CATARACT

Acquired cataract is due to the degeneration of lens fibres already formed. The reasons for the degeneration are not yet clear and probably vary in different cases; any factor, physical or chemical, which disturbs the critical intra- and extra-cellular equilibrium of water and electrolytes or deranges the colloid system within the fibres tends to bring about opacification.

Biochemically two factors are evident in this process. In the early stages of cataract, particularly the rapidly developing forms, hydration is a prominent feature so that frequently actual droplets of fluid gather under the capsule forming lacunæ between the fibres, and the entire tissue swells and becomes opaque (*intumescence*). To some extent this process may be reversible and opacities thus formed may clear up. Hydration may be due to osmotic changes within the lens or to changes in the semi-permeability of the capsule. The process is seen dramatically in traumatic cataract when the capsule is ruptured and the lens fibres swell and bulge out into the anterior chamber (*q.v.*). If, however, the proteins are denatured a dense opacity is produced, a process which is irreversible; opacities thus constituted do not clear up.

Such an alteration occurs typically in the young lens or the cortex of the adult where metabolism is relatively active. In the older and inactive fibres of the nucleus it is rarely seen. Here the usual degenerative change is rather one of slow sclerosis. Clinically, when the first process is predominant the condition is called a 'soft cataract'; the second is described as a 'hard cataract'.

Many factors lead to these changes. The most common is *age*; and it may be of significance that as age progresses the semi-permeability of the capsule is impaired, the inactive insoluble proteins increase, and the oxidation system is less effective. Experimentally, cataract can be produced in conditions of *deficiency*, either of amino acids (tryptophane) or vitamin B_2 (riboflavine), or by the administration of *toxic substances* (naphthalene, lactose, galactose, thallium, etc.). Dinitrophenol, used for slimming, and paradichlorobenzene, used as an insecticide, also produce lens opacities in the posterior cortex, as also do toxic products in the aqueous (as in cyclitis) (*complicated cataract*). *Hypocalcæmia* may lead to the same result perhaps by altering the ionic balance; this experimental finding is correlated with the cataract of parathyroid tetany. Cataractous changes may also follow the use of the stronger anticholinesterase group of *miotics* and after the prolonged systemic use of *corticosteroids*. Physical factors may also enter into the question — *osmotic influences* (as may be largely responsible for diabetic cataract), *mechanical trauma* (traumatic cataract), or *radiant energy* in any form.

Senile cataract

This is rare in persons under 50 years of age unless associated with some metabolic disturbance as diabetes, but is almost universal in some degree in persons over seventy. It occurs equally in men and women and is usually bilateral, but often develops earlier in one eye than the other. There is a considerable genetic influence in its incidence and in hereditary cases it may appear at an earlier age in successive generations.

Two types of senile cataract may occur — cortical cataract, wherein the classical signs of hydration followed by coagulation of proteins appear primarily in the cortex, and nuclear or sclerotic cataract wherein the essential feature is a slow sclerosis in the nucleus.

In the *cortical type of senile cataract*, pre-senile changes are the rule, the most characteristic of which is a demarcation of the cortical fibres owing to their separation by fluid. This phenomenon (*lamellar separation*) can only be seen with the slit-lamp and is invisible ophthalmoscopically. The general increase in the refractive index of the cortex in old people gives a grey appearance to the pupil in contradistinction to the blackness seen in the young; the greyness is due, not to cataractous changes, but mainly to the increase in reflection and scattering of light.

In the next stage of *incipient cataract* wedge-shaped spokes of opacity with clear areas between them appear in the periphery of the lens; they lie in the cortex, some in front of and some behind the nucleus (*lens striae*), and are preceded by sectorial alterations in the refractive indices of the lens fibres thus producing irregularities in refraction, some visual deterioration and polyopia. The bases of the wedge-shaped opacities are peripheral and they are most common in the lower nasal quadrant. At first they can only be seen with the pupil dilated, but as they develop their apices appear within the normal pupillary margin. With oblique illumination they appear grey; seen with the ophthalmoscope or mirror they are black against the red background of the fundus; and as they approach the axial area, vision becomes seriously disturbed.

Cuneiform opacities have a mean age of origin of 48 years corresponding with the period of maximum accommodative stress just before the onset of presbyopia.

As time goes on, opacification becomes more diffuse and irregular so that the deeper layers of the cortex become cloudy and eventually uniformly white and opaque. Meanwhile the progressive hydration of the cortical layers may cause a swelling of the lens, thus making the anterior chamber shallow (*intumescent cataract*). Eventually the entire cortex becomes opaque, the swelling subsides and the cataract is said to be ripe or *mature*. In the meantime the nucleus suffers little change except a progressive sclerosis.

As long as there is any clear lens substance between the pupillary margin of the iris and the opacity, the iris throws a shadow upon the grey opacity when light is cast upon the eye from one side (Fig. 19.3A). When the cortex is completely opaque the pupillary margin lies almost in contact with the opacity, separated only by the capsule; the iris then throws no shadow, and the cataract is known to be mature (Fig. 19.3B).

If the process is allowed to go on uninterruptedly the stage of *hypermaturity* sets in when the cortex becomes disintegrated and transformed into a pultaceous mass. The lens becomes more and more inspissated and

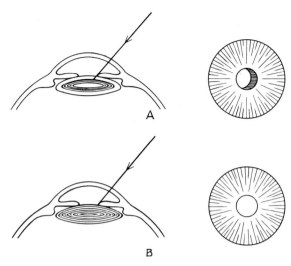

Fig. 19.3A and B. Diagnosis of the maturity of a cataract. (The pupil is illuminated from the right of the figure.) By courtesy of Hamblin

shrunken, sometimes yellow in appearance. The anterior capsule becomes thickened by proliferation of the anterior cubical cells, so that a dense white capsular cataract is formed at the anterior pole in the pupillary area. Owing to shrinkage the lens and iris become tremulous and the anterior chamber deep, and finally, degeneration of the suspensory ligament may lead to luxation of the lens.

Sometimes at the stage of maturity the cortex becomes fluid, and the nucleus may sink to the bottom of the lens. The liquefied cortex is milky, the nucleus appearing as a brown mass limited above by a semi-circular line, altering its position with changes in position of the head. Such a cataract is called a *Morgagnian cataract* (Plate 6, Fig. D).

The rate of development of senile cortical cataract varies greatly, sometimes occupying many years; indeed, the cataract may never reach maturity. Very rapid maturation in younger patients usually indicates some complication such as cyclitis or diabetes. The forms with fine radial lines evolve more slowly than those with cloudy opacities. It is best to examine every case periodically, a careful drawing of the opacities being recorded at each visit.

A second common type of cortical senile cataract is *cupuliform cataract*, consisting of a dense aggregation of opacities just beneath the capsule, usually in the posterior cortex. It is difficult to see with the ophthalmoscope but appears in the beam of the slit-lamp as a yellow layer. Examination with this instrument is important since, being near the nodal point of the eye, the opacity may diminish the vision considerably in older people.

In *senile nuclear sclerosis of the lens* the opposite process

occurs; the normal tendency of the central nuclear fibres to become sclerosed is intensified while the cortical fibres remain transparent.

This type of cataract tends to occur earlier than the cortical variety, often soon after 40 years of age. As time progresses the nucleus becomes diffusely cloudy, the cloudiness spreading gradually towards the cortex, and occasionally it becomes tinted dark brown, dusky red or even black owing to the deposition of melanins derived from the amino acids in the lens (*cataracta brunescens; black cataract*). In maturity the sclerosis may extend almost to the capsule so that the entire lens functions as a nucleus.

Initially little change may be seen with the ophthalmoscope except that the details of the fundus are hazy. Occasionally if there is much pigment the pupillary reflex may be entirely blackened. There is, however, considerable visual disturbance — at first a progressive myopia owing to the increased refractive index of the nucleus, and then general impairment of vision; but progress is usually very slow and hypermaturity does not occur.

Cataract associated with ocular disease

Complicated cataract

This results from a disturbance of the nutrition of the lens due to inflammatory or degenerative disease of other parts of the eye, such as iridocyclitis, choroiditis, high myopia, pigmentary retinal dystrophy or retinal detachment. After inflammations of the anterior segment, a nondescript opacification appears throughout the cortex which usually progresses and matures rapidly. In inflammations or degenerations affecting the posterior segment a characteristic opacification usually commences in the posterior part of the cortex in the axial region (*posterior cortical cataract*). Ophthalmoscopically it appears as a vaguely defined, dark area, and with the slit-lamp the opacity is seen to have irregular borders extending diffusely towards the equator and the nucleus; unlike developmental cataract it is not sharply confined to a particular zone. In the beam of the slit-lamp the opacities have an appearance like bread-crumbs and a characteristic rainbow display of colours often replaces the normal achromatic sheen (*polychromatic lustre*). Such a cataract may remain stationary in the posterior cortex for a long time or even indefinitely; in other cases the opacification spreads peripherally until all the posterior cortex is affected, and axially until the entire lens is involved. The total cataract formed in this manner is usually soft and uniform in appearance.

Even in the early stages vision is usually much impaired owing to the position of the opacity near the nodal point of the eye. The operative prognosis depends on the causal condition; but the presence of such a cataract without obvious cause should always call for a most minute examination of the eye for keratic precipitates or other signs of disease.

Cataract associated with systemic disease

Diabetic cataract

We have seen that in diabetic subjects senile cataract tends to develop at an earlier age and more rapidly than usual. *True diabetic cataract* is a rare condition occurring typically in young people in whom the diabetes is so acute as to disturb grossly the water-balance of the body. An immense number of fluid vacuoles appears under the anterior and posterior parts of the capsule, producing a diffuse opacity which at this stage is reversible.

Parathyroid tetany

Cataractous changes may occur when the parathyroid glands become atrophic or have been inadvertently removed in the course of a thyroidectomy; development may be prevented by the administration of parathyroid hormone and calcium. Clouds of small discrete opacities appear in the cortex separated from the capsule by a clear zone. These coalesce to form large, glistening, crystalline flakes and within six months the lens is usually opaque. The other ocular tissues are unaffected and the operative prognosis is good.

Myotonic dystrophy

Characteristic and somewhat similar cataracts may develop with myotonic dystrophy. In a sharply limited zone of the cortex underneath the capsule both anteriorly and posteriorly, fine dust-like opacities appear interspersed with tiny iridescent spots. The cataract may remain stationary; if it progresses the operative prognosis is good.

Galactosæmia

This a rare congenital disease characterised by an inborn inability of the infant to metabolise galactose. It is frequently associated with the development of bilateral cataract in early life, at first lamellar and eventually total. Recession may occur if milk and milk-products are eliminated from the diet in the early stages; otherwise if the patient survives, surgical treatment must be adopted.

Mongolian idiocy and cretinism

These may be associated with similar punctate subcapsular cataracts.

Atopic cataract

When this developes rapidly it appears frequently in sufferers from severe and widespread skin diseases — atopic eczema, poikiloderma vasculare atrophicans, scleroderma, keratosis follicularis, and others. The operative prognosis depends on adequate control of the allergic condition in eczematous cases.

Cataract due to radiant or other energy

Most types of radiant energy produce cataractous changes, particularly heat, X-rays and the γ-rays of radium or neutrons. Ultra-violet light has been implicated as a factor in the ætiology of senile cataract, a suggestion due largely to the common occurrence of this condition in tropical countries such as India and Northern Australia.

Heat (infra-red) cataract

This is a characteristic condition which may be induced experimentally in animals and occurs clinically in industry. The heat acts not directly on the lens but is absorbed by the pigment of the iris and ciliary body and thus influences the fibres of the lens indirectly; it has thus been found impossible to produce such cataracts experimentally in lightly pigmented or albino animals. The cataract is characteristic in appearance. In the early stages there is a small disc of opacity in the posterior cortex of the lens, thinner and more sharply defined than the posterior cortical opacity of complicated cataract, but it may extend throughout the cortex in the later stages. In addition, the zonular lamella of the capsule may be exfoliated, sometimes in large sheets which curl up in the pupillary area.

Such a cataract is seen industrially in two particular occupations. It is seen in *glass-workers* who have long been engaged in glass manufacture, particularly beer bottles and plate glass, but not in those who make flint-glass bottles or pressed glass articles since the heat of such furnaces is less. It also occurs in certain *iron-workers*, especially tin-plate millmen and chain-makers.

Irradiation cataract

This may be caused by X-rays, γ-rays or neutrons. The characteristic changes appear to be due to the direct action of the rays on the dividing cells and developing fibres of the lens itself. The initial changes are found near the equator shortly after radiation, and the first clinical evidences are apparent in the cortex near the posterior pole only after a period of one or two years when the equatorial cells have migrated posteriorly, where they resemble in appearance those of heat cataract. Maturation of the cataract may occur fairly rapidly. Technicians who have been inadequately protected may be thus affected, or patients treated for malignant conditions near the eye. Such cataracts have also developed in workers in atomic energy plants and occurred among the survivors of the atomic bombs released over Japan in the Second World War.

Electric cataract

This may develop rapidly after the passage through the body of a powerful electric current as from a flash of lightning or the short-circuiting of a high-voltage current. The cataract usually starts as punctate, subcapsular opacities and matures rapidly.

Ultrasonic radiation

Similarly this induces lens opacities, due to the effects of heat and concussion.

Traumatic cataract

May be due — either due to concussion or a perforating wound — see pp. 245, 248.

Symptoms of acquired cataract

These are entirely visual. Among the early complaints is that of seeing spots before the eye, not continually moving as in muscæ volitantes (*q.v.*), but stationary, retaining their relative position in the field of vision in different positions of the eye. Uniocular polyopia, another early symptom, is the doubling or trebling of the objects seen with the eye. It is due to irregular refraction by the lens so that several images are formed of each object; coloured halos may also be seen (p. 193). There may also be a change in colour values owing to the absorption of the shorter wave-lengths so that reds are accentuated.

As the opacity extends and becomes denser, the acuity of central vision suffers, the deterioration depending on the density and position of the opacity. If the opacities are peripheral, as in senile cortical cataract, serious visual embarrassment may be long delayed and the vision is improved if the pupil is contracted in bright light. If they are central, visual deterioration appears early, and the patient sees better when the pupil is dilated in dim illumination. Posterior cortical opacities often cause diminution of central vision apparently out of proportion to the amount of opacity observed. When nuclear sclerosis is prominent, the increasing refractivity leads to the development of a progressive myopia. It follows that with senile nuclear sclerosis a previously presbyopic patient may be able to read again without the aid of spectacles; he refers to his 'improvement' in vision as 'second sight'.

As opacification proceeds, vision steadily diminishes until only perception of light remains. In many cases of mature senile cataract fingers can still be counted at a few feet, or at least hand movements discerned. In all cases, however, light should be perceived readily and the direction of its incidence accurately indicated.

The treatment of cataract

No medical treatment by drugs or otherwise has been shown to have any significant effect in inducing the disappearance of cataract once opacities have developed. When the cataract is at the early stages of hydration and is due to general disease (as diabetes), control of the causal condition may result in a disappearance of the lens changes; if opacification has occurred, control of the general condition may stay its progress; but once the proteins of the lens have become coagulated, the change is immutable. In senile cataract the progress of opacification may cease spontaneously for many years, or refractive changes may result in temporary improvement of vision. From time to time these events have been seized upon as indicating a therapeutic effect of a particular remedy which may happen to be applied.

In all cases, however, a careful examination of the patient should be made to exclude any specific or constitutional cause of the disease; if any is found, it should be treated. This applies particularly to diabetes; the urine of all such patients should be tested.

In *incipient cataract* the condition of the patient may be much ameliorated during the tedious process of maturation. The refraction, which often changes with considerable rapidity, should be corrected at frequent intervals. There is no reason to restrict the use of the eyes in incipient uncomplicated cataract, but the patient may be much assisted by instructions as to the arrangement of illumination. If the pupillary area is free, brilliant illumination will be found best; if the opacities are largely central a dull light placed beside and slightly behind the patient's head will give the best result. In these cases, also, dark glasses are usually of great value and comfort when worn out-of-doors, an effect obtained with greater certainty by instilling a very weak mydriatic (atropine 0.05% every morning or cyclopentolate 0.5%), provided — owing to the risk of glaucoma — the angle of the anterior chamber is not narrow. Finally, in every case of incipient cataract the pupil should be dilated to allow a thorough examination of the fundus at the stage when it can still be seen.

When the cataract has become mature the only effective treatment is its operative removal. Before this is contemplated, however, a *general overhaul* of the patient should exclude the presence of serious systemic disease. A disease such as diabetes does not preclude operation but it should be adequately controlled before and after surgery.

A *thorough examination of the eye* is also a necessity, a routine particularly vital when the cataract appears to be of the complicated type, but eminently desirable in all cases. The retinal function must then be explored since, if it is defective, operation may be valueless and the patient warned of possible disappointment. In this respect the value of a thorough examination of the fundus in the incipient stage of cataract while the retina and optic disc are still visible is obvious. When it cannot be seen five tests are of value.

The detection of the *projection of light* is of the utmost importance. It is tested as follows in a dark room. The opposite eye is covered securely by the palm of the patient's hand. Light is then shone from the ophthalmoscope into the cataractous eye from various directions, the patient looking straight forwards. He is told to point with his other hand in the direction from which the light seems to come. He ought to do this readily and accurately.

The *macular function* can be vaguely assessed by asking the patient to look through an opaque disc perforated with two pin-holes close together behind which a light is held. If he can appreciate the presence of two lights, the central area of the retina is probably good. He should also be asked to look at a distant light through a Maddox rod (p. 294); if the red line is continuous and unbroken, macular function is probably good.

Ultrasonic investigation by the B-scan technique gives valuable information concerning the retina.

An *entoptic view of the retina* will often allow the patient to supply valuable information. If the eyes are closed and the globe is steadily and firmly massaged through the lower lid with the bare lighted bulb of an electric ophthalmoscope or torch, he will see clearly the entire vascular tree of the retina on an orange ground. An intelligent patient will describe any blanks or scotomata; particular attention should be given to the central area.

A foveal electroretinogram may give useful information of the functioning of this region.

If operation is considered worthwhile, disease in the anterior segment should be excluded. The pupil should react promptly and normally to light and it should dilate readily with mydriatics while the most careful search must be made for precipitates on the back of the cornea. When the cataract is complicated by intraocular disease, treatment must be directed in the first place to rendering it quiescent — often a tedious and sometimes an unsatisfactory procedure. Some cases are not suitable for operation, mostly on account of cyclitis or defective projection of light, but even in these, if there is a possibility of success, operation may be undertaken after warning the patient of the doubtful issue, for the loss of such an eye weighs little against a reasonable probability of improved vision. In such cases, also, wherein an inflammatory condition may be expected to flare up, the topical administration of steroids is often of great value in forestalling or controlling a relapse.

If operation is decided upon, the possibility of infective complications should be excluded as far as practicable. Gross focal sepsis, such as abscessed teeth, should be eliminated. The conjunctival sac should be examined, and any infection cleared up by suitable antibiotic treatment. Finally, the lacrimal sac should receive attention. If regurgitation is found on finger pressure (p. 325) or a mucocele is present, a nasal drainage operation should be performed.

The type of operation employed depends on the case. In young patients, the lens can be disposed of by *discission* and irrigation (p. 261). Such an operation is usually effective up to 30 years of age. In older people, the nucleus of the lens is hard and must be extracted. The extraction may be done by opening the capsule, expressing the nucleus and washing out the cortical substance, (*extra-capsular extraction*) (p. 263). Alternatively the nucleus may be emulsified by a phaco-emulsifier and the lens matter removed by suction while saline replaces the evacuated fluid under electronic control. When a complete iridectomy is performed during the operation to assist the removal of the lens the technique is termed *combined extraction*. Extracapsular extraction may have to be followed by a needling of the capsule. Alternatively, the entire lens including the capsule can be removed by rupturing the zonule (*intracapsular extraction*) (p. 263).

The treatment of *unilateral cataract* offers some difficulty when the vision is good in the fellow eye. Little advantage is gained by operating since the difference in refraction between the two eyes after operation will be so great that diplopia will result if the refraction is corrected with spectacles (p. 63), and if uncorrected the large blurred image formed by the eye may be a positive disadvantage. Binocular vision is often possible with a contact lens (*q.v.*), particularly in children, but their manipulation is difficult by the aged; and the technique of inserting a plastic lens into the eye (*vide infra*) may provide a way out of the difficulty. Neglecting these two expedients, the sole advantage gained from the extraction of a unilateral cataract is an increase of the field of vision on the affected side.

The presence of increased tension constitutes an anxiety in operating for cataract. The tension may be raised owing to the swelling of the lens in the incipient stage, or due to phacolytic glaucoma, in which case an extraction is indicated. On the other hand, simple glaucoma may be already present. If the glaucoma is medically controlled, the lens may be extracted and the treatment continued; if it is not, probably the best procedure is to perform a trabeculectomy followed later by cataract extraction or a combined procedure.

In some cases eyes with cataract have had surgery for simple glaucoma (p. 200). Theoretically it is obviously objectionable to make a cataract incision through a drainage area, but although such cases often do well it is probably better to make the incision in the upper part of the cornea in front of the drainage area; a safe alternative is to make the incision for the cataract extraction in an area separate from the filtering bleb as in the lower half.

The correction of the refraction after extraction of cataract is dealt with elsewhere (*see* Aphakia, p. 63).

After or secondary cataract

This is the opacity which persists or follows after extra-capsular extraction or discission of the lens. In both these operations the posterior and part of the anterior capsule remain in situ. In many cases these remnants are fine, forming a thin membrane which is difficult to see particularly following operation with modern suction and infusion devices. In other cases, especially when the cataract was not mature, some soft, clear cortex sticks to the capsule. This becomes partially absorbed by the action of the aqueous but often becomes shut off by adhesion of the remains of the anterior to the posterior capsule. In such cases the cubical cells which line the anterior capsule also persist; they continue to fulfil their function of forming new lens fibres, although those formed under the abnormal conditions are abortive and opaque. Sometimes these, enclosed between the two layers of capsule, form a dense ring behind the iris (*the ring of Sömmerring*) (Fig. 19.4); it may cause subsequent trouble by becoming dislocated into the anterior chamber. At other times, the subcapsular cells proliferate and instead of forming lens fibres, develop into large balloon-like cells which sometimes fill the pupillary aperture (*Elschnig's pearls*). If these remnants lie in the pupillary area a dense membrane is formed so that vision is impaired. If the previous operation has been followed by iritis, exudates also adhere to the lens remnants and organize, thus contributing a fibrous membrane in addition.

Treatment. Pupillary membranes if thin require dis-cission or they can be removed by a vitreous cutter alone (A) Tough and non-pliable membranes have first to be cut into smaller pieces before they can be aspirated into the cutting port. This can be done with a Zieglers' Knife (B), or by using vitreous scissor (C) (Fig. 19.5).

Dislocation of the lens
See p. 246.

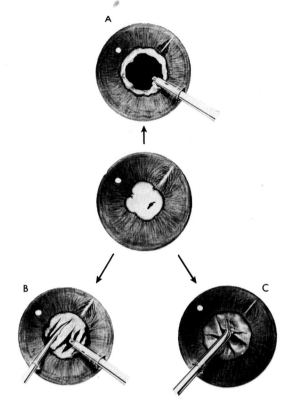

Fig. 19.5 Removal of pupillary membrane. (By courtesy of Kanski.)
A With a vitreous cutter.   B Preliminary discission with a Zeigler knife.   C Preliminary discission with vitreous scissors

CONGENITAL ABNORMALITIES OF THE LENS

Besides the various forms of *congenital cataract* (p. 171), abnormalities in the shape and position of the lens occur, often associated with other malformations of the eye.

Coloboma of the lens is the condition in which there is a defect usually in the inferior margin and notch-

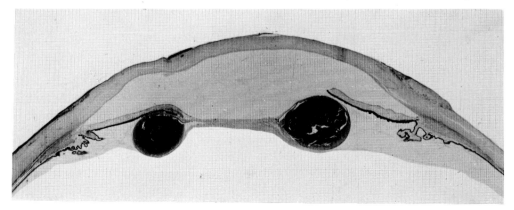

Fig. 19.4 Sömmerring's ring. (By courtesy of Ashton.)

shaped; less frequently it occurs in some other part of the margin. It is due to defective development of part of the suspensory ligament.

Ectopia lentis or congenital dislocation is a subluxation of the lens, usually upwards or up and in, and bilateral. The condition is often hereditary. The lens is small, but the edge is generally invisible until the pupil is dilated. The usual signs of subluxation (p. 246) are then seen. It is sometimes associated with arachnodactyly (*Marfan's syndrome*) or homocystinuria.

Homocystinuria. A deficiency in the enzyme cystathionine synthetase gives rise to excessive amounts of homocystine in the urine and wide-spread abnormalities characterized by dislocation of the lens and mental re-

tardation. Homocystine in the urine is detected by the cyanide nitoprusside test.

Ectopia lentis becomes more marked with age in this disease and gives rise to glaucoma. Such patients are poor operative risks because of the tendency to thromboses. Other signs include laxity of joints.

Homocystinuria is transmitted as an autosomal recessive disease.

Lenticonus, generally posterior, is an abnormal curvature of the lens, so that the surface is somewhat conical instead of spherical.

If these deformities cause great visual disability, treatment by discission of the lens is advisable.

20

Diseases of the vitreous

The vitreous humour is an inert, jelly-like structure which subserves only optical functions. It has all the properties of a hydrophilic gel, undergoing turgescence and deturgescence and readily becoming transformed into a sol when its protein basis becomes coagulated, a transformation which occurs with age and on the slightest insult, either mechanical or chemical. Hence 'fluid' vitreous is a common condition. It possesses no blood vessels in post-natal life and is incapable of becoming inflamed.

Age changes in the vitreous
Cloquet's canal which contains the primary vitreous at birth runs straight from the lens to the optic disc. In the young the vitreous gel is homogeneous but with age its fibres become coarser. The secondary vitreous eventually becomes liquified and shrinks producing a vitreous detachment in the latter third of life or earlier in myopes.

Vitreous detachment
Vitreous detachment occurs in three forms – posterior, basal and anterior.

Posterior vitreous detachment
The detachment occurs posterior to the vitreous base and is a senile phenomenon (although commoner in diabetics) appearing spontaneously and producing the sudden onset of photopsiae and floaters. The photopsiae are due to vitreo-retinal adhesions and are provoked by ocular movement. They are commonly noticed in the temporal field although they may be projected in the meridian opposite the site of retinal traction.

The upper part of the vitreous commonly collapses and as it occurs universally over the age of 65 years the incidence of retinal complications is low. The condition is benign unless it is associated with other pathological findings, such as retinoschisis, a rhegmatogenous retinal detachment or diabetic retinopathy.

Patients with posterior vitreous detachment must be carefully examined and if there is no evidence of vitreo-retinal adhesion or traction then they can be assured.

Basal and anterior vitreous detachment
Occur secondary to trauma and are accompanied by vitreous haemorrhage.

Opacities in the vitreous
1. Development opacities are located in Cloquet's canal and are remnants of the hyaloid system.
2. Degenerative.
a. Asteroid hyalosis is characterised by spherical white bodies in the vitreous cavity. There is a genetic relationship with diabetes and hypercholesterolaemia. It is unilateral in the majority of cases and affects both sexes, usually in the elderly. It is asymptomatic but it may make examination of the fundus difficult with the ophthalmoscope. Treatment is rarely required except in the one-eyed when vision may be reduced and a closed vitrectomy considered.

b. Synchisis scintillans. This degenerative condition leads to deposition of cholesterol crystals in the vitreous which are also found in the anterior chamber and subretinal space. It affects damaged eyes which have suffered trauma or inflammatory disease in the past. The crystals are multicoloured glittering particles which settle in the lower part of the vitreous cavity due to gravity but can be thrown up by eye movements to form a shower of iridescence. The vitreous in such cases is liquified and no treatment is indicated.

c. Amyloid degeneration. Amyloidosis is a rare systemic disease and amyloid material is deposited in the collagen fibres of the heart, thyroid, pancreas, peripheral nerves and muscles. It is a heredo-familial syndrome transmitted as a Mendelian dominant producing generalised weakness, loss of weight, peripheral neuropathy and symptoms related to the organs affected. It runs a long tedious course. The ocular signs consist of diplopia, loss of vision, external ophthalmoplegia, vitreous opacities, retinal haemorrhages and exudates. Both eyes are involved and the vitreous becomes opaque. The earliest lesion originates in the wall of a retinal vessel which has a cloudy margin and this slowly invades the vitreous body from behind forwards. Diagnosis is confirmed by biopsy of the conjunctiva, rectum, skin, or sternal marrow. Vitrectomy may be employed if the posterior vitreous is detached but the prognosis must always be guarded. The vitreous opacities themselves are linear with footplate attachments to the retina and posterior lens surface and this is a helpful diagnostic feature.

There are other causes of vitreous opacities. A senile eye produces opacities due to condensed vitreous fibres floating in areas of liquifaction. Similar opacities arise in the myope in the second half of life. Vitreo-retinal degeneration may form a part of other syndromes such as retrolental fibroplasia, Wagner's disease, Ehlers-Danlos syndrome and Marfan's syndrome. They can be formed by the inflammatory cells of cyclitis or be due to red cells secondary to diabetes, retinal vasculitis of subarachnoid haemorrhage and occasionally they are formed by neoplastic cells.

Vitreous bands and membranes

Vitreous bands or membranes often form after posterior vitreous detachment and originate from hyalocytes, fibrocytes or endothelial cells of the capillaries. If such a band is adherent to the retina producing retinal oedema, haemorrhage or a hole then it is likely to give rise to a detachment of the retina. A pre-retinal membrane lines the inner surface of the retina and if it is thin it looks like a sheet of cellophane and if thick it resembles a sheet of tissue. As the membrane contracts the retina wrinkles producing macular or extramacular pucker.

Signs of traction in the peripheral fundus are retinal areas of white-with-pressure, retinoschisis, detachment of the ora serrata or a U-shaped retinal tear with an operculum. In the posterior fundus they consist of oedema of the retina, haemorrhage, macular cystoid changes, heterotopia of the macula and tenting of the retina.

Persistent hyperplastic vitreous

In this condition there is a failure of the structures within the primary vitreous to regress. Shortly after birth a white pupil is noticed in the full-term infant. Other abnormalities such as cataract, glaucoma, long and extended ciliary processes, microphthalmos and intraocular haemorrhage may be found usually affecting one eye only.

The retrolental tissue contracts to pull the ciliary processes inwards. The lens becomes opaque and glaucoma intervenes.

If the condition is diagnosed at any early stage it may be possible to aspirate the lens with later excision of the retrolental membrane along with an anterior vitrectomy.

The posterior form of persistent hyperplastic vitreous includes a persistent hyaloid artery with a large stalk issuing from the optic disc for which little can be done.

Vitreo-retinal degeneration

Wagner's disease is a bilateral affection transmitted as an autosomal dominant. The fundus shows narrow and sheathed vessels, pigmented spots in the periphery or along retinal vessels, choroidal atrophy and optic atrophy. The vitreous is liquified with condensed membranes. Early in life during adolescence the vitreous shrinks and if attached to the retina may produce a tear. Cataract is a later complication. Extensive liquifaction of the central and posterior portions of the vitreous body takes place leaving a thin layer of formed cortex on the surface of the retina.

The management consists of regular examinations for retinal tears which should be treated with cryotherapy unless there is vitreous traction when plombage is indicated.

Goldmann–Favre's vitreo-retinal degeneration

This produces progressive loss of vision due to retinoschisis, pigmentary degeneration resembling retinitis pigmentosa and later cataract. The affliction is bilateral and familial, being transmitted as an autosomal recessive. Retinoschisis is both central affecting the macula and peripheral. When the pigment dispersal is marked the ECG is extinguished. The vitreous undergoes liquifaction. There is no satisfactory treatment.

Vitreous haemorrhage

Vitreous haemorrhage may occur as a preretinal phenomenon, or an intravitreous phenomenon or a combination of both.

There is a history of sudden onset of floaters and a fall in vision. Careful examination of the vitreous with the indirect ophthalmoscope is indicated and with the biomicroscope. Ultrasonography with a B-scan is particularly helpful. Haemorrhage within the vitreous cavity gives rise to scattered point-like echoes of varying amplitude. Sedimentation of haemorrhage within fluid vitreous produces a flat sheet of very high-amplitude echoes. A sheet of lower-amplitude echoes with more internal structure represents epiretinal fibrous tissue.

Posterior vitreous detachment is indicated by point-like echoes confined to the gel compartment or retrohyloid space. If incomplete, the detachment may cause only a single vitreal retinal adhesion often stalk-like in form. Retinal detachment produces membrane-like echoes of high amplitude which tether at the ora-serrata and the optic nerve head when total.

Extensive fibrovascular membranes on the retinal surface may be detected by ultrasound in proliferative diabetic retinopathy. Where the detached vitreous gel retains mobility, an apparent compaction of blood may be seen on the inner aspect of the posterior hyaloid interface ('Ochre membrane formation'). Diabetic traction detachment appears as an angular retinal elevation that is immobile on dynamic testing.

Sub-hyaloid blood remains unclotted and so moves about with gravity and tends to acquire a boat-shaped configuration which is red in colour. Blood in a lacuna of the vitreous tends to separate whereas blood in the gel clots and moves bodily with the gel itself. Blood of long-standing in the vitreous develops into a white opaque mass.

The common causes of vitreous haemorrhage are trauma, vitreous retraction and venous thrombosis.

Vitreous haemorrhage should be treated by bed-rest with the head elevated and the eyes padded so as to minimise dispersion of the blood within the gel. If the blood sinks under the influence of gravity it may be possible to discover a retinal hole which should be plombed or a new formed vessel which should be coagulated. If the vitreous fails to clear after a week then the patient is mobilised and seen at 2-monthly intervals. If the blood lasts 6 months closed vitrectomy should be considered in a patient with reasonable life expectancy provided the eye perceives light with an acuity of not greater than 6/60; the electroretinogram must indicate a live retina; ultrasonography should ensure that there is not a complete detachment of the retina and active treatment is particularly indicated if the fellow eye is similarly threatened.

Vitreous haemorrhage and retinal tears

This syndrome tends to occur in myopes and in those who have predisposing degeneration of the retina. It produces localised flashes and floaters before the onset of the haemorrhage itself and may be precipitated by mild ocular trauma.

The patient should be rested in bed with both eyes padded and with the head elevated. Scleral buckling with encirclement is usually indicated to close the hole.

Vitreous haemorrhage and posterior vitreous detachment

Bleeding in association with posterior vitreous detachment is due to retinal traction and a preretinal haemorrhage is always found which sinks to the lower part of the globe. The vessel affected is most readily closed by the argon laser.

Vitreous haemorrhage and retinal vein occlusion

Venous obstruction occurs at the lamina cribrosa or at the arterio-venous crossings and is prone to occur when the patient is hypertensive or arteriosclerotic. Venous collaterals form at the optic disc between the retinal and ciliary circulations and between branches of the obstructed vein and the adjacent patent venules particularly in tributory occlusion. Some 3 months after the occlusion capillary microaneurysms and fibro-vascular proliferation occur and vitreous haemorrhage may arise from the delicate new vessels. Photocoagulation has a part to play in this syndrome.

Eale's disease

Eale's disease may be a hypersensitivity reaction of the retinal vessels to tuberculoproteins and it develops when a protein of a similar nature is ingested. The retinal vasculitis leads to obliteration of the affected vessels, particularly the shunt capillaries of the peripheral retina which in turn produces hypoxia and finally vasoproliferation. The stages of development are periphlebitis leading to new vessel formation and eventually recurrent vitreous haemorrhages. They may be organised and give rise to retinal detachment and secondary glaucoma. Fluorescein angiography shows rapid leakage of dye from the peripheral venous vasculitis.

Treatment consists of systemic steroids which may be helpful in the early vasculitis stage. Abnormal vessels under traction should be destroyed by photocoagulation. Scleral buckling may be used in cases of marked vitreous traction. Closed vitrectomy may be employed in cases of long-standing vitreous haemorrhage.

Sickle cell retinopathy

Sickle cell haemoglobin is an abnormal haemoglobin found mainly but not exclusively in people of negro origin. When it is deoxygenated it becomes insoluble and distorts the normally discoid red cell into a characteristic sickle shape. Such sickled red cells tend to obstruct capillaries and this leads to infarction, particularly in the retinal periphery.

The globin of haemoglobin is a protein and consists of an assortment of 20 chemically distinct amino-acids linked to form a polypeptide chain in a genetically determined order. An alteration in the DNA of the determining gene will result in an alteration of the amino-acid composition of the polypeptide chain and an abnormal haemoglobin.

Normal adult haemoglobin is a tetramer formed from 4 haem/globin units each of the 4 globin units being a polypeptide chain of 140 amino-acids. Two of the globin units are so similar as to be called α, whereas the other two are called β; normal adult haemoglobin is called $\alpha2$ $\beta2$, different genes being responsible for the production of the α polypeptides chains and the β polypeptide chains.

Over 100 abnormal haemoglobins have been described and of these only four different types are common all of which have abnormalities in the β half of the haemoglobin molecules. In the case of sickle cell haemoglobin the molecule will be identical to normal haemoglobin except that in the sixth position in the β polypeptide chains the amino-acid valine will have been substituted for glutamic acid, the amino-acid normally present in the sixth position.

In the case of haemoglobin C the amino-acid lysine will have been substituted for the glutamic acid in the sixth position of the β polypeptide chains Patients with Sickle cell Haemoglobin C disease (SC disease) lack a normal B^a gene capable of producing normal β polypeptide chain genes. They therefore have no normal adult haemoglobin, their haemoglobins consisting of HbS and HbC produced by the $β^s$ and $β^c$ polypeptide chains, respectively. They suffer a little (if at all) from anaemia, the main clinical problem being infrequent but on occasions severe infarctive crises.

Although Sickle cell C disease does not occur as frequently as sickle cell anaemia or the sickle cell trait, it is the most important haemoglobinopathy in ophthalmology because its clinical manifestation is predominently in the eye consisting of retinopathy, angioid streaks, papilloedema, cataracts, glaucoma, and circumscribed dilatation and constriction of conjunctival capillaries.

Fundus findings are proliferative and non-proliferative. The former begin with occlusion of peripheral arterioles leading to neovascularisation and vitreous haemorrhage. Fibrovascular proliferation creates the form of 'sea fans' particularly in the superior temporal peripheral areas of the retina (Fig. 20.1A). The latter consists of vascular tortuosity, central retinal artery occlusion, central retinal vein occlusion, angioid streaks, sunburst spots (focal retinal pigment epithelial hypertrophy, hyperplasia and migration resulting from intraretinal and subretinal haemorrhages) and optic atrophy. Retinal detachment due to vitreous contraction is a late complication. Leakage of serum into the vitreous cortex which occurs near the vascular lesions causes vitreous organisation and this in turn may lead to traction (Fig. 20.1B).

Treatment consists of photocoagulation to destroy neovascular lesions and the feeder vessels. Scleral buckling may be required in the treatment of retinal detachment but anterior segment necrosis is a risk which must be borne in mind in such cases.

Vitreous haemorrhage due to ocular trauma

Trauma is commoner in young people and follows contusion or a perforating injury. Vitreous haemorrhage is usually intra-vitreous and the blood is clotted. An intra-ocular foreign body must be excluded or removed. The patient should be immobilised and the head elevated with padding of the eyes for 5–6 days. After 6 months closed vitrectomy may be considered. The closed surgical technique involves a water tight approach through the pars plana and illumination is provided from a slit lamp externally or a fibro-optic internally.

Closed vitreous surgery

Vitreous bands surrounded by liquified vitreous following intra-ocular foreign bodies or after vitreous loss during cataract extraction may be cut with vitreous scissors because they avoid retinal traction. Bands within the vitreous gel do not respond well to cutting with scissors and a vitreous tissue remover is required. Membranes which lie close to the retina have to be lifted forward before being cut and if vascularised the vessels are closed with intravitreous diathermy. Bullous keratopathy due to prolonged vitreous contact between vitreous and corneal endothelium following intracapsular extraction, is an indication for closed vitrectomy. Intermittent touch may be demonstrated by placing the patient on his back

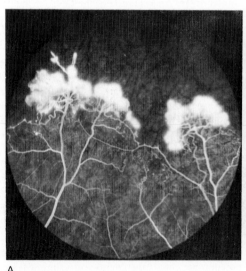 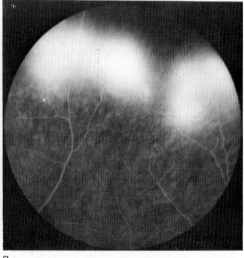

A   B

Fig. 20.1 Sea-fan: A, early fluorescein angiogram; B, late fluorescein angiogram. (By courtesy of Boase.)

since the vitreous moves posteriorly and the cornea clears. In time the endothelium undergoes metaplasia to form fibrocytes and keratoplasty plus vitrectomy is required.

Open sky vitrectomy is performed through a large corneal or trans-scleral incision. It necessitates removal of the lens. It is of value in vitreous loss occurring during lens extraction or aphakic keratoplasty and in removal of a dislocated lens and sometimes in removal of a large intra-ocular foreign body.

Pars plana vitreous surgery

Pars plana vitreous surgery is employed to restore the optical pathway of the eye. If the opacities are confined to the vitreous cavity the prognosis is good.

Intra-ocular membrane formation is an 'in vivo tissue culture'. The same applies to fibrovascular proliferation. The proliferating cells which form membranes are derivatives of the retinal pigment epithelium, by a process of metaplasia accompanied by retinal glial cells which grow through holes in the internal limiting membrane. The vitreous surgeon in order to produce long term effects must sever all connections between the vitreous base and the posterior vitreous to eliminate any scaffold along which cells could proliferate into the vitreous cavity. Membranes in the vitreous require complete removal to avoid further regrowth. Preretinal membranes must be hooked up before being cut and this is made easier if the membrane over the foveal area is not attached to the retina but bridges across it.

Any opacities in the anterior such as cataracts, after-cataracts and pupillary membranes eye can be adequately removed by vitrectors.

Vitrectomy can be employed in the management of intraocular foreign bodies. A cataract can be removed, the vitreous cavity emptied, the foreign body found and extracted and any retinal holes treated immediately.

A non-rhegmatogenous traction detachment responds to surgical removal of the intravitreal band. Small holes produced by a traction band may be closed successfully. Massive preretinal proliferation may also be treated by vitrectomy.

A patient should not be submitted to vitrectomy unless the visual acuity is at least Hand Movements. Accurate light projection is a comforting finding but can be misleading. Entoptic testing is a helpful method of evaluating macular function. Tests for retinal function of doubtful reliability are the two point discrimination test, the Maddox rod, laser interference fringes and pupillary reactions. Ultrasonography is a most valuable pre-operative investigation because it outlines the vitreous itself as well as the retina.

If the vitreous is densely opaque it is difficult to evoke an ERG. A light source 20 000 times brighter than the average stimulator can produce a recordable ERG from a functional retina. Increasing light intensities are employed on a logarithmic scale until a maximal response is recorded.

Iris angiography will reveal early rubeosis an important finding as two-thirds of diabetic patients with

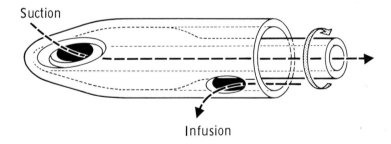

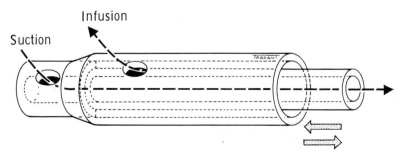

Fig. 20.2 A Vitreous infusion suction cutter; B, vitreous stripper

clinical rubeosis develop neovascular glaucoma after vitrectomy.

Vitreous instruments

In 1971, Machemer and his colleagues described vitrectomy through the pars plana. Their instrument was called the Vitreous Infusion Suction Cutter (VISC) consisting of a rotating cutting mechanism driven by a micromotor, a suction system and an infusion system (Fig. 20.2A). In 1974 Klöti designed a similar instrument with an oscillating vitreous cutter which he called a Vitreous Stripper the principles of which are shown in the diagram (Fig. 20.2B).

An operating microscope with a working distance of 125 mm is the preferred method of visualising the vitreous cavity during vitrectomy. The microscope should have X–Y coupling to permit the surgeon to move the position of the microscope field from one point to another. A slit illumination provides increased contrast and there should be a small angle between the reflected and illuminating light.

Removal of tissue near the retina requires a planoconcave corneal contact lens.

21

Glaucoma

Glaucoma is a symptomatic condition, not a disease *sui generis*. The characteristic physical sign is increased intra-ocular pressure. A sustained increase in intra-ocular pressure may be due to an increase in the formation of the aqueous humour, a difficulty in its exit or a raised pressure in the episcleral veins. Of these, the first and last are of little importance; it follows that glaucoma is essentially due to an obstruction to the circulation of the aqueous at the pupil or to its drainage through the angle of the anterior chamber. The importance of embarrassment of the drainage channels through the canal of Schlemm is thus obvious (p. 15). It must be remembered, however, that if they are blocked, some drainage occurs through the uveo-scleral outflow; such an alternative drainage is typically seen in cases of buphthalmos (*q.v.*). These alternative channels, however, are by no means efficient since the pressure remains higher than normal, and they are incapable of dealing with emergencies when sudden changes of pressure occur.

It is convenient to divide such clinical states into two classes — (1) primary glaucoma which comprises two separate conditions, simple and closed-angle glaucoma, and (2) secondary glaucoma due to a specific anomaly or disease of the eye.

Secondary glaucoma

Secondary glaucoma may show the characteristics either of closed-angle or simple glaucoma. The following are the more common causes, most of which are fully discussed elsewhere. The treatment of most is that of the primary cause.

1. *Inflammatory Glaucoma. Hypertensive uveitis* (p. 152), wherein the rise of tension is due to clogging of the drainage channels by the turbid aqueous and inflammatory exudates.

2. *Post-inflammatory glaucoma*, due to blockage of the circulation of the aqueous either at the pupil by annular posterior synechiæ (iris bombé) or at the angle of the anterior chamber by the formation of peripheral synechiae or organised exudative deposits. In *heterochromic cyclitis* there is a chronic uveitis associated with a pale depigmenting iris and often a posterior subcapsular lens opacity. In *glaucomatocyclitic crises* the patient suffers from symptoms of closed-angle glaucoma although the angle of the anterior chamber is open and inflammatory cells are present in the aqueous of the anterior chamber.

3. *Secondary glaucoma after perforation of the cornea* either by an ulcer or a traumatic or operative wound. The cause in these cases is the mechanical blockage of the drainage angle by anterior synechiae formed by adhesion either of the iris or lens capsule to the wound.

4. A massive *intra-ocular hæmorrhage* may cause glaucoma, particularly when following a concussion injury. If the ruptured vessel is large the intra-ocular pressure may be suddenly raised to that of the blood pressure. If the hæmorrhage is in the posterior segment of the eye, the lens-iris diaphragm may be pushed forward almost to touch the cornea, further occluding the drainage angle. As a rule in these cases vitrectomy is the treatment of choice.

A *neovascular glaucoma* may follow thrombosis of the central vein of the retina (*q.v.*); it is due to organisation of tissue at the drainage angle as is the glaucoma secondary to diabetic *rubeosis iridis*.

5. *Secondary glaucoma associated with the lens* may arise in two circumstances. If the lens becomes intumescent, either in the rapid development of cataract or after it has been wounded, the swollen lens obliterates the drainage angle by forcing the root of the iris against the sclera. Unless the condition is rapidly relieved by operation (p. 174), extensive peripheral synechiæ involving a permanent rise of tension will result even although the lens is subsequently removed or becomes absorbed. If the lens has been wounded, lens proteins escape into the aqueous, thus aiding the rise of tension by embarrassment of the filtration channels by phagocytes laden with lens matter (phacolytic glaucoma).

A dislocation of the lens acts similarly. If it is partial, a large segment of the angle of the anterior chamber may be compressed or blocked. In complete dislocation into the anterior chamber, the entire angle may be blocked especially if the iris becomes firmly contracted over the posterior surface of the lens. In *aphakia* glaucoma may arise due to pupillary block by the intact vitreous which also obstructs the peripheral iridectomy. It responds to a further peripheral iridectomy at the 6 o'clock meridian or to pars plana vitrectomy.

6. *An intra-ocular tumour* may cause a secondary glaucoma, not by its increase in volume, but by infiltration of the angle by neoplastic tissue (p. 238).

7. Secondary glaucoma is readily caused by *venous obstruction*, the drainage of aqueous being then impeded (p. 15). This occurs in such conditions as orbital inflammations, large orbital tumours, caroticocavernous communications, thyrotopic exophthalmos and orbital varices (*q.v.*).

8. *Obstructive glaucoma* may arise owing to an organic blockage of the angle of the anterior chamber. This may develop in inflammatory or neoplastic processes. Such an obstruction is present when *essential atrophy of the iris* or *airidia* is complicated by secondary glaucoma. A particularly intractable type of glaucoma results if the epithelium grows through a badly healed corneal wound and spreads round the angle onto the iris (p. 265). Such epithelial ingrowths may follow perforating injuries to the cornea or an operative section as for cataract.

Glaucoma capsulare is probably of obstructive origin. Depositions of an exudative material occur on the iris, the ciliary region and on the capsule of the lens. Clinically these appear as flakes on the anterior capsule of the lens which are particularly evident in the mid-peripheral region where it is rubbed upon by the iris; the axial region is usually free; they tend to collect in the angle of the anterior chamber and may obstruct the drainage of the aqueous humour. This material is evidence of a widespread degenerative change in the anterior uvea, particularly the ciliary region.

Pigmentary glaucoma is probably obstructive due to pigment dispersion in an eye with faulty trabeculae. It affects young male myopes who present with intermittent halos, an open angle and a Krukenberg's spindle of pigment on the corneal endothelium.

Infantile glaucoma (buphthalmos; hydrophthalmos)
This is usually of a simple obstructive type, due in most cases to a failure in the development of the tissues in the region of the angle of the anterior chamber; the iris may not completely separate from the cornea (p. 5) or be inserted more anteriorly than usual so that the angle remains closed by persistent embryonic tissue. Depending on the degree of obstruction the result is a permanent rise in the tension of the eye, but since the circulation of the aqueous is maintained, although at a lower rate, by the anterior ciliary veins and the uveo-scleral outflow, the rise in tension is usually neither marked nor acute. Both eyes are generally affected, and buphthalmos occurs in boys more often than in girls.

Owing to the extensibility of the sclera the eye be-haves differently from the adult organ under this increase of pressure. Not only does the lamina cribrosa give way, producing deep cupping (p. 196) but the entire cornea and sclera stretch so that the globe gradually enlarges; this stretching and expansibility may mask the increased pressure on clinical examination.

In early cases the first sign may be an oedema of the cornea with watering of the eyes and marked photophobia, occasionally with the development of corneal opacities. The picture may resemble that of a keratitis accompanied by photophobia and circumcorneal congestion, resembling an inflammatory condition or congenital obstruction of the lacrimal duct. At a later stage more discrete corneal opacities appear as lines with a double contour due to rupture of Descemet's membrane. As the disease progresses the entire globe stretches, the thinned sclera of the ciliary region becoming bluish in colour, owing to the uveal pigment showing through. The junction of the cornea and sclera also stretches, so that the cornea is forced forwards and assumes a globular shape resembling keratoglobus (*q.v.*); care should be taken to differentiate between the two conditions. The anterior chamber is therefore extremely deep (Fig. 21.1). The lens does not participate in the general enlargement; owing to the expansion of the ciliary region the suspensory ligament is stretched so that the lens is flattened and displaced backwards. This removes some support to the iris, which may become tremulous (iridodonesis). As a result of the expansion, the eyes are usually myopic, although much less so than might be

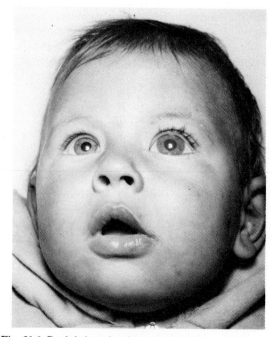

Fig. 21.1 Buphthalmos in a boy aged 8 months

anticipated from their length owing to the flattening of the lens and its displacement backwards. Equilibrium may be established with no further loss of vision but in other cases rapid deterioration occurs.

Sometimes in cases wherein the obstruction is incomplete, signs of raised tension may not appear until puberty. This may be called *juvenile glaucoma*. The type of *chronic glaucoma in young adults* which appears about the third or fourth decade and frequently shows hereditary tendencies may have the same basis.

Buphthalmos in relatively early life frequently occurs with more extensive congenital malformations, the most common of which are neurofibromatosis (p. 320) and the capillary nævus of the face associated with angiomatous conditions of the choroid and the brain (*Sturge–Weber syndrome*, p. 319).

Congenital or infantile glaucoma is transmitted as an autosomal recessive characteristic.

In the *treatment* of buphthalmos, miotics are obviously useless so that operative treatment has to be attempted. The standard drainage operations for simple glaucoma are unpredictable. More effective is the operation of *trabeculotomy (goniotomy)* (Fig. 21.2) wherein a specially constructed knife introduced at the limbus is swept round the angle of the anterior chamber in the opposite segment of the eye under direct gonioscopic observation. It is presumably effective by opening up the draining passages in those cases wherein the condition is due to the blockage of the corneo-iridic angle by persistent embryonic tissue, and may be supplemented by the operation of *gonio-puncture* whereby a puncture is made through the whole thickness of the trabecular region into the subconjunctival space.

Where goniotomy and goniopuncture fail then another form of trabeculotomy may be carried out by lowering a small flap of conjunctiva and a partial thickness flap of sclera at the upper limbus, exposing the canal of Schlemm by a vertical incision through the sclera and inserting a small trabeculotome shaped rather like a cyclodialysis spatula (Fig. 21.3). It is passed into the canal of Schlemm and then the trabeculotome is rotated so as to break the inner wall over one quarter of the canal. This is then repeated on the other side so that eventually the upper half of the canal wall is opened. The difficulty in this operation is the localisation of the canal itself.

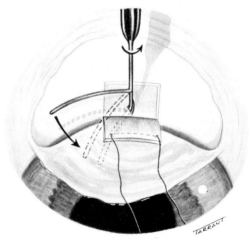

Fig. 21.3 Harms' trabeculotomy. The lower prong of a Harms' Trabeculotomy Probe is passed along Schlemm's canal to the right, the upper prong being used as a guide. (Reproduced from Miller S J H (ed) 1976 Eyes. In: Rob and Smith's Operative Surgery, 3rd edn. by courtesy of the publishers, Butterworths, London.)

If all forms of trabeculotomy fail then a trabeculectomy may be considered.

Primary Glaucoma

Two well-defined types of primary glaucoma exist which differ from each other in the type of patient affected, their clinical course and symptomatology, and in their prognosis and treatment — *closed-angle* and *simple glaucoma*. As a general rule, the first type is characterised by sudden episodic subacute attacks of raised tension, the most notable features of which are a diminution of vision and the subjective appearance of halos caused by corneal œdema. From the less severe of these attacks the eye may seem to recover to a considerable extent, but subsequent episodes tend to involve a

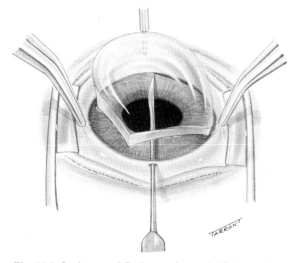

Fig. 21.2 Goniotomy. A Barkan goniotomy knife is passed obliquely through the limbus on the temporal side at 3 or 9 o'clock. Under gonioscopic control the knife is passed across the anterior chamber to the nasal part of the angle. An incision is made in the angle approximately mid-way between the root of the iris and Schwalbe's Ring through approximately 75°. The knife is then withdrawn. (Reproduced from Miller S J H (ed) 1976 Eyes. In: Rob and Smith's Operative Surgery, 3rd edn. by courtesy of the publishers, Butterworths, London.)

permanent raising of the tension (chronic congestive glaucoma) which may result in blindness (absolute glaucoma) or an acute attack may abolish vision. The second type, on the other hand, develops slowly, quietly and insidiously over many years with a characteristic triad of signs — raised tension, typical field defects and cupping of the disc — until in the 'absolute' stage the eye becomes intensely hard, all vision is lost and the disc develops a deep atrophic cup. It is to be noted that the differentiation between the two types is not based on tension, for an eye showing the picture of simple glaucoma may have a tension much higher than one with acute glaucoma. The differentiation depends on the mechanism of causation. In the closed-angle type the essential lesion is a closure of the angle of the anterior chamber during periods of raised tension leading to œdema of the tissues of the eye, while in the simple type the angle is clinically wide and open and signs of uveal congestion and œdema are replaced by optic atrophy and field loss.

Closed-angle glaucoma
This form of glaucoma occurs typically in persons, usually women, in the fifth or sixth decade; it may, however, occur earlier or later. It is seen particularly in those who are anxious in disposition.

The type of eye affected is characteristic. It is hypermetropic, the anterior chamber is shallow with the lens-iris diaphragm far forward and *its angle narrow*; the last feature is a constant characteristic. The narrowness of the angle may be due to the smallness of many of these eyes, the configuration of the ciliary body, and often to the relative size of the lens in comparison with the smallness of the eye so that this tissue crowds the root of the iris against the cornea, narrowing the filtration passages. Narrowness of the angle is often a hereditary characteristic but does not become apparent until the

fourth or fifth decade, a development typical of advancing years associated to some extent with the growth of the lens.

The mechanism of the closure of the angle of the anterior chamber varies. A common sequence of events follows pupillary dilatation. When the anterior chamber is of normal depth, the iris lies flatly in a transverse plane, its pupillary margin touching lightly the anterior surface of the lens (Fig. 21.4a). In an eye liable to closed-angle glaucoma with its shallow anterior chamber and anteriorly placed lens, the iris is closely apposed to the lens capsule over a wide area with a considerable component of force pressing it against the lens (Fig. 21.4b); communication between the posterior and anterior chambers is therefore difficult so that a condition of *blockage of the pupil* exists. In a state of semi-dilatation of the pupil the aqueous finds difficulty in passing forwards from the posterior chamber with the result that the relaxed iris bellies forward at its periphery resembling an iris bombé and its root approximates the inner surface of the cornea near the limbus, tending to cut off the filtration channels in the angle (Fig. 21.1). In other cases on dilatation of the pupil the iris may become crowded into the angle, or a swelling or anterior displacement of the ciliary body may produce the same effect.

It is possible that in some cases a mechanical occlusion of the angle by the iris is sufficient to block the drainage of the aqueous; for this reason *the instillation of atropine in an eye with a shallow anterior chamber or a narrow angle is dangerous* since it may precipitate an attack of raised tension. The administration of this drug, incidentally, is without danger in simple glaucoma when the angle is wide. It is to be remembered, however, that by no means every eye with a narrow angle develops glaucomatous attacks. Since both eyes usually

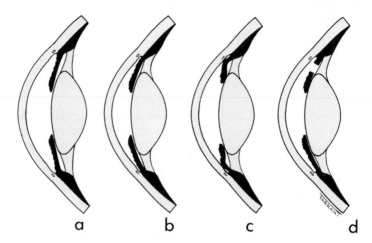

Fig. 21.4 The anterior chamber and its angle. (a) in a normal eye with a wide angle; (b) in an eye with a narrow angle; (c) physiological iris bombe with a semi-dilated pupil; (d) restoration of the patency of the angle after peripheral iridectomy

have a similar structure, this type of glaucoma is likely to be bilateral, but one eye is generally affected before the other.

The course of the disease may be divided into five stages. In the first or *prodromal stage*, occasional attacks of raised tension occur, characterised by some blurring of vision, the subjective appearance of halos around lights, and occasionally headache. In these attacks the eye remains white, without congestion, even although the tension may suddenly rise for a short period to heights of 40 or 60 mmHg. The characteristic symptom is the halos, due to corneal œdema. Such attacks may occur intermittently, being caused by such factors as over-work, anxiety, excitement, fatigue, and particularly by circumstances which cause a pupillary dilatation. At first, however, they are usually transitory and little attention may be paid to them; occasionally an acute attack may occur at an early stage, but in such cases it is rare not to elicit a history of previous attacks of halos on questioning.

A second *phase of constant instability* is reached when intermittency in these attacks is replaced by regularity. The normal diurnal variation of the ocular tension becomes exaggerated so that it may rise to very considerable heights, particularly in the late afternoon and evening; rest or sleep frequently induces a spontaneous fall in tension (Fig. 21.5).

Sooner or later, however, an *acute congestive attack* occurs, always associated with closure of the angle. This differs profoundly from the prodromal attacks in that the eye, instead of remaining white, becomes suffused and congested, there is acute pain and the tension remains up and, unless relieved by treatment, vision is gravely affected or lost. It is to be noted that although usually high, the tension in such an attack may be considerably lower than that found in the virtually symptomless prodromal attacks; the nature of the two is quite different. The clinical picture suggests that the crisis is due to acute ischaemia, perhaps associated with the liberation of prostaglandin-like substances.

An acute congestive attack presents a characteristic and dramatic picture. It starts suddenly, intense pain excited by stretching of the sensory nerves is felt in the eye and over the entire distribution of the fifth nerve. The pain is frequently so severe that it causes vomiting, and the attack is liable to be mistaken for a severe 'bilious attack' wherein the patient is prostrated and the pulse irregular and intermittent. The vision rapidly diminishes, so that in a few hours only hand movements can be recognised. In a considerable number of cases both eyes are affected, an attack in one eye being followed by a similar tragedy in the other.

Objective examination shows some œdema of the lids and conjunctiva; the latter is intensely congested and looks dusky red, owing to the dilatation of the veins. Ciliary congestion is marked; the cornea cloudy and insensitive; the anterior chamber very shallow; the iris discoloured, and the pupil moderately dilated and oval, generally with the long axis vertical. The reactions to light and accommodation are abolished. Ophthalmoscopic examination is impossible owing to the cloudiness of the cornea and the tension of the eye is considerably raised.

If the condition is not relieved by treatment, total abolition of vision may result due to acute ischaemic neuropathy. Spontaneous improvement, however, may occur, ushered in by diminution of pain; but considerable lowering of the visual acuity and, still more, irregular contraction of the field, follow every acute attack. Each attack also tends to produce a permanent adhesion of the root of the iris to the inner surface of the cornea forming *peripheral anterior synechiæ* (Fig. 21.6). These usually occur earliest and are most numerous in the upper part of the angle but gradually spread around the periphery; when three-quarters of the circumference has thus been obliterated, the eye reaches a precarious state, for the root of the iris becomes firmly adherent to the back of the cornea forming a 'false angle' and thus permanently embarrassing drainage. If these adhesions become sufficiently extensive the tension remains permanently slightly elevated even between attacks, and some congestion and irritability persist. This is the stage of *chronic closed-angle glaucoma*.

Up to the stage of the acute attack the visual acuity remains unimpaired; after an acute attack it is always depressed. Similarly, before an acute attack the visual fields remain normal; after an acute attack they become

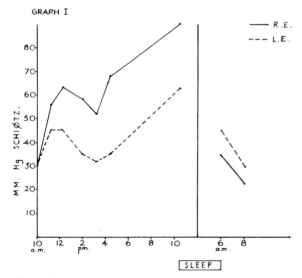

GRAPH I

Fig. 21.5 The diurnal variation of tension in closed-angle glaucoma, showing a tendency to rise progressively late in the evening, and to fall during sleep. The abscissa denotes the time of day; the vertical line indicates when the patient was asleep

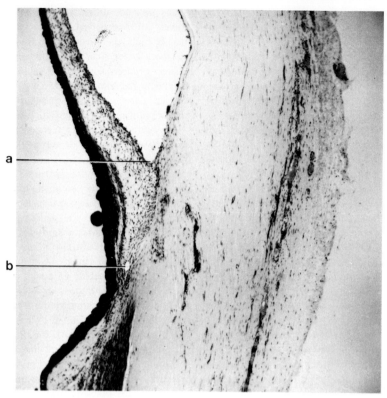

Fig. 21.6 The angle of the anterior chamber in advanced closed-angle glaucoma. (a) The level of the true angle (the line points to the canal of Schlemm); (b) the level of the false angle; (a) a peripheral anterior synechia. × 64. (By courtesy of Ashton.)

constricted irregularly as a result of anterior ischaemic optic neuropathy; but in the chronic congestive phase the typical scotomatous defects characteristic of simple glaucoma become evident (p. 197). At the same time, cupping of the disc (p. 195) appears for the first time, for the development of this phenomenon in this type of case is a late event depending on prolonged high tension.

The chronic phase, if untreated, with or without the occurrence of intermittent sub-acute attacks, gradually passes into the final phase of *absolute glaucoma* wherein the eye is completely blind. The anterior ciliary veins are dilated, and a reddish-blue zone surrounds the cornea. The cornea is clear, but insensitive; it may have vesicles (bullous keratopathy) or filaments (filamentary keratitis) upon it. The anterior chamber is very shallow. The iris is dilated, atrophic, and may have a broad zone of pigment around the pupil (ectropion of the uveal pigment). The pupil is grey in patches, instead of jet black. The optic disc is deeply cupped. The tension is high; usually the eyeball is as hard as stone. Such an eye is generally painful, with temporary exacerbations, and eventually suffers degenerative changes. The more important are due to a giving way of the sclera before the continued high intraocular pressure so that scleral

staphylomata are produced; they may be in the neighbourhood of the ciliary body (ciliary staphylomata) or at the equator (equatorial staphylomata). Such globes may eventually become enormous with walls as thin as paper and there is considerable danger of rupture from slight injury. Sooner or later the tension becomes normal or diminished, due essentially to degeneration of the ciliary body whereby its secretory functions are diminished or abolished; such an eye may even shrink and suffer widespread degenerative changes.

The *diagnosis* of closed-angle glaucoma in the prodromal stage is of immense importance. In the acute and congestive stages the nature of the condition is usually obvious. The only real difficulty which may arise is its differentiation from iritis; this has already been discussed (*q.v.*).

In the prodromal stages the diagnosis depends on the history of seeing *halos*, the presence of a narrow angle of the anterior chamber, and the observation or inducement of a rise of tension.

The early diagnosis of closed-angle glaucoma is unusually important since adequate treatment at this stage is easy and as certain of controlling the disease as in any condition in medicine; after an acute attack has occurred treatment is difficult and its results problematical. *A his-*

tory of halos, particularly if associated with periodic obscurations of vision, should therefore always excite the liveliest suspicion; this suspicion should not be diminished by the observation that in the early stages of the disease the eye (apart from its narrow angle) is normal, its tension between attacks is not raised, there is no cupping of the disc and its function (visual acuity and fields) unimpaired, while the facility of the drainage of the aqueous as measured tonographically (*q.v.*) is undiminished.

The halos are due to the accumulation of fluid in the corneal epithelium and to alterations in the refractive condition of the corneal lamellæ. They are seen as coloured rings around lights and are therefore usually observed after dark. The colours are distributed as in the spectrum with red outside and blue innermost. If the patient gives a vague history, their appearance can be demonstrated to him by his looking through a thin layer of lycopodium powder enclosed between two glass plates made up as a trial lens.

The only other condition which may commonly give rise to a similar appearance is early cataractous changes in the lens. The two may be differentiated by Fincham's test. A stenopæic slit is passed before the eye across the line of vision. As it passes, a glaucomatous halo remains intact but diminished in intensity, whereas a lenticular halo is broken up into segments which revolve as the slit is moved (Fig. 21.7).

The anatomical *configuration of the angle* is of immense importance in the diagnosis. Narrowness of the angle is almost invariably accompanied by shallowness of the anterior chamber which itself should give rise to suspicion. This can be seen by ordinary inspection. Examination with the slit-lamp provides a good index of the state of the angle since the degree of approximation of the optical sections of the cornea and iris in the periphery can be readily seen. A narrow periphery, however, may be assoicated with a wide angle, and the only conclusive evidence is obtained from gonioscopy (*q.v.*) which is invaluable in the diagnosis of the disease. The presence of keratic precipitates or other signs of iridocyclitis should always be excluded by slit-lamp examination to differentiate a primary glaucoma from a hypertensive iridocyclitic crisis (*q.v.*).

The demonstration of a rise in tension is often difficult in the prodromal stages since the hypertensive periods are temporary and often occur at inconvenient times. The patient should be instructed, however, to report to the surgeon whenever he sees a halo; if this cannot be arranged, *provocative tests* can be undertaken — but always with care in this type of the disease. These are designed to test the control of the ocular tension under conditions of stress.

In the *dark-room test* the patient is placed in a dark room for half an hour; he must remain awake so that the pupils dilate. Measurement of the tension before and after may show a rise which is pathological if greater than 8 mmHg (Schiötz). The dark room test may be re-

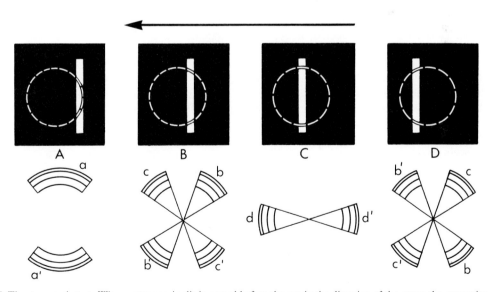

Fig. 21.7 The stenopaeic test. When a stenopaeic slit is passed before the eye in the direction of the arrow the successive appearances of the lenticular halo are represented. At A, when the lateral margin only of the pupil is exposed, and the horizontal radial fibres of the lens only are implicated, the horizontal portions a, a′, of the halo are visible. At B, when the oblique fibres are involved, the portions a, a′, appear to divide, forming b, c and b′, c′; as the slit is moved these rotate, b, b′ in a clockwise direction, and c, c′, anti-clockwise. When C is reached only vertical fibres are involved, and the portions appear to reunite in d, d′. On continuing the motion of the slit, the portions b′, c and c′, b, appear and revolve similarly, until finally, at the other extreme position, they become amalgamated as a, a′ in A. (By courtesy of Emsley and Fincham.)

inforced by placing the patient in a prone position while he remains in the dark. The effect of gravity on the lens tends to narrow the anterior chamber still further and give some idea of the vulnerability of the eye to spontaneous rises in tension. Nevertheless if the tension is found to be normal at all times and if the angle of the anterior chamber is open but narrow on gonioscopy then a positive provocative test does not constitute the diagnosis of closed angle glaucoma and in the absence of organic change in the eye or spontaneous symptoms, peripheral iridectomy is not justified.

Closed angle glaucoma is closely related to the degree of hypermetropia and the width of the angle of the anterior chamber. Such characteristics are genetically determined.

The *treatment* of this type of glaucoma is surgical. Whenever it is diagnosed — or suspected — the intermittent attacks of tension should be forestalled by a miotic such as pilocarpine 0.5 – 2.0% or one of its substitutes. This should be instilled, not necessarily in the morning when the tension in these cases is usually low, but before the halos habitually appear, that is, usually in the late afternoon or evening. The optimum time should be determined in each case by tonometric tests and, in addition, a prophylactic drop should be taken before any periods when fatigue, excitement or darkness is anticipated. Peripheral iridectomy (p. 258) should be performed without hesitation. In early cases before the development of peripheral synechiae, a peripheral (buttonhole) iridectomy is all that is required; on its performance, since free communication between the anterior and posterior chambers is now restored, the appearance of iris bombé at once disappears (Fig. 21.4d). Such an operation carried out on a quiet eye is practically without risk, involves no visual disability, and invariably results in a complete cessation of the disease. This is the only type of glaucoma wherein operative treatment can be counted on to be successful and the prognosis is good in both a surgical or laser approach.

Once an acute attack has developed the outlook is very different. If the case is seen early, every endeavour should be made to lower the tension before operating in order to avoid the difficulties of operation on a congested, chemosed eye, and the dangers of opening a globe the tension of which is high. Full sedation, should be attained. The pupil should be made small by Pilocarpine 1 or 2 % but once this has been accomplished there is no need for further use of a miotic. The more powerful cholinergic miotics such as DFP are dangerous since they may increase the congestion. At the same time, an attempt may be made to lower the tension by the systemic administration of carbonic anhydrase inhibitors in full doses (Diamox, Neptazane) which may well be supplemented by dehydration measures such as the intravenous injection of urea or mannitol or, more easily

and as effectively, by the oral administration of glycerol (1.5 g/kg body wt). Local heat by medical diathermy (p. 371) is frequently of benefit.

A further measure which is sometimes of great value in lowering the tension before operation is the retrobulbar injection of 1 ml of procaine (4 %) and adrenaline into the region of the ciliary ganglion (p. 255). Not only has this frequently a marked hypotensive effect within a quarter of an hour, but the accompanying anæsthesia relieves the patient's pain and anxiety. It is to be remembered, however, that since paralysis of the ciliary nerves stops the formation of acetylcholine, drugs such as eserine, which act by inhibiting cholinesterase, become ineffective.

Operation is most conveniently done under general anæsthesia, when the eye is less congested.

If the tension is relieved by medical treatment it is better to wait until the eye is quiet before operating, provided the angle of the anterior chamber has been opened. The choice of operation then depends on the state of the angle, which should be explored gonioscopically. If peripheral synechiæ are not extensive, an iridectomy will probably suffice; if they are, a filtration operation is advisable such as trabeculectomy (Chap. 27).

In all cases of acute glaucoma the other eye should be operated upon by a prophylactic peripheral iridectomy if the angle is narrow, even if the eye appears otherwise normal. The occurrence of acute glaucoma in the second eye within twelve months of an attack in its fellow is so common as to render this relatively safe procedure justifiable.

In absolute thrombotic glaucoma pain may be relieved by the exhibition of atropine 1% drops twice daily together with dexamethasone 0.1% topically twice daily. If the pain cannot be relieved it is best to excise the eye. If this is refused the tension may be lowered by the insertion of a silicone tube (0.12 mm in diameter) into the anterior chamber under a scleral flap with the distal end exposed in the superior fornix. The pain may be relieved for a time, varying in different cases, by a retro-ocular injection of 1.5 ml of procaine (4%) followed 7 min later by alcohol (80%) (p. 255); a firm pad and bandage are applied for 24 hours. If the pain recurs this treatment can be repeated. In such eyes a filtration operation is rarely effective, and the frequency with which a blind painful eye with high tension contains a malignant growth justifies its removal.

Simple glaucoma

This presents an entirely different clinical picture from the acute form. While the latter occurs preferentially in women in the fifth and sixth decades, of an excitable habit and with an unstable vasomotor system, simple glaucoma occurs in either sex a decade later, affecting people who are of no specific psychological pattern. While closed-angle glaucoma is characterised by premonitory symptoms and a turbulent course, simple glaucoma is quietly and slowly progressive and practically symptomless. The first type always occurs in a specific type of eye with a narrow angle of the anterior chamber. The second occurs with any type of angle; this, as is found in the population generally, is therefore usually wide. In the first type, field-defects and cupping of the disc appear late and develop rapidly; in the second, early and insidiously. Both forms of the disease, however, lead to the same end — a stage of permanent congestion, absolute glaucoma and blindness. In both types the condition is almost always eventually bilateral.

The clinical course of simple glaucoma is characteristic. No symptoms are generally experienced although mild headaches and eye-aches may occur. An observant person may notice a defect in the visual field; while reading and close work often present increasing difficulties due to accommodative failure owing to pressure upon the ciliary muscle and its nerve supply. An increase in the strength of presbyopic glasses is therefore often required. On the whole, however, the disease is so insidious that it is often not noticed until the vision of one eye is almost lost and that of the other seriously impaired, when it may be discovered only by accident. This constitutes one of the main reasons why periodic eye examinations by an expert are advisable after midlife, *particularly for those with a family history of glaucoma* and certainly whenever visual symptoms require a change of spectacles. Central vision usually remains unaffected until a late stage and is no guide to the extent or progress of the disease.

Defective light sense is often an early feature of simple glaucoma. The light minimum is raised and dark adaptation is slowed, so that patients take longer to get used to the lower degree of illumination in passing into a dimly lighted room, a disability which becomes increasingly disturbing in the later stages.

The diagnosis therefore depends on the three objective signs — raised tension, cupping of the disc and field defects.

The *tension* in simple glaucoma requires careful study and repeated observation; hospitalization of the patient may be advisable over 24-h periods, at any rate in the early stages. The initial change is not so much a rise of tension as an exaggeration of the normal diurnal variation (p. 15) to form a rhythmic swing. During the rising phase of tension the venous pressure in the episcleral veins may increase above the pressure in the anterior chamber as is seen by the blood influx into the aqueous veins (p. 15). Before a fall of tension, whether it occurs naturally or is induced by miotics, the opposite phenomenon is seen; the venous pressure falls and the aqueous veins fill with clear fluid. Moreover, the entire cycle is abolished by cholinergic drugs (miotics).

In most patients however, contrary to what happens in closed-angle glaucoma, the tension falls during the evening. At first, between its phasic rises, the tension usually returns to normal; as time goes on the variation increases and the normal level is no longer attained. The difference between the "peak pressure" and the "base pressure" thus diminishes and a permanent elevation occurs, usually, however, retaining some of the phasic element. In many cases, if this raised tension is prolonged, the eye goes quietly blind owing to atrophy of the optic nerve fibres; in other cases, if the tension is sufficiently high, a congestive phase develops particularly in young people; and in all cases the natural result is a condition of absolute glaucoma similar to that occurring in the acute form of the disease (*q.v.*).

It must be stressed that in the initial stages the tension is not necessarily permanently raised; the important feature is its variability. A single reading of the tension is therefore valueless if it is found to be normal since this may coincide with a temporary fall to a base pressure which may not be elevated. *A variation in the ocular tension of over 5 mmHg (Schiötz) should always excite suspicion of glaucoma even although the whole excursion lies under the limits generally accepted as normal (20 mmHg).* This constant variation in tension can cause grave damage to the eye and produce field defects and cupping of the disc, particularly when the lamina cribrosa is weak.

Cupping of the optic disc, is an essential feature of simple glaucoma (Figs 21.8–21.9). The process frequently starts segmentally often in the lower temporal quadrant, to produce an increase in size of the vertical diameter of the excavation and essentially an oval cup. The thinning

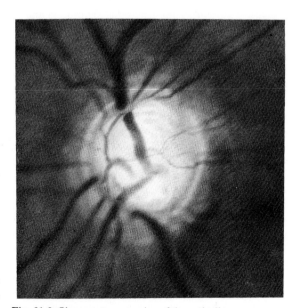

Fig. 21.8 Glaucomatous cupping of the optic disc

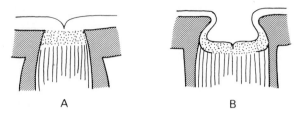

Fig. 21.9 A, diagram of meridional section of normal disc; B, diagram of meridional section of glaucomatous cupped disc. Note the displacement backwards of the lamina cribrosa

of the rim at the lower border of the cup in the 6 o'clock periphery corresponds with the early appearance of an upper arcuate scotoma. When fully developed it differs in ophthalmoscopic appearance from a deep physiological cup, with which it is most likely to be confused, in that the excavation reaches to the edges of the disc and the sides are steep, not shelving. The retinal vessels have the appearance of being broken off at the margin of the disc. If they are accurately focused here their continuations upon the floor of the cup are slightly out of focus and look broader and paler. When the edges overhang, as is often the case, the course of the vessels as they climb the sides of the cup is hidden. By the indirect method of ophthalmoscopy slight lateral movement of the condensing lens causes a distinct parallax (p. 86), which is more marked the deeper the cup. By the direct method the difference in level between the vessels at the edge and on the floor can be measured (p. 87). When the tension is high pulsation of the arteries may be seen — always a pathological phenomenon (p. 95) (Plate 3, Fig. E).

There is always some atrophy of the optic nerve when the disc is cupped by the glaucomatous process and as the fibres degenerate the structure of the lamina may become exposed at the bottom of the cup; it is therefore not surprising that there may be great difficulty in distinguishing a shallow glaucomatous cup from the slight depression which follows simple atrophy of the nerve without increase of tension (p. 195). In shallow glaucomatous cups the disc has a pink colour, whereas the atrophic cup is white. In many early cases all the conditions have to be weighed carefully before it is possible to come to a definite conclusion; and in early cases progressive changes should be carefully noted and periodically described and drawn or photographed so that any progress may be recorded rather than left to memory. The vertical diameter of the cup should be expressed as a decimal fraction of the vertical diameter of the disc. If this factor — the cup/disc ratio increases with time glaucoma simplex is suspected.

Cupping of the disc is due to two factors. To some extent the raised pressure may act mechanically, forcing the lamina cribrosa backwards and squeezing the nerve

fibres within its meshes to disturb axoplasmic flow. A further factor, however, is glial atrophy due to anoxia. The characteristic pathological feature of the optic nerve in such cases is the disappearance of the nerve fibres without a corresponding increase in the supporting glial tissue (as occurs in primary optic atrophy) so that large caverns or lacunæ are formed (*cavernous optic atrophy*). Such a histological picture develops typically in any organ when the blood supply is gradually cut off; the more highly differentiated elements degenerate and disappear and, owing to lack of nutriment, the supporting elements do not proliferate but eventually also degenerate (Fig. 21.10).

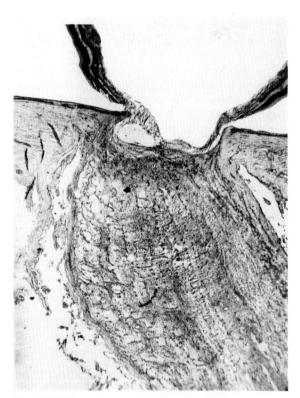

Fig. 21.10 The optic nerve in a case of advanced simple glaucoma. Note the cavernous atrophy towards the left of the figure. × 25. (By courtesy of Ashton.)

Such a condition may occur in the optic nerve without any irregular variation or rise in tension. These cases show the same appearance of the disc and the same field defects as characterise simple glaucoma; but they should be designated as low-tension glaucoma due to a weak lamina cribrosa.

The *field defects* in simple glaucoma usually run parallel to the changes in the optic disc. The careful and repeated charting of the fields — particularly the central fields by the Bjerrum screen (p. 197) — is of unusual importance owing to the retention of central vision until the disease is at an advanced stage (Figs 21.11–21.14).

The earliest sign is said to be a localised constriction of the central field to very small test objects (1/2000) so that instead of skirting the 30° isopter concentrically, the field becomes deformed, curving inwards to exclude the blind-spot (baring of the blind-spot) (Fig. 21.11). This sign is not pathognomonic of early glaucoma simplex. It may be manipulated by change in illumination or size of pupil. The earliest sign is the appearance of

one or more small scotomatous areas, initially a relative defect, in the same isopter as the blind-spot and usually above the disc. Ocassionally there is a sickle-shaped extension of the blind-spot above or below, or both, with the concavity of the sickle directed towards the fixation point (*Seidel's sign*); this is of more significance. At a later stage a considerable area of relative defect can frequently be traced in direct continuity with the blind-spot (*Bjerrum's scotoma*). The scotoma may pass in an arc from the blind-spot above or below the

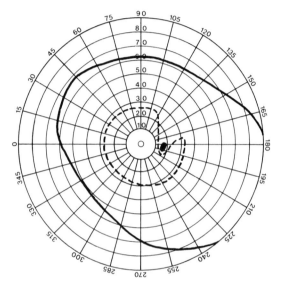

Fig. 21.11 Baring of the blind-spot (5/330, 1/2000)

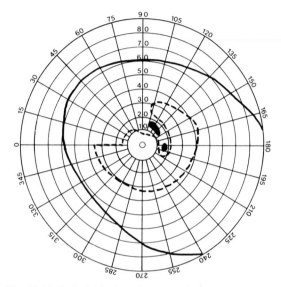

Fig. 21.12 Early sickle-shaped scotoma (5/330, 1/2000)

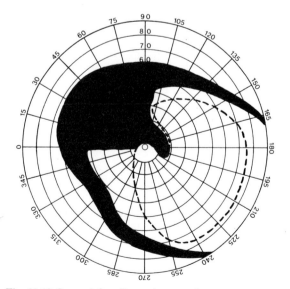

Fig. 21.13 Sector defect, Roenne's step and arcuate scotoma (5, 2/330)

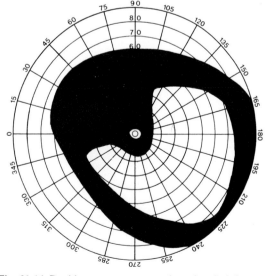

Fig. 21.14 Double arcuate scotoma and quadrantic defect (5/330)

Figs. 21.11–21.14 Changes in the visual fields in glaucoma

fixation point, or may form a complete annular scotoma. Sometimes at an early stage and sometimes only late in the disease, defects appear in the peripheral field. The upper or sometimes the lower nasal field particularly tends to show sectorial defects which have a characteristically sharply defined horizontal edge (*Roenne's step*). In the later stages the general contraction is more marked, and eventually only a paracentral patch of the temporal field persists, central vision being abolished. The early changes are characteristic *nerve-bundle defects* and their distribution may be due to premature destruction of the thick bundles of arcuate fibres that crowd on the temporal side of the disc and run an arcuate course above and below the macula (Figs 21.15–21.16).

Pathologically, little is evident in such eyes except the effects of generalised sclerosis and pressure. We have already noted the peculiar type of atrophy of the optic nerve. In the later stages the entire uveal tract may become extremely atrophic, only the larger vessels remaining. The angle of the anterior chamber is usually wide and peripheral synechiæ are not usually found; but the trabeculæ are sclerosed and thickened and often heaped with pigment derived from the degenerated uvea and there is an absence of giant vacuoles in the cells lining the canal of Schlemm.

The cause of the disease is unknown but it may be presumed in general to be due to inefficiency of the drainage channels so that they are permeable with difficulty and the base pressure rises.

The *diagnosis* of simple glaucoma depends, as we have seen, on a close investigation of the tension — initially of its variations, eventually of its permanent elevation — and on the presence of atrophic cupping of the disc and the typical field defects, particularly in the early stages those in the paracentral area, which should be repeatedly explored in doubtful cases.

A test of doubtful value in assessing the progress of the disease, or the extent of embarrassment to drainage, is the technique of *tonography*. In this the standard Schiötz tonometer may be used or a graphic record may be obtained with the electronic tonometer. If the normal eye is compressed by a weighted tonometer for four minutes, aqueous and choroidal blood are expressed so that the ocular tension gradually falls while the compression is maintained, and when the weight is lifted the tension is considerably less than it was originally. In simple glaucoma, similar compression leads to a smaller fall during the period of compression since the aqueous cannot easily escape, and when the weight is removed the tension of the eye remains relatively high. The extent of the fall in tension gives an approximate estimate of the facility of the outflow of aqueous.

The estimate is only approximate because no measurement can be made of how much aqueous or how much choroidal blood has been expressed. Until this is known it is impossible to assess to what extent the fall in tension is due to a poor facility of aqueous outflow. Unfortunately tonography fails to give help in the clinically doubtful case of glaucoma.

Primary open angle glaucoma has a polygenic inheritance and it would seem that patients who develop the frank disease must inherit a number of abnormal genes. Such genes influence the height of the intraocular pressure, the facility of outflow and the cup/disc ratio. Diabetes mellitus and myopia are also accompaniments which occur more frequently in a glaucomatous population than in the general population.

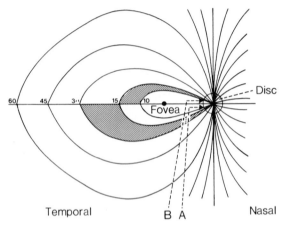

Fig. 21.15 The course of the nerve fibres in the retina: showing the fibres involved in field defects, A and B, in Figure 21.16

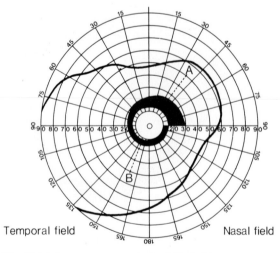

Fig. 21.16 Arcuate scotomata in the field of vision corresponding with lesions A and B in Figure 21.15

Open angle glaucoma
The treatment of this form of glaucoma is, in the first place, always medical, with operation as a last resort.

The aim is to prevent field loss which results from too high an intra-ocular pressure. Optic nerve heads vary in susceptibility to pressure damage (optic discs which are cupped are particularly susceptible), so that the danger-level of tension varies from patient to patient. Management requires continued supervision by an ophthalmologist because it may involve periodic tonometry and regular fundus photography as well as careful and repeated mapping of the fields of vision. These are time consuming tests which can, however, be delegated to suitably trained staff.

Pilocarpine is still the sheet anchor of treatment administered at six-hourly intervals as drops which constrict the pupil (miosis). It may be administered in soaked hydrophilic contact lenses or slowly released by 'ocuserts'. Long-acting anti-cholinesterase drugs require instillation less frequently — once or at most twice daily. The drugs of this group in common use are demecarium bromide ('Tosmilen Eye Drops') and ecothiopate iodide ('Phospholine') both of which produce a marked miosis, so much so that patients with lens opacities often find their vision too restricted. Adrenaline drops may be employed alone in early cases, particularly in the younger age groups in whom accommodation is active.

In general it may be stated that in established glaucoma simplex under the age of 45 an attempt should be made to control the ocular tension with adrenaline drops. If adrenaline fails then Timoptol (Timolol Maleate) 0.25 or 0.5% drops 12-hourly should be tried. Timolol Maleate is a topical non-selective beta$_1$ and beta$_2$ adrenergic blocking agent with little significant intrinsic sympathomimetic, direct myocardial depressant or local anesthetic (membrane stabilising) activity.

It lowers intraocular pressure by reducing the rate of aqueous formation as a result of direct action on the secreting epithelium of the ciliary body. It is used every 12 h and produces no significant change in pupil size, accommodation, visual acuity or tear production.

It should not be used in patients who have previously experienced asthma. It should be used with caution in patients with cardiovascular problems because of the possibility of inducing systemic vascular hypotension and bradycardia and in patients using adrenergic-augmenting psychotropic drugs. Patients taking oral beta-adrenergic blocking agents must be watched for potential additive effects. Timilol produces occasional disturbances of the central nervous system consisting of disorientation, and confusion. Eye complications are minor.

If Timoptol alone fails Adrenaline 1% drops or Dipivalyl Epinephrine 0.1% may be added twice daily although the pupils may become dilated on this combination. If this fails, then pilocarpine in various strengths should be employed or resort should be had to the combination of pilocarpine with adrenalin. If this fails then a systemic carbonic anhydrase inhibitor such as acetazolamide ('Diamox') or dichlorphenamide ('Daranide') must be added.

The combination of an anti-cholinesterase drug with adrenaline or timoptol and a carbonic anhydrase inhibitor produces maximal reduction in pressure. If tension is uncontrolled on such therapy, operation should be undertaken; unjustified delay accounts for more blindness than the complications of surgical decompression. Details of the use of the drugs mentioned above are as follows:

Adrenaline diminishes the aqueous inflow and reduces the intraocular pressure. Combined with pilocarpine, which increases the outflow, the pressure reducing effect is additive. This also applies to adrenaline combined with the systemic carbonic anhydrase inhibitors. When it has been used for some time adrenaline also increases aqueous outflow, an action which is difficult to explain. Adrenaline is given as drops of the bitartrate, hydrochloride or borate in concentrations of 1–2%. The maximal effect is exerted in about 12 h but it remains appreciable for at least 48 h. After use for some months many patients develop conjunctival irritation and hyperæmia. Black spots formed by the oxidation of adrenaline to melanin may appear in the conjunctiva but these are without serious significance. Adrenaline may be used topically along with guanethidine in various strengths (3% guanethidine and 0.5% adrenaline or even weaker concentrations (1 : 0.2)). Occasionally patients suffer from hyperaemic conjictivae and a corneal epitheliosis.

Pilocarpine is a miotic which only rarely produces irritation or allergic reactions and is one of the safest drugs in the pharmacopœia. For eye drops it is used as a nitrate in concentrations of 0.5–4%; its action when placed in the conjunctival sac lasts for about 8 h. It reduces ocular tension by facilitating aqueous outflow.

Demecarium bromide is a synthetic carbamate which reacts irreversibly with cholinesterase. It is water soluble and stable at room temperature and is used in concentrations of 0.25–0.5%. It can be given once or twice daily but once or twice weekly may suffice.

Ecothiopate iodide is an organo-phosphate and reacts with cholinesterase to form a phosphorylated enzyme. It is a water-soluble long-acting miotic reaching its maximal effect 24 h or so after instillation. In some patients 0.06% ecothiopate twice daily is more effective than 4% pilocarpine four times daily. It is employed in concentrations of 0.03–0.25%.

These two anti-cholinesterase drugs are tending to lose their popularity because of their side-effects which include a profound miosis, ocular discomfort, myopia from ciliary spasm, occasional uveitis if used over a long period and sometimes in myopes the production of detachment of the retina. The report of induced lens opacities after prolonged use has also seeded doubts in the minds of prescribers. Systemic side effects are sometimes met consisting of nausea, vomiting, diarrhœa, hypotension and general weakness. In some patients there is an associated depression of red cell and plasma cholinesterase.

Acetazolamide and *Dichlorphenamide* are carbonic anhydrase inhibitors. The former is given orally in doses of 125–250 mg and the latter in doses of 50 mg one to four times daily. Sustained action capsules of 500 mg ('Diamox Sustets') have a more prolonged effect and are given twice daily. These drugs reduce the formation of bicarbonate so that the volume of aqueous humour is lessened. Acetazolamide may produce tingling of the fingers and if used over a long period in elderly patients may cause indigestion, diarrhœa and loss of appetite and weight. Renal colic is another complication to which it may give rise and this constitutes a contraindication to its further use. As diamox leads to the renal excretion of potassium, Slow K is usually prescribed in dosages of 1 gm daily.

Several operations may be employed to control the tension by the establishment of a 'filtering scar'. The scar in these cases is composed of spongy tissue, through the interstices of which the intra-ocular fluid is able to make its way into the subconjunctival tissue, where it is absorbed; instead of the normal drainage into the episcleral veins, the aqueous thus drains to the atmospheric level of this tissue. In an ordinary corneo-scleral section the lips of the wound are in good apposition and sound healing rapidly takes place. This is much less likely to occur if there is a gap between the lips of the wound which becomes filled with loose scar tissue so that a filtering cicatrix results. Various operations have been based upon this principle. A circular wound in the sclera minimizes this tendency and is the basis of the operation of *trephining* (p. 259). In *Lagrange's operation* (p. 259) a piece of sclera is excised; in *Scheie's operation* (p. 259) this is combined with cauterisation of the lips of the wound; in *Preziosi's operation* a fistulous track is made into the angle of the anterior chamber underneath a conjunctival flap by an electrocautery. The incarceration of a piece of iris in the wound to maintain a channel is the basis of *iridencleisis* (p. 260). Trabeculectomy involves excising a piece of tissue which includes a short length of the canal of Schlemm. This gap produces two new entrances into the canal itself. Such an operation also forms a filtering channel to the sub-conjunctiva so that its effectivity depends upon two ways of escape of aqueous, one by the canal of Schlemm and the other by a transcleral route to the subconjunctival spaces. Other surgical alternatives are available. A communication between the anterior chamber and the suprachoroidal space, which also may lower the tension by inhibiting

secretion by the ciliary body, comprises the operation of *cyclodialysis* (p. 260); it is of particular value in aphakic eyes. A very effective procedure is the combination in *Stallard's operation* of a flap-sclerotomy hinged on the limbus, with a small cyclodialysis and a basal iridencleisis wherein a tongue of the peripheral part of the iris is included within the lips of the scleral flap. A generalised atrophy of the ciliary body may be induced by a *cyclodiathermy* (p. 260), or cyclocryopexy. Finally the inner wall of the Canal of Schlemm may be punctured by the Argon Laser and outflow thereby is increased by trabeculoplasty.

Some of these operations — particularly the most effective — are not without their dangers. The presence of a draining bleb covered with thin conjunctiva may lead to the subsequent development of *secondary infection* — a serious complication, now less catastrophic if it is treated early and intensively with antibiotic drugs (Chapt. 14). This is most common after a trephining operation. *Cataract* is a more common sequel, particularly if early changes are present in the lens when surgery is undertaken. If such opacities exist, a drainage operation can be done first and an extraction of the cataract performed at a later date when the section is made at the lower limbus.

In very advanced cases the field of vision may be found reduced almost to the fixation point. If, the tension is not controlled, it is advisable to operate, but in such cases every attempt should be made to lower the tension before operation.

On the whole, it is to be remembered that more eyes are lost by delay in undertaking surgery than by surgical intervention.

All these operations undertaken for the control of simple glaucoma are uncertain in their results, for they can control the factor of tension only. In general it may be said that if the deterioration of vision is due essentially to a raised tension, its surgical relief will usually prevent further loss; if the tension is low and the deterioration is essentially due to a trail lamina cribrosa, the vision will probably continue to fall in spite of the operation. Unfortunately cases of this type are not uncommon. *The prognosis of simple glaucoma is good only if the case comes under adequate control early, if operation is undertaken before raised tension has had serious effects, and if the lamina cribrosa is tough.* In practically all cases wherein treatment has not been instituted until a late stage, the outlook is bad. The prognosis thus depends largely on early diagnosis and the institution of early and adequate treatment to forestall cupping of the optic disc and field loss.

Plate 1

Plate 2

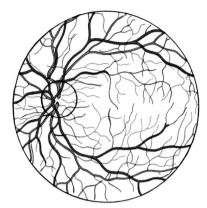

A. The retinal circulation

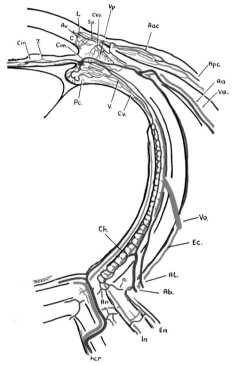

The ciliary circulation

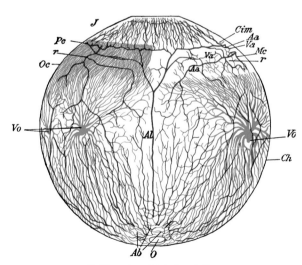

B. The choroidal circulation

Aa, anterior ciliary arteries; Ab, short posterior ciliary arteries; Al, long posterior ciliary arteries; Ch, choroid; Cim, circulus iridis major; J, vessels of the iris; Mc, ciliary muscle; O, optic nerve; Oc, orbiculus ciliaris; Pc, ciliary processes; r, recurrent ciliary arteries; Va, anterior ciliary veins; Vo, vortex vein.

Aa, anterior ciliary artery; Aac, anterior conjunctival artery; Ab, short posterior ciliary artery; Acr, central artery of the retina; Al, long posterior ciliary artery; An, anastomosis of choroidal vessels with those of the optic nerve; Apc, posterior conjunctival artery; Av, aqueous vein; C, canal of Schlemm; Cev, ciliary efferent vein; Ch, choriocapillaris; Cim, circulus iridis major; Cin, circulus iridis minor; Cv, recurrent choroidal veins; Ec, episcleral artery; En, vessels to the outer sheath of the optic nerve; J, radial vessels of iris; In, vessels to the inner sheath of the optic nerve; L, limbal vessels; n, branch of short posterior ciliary artery to optic nerve; Pc, ciliary plexus; Sp, scleral plexus; V, branch of vena vorticosa from ciliary system; Va, anterior ciliary vein; Vo, vortex, vein; Vp, ciliary venous plexus.

Plate 3

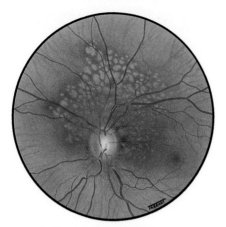

A. Drusen of the posterior pole

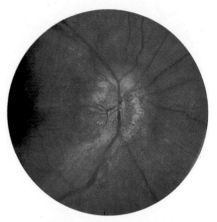

D. Plerocephalic disc oedema

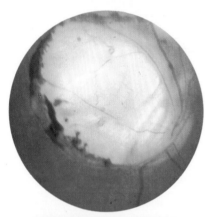

B. Coloboma of the optic disc

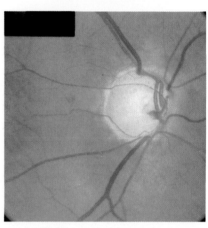

E. Glaucomatous cupping

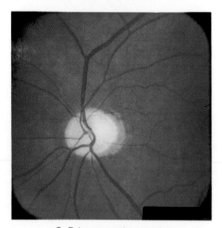

C. Primary optic atrophy

Plate 4

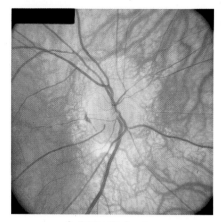

A. Albinotic fundus

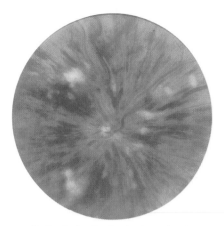

C. Central retinal vein thrombosis

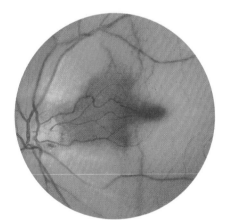

B. Central retinal artery occlusion with a cherry red spot and sparing of a temporal cilio-retinal vessel.

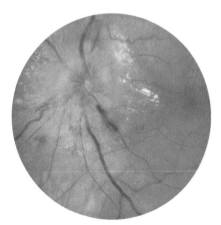

D. The fundus in accelerated hypertension with disc oedema

Plate 5

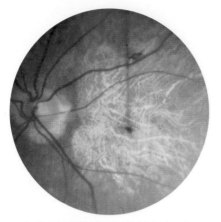

A. Central areolar choroidal atrophy

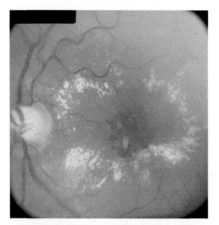

B. Circinate retinopathy

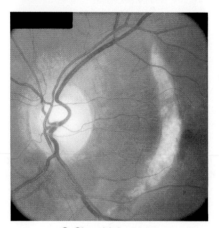

C. Choroidal rupture

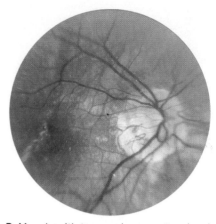

D. Myopia with temporal crescent and early maculopathy

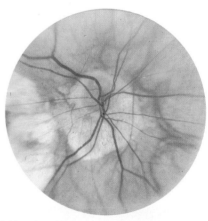

E. Myopia with extensive retinal degeneration

Plate 6

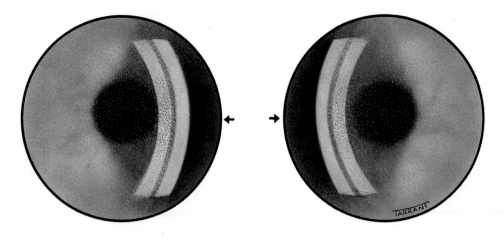

R.E.   L.E.

A. Fuch's endothelial dystrophy

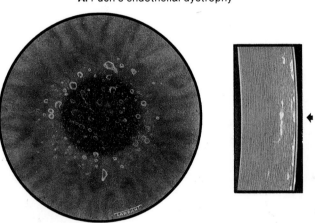

B. Reis-Buckler's corneal dystrophy

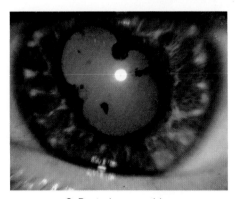

C. Posterior synechiae

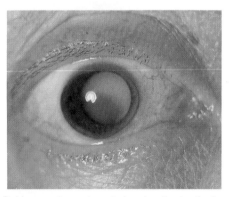

D. Morgagnian cataract showing the lenticular nucleus

Plate 7

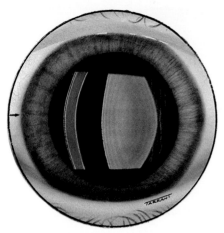

A. Optical section of the normal eye, as seen with the slit-lamp. The light (arrowed) comes from the left and in the beam of the slit-lamp the sections of the cornea and the lens are clearly evident

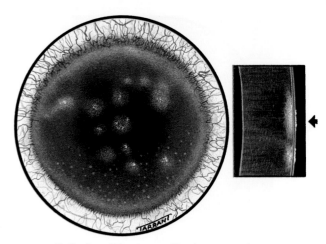

B. Zoster of the cornea. The large maculae are zoster lesions; the small dots below are keratic precipitates

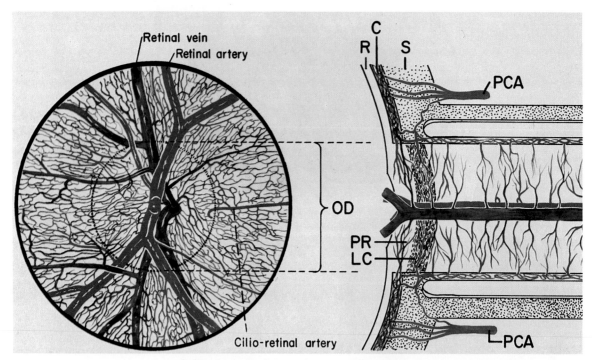

C. Blood supply of the optic nerve. OD — optic disc; R — retina; C — choroid; S — sclera; PCA — posterior ciliary artery; LC — lamina cribrosa; PR — prelamina. Reproduced from Hayreth S S 1977 Archives of Ophthalmology 95: 1560, with kind permission

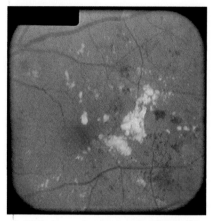

A. Diabetes — background retinopathy

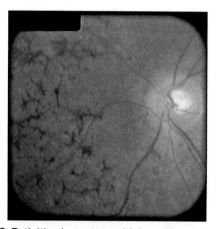

C. Retinitis pigmentosa with bone corpuscle formation, attenuated retinal arterioles and a yellowish disc

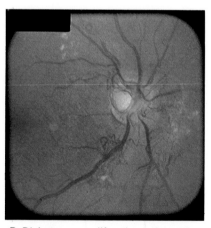

B. Diabetes — proliferative retinopathy

22

Diseases of the retina

Primary affections of the retina are almost always the result of some general disease, and should therefore be properly regarded as symptomatic diseases to which the term 'retinopathy' is usually more applicable than the classical term 'retinitis'. For this reason most of these conditions are bilateral.

These affections in general give rise to the following symptoms, only some of which need be present in individual cases. There is usually some diminution in visual acuity. There may be concentric constriction of the field of vision, or scotomata may be present corresponding with the areas especially affected. There may be metamorphopsia, micropsia, or macropsia (p. 156). The light sense is diminished, and photophobia may be present but pain is almost invariably absent, although discomfort may be experienced.

VASCULAR DISORDERS OF THE RETINA

The blood vessels of the retina are peculiarly subject to disease, sometimes in association with inflammation but more usually as a concomitant of general systemic disease.

Hyperaemia
This may be arterial or venous. Arterial hyperaemia, characterized by fulness and tortuosity of the arteries, accompanies not only inflammation of the retina but also inflammation of neighbouring structures, especially the uveal tract. Venous hyperæmia, characterized by dilatation and tortuosity of the veins, is the result of impeded return of blood to the heart. It may be due to general venous congestion, seen in its most extreme form in congenital malformation of the heart (*cyanosis retinæ*), or to local causes. The latter most commonly affect the veins at the optic disc, as is seen in moderate degree in glaucoma and optic neuritis, and in extreme form in thrombosis of the central vein of the retina. Increased intra-orbital pressure, as from a tumour, may also impede the exit of blood from the eye. The veins are much enlarged and dark in colour in polycythæmia and engorged in leucaemia.

Anaemia
Anaemia may be part of general anaemia or due to local causes. It may be sudden or slow in onset. Sudden anaemia is seen in obstruction of the central artery of the retina (*q.v.*) and in quinine amblyopia (*q.v.*) when the retinal vessels are attenuated and the optic disc is pale. The retinal vessels constrict when the oxygen concentration in the blood is high, and dilate in anoxaemia.

Oedema of the retina
This may be diffuse or localised. There may be general oedema, manifesting itself as a faint, diffuse haze, obscuring details so that the normal bright red appearance is replaced by a paler cloudiness. In the macular region, owing to the arrangement of the nerve fibres, œdema tends to throw the retina into radiating folds arranged like the rays of a star; such an appearance may be very dramatic in hypertensive retinopathy and papilloedema.

Macular oedema
Extra cellular fluid may accumulate in the foveal region by leakage from the local capillaries. Fluorescein angiography demonstrates that there are two forms of macular œdema: (1) cystoid which signifies a simple disturbance of the blood-retinal barrier without a structural alteration of the foveal tissues as occurs after cataract extraction and (2) non-cystoid or amorphous œdema when the normal capillary architecture at the macula has become distorted either by traction forces or by the development of neo-vascularization. Such an appearance is common after branch vein occlusions affecting the macula and also in the presence of pre-retinal membranes secondary to posterior detachment of the vitreous. In general the visual prognosis in the cystoid type is better since it tends to represent the result of an underlying disturbance of perfusion which may respond to medical treatment or may reverse spontaneously.

Central serous retinopathy

This presents a characteristic clinical picture of an oedema limited to the macular area; it is caused by exudation from the parafoveal or choroidal capillaries. It occurs preferentially in young adult males, appearing as a circular dark swelling, usually about the size of the optic disc or somewhat larger. The oedema may be pre- or sub-epithelial so that the affected area is raised above the level of the retina and is surrounded by a characteristic ring-shaped reflex. The condition is usually transient and tends to resolve leaving, however, a few exudative dots and usually impairing the central vision to some extent (often to 6/9 or 6/12). Recurrences are frequent. Intravenous fluorescein injections have shown that it is sometimes due to a leakage of fluid through a pin-point defect in Bruch's membrane. Argon laser burns may be applied to coagulate this spot. The aim of treatment is to produce a burn just sufficient to blanch the pigment epithelium if it is not too near the fovea and if the oedema has persisted for 4 months or longer. A good prognosis in serous detachment of the pigment epithelium depends on age (under 55 years) a detachment less than one disc diameter in size and non-involvement of the fovea. Serous detachment of the macula in young patients with a demonstrable leak flattens more rapidly after argon laser treatment but the prognosis of ultimate visual acuity is not improved.

Haemorrhages

Haemorrhages from the retinal vessels, when small, are contained within this tissue (*intra-retinal haemorrhages*). They assume a characteristic appearance according to their location, conforming to the anatomical configuration of the layer in which they lie. When they lie superficially in the nerve-fibre layer they are striate or flame-shaped; rounded or irregular when in the deeper layers. Intra-retinal haemorrhages are absorbed very slowly, gradually becoming white, rarely pigmented.

When the bleeding arises from a large vessel it spreads between the surface of the retina and the vitreous (*pre-retinal or subhyaloid haemorrhages*); such haemorrhages usually occur in the neighbourhood of the macula, and may be large. At first they are round but quickly become hemispherical, the upper margin being straight owing to the effect of gravity. The retinal vessels are hidden from view in the affected area. The upper part gradually becomes lighter in colour, an appearance generally attributed to the sinking of the red corpuscles, and the blood slowly becomes absorbed, usually in a patchy manner, but finally disappears. In this event vision is restored, but if the underlying vascular condition persists, recurrences are not uncommon. Large haemorrhages tend to break into the vitreous rendering it opaque so that the fundus reflex is lost; blood in the vitreous body clots and is slow to absorb; a proliferation of fibrous tissue may result (proliferative retinopathy, *q.v.*).

Exudative retinopathy of Coats

This presents a characteristic monocular ophthalmoscopic picture seen usually in boys, otherwise apparently healthy. The retinopathy may form a manifestation of the 'battered baby' syndrome. There is usually a large raised yellowish white area or several smaller areas posterior to the vessels; detachment of the retina, cataract or glaucoma may occur in the late stages. There is always evidence microscopically of haemorrhage between the retina and choroid and in the deep layers of the retina, and the ophthalmoscopic appearance is usually characterised by a number of small aneurysms and a varying amount of exudate, sometimes with masses of cholesterol crystals embedded in it; the choroid is at first healthy. A very similar picture may be produced in angiomatosis. A somewhat similar disease may occur in older patients. No treatment is effective.

Proliferative retinopathy

When a haemorrhage occurs into the vitreous, the blood clot is usually slow to absorb. In some cases, however, especially in the presence of diabetes when the haemorrhage has been large it may become organized by fibrous tissue derived from the mesoblastic elements associated with the retinal vessels or on the optic disc. In this way large sheets of tissue are formed which may proliferate widely into the vitreous (Plate 8, Fig. B). Owing to the loss of vision and the liability to retinal detachment, the prognosis is often serious.

Retrolental fibroplasia

This is a disease which is generally noted some weeks after birth in premature infants who have been given high concentrations of oxygen, and is usually confined to those under four pounds in weight at birth. The earliest signs are dilatation of the retinal veins and the appearance of hazy white patches in the periphery of the retina which shortly show an indefinite proliferation into the vitreous. This is due to the formation of new vessels in the retina itself which bud into the vitreous. Their appearance is followed by the development of fibrous tissue which eventually proliferates to form a continuous mass behind the lens, appearing as a type of pseudoglioma (p. 241). Activity may cease spontaneously at any stage so that some vision may be retained, but in many cases it progresses so that the retina is detached and the eye becomes microphthalmic. In this case, of course, vision is lost. The condition is usually bilateral.

Retrolental fibroplasia was not diagnosed as such until the late 1930s, whereafter it occurred commonly in hospital clinics dealing with premature infants, to such an extent that it became the commonest cause of bilateral blindness in children. It has been shown to follow excessive oxygenation in the nursing of premature infants in the early stages of their lives. As a result the retinal arteries and eventually the veins are obliterated, a phase followed by neovascularization. Prophylaxis is thus important. In the management of premature infants weighing less than 200 gm the PaO_2 of blood from the umbilical artery should be monitored, levels of 50–100 mmHg being regarded as unlikely to produce constriction of immature retinal vessels. Unsatisfactory guides include 'pinkness', oxygen under 40% in the tent and vascular constriction as seen by the ophthalmologist. Before the child is discharged from the hospital the temporal periphery of each retina should be examined with the indirect ophthalmoscope. If minor signs of retrolental fibroplasia are noticed examination should be made at the age of one, three and six months and every four months upto the age of four years with the object of diagnosing early retinal holes or localized detachment of the retina. Treatment by photocoagulation or cryotherapy of one eye should be considered only when *definitely progressive* bilateral proliferative lesions are noted in the vitreous. The presence of mild intravitreal neovascularisation warrants delay in consideration of photocoagulation therapy since spontaneous resolution occurs in a high percentage of patients (80%). Once the condition has fully developed treatment is ineffective, for removal of the fibrous mass has been found to be surgically impossible.

Retinal changes in diseases of the blood

Retinal haemorrhages, often of a characteristic type, may occur in many blood diseases. It seems probable that in such diseases deficient oxygenation may lead to an increase of capillary permeability and consequent increased diapedesis.

Anaemia

In severe *anaemia*, whether of the secondary or primary pernicious type, the veins are frequently engorged and in the posterior half of the retina haemorrhages appear, often with characteristic white centres, consisting of leucocytes centrally and erythrocytes peripherally.

Sickle cell haemoglobin is an abnormal haemoglobin found mainly but not exclusively in people of negro origin. This particular abnormal haemoglobin has an unusual property in that, when it is deoxygenated, it becomes insoluble and distorts the normally discoid red cell into a characteristic sickle shape. Such sickled red cells tend to obstruct capillaries and this leads to infarction, especially in areas of vascular stasis such as the spleen and the bone marrow. The periphery of the retina may also be affected.

Sickle cell haemoglobin

Patients with S.C. disease have no normal adult haemoglobin, the haemoglobin consisting of haemoglobin S and haemoglobin C. They are not anaemic but on occasions develop severe infarctive crises. Peripheral arterioler occlusions are common in the retina and retinitis proliferans develops. In children there is an unequivocal progression of severity of the retinopathy. Photocoagulation attacking the feeding arterioles before treatment of new vessels is the therapy of choice.

Leucaemia

Leucaemia provides the most characteristic ophthalmoscopic picture among the blood diseases. The fundus is pale and orange-coloured. The veins are dilated and tortuous, often with white lines along them, and are bright red, not dark; the arteries are small and pale yellowish red. Typical hæmorrhages occur with white centres, most commonly in the peripheral retina.

Haemorrhages also appear in all the *purpuras*. Similar haemorrhages may occur in *polycythaemia vera*; in this disease, although the arteries appear normal, the veins are enormously dilated and tortuous and the congestion may lead to the development of papilloedema and venous thrombosis due to plasma hyperviscosity.

Obstruction of the retinal vessels

An obstruction, complete or partial, permanent or temporary, may affect either the retinal arteries or veins.

Obstruction of the arterial circulation

Obstruction of a retinal artery is usually due to an embolus; the factor of spasm is often added which completes the occlusion. It may occur without obvious general vascular disease or when this is widespread as in arteriosclerosis, hypertension or Buerger's disease. Obstruction by an embolus is often secondary to a plaque of atheroma situated at the bifurcation of the common carotid artery in the neck, or occasionally to a diseased mitral or aortic valve.

The obstruction may affect the central artery itself when the entire retina is involved or a peripheral branch when the effects are localized. *Obstruction of the central retinal artery* is nearly always at the lamina cribrosa, where the vessels normally become slightly narrowed (Fig. 22.1). Such an accident causes sudden and complete retinal anæmia and this tissue rapidly dies. The eye becomes suddenly blind, although when minute emboli are a factor premonitory obscurations of vision may occur. Examination of the fundus reveals a very typical picture (Plate 4, Fig. B). The larger arteries are reduced to threads, the smaller are invisible but the veins are little altered except on the disc where they are contracted. Within a few hours the retina loses its transparency, becoming opaque and milky-white, especially

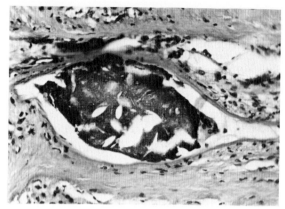

Fig. 22.1 Embolic occlusion of the central retinal artery. (By courtesy of Wolter.)

in the neighbourhood of the disc and macula. At the fovea centralis, where the retina is extremely thin, the red reflex from the choroid is visible and appears as a round 'cherry-red' spot, presenting a strong contrast to the cloudy white background.

When the obstruction to the blood flow is not complete, the flow may be partially restored in the course of a few days in which case gentle pressure upon the globe may break up the column of venous blood into red beads separated by clear interspaces. The beads move in a jerky fashion through the vessels, sometimes in the normal direction of blood flow, sometimes in the opposite direction (the 'cattle-truck' appearance). If the veins are easily emptied of blood or arterial pulsation is produced by slight pressure on the eyeball, it is evidence of incomplete blockage.

The white appearance of the retina takes several weeks to clear up but eventually the membrane regains its transparency and appears normal; it is, however, completely atrophic apart from the outer layers which receive their nourishment from the choroid. The vessels are contracted or reduced to white threads although some of them refill at a later stage due to the establishment of a feeble collateral circulation through the anastomoses with the ciliary system round the disc. The disc is atrophic. There is no direct pupillary reaction and light perception is lost.

In some cases a certain degree of central vision persists in spite of apparent complete occlusion of the central artery. It is due to the presence of cilio-retinal arteries which, when present, always supply the macular region and naturally escape occlusion; or to a macular branch of the central artery given off proximal to the block. The remainder of the field of vision is lost. In rare cases a cilio-retinal artery alone becomes blocked.

In *obstruction of a branch of the retinal artery* the area supplied by this branch is then affected alone. In the early stages the corresponding scotoma is usually some-

what indefinite, but later it settles down to form a permanent sector-shaped defect.

Treatment is seldom of any avail, but attempts should be made to relieve any spasm or drive an embolus into a less important branch if the case is seen early. Massage of the globe is probably the most effective method but paracentesis has been employed for this purpose; to be effective such measures must be adopted without delay. Inhalation of amyl nitrite is generally useless, but a return of vision has been reported following the injection into Tenon's capsule of acetylcholine which produces vasodilatation. Branch occlusion may be relieved in this way. The normal result of an occlusion of the central artery, however, is blindness.

Obstruction of the venous circulation

Benign vascular retinopathy is a well-defined clinical entity that consists of unilateral disc oedema with variable retinal vascular changes in young healthy adults. The individual is usually aged 20–40 years and the initial symptom is a vague unilateral fogginess of vision. The retinal vascular abnormality may be minimal or present markedly engorged dilated tortuous veins and haemorrhages at the posterior pole extending into the retinal periphery. Visual acuity remains good and vitreous haemorrhage is never present. Neuro-ophthalmological examination is negative and fluorescein angiography shows venous stasis with delayed venous drainage. The syndrome lasts about 18 months with no permanent visual defect. Systemic corticosteroids are occasionally used but the disease can safely be followed without neuro-diagnostic studies in a healthy young adult where there are no abnormal systemic or neuro-ophthalmological findings. Steroids should be withheld unless there is macular oedema. The fundus picture simulates that of central venous thrombosis and probably results from phlebitis affecting the central vein within the optic nerve head. The cause is unknown although increased levels of circulating IgM have been reported in a significant number of patients.

Venous thrombosis usually occurs in elderly people with cardio-vascular disease. In these cases the obstruction is usually in the central vein just behind the lamina cribrosa where the vein shares a common sheath with the artery so that the two are affected by the same sclerotic process (Fig. 22.2). At other times in arteriosclerotic patients the block may be peripheral, usually at a bifurcation or where a sclerosed artery crosses a vein, an event which is particularly prone to occur in the superior temporal vein. In young people it may be due to an infective periphlebitis (*q.v.*) in which case a branch of the central vein is affected. Thrombosis may also be due to local causes, such as orbital cellulitis or facial erysipelas. In all cases the condition is to be regarded as a danger signal and constitutional investigation and treat-

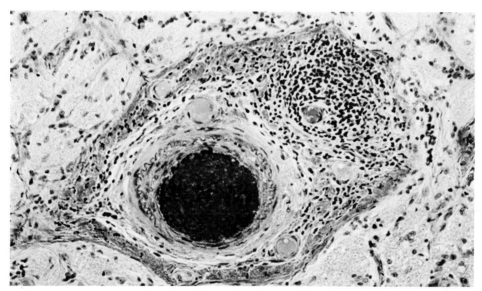

Fig. 22.2 Inflammatory venous occlusion at the disc. Section through the central vessels, close to actual venous occlusion. CRA normal, but lumen of vein (above right) extremely narrowed by dense lymphocytic infiltration of wall. (By courtesy of Klien.)

ment should be assiduously undertaken.

In *central vein thrombosis* all the veins of the retina become enormously engorged with blood and extremely tortuous, and the retina is covered with haemorrhages (Plate 4, Fig. C). Sight is much impaired although not so rapidly as in obstruction of the central artery, but recurrent extravasations usually destroy it. In many cases bunches of tortuous new vessels are formed upon the optic disc; in others a collateral circulation is effected by similarly tortuous new vessels in the retina. Eventually the affected retina becomes atrophic with fine pigmentary changes. The prognosis is rendered worse by the fact that secondary glaucoma ensues in two to three months in a considerable number of cases, due to sclerosis and neovascularization at the angle of the anterior chamber.

In *branch thrombosis* when a single branch of the central vein is blocked, the oedema and haemorrhages are limited to the area supplied by the vein. In these cases the visual defect is not sectorial as in the case of occlusion of a branch of the artery; the prognosis for central vision is better, but unfortunately blockage of the superior temporal vein frequently involves the macula. Eyes with intact or complete perifoveal capillary arcades have a better visual prognosis than eyes with incomplete arcades as demonstrated angiographically. In branch thrombosis secondary glaucoma rarely occurs (Fig. 22.3).

No *treatment* is effective in cases of venous occlusion once the blockage has become complete. If there is widespread capillary occlusion pan-photocoagulation of the retina (or cryo applications if the media are hazy) may forestall neovascular glaucoma and rubeosis iridis. Widespread capillary occlusion is associated with cotton-wool spots, delayed arteriovenous transit time, large vessel leakage and retinal oedema. In branch occlusion destruction of areas of poor perfusion as seen by closure of retinal capillaries in the angiogram may relieve persistent oedema and inhibit neo-vascularisation. Secondary glaucoma is difficult to treat.

Vascular sclerosis

Close observation of the retinal vessels is important since, being derived from the cerebral vessels, they mirror the condition of the circulation in the brain. Since they are the only vessels in the body of arteriolar calibre accessible to direct observation wherein early pathological changes can be seen, their study is of great value as a guide to the state of the circulation. Apart from their interest as a local manifestation of disease, degenerative changes in the retinal vessels are thus of the utmost importance in general medicine. Disease of the retinal vessels is almost invariably associated with disease of the cerebral vessels, but disease of the latter may be present when there are no ophthalmoscopic signs of disease of the retinal vessels. Moreover, if marked organic changes occur in the retinal vessels, other organs, as the kidney, are probably also affected.

Before discussing the appearance of the vessels in the different types of vascular sclerosis, a summary of the most important changes may be useful.

Tortuosity of the vessels is common and may be particularly evident in the small arteries near the macula which assume a cork-screw shape particularly when involved with pre-retinal fibrosis. This change is of little systemic significance unless accompanied by other abnormalities.

Alterations of the lumen may occur, appearing as irre-

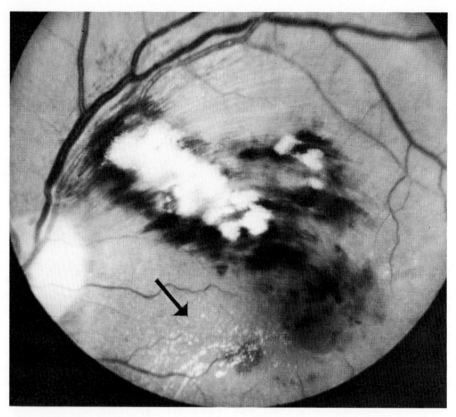

Fig. 22.3 Tributary venous occlusion affecting macular branch of upper temporal vein with gross exudates, flame-shaped haemorrhages and circinate retinal changes (arrowed). (By courtesy of Raitta.)

gularities in the size and breadth of the arteries so that stretches of the vessel are constricted, alternating with normal or dilated portions. These changes are due to endothelial proliferation in the intima.

Changes in the light reflex, an increase of brightness and width, are important. As we have seen (p. 94), the normal streak is due to the reflex of the blood-column seen through the transparent artery walls. When the wall becomes thickened and also reflects light, the streak becomes wider and appears as burnished copper ('copper-wire' arteries). When the wall becomes so thick as to reflect all the light, the reflex becomes brilliantly white ('silver-wire' arteries).

Sheathing of the vessels appears when thickening of the walls as in vasculitis makes the sides of the arteries visible as white lines.

At the *arterio-venous crossings* these phenomena are more marked. Normally it is possible to see a vein through an artery at a point of crossing; in sclerosis the artery loses its translucency so that the vein is obscured. Moreover, the hard artery exerts pressure on the vein so that the blood flow is obstructed; the vein seems therefore to stop at the crossing and is more distended on the distal side than on the side towards the disc (the

phenomenon of *nicking*). Sometimes the vein appears to be pushed aside by the crossing artery; in severe cases the vein, whether crossing above or below the artery, is diverted so that it crosses at right angles, the shortest possible route.

Minute miliary aneurysms are sometimes seen.

The various types of sclerosis seen in the retinal vessels may be classified as occurring in the arteriosclerosis of old age, and in atherosclerosis.

Involutionary (senile) arteriosclerosis (affecting primarily the muscular layer), occurs usually in patients over fifty years of age. The retinal arterioles exhibit alterations in calibre and lose their transparency. In the absence of raised arterial tension, however, progress is slow and the prognosis relatively good.

Atherosclerosis (affecting primarily the intima) is not seen in the retinal vessels beyond the central artery and its larger branches where atheromatous plaques occasionally appear. Atherosclerotic changes in the central vessel, however, may cause an alteration in the course of the retinal vessels so that they appear to be drawn backwards into the disc; they lose their normal tortuosity and become straight while the angulation of their branching is increased.

THE VASCULAR RETINOPATHIES

The vascular retinopathies occurring in general disease — hypertension, diabetes and the late toxæmia of pregnancy — are usually (with the exception of diabetes) associated with raised blood pressure and always with pronounced degenerative changes in the retinal vessels. The retinal changes probably originate from a state of anoxia which results in an increased permeability of the capillaries, the formation of multiple micro-aneurysms, and local degenerative changes in the tissues of the retina.

These circulatory changes lead to the development of retinal œdema (q.v.) but, since in these cases the extravasated fluid is rich in fibrin and proteins which readily coagulate, a characteristic feature is their deposition as masses of 'exudates'. The most common form is due to swelling of the nerve fibres, giving the appearance of cloud-like, 'soft' aggregates with ill-defined margins (cotton-wool patches), usually seen in the superficial layers of the retina. They are commonly small, but may form accumulations larger than the disc, and, since they may disappear rapidly, they frequently change their shape. They are formed by the arrest of axoplasmic flow arising at the edge of an ischaemic area where nerve fibres cross the boundary. Other degenerative changes in the neural elements result in the formation of hyaline or lipid deposits which appear as discrete, 'hard', yellowish or white deposits. These are seen as round patches, and in the macular region, as with œdematous accumulations, they tend to be thrown into radiating folds following the arrangement of the nerve fibres to form a fan- or star-shaped figure (the macular star).

The treatment of all these retinopathies is confined to that of the general disease, but their presence — or the suspicion of their presence — should at once call for a medical overhaul with an examination of the blood pressure and of the urine for albumin and sugar.

Hypertensive retinopathy

This may occur in four circumstances. In simple hypertension without sclerosis, seen in young patients, the retinal signs are few: a constriction of the arterioles which appear to be pale, unduly straight with acute-angled branching, while haemorrhages may occur and exudates are absent (Plate 4, Fig. D). In hypertension with involutionary sclerosis, occurring in older patients, the picture of arteriosclerotic retinopathy appears. The vascular signs just described are augmented by localised constrictions and dilatations of the vessels with sheathing of the vessels and the deposition of 'hard' exudates and sometimes of haemorrhages without any œdema. Although the vascular changes are bilateral, the retinopathy may remain confined to one eye due to carotid insufficiency on

that side and the ocular prognosis is relatively good.

In arteriolar (diffuse hyperplastic) sclerosis occurring in younger patients, the relatively youthful arterioles respond to the hypertension by proliferative and fibrous changes mainly affecting the media. In the kidneys there is a chronic glomerulo-nephritis and the ophthalmoscopic picture classically known as 'albuminuric' or 'renal' retinopathy arises (Plate 4, Fig. D). The vessels show evidences of hypertension. They are narrow and tortuous with nicking at the arterio-venous crossings; multiple haemorrhages are present with, in the early stages, œdema and cotton-wool patches and, in the later, 'hard' exudates scattered diffusely but usually forming a macular star. If the patient survives, these changes in the fundus may regress and although blindness does not occur the vision may be seriously impaired; the usual outcome is death from uraemia.

Malignant hypertension is an expression of accelerated progression of the hypertensive state in a patient with relatively young arteries, undefended by sclerosis. It is associated with renal insufficiency and the picture of the fundus is known as hypertensive neuroretinopathy, dominated by the appearance of œdema (Plate 4, Fig. D). The entire retina may be clouded by a generalised oedema which may be particularly accentuated at the disc, resulting in a marked degree of papillœdema with multiple cotton-wool patches; 'hard' exudates may be so profuse that the patches form enormous masses among which a marked macular star is usually prominent. Vision is usually gravely affected. In such cases, particularly when papilloedema is marked, the prognosis is grave and unless the hypertension can be controlled by medical or surgical methods, life is not usually prolonged more than two years. If general treatment is successful, the ophthalmoscopic appearances may ameliorate dramatically and the vision improve; but the ultimate prognosis is unsatisfactory.

Retinopathy in the toxaemia of pregnancy

This occurs late in pregnancy, exceptionally before the sixth and practically always in the ninth month. It has many of the characteristics of hypertensive retinopathy. Initially there is narrowing of the retinal arteries, usually the nasal branches first which in any event are the smaller; and this is followed by spasmodic contractions. As the blood pressure rises, œdema makes its appearance resembling hypertensive retinopathy in its most marked forms, and the exudation may be so profuse and generalised as to cause a retinal detachment.

The occurrence of this disease puts a peculiar responsibility on the ophthalmologist, and any visual symptoms occurring in the later stages of pregnancy must be thoroughly investigated. Constriction, particularly of the nasal branches of the retinal artery, should at once call for extreme care in the general treatment of the case; the occurrence of arterial spasms together with an increase in weight indicating the systemic retention of fluid, are ominous signs; while the advent of retinopathy should call for a termination of the pregnancy, since its continuance will probably result in the loss of vision and perhaps of the life of the mother as well as in the birth of a still-born fetus. Timely induction of labour, however, as well as adequate general care, usually lead to recovery provided gross organic changes have not occurred in the retina; even the retinal detachment will resolve in these circumstances. The retinopathy of a pheochromocytoma has similar features in that it usually affects a healthy retinal vascular system and the changes are reversible provided they have not been present for too long a period.

Lupus erythematosis retinopathy

Retinopathy occurs in about 10% of patients suffering from lupus erythematosis. Cottonwool spots in the posterior retina associated with flame-shaped haemorrhages occur sometimes with minor papilloedema. If there is renal involvement the picture may be complicated by the super imposition of a hypertensive retinopathy.

Other associations are kerato-conjunctivitis as part of a Sjögren's syndrome, nodules in the sclera and episclera, anterior uveitis and a butterfly skin eruption over the nose and cheeks involving the lower lids.

Such patients demonstrate the LE cell phenomenon whereby leucocyte nuclei undergo spontaneous denaturation and phagocytosis. Antinuclear factors are demonstrated by immunofluorescence and are present in 95–100% of patients.

The tissue lesions of this disease are due to deposition of antigen–antibody complexes. IgG and complement have been demonstrated in the glomeruli of lupus erythematosis patients.

Systemic lupus erythematosis affects young women nine times more commonly than men. It may be due to an innate tendency to produce auto-antibodies because defective T-lymphocytes fail to exercise their restraining influence on B-lymphocyte function.

Diabetic retinopathy

It is not necessarily associated with hypertension. It is frequently so accompanied, in which case the ophthalmoscopic picture may be complicated, particularly in elderly subjects, by arteriosclerosis and hypertension or even renal disease; but in the absence of these complications a characteristic picture is seen in the fundus, particularly in young people. The causal factor is unknown; it is not hyperglycaemia, for retinopathy occurs as frequently when the blood-sugar is relatively low as when it is high. The frequency of its incidence increases with the length of time the patient has had diabetes, even

although the general disease is mild or has been well controlled; for this reason it usually occurs in elderly patients and has become much more common since the general use of insulin which has prolonged the life of diabetics. Retinopathy is common after the disease has lasted ten years and affects the majority of patients after twenty years; but it is not invariable. It affects young and old, for it is the diabetic age, not the chronological that is important. Nor does the presence of retinopathy bear any relation to the prognosis of the diabetes or the expectancy of life; visual damage, however, is frequently great and permanent, a calamity since the disease is bilateral.

Ophthalmoscopically the earliest changes of *background retinopathy* characteristically affect the smaller blood vessels. Small dot and blot haemorrhages are common, and the degeneration of the vessel walls leads to the development of micro-aneurysms, sometimes in vast numbers, which appear as minute round dots sometimes arranged like clusters of grapes at the ends of small vascular twigs; these may appear as an early sign in the macular area (Fig. 22.4 and Fig. 22.5). Oedema is not marked, but all over the posterior pole there tend to gather hard, white or yellow, waxy-looking patches of exudates with clearly cut, often serrated margins, which occasionally coalesce into extensive plaques (Plate 8,

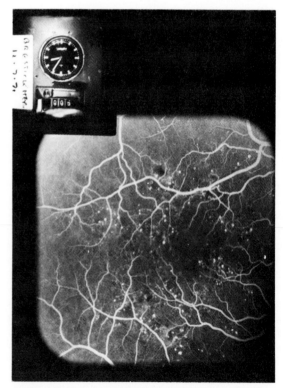

Fig. 22.4 Fluorescein angiogram outlining the aneurysms

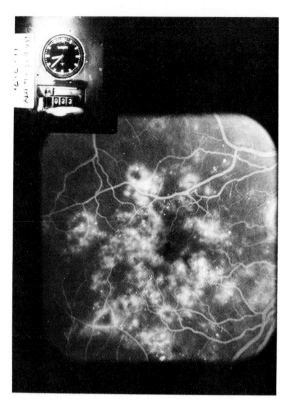

Fig. 22.5 Fluorescein angiogram to show leakage from the aneurysms into the retina

Fig. A). The fully developed ocular picture with micro-aneurysms is often associated with evidences of glomerulosclerosis in the kidney (Kimmelsteil–Wilson nephropathy). When these changes involve the macular area the central vision is profoundly affected.

Proliferative or neovascular retinopathy

This is the commonest cause of spontaneous vitreous haemorrhages. The neovascularisation arises from the optic nerve head and along the large vessels. It appears in areas of capillary closure and the accompanying fibrous tissue varies in extent. Such tissue lies flat on the retina or may attach itself to the posterior vitreous face leading later to vitreous traction, retinal separation and the tearing of blood vessels with haemorrhages.

Four retinopathy factors have been identified which increase the risk of severe visual loss over a 2 year period. They are the presence of vitreous or preretinal haemorrhage and new vessels especially if near the optic disc and if prolific. Rapidly developing cataract of the senile type is also frequent. From these complications many patients become blind.

The only ocular treatment available is light-coagulation of new vessels to prevent their progression and inhibit hæmorrhages and the conversion of hypoxic foci into inert scars thus relieving the retina of oedema and hard yellow exudates and improving its function. Patients who have neovascularisation emanating from the optic nerve head require panretinal photocoagulation. A circular area of radius 2½ disc diameters with the fovea at its centre is left untouched. Photocoagulation burns are applied within the vascular arcade above and below the macula using 200 μm spot burns. In all meridians photocoagulation is extended anteriorly to the equator using 500 μm spot burns. A range of 800–3000 spot burns is needed to complete the treatment in each patient administered in six sittings over a period of a week. It it fails to involute, direct treatment may be applied to the new disc vessels using the 50 μm spot size of the argon laser with an intensity not greater than 250 milliwatts. Peripheral retinal neovascularation if not too widespread may be treated directly by a Coherent 800 gas-argon laser using a 3-mirror Goldmann lens.

In more advanced fibro-proliferative retinopathy or with vitreous haemorrhage that does not clear vitrectomy is the treatment of choice. (see Vitrectomy p. 185).

Destruction of the pituitary by radiation or otherwise may result in (temporary) amelioration of the ocular condition in relatively young people with no gross renal involvement when the retinopathy is of the vascular but not of the exudative type; the operation, however, is severe and the necessity for the continuous administration of systemic corticosteroids throughout life must be weighed against the possible visual advantage. Reduction of animal fats in the diet and their replacement by vegetable oils may be of some value.

A peculiar feature sometimes met with in diabetes is *lipaemia*. It occurs especially in young patients when the triglyceride concentration of the blood exceeds 2000 mg/100 ml. The condition occurs in growth onset diabetes associated with marked acidosis. The ophthalmoscopic appearances are striking. The retinal vessels contain fluid which looks like milk, the arteries being pale red, the veins having a slight violet tint. The general fundus has a relatively normal coloration. Lipaemia responds rapidly to insulin treatment.

INFLAMMATION OF THE RETINA: RETINITIS

Most of the inflammations of the retina are associated with inflammation of the choroid, the inflammatory process involving both tissues to form a chorioretinitis: these have already been discussed (*q.v.*). Inflammations may be primarily retinal. These may be divided into purulent inflammations caused by the pyogenic organisms and granulomatous inflammations caused by specific infections. In all cases, *treatment* is that of the general condition.

Cytomegalic inclusion disease

Human cytomegalo-virus infection is characterised by distended tissue cells in which nuclei contain large acidophilic inclusion bodies. The majority of the population is infected and has no symptoms but in patients with impaired lymphoid function the disease may become manifest as in patients who have received organ transplants followed by massive doses of immunosuppressive agents.

The eye may be affected by an isolated macular lesion or by a severe chorio-retinitis with exudates.

Purulent retinitis

This may be either acute or subacute. The acute forms, due to the lodgment of organisms in the retina in the course of a pyæmia, lead to metastatic endophthalmitis or panophthalmitis (*q.v.*).

Subacute infective retinitis (Septic Retinitis of Roth)

This occurs in less virulent infections of a metastatic nature, typically in bacterial endocarditis and sometimes in puerperal septicæmia. The posterior part of the fundus is generally affected. Here numerous recurrent haemorrhages of embolic origin appear, some of them with white centres as in the anæmias (*q.v.*). The characteristic feature is the presence of round or oval white spots (Roth's spots), many of which are cytoid bodies. There is little general reaction in the retina although some œdema and papillœdema may occur, but the disease is frequently fatal and vision may be seriously impaired before death.

Syphilis

Most syphilitic retinal affections are secondary to choroidal inflammations, but certain vaguely defined changes may occur primarily in the retina. *Congenital syphilitics* occasionally show a dusty discrete pigmentation of the retina at the periphery where a multitude of black and white spots appear ('pepper-and-salt' fundus). In the more definite forms there are larger atrophic and pigmented areas at the periphery (anterior retinitis), a condition often seen in interstitial keratitis (p. 142).

In *acquired syphilis* endarteritis may be prominent with whitish exudates along the course of the vessels. A diffuse retinitis may occur particularly in the secondary stage of the disease wherein the retina, especially in the central area, becomes grey and cloudy. As the condition subsides the typical picture which develops consists of an atrophic optic disc, attenuated vessels, and a generally depigmented retina with the pigment aggregated in corpuscles particularly at the periphery in a distribution resembling pigmentary retinal dystrophy (p. 211).

The subjective symptoms are defective central vision, night-blindness, irregular and concentric contraction of the field with or without central, paracentral, or ring scotomata, and metamorphopsia.

Sarcoidosis

The characteristic histological lesion in sarcoidosis is an epithelioid cell granuloma, similar to tubercle without caseation. The mediastinal lymph nodes are a common site of such lesions but the lungs, liver, spleen, skin and eyes together with the parotid glands are also affected.

ESR is usually elevated with a slight leucopenia. The serum albumin globulin ratio is disturbed. There may be a hypercalcæmia. The tuberculin test is usually negative but the Kveim reaction, which is a test for skin sensitivity to sarcoid material, may be useful. X-rays of the chest may show bilateral lymph node involvement in the hylar region of the lungs and this may lead eventually to pulmonary fibrosis. Occasionally the bones of the hand are affected so that the phalanges show cystic areas. When the retina is involved there is often an associated affection of the central nervous system. A widespread retinopathy may develop consisting of candle-wax spots and small whitish areas which have been shown to be granulomata. The optic nerve head may be œdematous and also be affected by nodular granulomata leading to atrophy. There may be patches of chorio-retinitis and peri-phlebitis in association with posterior uveitis. Twenty-five per cent of patients with ocular sarcoid show evidence of posterior segment involvement during their illness.

Toxoplasmosis

See p. 160.

Toxocara

When tissues other than the skin are invaded by nematode larvae the condition is referred to as visceral larva migrans. *Toxocara canis* and *Toxocara cati* are round worms and are common causes of ocular disease.

Children eat infected material so that the eggs hatch in the duodenum and the larvae then penetrate the intestinal wall, enter the venous circulation and migrate across the pulmonary capillary bed to reach the respiratory tree and are swallowed to reach the jejunum. If the infection is heavy the children suffer from fever, anorexia, eosinophilia and hepatomegaly. The larvae may lodge in the eye without systemic signs.

The larvae produce an intra-ocular granuloma consisting of eosinophils and IgE which is situated centrally or peripherally in the retina as a white lesion. It protrudes into the eye from the retinal tissues and occasionally an endophthalmitis develops.

During the acute stage antibody titres rise in the blood stream and a skin test with antigens may produce a reaction. No eggs are found in the stool because no adult worms develop systemically. A skin test is made with an antigen of the adult worm. Testing with larval antigens is more sensitive as in the enzyme-linked immunosorbent assay (ELISA).

Vitreitis may respond to topical steroids which may be supported by thiabendazole and systemic steroids.

Ascaris lumbricoides may also produce ocular inflammation as a result of larval migration.

Periphlebitis retinae
This is a relatively common disease which manifests itself clinically by repeated hæmorrhages into the vitreous. It occurs typically in apparently healthy young adults, usually males (*Eales's disease*).

Retinitis from bright light (photo-retinitis)
This occurs after exposure of the eyes to bright sunlight, as in looking at an eclipse of the sun with inadequately protected eyes ('eclipse blindness'), or exposure to the flash of the short-circuiting of a strong current. Practically all the visible rays and many infra-red rays pass unimpeded to the retina (p. 31) and these are absorbed by the pigmentary epithelium; the pathological changes are produced by the resultant heating effect. The lesion is, in fact, a burn of the retina.

The symptoms are persistence of the after-image, progressing later into a positive scotoma, and metamorphopsia. Ophthalmoscopically there may be no signs at first, or a pale spot is seen at the fovea with a brownish red ring round it. Later there are usually deposits of pigment and small grey punctate spots around the fovea or even the formation of a retinal hole. Prognosis must be guarded; although improvement often occurs, some defect usually remains and the scotoma may persist permanently.

No treatment is effective. Glasses impervious to infra-red rays should be used prophylactically on such occasions or preferably the light source may be viewed by reflection from a mirror or not at all.

DEGENERATIONS OF THE RETINA

Senile macular degeneration
This is usually due to a hereditary dystrophy (p. 167).

Circinate retinopathy
This is due to chronic oedema involving a considerable area of the retina at and around the macula, with massive changes in the retina itself. It occurs in elderly people and may form part of a diabetic or hypertensive retinopathy. A girdle of bright white patches with crenated borders appears around the macula made up of aggregations of macrophages full of lipids (Plate 5, Fig. B). The diameter of the girdle, which is usually an imperfect circle or ellipse or horseshoe-shaped open towards the temporal side, is generally considerably greater than a disc diameter, and follows the larger temporal branches of the superior and inferior temporal vessels. The vessels pass over the spots. The macula shows yellowish white areas, slight pigmentation and usually œdema. The patches develop slowly and are usually well advanced before they are noticed. The disease is unilateral in about half the cases. Central vision is much reduced, but the field remains full. The patches sometimes disappear slowly and vision improves. Treatment may be effective if the source of vascular leakage can be localised and destroyed by photo-coagulation.

Benign peripheral retinal degenerations
There are a number of retinal degenerations which do not threaten the retina or lead to retinal breaks. Such lesions are *snowflakes*, so called because of the dotted white appearance which occurs close to the ora serrata; *paving stone degeneration* which is due to focal chorioretinal atrophy and is present in a high percentage of normal eyes; *reticular pigmentary degeneration* which looks rather like a honeycomb with each cell outlined by pigment; *equatorial drusen* which is commonly found in elderly people and *peripheral cystoid degeneration* which is present in all adult eyes and is a regular accompaniment of the ageing retina.

Angioid streaks
Dark brown or pigmented streaks which anastomose with each other and may be mistaken for blood vessels, are sometimes seen ophthalmoscopically. They differ in distribution from any normal set of vessels, are usually situated near the disc, at a deeper level than the retinal vessels, and are very irregular in contour. They are due to changes in the elastic tissue of Bruch's membrane, and are frequently associated with more widespread degeneration of a similar nature, as in the elastic tissue of the skin (*pseudo-xanthoma elasticum*) or of the arterial walls. Vascular and degenerative choroidal lesions elsewhere in the fundus, particularly at the macula, are common developments. Paget's disease of bone, Ehlers–Danlos syndrome and sickle cell disease may be associated with angioid streaks.

Pigmentary retinal dystrophy (Retinitis Pigmentosa)
This is a slow degenerative disease of the retina almost invariably occurring in both eyes, beginning in childhood and often resulting in blindness in middle or advanced age. The degeneration affects primarily the rods and cones, particularly the former, and commences in a zone near the equator of the eye gradually spreading both anteriorly and posteriorly. The macular region is not affected until a late stage.

The symptoms are characteristic, the most prominent

being defective vision in the dusk (night-blindness) (p. 18). This symptom may be present several years before pigment is visible in the retina and is due to the degeneration of the rods which are primarily responsible for vision in low illumination. The fields of vision show concentric contraction, especially marked if the illumination is reduced. In early cases a partial or complete annular or ring scotoma is found corresponding with the degenerated zone of retina (Fig. 22.6). As the case progresses the field becomes gradually smaller until at last it is reduced to a restricted area round the fixation point. Even although the central vision may be retained for a long time, such patients with 'tube vision' have great difficulty in getting about, for they are in much the same condition as a person looking down two long tubes seeing only the thing they are actually looking at and nothing around it. Loss of central vision does not usually occur until fifty or sixty years of age, although cataractous changes may cause earlier deterioration.

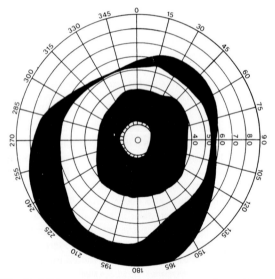

Fig. 22.6 Ring scotoma in a case of pigmentary dystrophy

Ophthalmoscopic examination shows a characteristic picture (Plate 8, Fig. C). Initially the equatorial region is affected and the posterior pole and the periphery are normal, but as the disease progresses the entire retina may become involved. In the zone affected the retina is studded with small jet-black spots resembling bone corpuscles with a spidery outline. The retinal veins, never the arteries, often have a sheath of pigment for part of their course. As the pigment from the retinal pigmentary epithelium migrates into the retinal layers, the epithelium itself becomes decolorised so that the choroidal vessels become visible and the fundus appears tesselated. The pigment spots which lie near the retinal vessels are seen to be anterior to them, so that they hide

the course of the vessels. In this respect they differ from the pigment around spots of choroidal atrophy (p. 165) in which the retinal vessels can be traced over the spots. The number of pigment spots differs much in individual cases, and they are often very scanty in the early stages.

The retinal blood vessels, both arteries and veins, become extremely attenuated and thread-like. As the disease progresses and the ganglion cells become degenerate, optic atrophy sets in and gradually increases. The disc exhibits the characteristics of primary optic atrophy (p. 229), but is not quite typical of this condition for, although pale, it has a wax-like yellowish appearance. In the later stages a progressive posterior cortical cataract is formed, leading ultimately to complete opacification of the cortex.

The electroretinogram and particularly the electro-oculogram in such cases are markedly subnormal or completely extinguished early in the disease before subjective symptoms or objective signs appear, a point of great prognostic importance in assessing the future of a young child in an affected family. In secondary retinitis pigmentosa, a sequel to an inflammatory retinitis, on the other hand, often ophthalmoscopically indistinguishable from the primary condition, the response is only slightly subnormal unless the condition is very advanced.

The condition is abiotrophic in nature and is genetically determined. In the majority of families it appears as a recessive trait and consanguinity of the parents is not infrequent. Occasionally it shows a dominant heredity when the disease may be transmitted through several generations but is the mildest form of the disease. Exceptionally it is sex-linked and clinically the prognosis for vision is poor. No advice can therefore be given as to the likelihood of transmission in any particular case unless the individual pedigree has been investigated.

Other defects elsewhere may be associated with the condition, the most common of which is a syndrome of obesity, hypogenitalism, mental defect and polydactyly (*Laurence–Moon–Biedl Syndrome*).

Congenital syphilis may produce a similar picture, although the distribution of the pigment spots is seldom typical (p. 156).

Treatment is eminently unsatisfactory since, despite many claims, nothing appears to have a decided influence upon the course of the disease.

Retinitis pigmentosa sine pigmento is a variety of the disease with the same symptoms, but without visible pigmentation of the retina. It is probably only the early stage of the more common dystrophy. It is progressive and leads to optic atrophy, therein differing from *congenital night-blindness*, which is a rare hereditary disease without ophthalmoscopic signs, remaining stationary throughout life.

Retinitis punctata albescens is an allied condition in which, with the same history and symptoms, the retina shows hundreds of small white dots distributed fairly uniformly over the whole fundus. A stationary form exists; but other cases are progressive and almost certainly represent atypical varieties of the pigmentary dystrophy. In the first case the electroretinogram is normal; in the second subnormal or extinguished.

HEREDITARY DYSTROPHIES OF THE CENTRAL RETINA AND CHOROID

Hereditary dystrophies of the posterior pole of the eye produce a bilateral and usually symmetrical lesion in the absence of general physical disturbance. The fundus picture in individuals of the same family is often similar and examination of relatives may lead to a diagnosis.

Classification

Nerve fibre layer	Sex-linked juvenile retinoschisis.
Neuro-epithelium	Stargardt's disease.
	Dominant foveal dystrophy.
	Inverse retinitis pigmentosa.
	Progressive cone dystrophy.
Pigment epithelium	Vitelliform dystrophy of the fovea.
	Reticular dystrophy of the retinal pigment epithelium.
	Butterfly-shaped pigment dystrophy of the fovea.
	Fundus flavimaculatus.
	Grouped pigmentation of the foveal area.
Choroid	Central areolar choroidal atrophy.

Sex-linked juvenile retinoschisis

This is a common dystrophy of the central retina. The fovea displays a cystoid structure with a radiating striation of the superficial retinal layers. In 50% of cases a peripheral retinoschisis is found in the temporal inferior quadrant. ERG is subnormal. EOG is normal. It is due to a splitting of the sensory retina, predominantly within the nerve fibre layer.

Stargardt's disease

Stargardt's disease is a recessive, progressive tapeto-retinal dystrophy of the central retina and develops between the ages of eight and fourteen. In the early stages the fovea appears normal but in the advanced stages a demarcated focus of 'beaten bronze atrophy' is seen in the foveal region. Whitish flecks surround the ovoid zone of atrophy, when differential diagnosis from fundus flavimaculatus, which is often accompanied by a foveal dystrophy, may be impossible. In the final stages the posterior pole shows an extensive chorioretinal atrophy with poor vision. Dark adaptation, ERG and EOG are subnormal while the visual fields may become slightly restricted. Fluorescein angiography shows defects in the pigment epithelium. There is no leakage of dye. The final result is the complete disappearance of the visual elements and the pigment epithelium in the centre of the retina.

Dominant foveal dystrophy

This is a progressive tapeto-retinal dystrophy of the central retina. It starts later in life and runs a milder course than Stargardt's disease.

Inverse retinitis pigmentosa

Bone corpuscles are visible in the perifoveal area while the retinal periphery is normal. True bone corpuscles are never found in the fovea itself. Histological studies show a progressive degeneration of the neuro-epithelium and pigment epithelium. Later there is a general atrophy of the whole retina. Heredity is autosomal recessive.

Progressive cone dystrophy

Progressive cone dystrophy is a dominantly inherited condition characterised by a bilateral progressive loss of visual acuity with extreme photophobia. Visual fields reveal a central scotoma and colour vision is absent. Ophthalmoscopy may only show a moderate foveal change but later a bull's eye pattern of depigmentation develops with a central hyperfluorescent spot. Cone components of the ERG are reduced or absent while the rod components are normal. The EOG is unaffected. It is due to a primary dystrophy of the retinal cone.

Vitelliform dystrophy of the fovea

Vitelliform dystrophy of the fovea is known as Best's disease. It is characterised by a sharply delimited, usually bilateral organge-yellow disc in the foveal region resembling the yolk of a fried egg. Visual acuity remains good while the neuro-epithelium is unaffected. Serious loss of vision occurs only after transition to an irregular pigmented lesion, after the egg has become 'scrambled' or after haemorrhages. This leads to a polymorphous foveal dystrophy. The vitelliform disc is probably situated in the pigment epithelium and contains homogeneous viscous material. Visual fields are normal with the exception of a central scotoma. Dark adaptation and the ERG are normal but the EOG is definitely pathological.

Reticular dystrophy of the retinal pigment epithelium

Reticular dystrophy of the retinal pigment epithelium is characterised by a peculiar defined network built up of black pigmented lines consisting of closely packed pigment granules at the posterior pole. The fovea itself displays a black spot of about one disc diameter situated at the level of the pigment epithelium. The condition is due to an autosomal recessive gene.

Butterfly-shaped pigment dystrophy of the fovea
This is a rare dystrophy with a pigmented butterfly-shaped structure at the level of the pigment epithelium at the fovea. Visual acuity is only slightly diminished. The ERG is normal while the EOG is found to be subnormal in most cases. The affection is inherited dominantly.

Fundus flavimaculatus
Fundus flavimaculatus is a flecked retinal dystrophy affecting both eyes and appears usually in the third or fourth decade of life. White or yellowish-white deep retinal flecks resembling fish tails with fuzzy or medium-sharp outlines are characteristic as seen with the ophthalmoscope. The flecks never extend beyond the equatorial retinal zone. 50% of affected individuals have macular affections. The central vision falls when the macula is affected. Dark adaptation and the ERG are normal but EOG is mostly pathological indicating a diffuse involvement of the retinal pigment epithelium. Histology reveals a primary abnormality of the pigmentary epithelium due to an accumulation of lipofuscin-like substance while the neuro-epithelium, Bruch's membrane and choroid are normal. It is now considered to be part of Stargardt's disease.

Grouped pigmentation of the foveal area
Grouped pigmentation of the foveal area has been described rarely. Round pigmentary spots are present in the foveal area. Visual acuity is normal or slightly diminished. Visual fields, dark adaptation and ERG are normal.

The hyaline dystrophies
The hyaline dystrophies have been described under several names — Doyne's honeycomb dystrophy or Hutchinson–Tay's choroiditis. It is due to an enzymatic defect in the pigment epithelium. Initially tiny round white flecks appear in the posterior pole of the eye. White colloid bodies on the nasal side of the optic disc may be regarded as pathognomonic of this affection. The dystrophy is first seen between the ages of 20 and 40 and initially is without symptoms. The colloid bodies increase and coalesce and eventually visual acuity may be disturbed. In advanced stages a central scotoma is found. Dark adaptation, ERG and EOG are normal. Fluorescein angiography shows multiple round fluorescent spots with sharp borders. There are also abnormal areas with fluorescein angiography indicating a disturbance in the pigment epithelium overlying the drusen. Histology reveals a deposition of a mosaic of colloid excrescences on the cuticular lamina of Bruch's membrane

and an absence or deficiency of the pigment epithelium over each hyaline deposit. Inheritance follows a regular dominant pattern.

Pseudo-inflammatory foveal dystrophy (Sorsby)
This is a rare hereditary dystrophy characterised by bilateral inflammatory signs in the posterior pole. Haemorrhages, exudates, oedema and pigmentary proliferation are manifestations of this disease starting between the ages of 30 and 50. Later a generalised choroidal atrophy develops. Histology presents degeneration in the elastic layer of Bruch's membrane and a choroidal atrophy. The defects in Bruch's membrane are regarded as a primary causal agent. Hereditary is usually autosomal dominant.

Central areolar choroidal atrophy
Central areolar choroidal atrophy is a disease primarily affecting the posterior pole appearing over the age of 40 years. A progressive atrophy of the choroidal vessels is found and the choriocapillaris, pigment epithelium and outer retinal layers gradually disappear. A central yellowish-white area of chorioretinal atrophy evolves and eventually central vision is lost. Colour vision is affected. Dark adaptation, ERG and EOG are mostly normal. Fluorescein angiography shows intense fluorescence in the area of the visible choroid where the retinal pigment epithelium has disappeared. Histology shows a central area of chorioretinal atrophy. Heredity is usually autosomal recessive but autosomal dominant inheritance has been described.

The amaurosis of Leber
Leber described a pigmentary retinitis with congenital amaurosis in which blindness occurred in early infancy. The essential features are bilateral blindness as soon as this can be registered, with course nystagmus and some retention of the pupillary reflexes and the eventual appearance of pigmentary degenerative changes in the fundi. It is a relatively common cause of blindness in infants, male and female alike and is transmitted as an autosomal recessive trait. Initially the fundi may appear normal and may remain so in the first few months of life. Soon various polymorphic lesions appear the most typical of which are small white spots in the periphery of the fundus to be followed by pigmentation, at first punctate of the 'pepper and salt' variety and later being aggregated until eventually the typical bone-corpuscular form of pigmentary dystrophy develops. The optic discs become pale, the retinal vessels attenuated and the macula affected. The ERG is absent and the EOG defective.

A juvenile form of the disease affecting vision in the sixth or seventh year of life leading to blindness at the age of 30 has also been described.

Familial lipid degenerations

Three familial syndromes characterised by lipid degeneration and the formation of large vacuolated 'foam' cells may affect the retina. In two of them the ganglion cells of the central nervous system and retina only are affected (Tay–Sachs disease and Batten–Mayou disease), while the other has a more general distribution (Niemann–Pick disease).

Amaurotic family idiocy (Tay-Sachs Disease)

This is an autosomal recessive abnormality which occurs most commonly in Jewish children, and commences during the first year of life. Several members of a family may be affected. The apparently healthy child becomes gradually blind, with muscular weakness and wasting, and mental apathy progressing to idiocy. Death follows in from one to two years. The ophthalmoscopic picture is very characteristic and the same in every case, resembling that of embolism of the central artery but of a quite different origin. There is a round brilliantly white area at the macula, fading off peripherally into the normal fundus. In the centre of thé patch is a cherry red, circular spot at the fovea (Fig. 22.7). In the later stages there is optic atrophy. It is always bilateral. The disease is due to an absence or deficiency of hexosaminidase A enzyme leading to storage of ganglioside G_{m2} in the central nervous system including the ganglion cells of the retina. The heterozygote may be detected by decreased enzyme activity in the serum. Prenatal diagnosis is possible by amniocentesis.

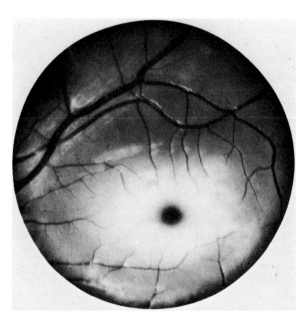

Fig. 22.7 Amaurotic familial idiocy with cherry-red spot at the macula (Banks Anderson)

Maculo-cerebral familial degeneration (Batten–Mayou Disease)

It is a familial disease exhibiting an autosomal recessive pattern, occurring in other than Jewish children, and commencing at a later age, usually at about six or eight years. Defective vision with a central scotoma is accompanied by weak intellect, and later convulsions and spasticity. Ophthalmoscopically the discs are pale and the vessels small. At the macula there are yellowish-grey spots and granular pigmentation, and there may be pigmentation in other parts of the retina of the pepper-and-salt type. The ophthalmoscopic picture varies much in different cases. A cherry-red spot never develops. Thirty per cent of lymphocytes in the peripheral blood are vacuolated. Autofluorescent material is deposited intracellularly throughout the body-possibly ceroid and lipofuscin. The syndrome is eventually fatal and there is no method of prenatal diagnosis.

Lipid histiocytosis (Niemann–Pick Disease)

This is characterised by similar but much more widespread changes of lipid storage; the spleen and liver are particularly affected. Sphingomyelin and cholesterol accumulate in the reticuloendothelial and nervous systems and in the parenchymal cells of many organs. Late in the course of the disease the retina may be involved when changes similar to those in Tay–Sachs disease may be found. Conjugate gaze palsies are common.

NEW FORMATIONS IN THE RETINA

The phakomatoses comprise a group of diseases with a familial incidence and a congenital basis with a tendency for the development of neoplasias in the central nervous system and elsewhere. In this the retina and optic nerve may be involved.

Angiomatosis of the retina (the von Hippel–Lindau Disease)

This is a rare familial disease which generally becomes manifest in the third and fourth decades of life, more frequently in males than females. The cerebellum, medulla, spinal cord, kidneys and adrenals are also affected with angiomatosis and cysts. The ocular lesions are often bilateral, slowly progressive, and may precede a fatal cerebellar lesion by 10 to 15 years. The ophthalmoscopic appearances vary; the most common is a great tortuosity and dilatation of the vessels together with the presence of aneurysms. Sometimes they are large like balloons; at other times small and miliary (Fig. 22.8). The condition is progressive and eventually the increased permeability of the vessels leads to the deposition of enormous quantities of exudates which appear in great masses in the fundus, resembling eventually the exuda-

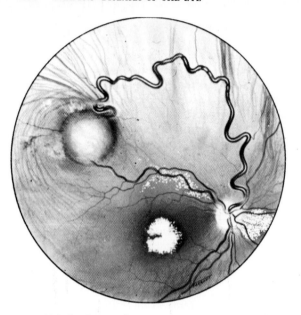

Fig. 22.8 Angiomatosis retinae or von Hippel disease of the retina.

tive retinopathy of Coats (*q.v.*). A retinal detachment is a frequent sequel.

Treatment is unsatisfactory, but in the early stages the cryo destruction or light-coagulation of a localised aneurysm as in the operation for retinal detachment (*q.v.*) may have a beneficial effect.

Tuberous sclerosis (Bourneville's Disease)
When this occurs in young individuals, it is associated with nodular lesions in the central nervous system and the skin, particularly on the face (adenoma sebaceum). Similar nodular tumours about the size of the disc occur in the retina particularly near the optic-nerve head. The cerebral lesions frequently lead to epilepsy and mental deficiency.

Neurofibromatosis (v. Recklinghausen's Disease)
This may be associated with somewhat similar tumours in the retina, corresponding to those related to the nerves of the lids and orbit (p. 320).

Cysts of the retina
These are commonly found in the microscopic examination of degenerated eyes, especially near the ora serrata in old people. Larger cysts occur below and on the temporal side of the retinae and are a form of retinoschisis. In rare cases a large cyst may clinically simulate a detached retina.

Tumours of the retina
See p. 240.

DETACHMENT OF THE RETINA (SEPARATION OF THE RETINA)

The two retinal layers — the retina proper and the pigmentary epithelium — normally lie in apposition, the potential space between them representing the original primary optic vesicle (p. 3). It is understandable that the two layers can readily become separated; such an event is called a *detachment* or (since only the inner layer of the embryonic retina is involved) a *separation* of the retina.

Detachments of the retina can conveniently be divided into two classes from the clinical point of view — *secondary detachments* due to an obvious mechanical cause when the detachment is a subsidiary event to other happenings in the eye, and *simple detachments* due to the development of a hole in the retina, in which case the state of this tissue occupies primary attention.

Secondary detachments may be due to the retina being pushed away from its bed by an accumulation of fluid or a neoplasm. The fluid may be blood (as from a choroidal haemorrhage) or exudate; we have already considered many examples of the latter (exudative choroiditis or retinopathy, angiomatosis, the late toxæmia of pregnancy, etc.). If such an exudate is absorbed, the detached retina may well become spontaneously replaced. Tumours of the choroid (*q.v.*) have a similar effect, partly by lifting up the retina mechanically, partly by the transudation of fluid due to the circulatory disturbances caused by the mass of the neoplasm; for this reason such detachments habitually cause an extensive separation of the retina, particularly in the lower part of the eye where the fluid tends to gravitate. The diagnostic features of such a detachment are obviously important and will be considered in the chapter on intra-ocular tumours (p. 238). Alternatively, a secondary detachment may be due to the retina being mechanically pulled away from its bed by the contraction of fibrous tissue in the vitreous, such as occurs in plastic cyclitis, proliferative retinopathy or retrolental fibroplasia (*q.v.*). The prognosis in such cases is, of course, less good.

Simple detachment of the retina is probably always due to the formation of a hole in the retina which allows fluid from the vitreous to seep through and raise the retina from its bed. It is probable that if the vitreous gel is healthy and solid such a detachment rarely occurs; if it is fluid or detached, and particularly if it is adherent to the retina so that with movements of the eye it continually drags upon the torn area, a detachment readily develops, which is known as rheqmatogenous.

Retinal holes or tears result from various causes. A normal fundus when viewed with the indirect ophthalmoscope by scleral indentation reveals a reddish chorio-retinal elevation but in *retinal white-with-pressure* the fundus coloration over the indented area becomes greyish. *Retinal white-without-pressure* is an exaggeration of this phenomenon and is present without indentation. Such areas are located in the peripheral fundus and may be associated with lattice retinal degeneration. It would seem that vitreous traction is the cause of this retinal finding and a posterior vitreous detachment often terminates at the posterior border of the retinal white-with- or white-without-pressure. Retinal tears may develop along the posterior margin of such areas. The loss of transparency is caused by intra-retinal oedema, disorganised retinal tissue or fibrous condensation of the vitreous cortex resulting from vitreous traction.

Lattice retinal degeneration
Lattice retinal degeneration is recognizable by white arborising lines arranged in a lattice pattern occurring in the upper peripheral fundus near the equator with the long axes parallel to the ora serrata. Retinal thinning is a constant feature and abnormal pigmentation is often present. The degeneration is slowly progressive and retinal tears are common in association with vitreous liquefaction.

Focal pigment proliferation or clumping
This occurs in the equatorial region or near the ora serrata. The pigment may be in the retina, choroid or both. In the equatorial region focal pigment proliferation may be found with a retinal tear. Posterior vitreous detachment is common with adhesions to the area of affected retina.

Diffuse chorio-retinal degeneration
This is often found in myopic eyes. The choroid is depigmented and the retina thin and this may lead to the development of a retinal hole. Chorio-retinal scars from old inflammatory processes particularly if they are peripherally situated are prone to produce retinal tears.

Cystoid retinal degeneration of the peripheral retina
This type of degeneration is present in varying degrees in all eyes but tends to increase with age and in the very old may predispose to retinal detachment.

Senile retinoschisis
This is characterised by splitting of the retina at the level of the inner nuclear and outer plexiform layers. It is symmetrical occurring in the lower temporal quadrants and progressing slowly. It produces an absolute field defect starting in the upper nasal field and enlarging towards the fixation point. When retinoschisis affects the macula the central field is certainly lost. Breaks may occur in the inner or outer layers of a retinoschisis.

Retinoschisis can be confused with retinal detachment and is differentiated from it by the presence of an absolute field defect as well as by the immobility and transparency of the inner layer. No treatment is indicated unless breaks appear in the outer layer or the condition is threatening macular vision. Progression may be halted by the use of photocoagulation placed in healthy retina on the disc side of the retinoschisis. Breaks in the outer layer of the retinoschisis must be closed whereas inner layer breaks are unimportant. When schisis is accompanied by rhegmatogenous retinal detachment scleral buckling with encirclement is the operation employed.

Retinal holes are frequently very difficult to find, but to find them is extremely important. In the first place, the presence of a hole designates a detachment as 'simple'; in the second, cure depends on its occlusion. The shape of such holes varies; some are horse-shoe or arrow-shaped with a lid-like tongue or operculum sometimes pulled inwards by the vitreous (Fig. 22.9A); they are most frequent at the periphery and commonest in the upper parts of the retina where the vitreous drags if it is adherent. Others are rounded (Fig. 22.9B); usually these are less peripheral and they sometimes occur at the macula. Occasionally great and extensive tears occur; an anterior dialysis may be large in which case the choroid is seen through it and the edge of the detached retina is sharply defined (Fig. 22.9C).

The clinical picture of a detached retina is characteristic, but the diagnosis may be difficult in the case of shallow detachments. Failure in diagnosis is almost always due to the omission of a proper routine examination of the eye. The observer often employs the direct method of ophthalmoscopy only, with which a shallow detachment appears little altered from the normal fundus. By preliminary examination with the mirror alone, a difference in the nature of the reflex as the eye is turned in various directions will at once arrest attention, while ophthalmoscopic examination with the indirect binocular method will make the matter clear.

In the early stages, and sometimes for a long period in shallow detachments, the colour of the detached portion differs little from the normal. Eventually, and sometimes rapidly, the detached portion of retina assumes a different tint from the normal fundus; in the most typical condition it is white or grey, with folds which show a bright sheen at the summits and appear greenish grey in the depressions. During slight movements of the eye the folds show oscillations and the retinal vessels are seen coursing over the surface, following all the curves of the folds. Owing to the fact that they are separated from the choroid, they cut off the light reflected from this membrane and therefore look much darker than usual, and may be almost black showing no central light streak. When the detachment is very extensive great balloon-like folds may be seen, and these may cut off all view of the disc. At the edges of the detachment a considerable degree of

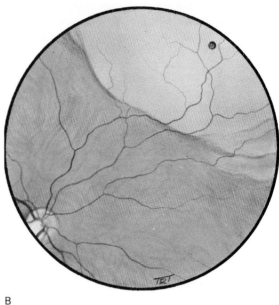

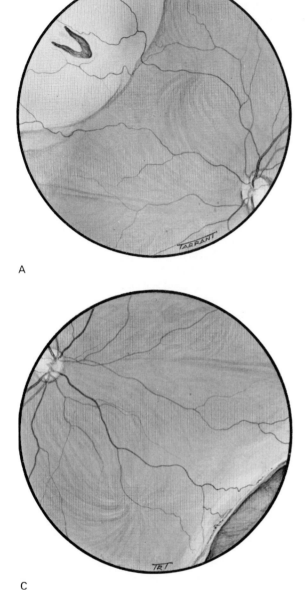

A

B

C

Fig. 22.9 Holes in the retina. (By courtesy of Shapland.)
A Arrow-head rent. B Round hole. C Anterior dialysis

pigmentary disturbance may appear as well as white spots of exudate, hæmorrhages, and greyish-white lines due to retinal folds. In total detachment the retina is funnel-shaped, remaining attached at the disc and at the ora serrata. Still later it becomes largely bunched behind the lens, the part attached to the disc being pulled out into a straight cord. In these cases the disturbance to nutrition of the eye leads to the development of a com-

plicated cataract (*q.v.*) so that ophthalmoscopic examination becomes impossible.

The symptoms in the initial stages of a shallow detachment may be indefinite, for the retina may obtain sufficient nourishment from the fluid which underlies it to retain its functions only partially impaired for a considerable period. Sometimes the first symptom observed is transient flashes of light (photopsiæ) in a particular part of the visual field, due to slight traction of the retina which irritates the neuro-epithelium. They should always be regarded with serious attention, particularly if they appear in the nasal field and if followed by an increase in muscae volitantes but they not infrequently occur, especially in myopic eyes, without being followed by detachment.

Usually, however, the patient complains that there is a cloud in front of one eye, so that parts of objects, generally the upper or lower parts, are not seen; a scotoma is confirmed by making a chart of the field of vision. The scotoma corresponding with the detached area is usually absolute, but in shallow detachments some vision may persist. As a rule central vision is intact at first, but all detachments of the retina tend in time to be complete; when the macular region becomes affected central vision is lost and, when the detachment is total, visual disability becomes complete.

The *treatment* of a simple detachment of the retina is by operation; either by approximating the torn part of the retina to an area of the choroid in which an aseptic inflammation has been excited by, light-coagulation or cryosurgery, or approximating the choroid to the retina in this region by scleral resection, or alternatively, buckling so that in either case adherence between the two tissues results and therefore obliteration of the hole (pp. 218); traction bands in the vitreous which pull on the retina must be obliterated by vitrectomy; but before this can be done the traction bands and retinal holes must be accurately located.

Since more than one hole may exist, this must involve a thorough and painstaking examination of every part of the fundus in every case; this may be time-consuming but it is necessary. Since many holes are in the extreme periphery, full mydriasis is necessary, and for this purpose the indirect method of ophthalmoscopy, using strong illumination, is more useful and effective than the direct. Sometimes such a lesion is rendered visible only by pressing gently on the sclera near the ora serrata with a strabismus hook. The retinal periphery should also be examined using a Goldmann 3 mirror fundus lens which provides a magnified view of the ora and its environs through the slit-lamp microscope. A careful drawing, showing the position of retinal holes, pathological lesions, retinal vessels and other landmarks, is made of the fundus. Several examinations should be made with the patient in different postures — sitting, supine, lateral, and so on; of these the supine is most important, since this is the position in which the operation is usually performed. Changes in posture may reveal a retinal tear which has hitherto been hidden by a retinal fold. Accurate localisation of the retinal tear or holes in relation to the outside of the sclera is essential; it is done by assessing in terms of the clock-face the meridian in which the hole lies. Its distance from the ora serrata is judged ophthalmoscopically in terms of optic disc diameters (= 1.5 mm).

The prognosis in simple detachment of the retina, untreated by operation, is unfavourable. The detachment becomes total, and complicated cataract and iridocyclitis follow. The results of surgical treatment are good in 80–90% of cases due to trauma with a retinal dialysis at the ora serrata in the lower temporal quadrant. In healthy patients whose vitreous, retina and choroid show no disease other than changes at the site of the retinal hole the prognosis is good in about 75% of cases if operated on early. The prognosis is bad in the aged; if the holes are large or multiple; when the vitreous, retina and choroid are grossly degenerated especially in the presence of multiple vitreous bands and when there is high myopia and if the detachment has been present for nine months or more. Massive vitreous retraction or massive periretinal proliferation is a bad prognostic sign leading usually to a totally detached funnel shaped retina. Metaplasia of the retinal pigment epithelium and proliferation of retinal glial cells leads to complications varying from a cellophane maculopathy to massive vitreous retraction. The only possible therapy is by a combination of pars plana vitrectomy, peeling away of retinal membranes and buckling procedures. Silicone oil injection has nothing to offer.

CONGENITAL ABNORMALITIES OF THE RETINA

Congenital pigmentation of the retina

Small oval grey spots or groups of polygonal greyish-black spots are occasionally seen in the retina in routine examination of the fundus. They are flat, lie below the vessels, and remain unchanged indefinitely. They are congenital and due to heaps of retinal pigment and epithelium similar to those forming melanomata in the iris (q.v.). (See also Nævus of the Choroid, p. 238.)

Medullated nerve fibres

The medullary sheaths of the fibres of the optic nerve cease normally at the lamina cribrosa. Occasionally patches of fibres regain these sheaths after they have passed through the lamina cribrosa. They appear ophthalmoscopically as white patches, the peripheral edges of which are radially striated, looking as if frayed out (Fig. 22.10). Usually the patches are continuous with the disc; occasionally they are isolated, but rarely far from the disc. Usually the retinal vessels are covered in places by the opaque fibres. When present the blind spot is enlarged, or a scotoma corresponds with the position of the patch. Very rarely the patch is large and involves the macula, so that central vision is abolished. If

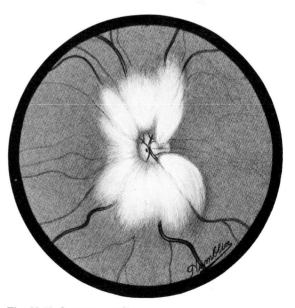

Fig. 22.10 Opaque nerve fibres

glaucoma or optic atrophy causes the fibres to degenerate the medullary sheaths disappear and no trace of the abnormality remains. It is important to be able to diagnose such fibres, since they may be mistaken for exudates, as in hypertensive retinopathy. They not infrequently occur in both eyes. They are not strictly speaking congenital, for myelination of the optic nerve progresses from the brain towards the periphery, and is not completed until shortly after birth. No treatment is required.

Coloboma of the retina and choroid
See p. 169.

Albinism
See p. 170.

23

Diseases of the optic nerve

Before discussing diseases of the optic nerve it is well to repeat that it has the structure and shares the diseases of a neurone of the second order of the central nervous system, rather than of a peripheral nerve (p. 20). The fibres (derived from the ganglion cells of the retina) have myelin sheaths normally proximal to the lamina cribrosa; these sheaths are separated by glial tissue and a neurilemma is absent. For this reason, like tracts in the central nervous system, they do not regenerate after section.

Disturbances of the circulation

Papilloedema (plerocephalic oedema: choked disc)
Since the optic nerve is enclosed up to the lamina cribrosa within meningeal sheaths common to the brain, and since the subarachnoid and subdural spaces around the nerve are freely continuous with those around the brain, any rise in the intracranial pressure becomes equally evident around the nerve as within the cranium. When this occurs the subarachnoid space may sometimes become so distended that it is ampulliform just behind the globe.

As a result, oedema develops at the optic disc; this is a purely hydrostatic, non-inflammatory phenomenon. Its cause has been in dispute. The oedema has been ascribed to several factors. It was thought to be due to compression of the central retinal vein as it crosses the subdural and subarachnoid spaces, causing its collapse, whilst the thicker-walled artery continued to transmit blood. Elevated cerebrospinal fluid pressure produces axoplasmic stasis in the optic nerve head leading to optic disc swelling and secondary vascular changes at the disc surface as demonstrated angiographically. The degree of papilloedema varies with the ease of access between the meningeal spaces within the cranium and around the optic nerve, and if the optic nerve-sheath is opened in patients with increased intracranial pressure, papilloedema is relieved.

The clinical appearance of papilloedema is ushered in by blurring of the margins of the optic disc. The blurring starts at the upper and lower margins and extends around the nasal side, while the temporal margin is usually still visible and sharp. As time goes on, progressive oedema extends over the surface of the disc reducing the size of the physiological cup, blurring the temporal margin and spreading into the surrounding retina. As the disc swells the veins become congested and turgescent, their pulsation may be absent even on pressure upon the globe, while the small arterioles also become prominent, appearing as red streaks on the swollen disc, sometimes giving it a striated appearance. Eventually the disc becomes elevated into a mound high over the surrounding retina and mushrooms out so that the vessels bend sharply over its margins; with the indirect method of ophthalmoscopy a definite parallax may be elicited between its summit and the retina beneath, and by the direct method a difference of 2–6 dioptres may be found between the focus of the vessels at the top of the disc and those on the retina a little way off (p. 87).

Meantime, the vascular engorgement and stasis result in the appearance of numerous haemorrhages on the disc and in the retina where they may be both flame-shaped and punctate, the oedema of the retina spreads so that this tissue is thrown into traction folds, and the veins, now tortuous and enormously dilated, may be buried for large tracts of their course in the swollen and oedematous retina (Plate 3, Fig. D). The surface of the disc has now lost its reddish hue and has become opaque, and exudates begin to appear upon it and in the retina itself; the radiating, oedematous folds around the macula take on the appearance of a macular star, usually incomplete so that it takes on a fan-shape on the side towards the disc, and fluffy patches (cotton-wool spots) appear scattered throughout the posterior half of the fundus. At this stage the ophthalmoscopic picture may be indistinguishable from that of the retinopathy of malignant hypertension (p. 207).

Frequently the swelling begins to subside before this final stage is reached; but in all cases subsidence eventually occurs, a process preceded by atrophic changes when the nerve fibres become unable to withstand the pressure and degenerate. When this process commences, the vascularity of the disc diminishes so that it appears a pale grey; and eventually, even although the increase in intracranial pressure remains unrelieved, the disc becomes flat and atrophic. This appearance of '*post-neuritic*' *atrophy* is characteristic, depending on the fact that the absorption of the exudates is accompanied by a certain amount of organisation with the formation of a variable quantity of fibrous tissue on the disc. This tissue obscures the lamina cribrosa and fills in the atrophic cup. It extends over the edges, which are thus indefinite, and along the vessels as a thickening of the perivascular sheaths. Further, it throttles the vessels, so that they become markedly contracted, especially the arteries. Meantime, owing to the widespread exudative deposits, the surrounding retina often shows permanent changes, chiefly manifested by pigmentary disturbances which are most common at the macula. The amount of reactionary organisation varies greatly in different cases, and the tissue laid down is in the course of time gradually absorbed to some extent. When such changes are marked they suggest the previous occurence of papilloedema but in their absence the conclusion that there has not been papilloedema is not justifiable.

After any considerable papilloedema the disc rarely regains its normal appearance, but after timely relief of the intracranial pressure the changes may disappear leaving an apparently normal disc.

The pathology of papilloedema shows signs of passive oedema without evidence of inflammation; the oedematous changes are located in the optic nerve head in front of the lamina cribrosa. The nerve fibres in the optic nerve head are swollen and axoplasmic stasis is noted in them. The physiological cup becomes filled in and the internal limiting membrane raised (Fig. 23.1). The nerve-fibres become swollen and varicose, ultimately degenerating; they show numerous cytoid bodies, in front of but not behind the lamina cribrosa. The neuroglia proliferates and the mesoblastic tissue around the vessels becomes thickened; there is subpia-oedema distal but not proximal to the site of entry of the central vessels, and the subarachnoid space is frequently distended.

The macular fan is caused by oedema in the nerve-fibre layer raising the internal limiting membrane in folds; the outer plexiform layer may be oedematous, but there are no large cystic spaces as in hypertensive retinopathy.

Symptoms are generally absent or vague and for long the vision may be unimpaired. This particularly applies to the central vision which may be unaffected even in the presence of a macular fan. Transient attacks of blurred vision, lasting for a few minutes up to an hour or so, are not uncommon in the early stages. As the condition progresses, however, two additional signs may be found — an enlargement of the blind-spot owing to separation of the retina around the disc by the oedema, and a progressive contraction of the visual field due to atrophy of the nerve. At this stage relative scotomata first to green and red may be present. If the condition persists, however, the vision slowly diminishes but the loss bears no relationship to the amount of swelling of the disc. As atrophy sets in, complete blindness ensues; the pupils, hitherto normal in size and reactions, are then large and immobile.

The diagnosis is easy in severe cases; it may be very difficult in slight cases for the colour of the disc is no sure

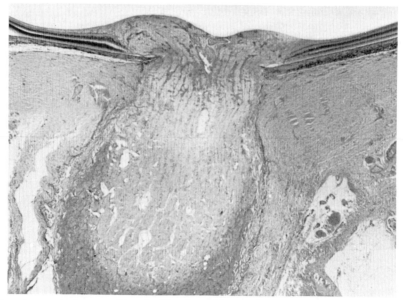

Fig. 23.1 Papilloedema in a cerebral tumour. Note the dilatation of the central vein. (By courtesy of Paton)

guide unless there is an undoubted difference between the two eyes. Fluorescein angiography, however, demonstrates dilatation of surface capillaries and leakage of dye which accummulates 10 min after intravenous injection as a vertically oval pool surrounding the nerve-head. Attention should be directed to the edges of the disc; if these can be seen clearly defined with any lens in the ophthalmoscope there is no papilloedema, but it does not follow that there is papilloedema if they appear blurred. Astigmatism, for example, causes apparent blurring of the disc margin. Moreover, the appearances of papilloedema may be stimulated in 3 conditions — pseudoneuritis, drusen of the nerve-head and a true optic neuritis. In some cases it is necessary to keep the patient under careful observation for a considerable period before a certain diagnosis can be made, while due attention should be paid to other signs and symptoms in the central nervous system.

Pseudo-neuritis is a condition occurring usually in hypermetropic eyes when the lamina is small and the nerve fibres are heaped up as they debouch upon the retina. The ophthalmoscopic appearance of swelling and blurred margins is largely due to reflexes. The swelling is never more than 2 dioptres, there is no venous engorgement, oedema or exudates, and the blind-spot is not enlarged. A fluorescein angiogram reveals no leakage.

In optic neuritis due to inflammation the appearance of the disc is often ophthalmoscopically indistinguishable from that in papilloedema. The swelling, however, is usually moderate — 2 or 3 D — shelving off gradually into the surrounding retina. Vitreous opacities are usual although they may be very fine. The visual symptoms, however, are usually marked, and the acute depression of central vision and the absence of signs of an intracranial space-occupying lesion form the most important differential features (Fig. 23.2).

Drusen of the optic disc occurs in families and is typically bilateral, inherited as an irregular dominant trait. The drusen bodies evolve slowly over many years and the appearance may mimic papilloedema associated with visual defects which do not correspond to the position of the drusen. Drusen is often associated with rather small optic nerve heads. They are composed of calcified concentrically laminated globular aggregates. Drusen may form as a result of altered axoplasmic transport at the optic disc secondary to local obstructing factors. Angiographically the vessels of the optic nerve head are normal in pseudo-neuritis and drusen.

Ætiology. In the vast majority of cases papilloedema is due to an increased intracranial pressure. Any intracranial tumour in any position, with the exception of the medulla oblongata, may induce it, the highest percentage being found with tumours of the mid-brain, parieto-occipital region, and cerebellum (p. 349). Tumours of the anterior fossa produce papilloedema more rarely and late. In general those tumours which tend to produce internal hydrocephalus are most certain to cause papilloedema. The site of the tumour is of more importance than its nature, its size or its rate of growth. Other intracranial causes — abscess, thrombosis of the cavernous sinus, aneurysm, subarachnoid haemorrhage, hydrocephalus — are more rare; malignant hypertension is common.

In intracranial disease papilloedema is usually bilateral, although not necessarily equal on the two sides. The

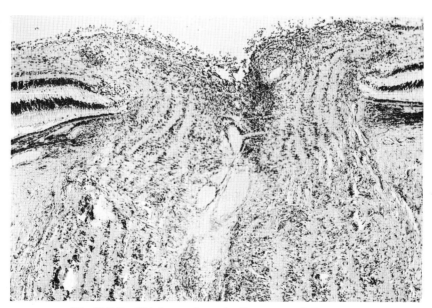

Fig. 23.2 Papillitis in toxoplasmosis. (By courtesy of Zimmerman.)

relative amount of swelling may be of localising significance in these cases but its value has been over-estimated; in frontal tumours and middle ear disease, however, the swelling is usually greater on the side of the lesion. The time of onset is a more important indication than the amount of swelling, the localising value being attached to the side first affected. Thus the swelling may be actually less on the side first affected owing to subsidence associated with commencing atrophy. Unilateral papilloedema, with or without 'secondary' optic atrophy on the other side, suggests a tumour of the opposite olfactory groove or orbital surface of the frontal lobe or of the pituitary body (the *Foster–Kennedy syndrome*, p. 349).

Table 23.1

Causes of unilateral disc edema	
Ocular orbital	*Mixed intracranial and orbital*
1. Papillitis	1. Unilateral optic atrophy and true papilloedema (Foster-Kennedy syndrome)
2. Drusen of the nerve head	
3. Ischaemic optic neuropathy	
4. Postcataract extraction (Irvine-Gass syndrome)	2. Unilateral high myopia and true papilloedema
5. Ocular Hypotony	3. Unilateral glaucoma without atrophy and true papilloedema
6. Central retinal vein occlusion	
7. Metastases to the optic nerve head	4. Cavernous sinus thrombosis
8. Ocular inflammatory disease	5. Carotid cavernous fistula
9 Optic nerve glioma or meningioma	*Pure intracranial*
10. Primary or metastatic compressive orbital masses	1. Posterior fossa tumour
	2. Pseudotumour cerebri
	3. Brain abcess
	4. Subarachnoid haemorrhage
11. Orbital cellulitis	5. Optochiasmatic arachnoiditis
12. Thyroid eye disease	

Giant cell arteritis and papilloedema. Giant cell arteritis or temporal arteritis is a self-limiting disease of large and medium-sized arteries affecting people over the age of 55 particularly women. Other vessels such as the coronary or the renal arteries may also be involved.

The typical features are constant headaches which may be unilateral or bilateral in the temporal area with prominent vessels which are tender. Pulsation in the temporal artery is often absent. There may be intermittent claudication of the jaw. The syndrome is self-limiting but may lead to blindness due to vascular occlusion often heralded by intermittent attacks of loss of vision in one eye or an extra-ocular muscle palsy.

The arteritis is granulomatous with infiltration of the full thickness of the vessel wall by lymphocytes, plasma cells and macrophages. Multinucleated giant cells are often conspicuous.

Ischaemic optic atrophy is a common ocular lesion due to involvement of the ophthalmic artery leading at first to swelling of the optic nerve head and later to atrophy and cupping.

Corticosteroid therapy should be begun as soon as possible when the headache will be promptly relieved. High dosages of 60–80 mg of oral Prednisolone should be given daily for the first week. The dosage can be reduced as the erythrocyte sedimentation rate falls. A maintenance dose of 5–15 mg is continued for at least 6–12 months.

Orbital lesions and papilloedema. As rarities, conditions of stasis in the orbit may produce papilloedema — tumours of the optic nerve, a meningioma near the apex of the orbit, venous thrombosis, cellulitis or pseudo-tumour of the orbit, or haemorrhage into the optic nerve sheath.

Treatment of papilloedema is essentially the relief of the causal pressure; if this cannot be relieved, the prognosis is bad and blindness the normal result. If, however, timely decompression or removal of the tumour is successfully performed, the effect is remarkable. Along with the relief of the general symptoms of intracranial pressure (headache, vomiting, stupor, etc.), vision improves rapidly unless the nerves have been irretrievably damaged, and the papilloedema quickly subsides; the recovery of vision, indeed, may be more rapid than the subsidence of the papilloedema. On the other hand, vision may deteriorate after operation, probably owing to progressive sclerosis at the disc, especially if surgical intervention has been delayed; if signs of subsidence and commencing atrophy are present, further diminution of vision is to be anticipated. Subsidence of the papilloedema is usually rapid after operation, a decided change being seen in a week to a fortnight, but there is considerable variation in different cases.

In all cases the visual fields should be carefully watched and decompression should be urged from the ophthalmological point of view before peripheral constriction becomes evident. As we have seen, this indicates that the optic nerve fibres have reached the stage when they are unable further to withstand the effects of compression; once atrophy becomes clinically visible at the disc, further visual deterioration will probably follow even if surgical relief is successfully accomplished. Local decompression through the vaginal sheaths in the orbit is occasionally practised for benign intracranial hypertension.

Anterior ischaemic optic neuropathy (AION)

Ischaemic optic neuropathy producing an altitudinal field defect has been recognised for many years as a complication of severe anaemia or after a massive haemorrhage. Patients suffering from a neglected acute attack of closed angle glaucoma are also likely to develop ischaemic neuropathy with subsequent optic atrophy.

The condition however may arise spontaneously and the clinical entity comprises sudden loss of vision, initially associated with swelling of the optic disc which resolves to optic atrophy within a month or two leaving a permanent visual defect. It is due to interference with the posterior ciliary artery supply to the anterior part of the optic nerve producing a post-laminar infarct without necessarily involving the central retinal artery Fig. 23.3A and B).

In AION due to temporal arteritis many of the patients show pallid swelling of the optic disc often without haemorrhages while others show pink oedema of the optic disc with flame-shaped haemorrhages. The latter is the common clinical picture in the absence of arteritis. The nature of the ophthalmoscopically visible pre-laminar swelling has been variably interpreted as an infarct of the disc or due to an accumulation of opaque axoplasmic debris in the optic nerve head. The majority of optic discs with AION due to temporal arteritis develop cupping. If a cilio-retinal or central retinal artery is compromised then there may be an associated infarction of a sector or of the entire retina.

The triggering factor for an attack of acute ischaemic neuropathy even in the presence of arterio-sclerosis or other recognizable cardiovascular anomaly is rarely identified. Management, therefore, presents complicated problems because ischaemic optic neuropathy is not a diagnosis but merely a recognition of local anoxia of the anterior region of the optic nerve and the causes are both multiple and complex.

Investigations should include assessment of the circulatory and micro-circulatory systems, specific examination to exclude any form of arteritis and sophisticated immunological, haematological and rheological tests. In the presence of temporal arteritis systemic steroids are mandatory and in large doses gradually tailing off to a maintenance dose. The eye itself should be carefully assessed for raised intraocular presure and for a low ophthalmodynamometric reading in the ophthalmic artery. Patients with arterio-sclerotic disease may have an optic nerve head which just survives despite minimal perfusion from the posterior ciliary arteries. A subtle change such as mild polycythaemia or anaemia or slight elevation of intraocular pressure may suffice in combination to impair disc perfusion and precipitate an attack of anterior ischaemic optic neuropathy.

Inflammations of the optic nerve: optic neuritis

The optic nerve may be affected by inflammation in any part of its course, but for clinical convenience it is usual to divide inflammatory conditions into two categories — those affecting the part of the nerve ophthalmoscopically visible at the disc and therefore showing obvious signs of disease (*papillitis*), and those which attack the nerve proximal to this region and therefore show no ophthalmoscopic changes so that the diagnosis has to be

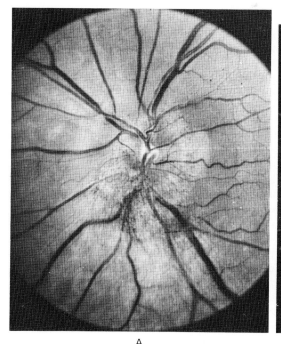
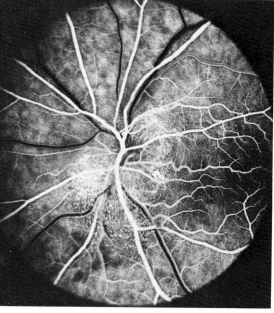

A   B

Fig. 22.3 A, Swollen disc with poor filling of the vessels above, irregularity of the arterioles and dilated capillaries below; B, Fluorescein angiogram of A. (By courtesy of Eagling.)

made on the basis of symptoms alone (*retrobulbar neuritis*). Retrobulbar neuritis is usually divided into an acute and a chronic form; the latter is the condition which is described as toxic amblyopia (*q.v.*) and may be due to a primary retinal lesion.

Papillitis

This may be ophthalmoscopically indistinguishable from papilloedema (*q.v.*). The disc is at first hyperaemic, the margins become blurred, swelling and oedema ensue which spread onto the retina, the retinal veins become tortuous and much distorted, exudates accumulate upon the disc and in the retina sometimes forming a macular fan, and there are fine vitreous opacities. When the retina is seriously involved, the condition is called *neuroretinitis*. Even in the most severe cases, however, the swelling of the disc rarely exceeds 2 to 3 dioptres.

If the inflammation has not been severe, the optic disc may appear normal on its subsidence; but if it has been sufficiently serious to destroy the nerve fibres, the picture of *post-neuritic atrophy* results. Here again, the ophthalmoscopic picture is indistinguishable from that following papilloedema — the disc margins are blurred and the floor has a dirty grey colour and is filled in with organised tissue which is continued onto the constricted arteries as perivascular sheaths.

Acute retrobulbar neuritis

On the other hand, *acute retrobulbar neuritis* produces no ophthalmoscopically visible changes, unless the lesion is near the lamina cribrosa when slight evidences of papillitis may be seen with some distension of the veins and attentuation of the arteries. If atrophic changes follow, the degeneration extends not only towards the brain but also towards the eye. In the milder cases pallor of the disc may be limited to the temporal side.

The symptoms and clinical course of both types of optic neuritis are, however, very different from papilloedema, and are typical. The disease is usually unilateral and of sudden onset, when the visual loss is profound. Even in cases of papillitis it is usually much greater than the objective signs would seem to warrant; in both types it may rapidly progress during one to eight days when blindness may be complete. In retrobulbar inflammations, this rapid deterioration of vision in the presence of a normal fundus may suggest hysteria. In these cases the diagnosis depends on the presence of local tenderness, the pupillary reactions and abnormalities in the visual fields. Recovery is often equally rapid, but the disease has a habit of showing remissions.

Local pain in retrobulbar neuritis may be felt on moving the eye. The pain is increased by pressure upon the globe, and neuralgia and headache may be present. The tenderness of the eyeball to digital pressure is limited to a small area corresponding roughly with the site of attachment of the superior rectus tendon. This sign is present only in the early stages of the disease and disappears in a few days. At first glance the pupillary reactions will be apparently normal both directly and consensually to light, as well as to convergence. More minute inspection will show, however, that although the pupil of the affected eye reacts to light, the contraction is not maintained under bright illumination so that instead of remaining contracted the pupil slowly dilates while the light is still kept on the eye. *Lack of sustained constriction of the pupil to light*, if it can be placed beyond dispute, *is of the greatest diagnostic significance*. A Marcus Gunn pupil is also of diagnostic significance indicating an afferent pupillary defect due to a pathological lesion in the optic nerve.

The field of vision may show a central scotoma which may be relative for colours or absolute. It is not always quite central, but may be paracentral or sectorial or in the form of a ring around the fixation point. There is usually some peripheral loss of the field and there may be complete blindness. Loss of contrast sensitivity is an early sign in optic neuritis.

The aetiology of optic neuritis is composite and it is usually impossible to deduce the cause of the disease from local signs and symptoms; reliance must be placed on a systemic examination and even then a definite ætiological diagnosis is frequently impossible.

Much the most common cause is a demyelinating affection of the nerve as occurs in other tracts of the white matter of the central nervous system. (*q.v*). The occurrence of retrobulbar neuritis should always excite suspicion of the presence of multiple sclerosis, of which it frequently forms a first symptom. In these cases the habit is for recurrences to appear in either eye from time to time, occasionally at considerable intervals; but it may be many years before more widespread signs of the disease occur.

Other diseases of the central nervous system wherein optic neuritis occurs are neuromyelitis optica (of Devic) (*q.v.*), acute disseminated encephalomyelitis, zoster, epidemic encephalitis and poliomyelitis. The more important of these will be noted in Chapter 34 but one condition wherein the optic nerve is primarily affected without other obvious central nervous involvement, deserves mention — Leber' disease.

The local causes of optic neuritis are relatively unimportant — a uveitis or a retinitis may spread onto the disc; among the former, sympathetic ophthalmitis is prominent. Similarly, a meningitis may affect the nerve, causing primarily a perineuritis. Both syphilis and tuberculosis may act in this way. Sinus disease, particularly sphenoid and ethmoid affections and orbital cellulitis, may act similarly; but such a sequence is probably rare.

Finally, endogenous infections may also produce an optic neuritis — acute infective diseases (influenza, malaria, measles, mumps, etc.), or metabolic dyscrasias (diabetes, anæmia, pregnancy, avitaminosis, starvation). The effect of exogenous toxins will be discussed under the toxic amblyopias.

Hereditary optic neuritis (hereditary optic atrophy, Leber's Disease)

This is a form of retrobulbar neuritis, usually commencing at about the twentieth year of life. Descent is generally through an unaffected female to males, although females are also sometimes affected. Vision generally fails rapidly at first, then gradually, but remains stationary or slowly improves after six months. Both eyes are always involved, although one may precede the other by a period varying from a few days to eighteen months. In two-thirds of the cases there is a central or centro-caecal scotoma, either partial for colours or also for white. The peripheral field is usually normal, but concentric contraction or sector-shaped defects may occur. Total and permanent colour-blindness has been known to follow. The central scotoma generally persists, but progressive constriction of the field to complete blindness is rare. Members of the same family often show identical peculiarities in the progress of the disease. The fundus is at first normal or there is slight blurring of the edges of the disc. In later stages, after several months, optic atrophy ensues, with pallor confined to the temporal side or involving the whole disc. Apart from headache, the general health is good. The ætiology is unknown although cyanide intoxication may play a part. There are numerous signs indicating an X chromosomal hereditary association.

Treatment of optic neuritis is essentially directed to the cause, if that can be found. ACTH has recently been advocated. It shortens the course of the disease without influencing the end-result. Hydroxocobalamine may be given by injection as a detoxicating agent.

The toxic amblyopias

The toxic amblyopias include a number of conditions in which the optic nerve fibres are damaged by exogenous poisons. The most common of these are tobacco, ethyl alcohol, methyl alcohol, lead, arsenic, thallium, quinine, ergot, filix mas, carbon disulphide, stramonium and cannabis indica. In some of them (tobacco, methyl alcohol) the disease is primarily retinal and follows poisoning of the ganglion cells of the retina which results in degeneration of the nerve fibres, demonstrable only after they have obtained their medullary sheaths behind the lamina cribrosa. Others are due to a direct effect on the nerve fibres themselves.

Tobacco amblyopia

This results from the excessive use of tobacco, either by pipe smoking or chewing; and also occasionally from the absorption of dust in tobacco factories. Smokers of shag and strong tobacco mixtures or cigars suffer most; cigarette smokers are rarely affected. In many cases there is also over-indulgence in alcohol but this is not invariable. The patients, usually 35–50 years of age, may have smoked excessively for years with impunity, the attack coinciding with some intercurrent cause of debility or digestive disturbance. Various substances have been regarded as the toxic agent, but a potent factor may be poisoning with the cyanide in tobacco smoke associated with a deficiency of vitamin B_{12}.

The patient complains of increasing fogginess of vision, usually least marked in the evening and in a dull light. Central vision is greatly diminished, so that reading and near work become difficult; although the condition is bilateral, one eye is usually more affected.

The fundus is normal or a slight temporal pallor may be seen in the disc; but the diagnosis is made from the characteristic defects in the central fields. These involve primarily the centrocæcal area between the fixation point and the blind-spot. Here, occupying a horizontally oval area, there is a relative scotoma to white and colours, particularly for red, and in it, on the horizontal meridian, there are one or more islands of complete visual loss. The scotoma gradually extends to involve the fixation area itself so that central vision may be lost but the peripheral field remains unaffected.

Pathologically the condition is due to degeneration of the ganglion cells of the retina, particularly of the macular area where the cells show vacuolation and Nissl degeneration. In the nerve the papillomacular bundle is degenerated.

Treatment consists of abstention from or severely curtailing the use of tobacco and alcohol. If this is done the prognosis is eventually good although visual improvement may be not be evident for a period of some months; thereafter it may be slow. Improvement may be hastened by injections of hydroxocobalamin 1000 μg intramuscularly. This dose should be repeated 5 times at intervals of 4 days and then at 2 weekly intervals for some months. Recovery may be monitored by the VEP. Recurrences are very rarely seen even if tobacco is resumed in strict moderation, but this is perhaps unwise.

Ethyl alcohol

Although alcohol is usually an adjuvant in tobacco amblyopia, it may cause a similar amblyopia in the absence of the latter. Such patients frequently suffer from alcoholic peripheral neuritis. The disease, characterised by a central scotoma, may be due essentially to avitaminosis owing to chronic lack of nourishment (*q.v.*).

The amblyopia produced by *diabetes, carbon disulphide* (seen in the rayon industry), and *iodoform* resembles that of tobacco.

The amblyopias produced by *methyl alcohol, lead, nitro-*

and *dinitro-benzol*, differ from the above type in the more serious optic atrophy which generally ensues. There is probably always a stage at which a central scotoma is present, but it is often missed.

Methyl alcohol

Poisoning from drinking wood-alcohol has always been common in countries during prohibition, and occurs sporadically from drinking methylated spirit. Individual susceptibility is marked. It may occur in an acute or chronic form. In the acute form nausea, headache and giddiness are followed by coma. If the patient survives, vision very rapidly fails, passing through the stages of contracted fields and absolute central scotomata to blindness. The vision may improve, but usually again relapses, becoming gradually abolished by progressive optic atrophy. Restoration is rarely complete. Ophthalmoscopically there may be blurring of the edges of the discs and diminished size of the vessels in the early stages. Later there are signs of optic atrophy, usually of the primary type (p. 229). Pathologically there is widespread degeneration of the ganglion cells of the retina.

Arsenic

This is specially liable to cause optic atrophy, usually total, when administered in the form of pentavalent compounds such as atoxyl or soamin. These were used for attacking the trypanosome of sleeping sickness, but have now been abandoned.

Lead

Lead poisoning is rarely seen since precautions have been taken to eliminate salts of this metal from pottery glazes, etc. The ocular signs are optic neuritis or optic atrophy, which may be primary or post-neuritic. Some cases develop a retinopathy which may be due directly to lead or be of the renal type, secondary to lead nephritis.

Quinine amblyopia

This differs in some striking characteristics from tobacco amblyopia. Here total blindness (amaurosis) may follow the use of the drug, even in such small doses as 60 mg in susceptible persons; 150 mg is the maximum amount of sulphate of quinine which should be given within 24 hours. The largest doses are usually taken for malaria, but quinine is also used as an abortifacient. The pupils are dilated and immobile. Deafness and tinnitus are present. Ophthalmoscopically the retinal vessels are extremely contracted and the disc is very pale; oedema of the retina has been described in the early stage. Occassionally blindness is permanent and optic atrophy ensues. In less marked cases or at a later stage the fields of vision are much contracted but central vision may be completely restored so that tube-vision results. The discs may remain pale for years or become normal.

Filix mas (used as an anti-helminthic) may cause amblyopia in excessive doses, especially if given with castor oil; optic atrophy may supervene.

Ethambutol

This is an oral chemo-therapeutic agent used in the treatment of tuberculosis and may produce an optic neuritis resulting in reduced visual acuity and colour vision and eventually a central scotoma. The neuritis is reversible when the drug is discontinued but patients should be examined monthly during the early stages of therapy. 15 mg ethambutol per kg per day is the upper limit of safety with regard to eye complications.

Optic atrophy has been reported following the use of chloramphenicol, streptomycin, sulphonamides and isoniazide.

Chloroquine

This is an anti-malarial drug used in the treatment of lupus erythematosus and arthritis. Prolonged administration may give rise to a keratopathy, myopathy or retinopathy. The retinopathy is a serious pigmentary degeneration of the retina which may lead to loss of vision. A mild pigmentary disturbance in the macular area leads to a characteristic 'bull's-eye' retinal lesion and eventually there is a widespread retinal atrophy with pigment clumping and attenuated retinal vessels. Few cases of retinopathy have been reported in patients receiving a total dose of less than 300 gm. Patients with lupus erythematosis are more susceptible to chloroquine toxicity. Careful perimetry, preferably static, with determination of threshold sensitivities within 5 degrees of the fixation point with red stimuli is a reliable method of detecting early signs of chloroquine retinal toxicity.

Oral contraceptives

These are usually a combination of progestogens and oestrogens. They may play a part in the production of occlusive vascular disease, particularly in women who suffer from vascular hypertension, migraine or other vascular syndromes. Infarction of the brain or of the optic nerve head occurs more commonly in women using contraceptive therapy. Occasionally contact lens wearers develop an intolerance to their lenses when taking oral contraceptives. Their symptoms are photophobia and irritation together with mild oedema of the conjunctiva.

Treatment of these amblyopias is cessation of the drug.

Deficiency amblyopia

A deficiency of vitamins in the diet, particularly of thiamine, may be responsible for the development of an optic neuritis usually of the axial type, resulting in the loss of central vision; similar lesions in the mid-brain cause various types of ophthalmoplegia (acute hæmorrhagic anterior polioencephalitis of Wernicke.

Such an amblyopia is seen in extreme degrees of pellagra. An optic atrophy, usually partial but occasionally apparently complete, may eventually develop and in severe cases the prognosis is bad. An efficient diet, if resumed before atrophy develops, is curative; after atrophy has set in the visual defect is permanent.

Degenerations of the optic nerve: optic atrophy

Optic atrophy
This is the term usually applied to the condition of the disc when the optic nerve is degenerated. It has been pointed out that injury to the nerve fibres in any part of their course from the retina to the lateral geniculate body leads to degeneration not only on the proximal (cerebral) side — as might be anticipated for afferent fibres — but also on the distal (ocular) side (p. 221). Optic atrophy therefore follows extensive disease of the retina from destruction of the ganglion cells, as in pigmentary retinal dystrophy or occlusion of the central artery; these cases are sometimes called *consecutive atrophy*. The break in continuity of the fibres may be at the disc itself, such as results from the strangulation occurring in papillitis, neuro-retinitis or papilloedema. These cases are distinguished as '*post-neuritic*' atrophy. It also follows destruction of the nerve in the orbit, as in fracture of the base of the skull or severe retrobulbar neuritis. In addition there is a group of cases in which optic atrophy occurs without local disturbances but associated with general disease, usually of the central nervous system, or without discoverable cause. Such cases are described as *primary atrophy*. *Toxic atrophy* has already been discussed, as well as *glaucomatous atrophy*.

The essential ophthalmoscopic features of optic atrophy in general are an alteration in the colour of the disc and changes in the blood vessels. The disc is always pale, but may show varieties of tint especially associated with various types of atrophy. The pallor affects the whole disc and must be carefully distinguished from the white centre, often encroaching upon the temporal side, due to physiological cupping. The pallor is not due to atrophy of the nerve fibres, but to loss of vascularity owing to obliteration of the vessels; it is thus an uncertain guide to visual capacity.

When the atrophy is due to disease or poisoning of the second visual neurone proximal to the disc so that there are no ophthalmoscopic evidences of previous local inflammation, it is called *simple or primary atrophy*. In such cases the disc is grey or white, sometimes with a greenish or bluish tint (Plate 3 Fig. C). The stippling of the lamina cribrosa is seen; the edges are sharply defined and the surrounding retina looks normal. Owing to the degeneration of the nerve-fibres there is slight cupping (atrophic cupping) which must be carefully distinguished from glaucomatous cupping; it is shallow and

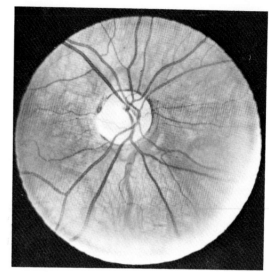

Fig. 23.4 Syphilitc optic atrophy

saucer-shaped, as shown by the slight bending of the vessels, but is scarcely measurable with the ophthalmoscope. These is no retraction of the lamina cribrosa. The vessels are only slightly contracted (Fig. 23.4).

The classical cause of primary atrophy is tabes (*q.v.*) in which the degeneration is due to a chronic inflammation of the pia which causes a secondary degeneration of the nerve fibres commencing in the optic nerve in the neighbourhood of the chiasm. Tabetic optic atrophy is slowly progressive and the prognosis is bad, but owing to efficient anti-syphilitic treatment, the disease has now become relatively rare. The same applies to the atrophy of general paralysis. The most common cause to-day is multiple sclerosis wherein recurrent attacks of transient demyelination cause an increasing degree of atrophy, but in this disease it is rarely complete (Fig. 23.5). Other causes are the demyelinating diseases already noted in the ætiology of optic neuritis (p. 226), Leber's disease, and the many exogenous poisons which give rise to toxic amblyopia.

Secondary atrophy which has exactly the same ophthalmoscopic picture as the primary variety, follows any injury or direct pressure affecting the visual nerve-fibres in any part of their course from the lamina cribrosa to the geniculate body. It is noteworthy that a brain tumour will produce a secondary atrophy if it presses upon the chiasm or optic nerve, and a post-neuritic atrophy if it causes papilloedema by increased intracranial pressure. The differentiation does not indicate the nature or site of the pressure; it merely differentiates whether the atrophy has affected a normal disc or one which has been choked.

The characteristic ophthalmoscopic picture of *post-neuritic atrophy* has already been described (p. 226).

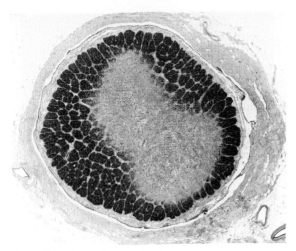

Fig. 23.5 Optic atrophy showing demyelination of the papillo-macular bundle

In the *'consecutive'* atrophy of retinal and choroidal disease, the disc has a yellowish waxy appearance, the edges are less sharply defined, and the vessels are very markedly contracted, sometimes almost to the point of disappearance.

In total optic atrophy the pupils are dilated and immobile to light and the patient is blind; when unilateral the consensual reaction to light is exaggerated. In partial optic atrophy central vision is depressed and there is concentric contraction of the field, with or without scotomata, relative or absolute, according to the cause. It is important to note that no deduction as to the amount of vision can be made from the ophthalmoscopic appearances for the presence of all the signs of atrophy is not inconsistent with a certain, sometimes a considerable, amount of vision.

No *treatment* is effective for optic atrophy; the prognosis depends on the possibility of controlling the causal factor.

Tumours of the optic nerve
See p. 335.

Congenital abnormalities of the optic disc

Coloboma of the optic disc
This occurs in two forms, one of which is common, the other rare. The common form is due to incomplete closure of the embryonic fissure, and manifests itself as an *inferior crescent*, much resembling the myopic cresent (*q.v.*) but situated at the lower edge of the disc. It occurs most commonly in hypermetropic and astigmatic eyes, which are often found to have slightly defective vision in spite of the correction of any error of refraction. It is often slightly ectatic (*conus*).

In what is commonly known as *coloboma of the disc* (or nerve sheath) there is greater failure of the embryonic fissure to close. The disc looks large and the vessels have an abnormal distribution, appearing only above or irregularly round the edges. The apparent disc is really the sclera and the inner surface of the sheath of the nerve, the nerve itself being usually spread out as a pink horizontal linear band at the upper part. The floor of the coloboma is white and measurably depressed, often quite ectatic. The eye usually has defective vision.

Rarer anomalies allied to coloboma are round cavities (*'holes'*) on the disc, generally situated in the temporal portion; they usually look grey or black owing to shadow and patches of *pigment* due to the inclusion of retinal pigmentary epithelium. They may be associated with œdema of the macula.

Mention has already been made of an excess of *fibrouslike tissue on the disc* and extending a short distance along the vessels, the remnants of the sheaths of the hyaloid vessels (p. 181). Sometimes the fibrous tissue takes the form of a delicate semi-transparent membrane covering the disc and appearing to be slung from the vessels.

Hypoplasia of the optic nerve
The diagnosis of hypoplasia presents little difficulty in the extreme case. The disc is small with slightly tortuous and occasionally small vessels and is surrounded by a yellowish mottled peri-papillary halo with a pigmented rim approximately corresponding to the size of a normal disc. The retinal nerve fibre layer is thin. The condition is often bilateral but may be asymmetrical and central vision is usually involved.

There is an important association between hypoplastic discs and cerebral malformation which may include absence of the septum pellucidum, congenital hypopituitarism and agenesis of the corpus callosum. This condition has been described following the maternal ingestion of an anticonvulsant with known teratogenic properties — phenytoin.

24

Symptomatic disturbances of vision

Apart from the disturbances of vision which have already been considered and have their origin in the eye itself, there are others dependent upon lesions in the visual nervous paths. Since they not infrequently closely simulate the disorders due to peripheral causes or are early evidence of disease, they lead the patient to consult an ophthalmic surgeon. There are also visual defects the cause and seat of which are imperfectly elucidated; although some are probably peripheral in origin, it will be convenient to consider them here.

Hemianopia

Hemianopia denotes loss of half of the field of vision. The commonest clinical form is *homonymous hemianopia*, in which the right or left half of the binocular field of vision is lost, owing to loss of the temporal half of one field and the nasal half of the other, a condition due to a lesion situated in any part of the visual paths from the chiasma to the occipital lobe. A focus of disease in this area causes loss of vision of the corresponding halves of each retina (hence the designation homonymous) and therefore loss of the opposite halves of the visual fields (Fig. 24.1). Right hemianopia is more quickly discovered than left owing to the fact that reading is impossible; left hemianopia is often discovered when the patient does not see food on the left side of the plate.

In many cases of hemianopia the fixation area in each field escapes, especially if the lesion is near the occipital cortex; in infra-geniculate lesions the fixation point is usually bisected. In a number of cases it is probable that the macular fibres are in fact spared owing to their widespread but segregated course in the optic radiations and their separate representation in the occipital pole. The immunity of the macula in vascular lesions of the cortex is attributed to the fact that the occipital pole is supplied by the posterior and middle cerebral arteries both of which are seldom blocked at the same time. The explanation in other cases is not so obvious. In certain cases the sparing of the macula may be only apparent owing to a functional shift of fixation towards the seeing part of the retina, while in other cases a possible ex-

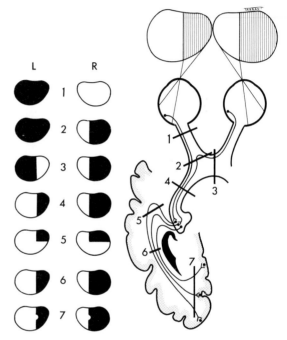

Fig. 24.1 Diagram of the visual paths, showing sites of lesions and the corresponding field defects: 1, lesion through optic nerve — ipsilateral blindness; 2, lesion through proximal part of optic nerve — ipsilateral blindness with contralateral hemianopia; 3, sagittal lesion of chiasma — bitemporal hemianopia; 4, lesion of optic tract — homonymous hemianopia; 5, lesion of temporal lobe — quadrantic homonymous defect; 6, lesion of optic radiations — homonymous hemianopia (sometimes sparing the macula); 7, lesion of occipital lobe — homonymous hemianopia (usually sparing the macula)

planation may be sought in the integrative powers of the central visual mechanism.

Lesions of the lateral geniculate body cause homonymous hemianopia (Fig. 24.1); those limited to the pulvinar and superior colliculus do not.

Cortical and sub-cortical lesions. The majority of cases of hemi-anopia is due to lesions above the primary visual centres, usually in the occipital lobe or optic radiations (Fig. 24.1: 6, 7). The chief causes are injury by falls on the back of the head or gun-shot wounds, cerebral tumour, or cerebral softening due to disease of the blood vessels. In gun-shot wounds both occipital lobes are not infrequently injured; there is usually unconsciousness from concussion at first and the hemianopia becomes manifest with the gradual recovery. If both lobes are extensively injured there is complete blindness; often, however, some portion of the cortex of one or other calcarine fissure escapes, and in these cases some measure of central vision is regained.

In less extensive injury the hemianopic symptoms may gradually improve. The first sign of improvement is the perception of the movement of objects in the affected field without recognition of their nature and details. The onset of hemianopia due to disease of the cortex is more gradual, and careful investigation with the perimeter shows that the colour fields are often lost before the field for white light, although this is always contracted. This *hemiachromatopsia* is itself of gradual onset. In cortical and sub-cortical lesions the pupillary reactions are normal (p. 26), and the fundi reveal no ophthalmoscopic changes, except in the case of tumours which may be associated with bilateral papillœdema. Cortical lesions are liable to be accompanied by word-blindness, usually due to involvement of the angular gyrus. When the lesion is in the posterior part of the internal capsule hemianaesthesia, with or without hemiplegia, is likely to be present. Optokinetic testing in occipital lobe hemianopias should elicit a normal response to each side. A depression of the response toward the side of the lesion implies involvement of the parietal lobe and indicates the possibility of a neoplastic aetiology rather than a vascular cause.

Occipital lobe hemianopias are extremely congruous with a homogeneous density with macular sparing. Riddoch's phenomenon wherein appreciation of a dim kinetic target is retained within the defective visual field with loss of appreciation of a static bright target is typical of an occipital lesion.

Rare cases of homonymous *quadrantanopia* have been reported, in which corresponding quadrants of each field — the upper or lower half of one temporal, and the upper or lower half of the other nasal — have been lost. These may be caused by cortical or sub-cortical partial lesions of one occipital lobe, destruction of the part above the calcarine fissure leading to loss of the lower quadrants and *vice versa* (Fig. 4.5A and B). A similar quadrantic defect occurs in lesions of the temporal lobe owing to the fact that a ventral band of the optic radiations passes first forwards and then backwards in the temporal lobe in its course from the lateral geniculate body to the occipital lobe (Fig. 24.1:5). Partial hemianopia of a quadrantic type is then commoner than the typical homonymous defect, usually greater on the

side of the lesion. Subjective sensations of smell occur in some of these cases, due to the involvement of the uncinate process of the hippocampal gyrus.

Lesions of the optic tract. In these cases, since the afferent pupillary fibres part company with the visual fibres before the latter enter the lateral geniculate body (p. 26), Wernicke's hemianopic pupil reaction should be present (p. 76); but the reaction is always difficult to elicit. More assistance in diagnosis is afforded by collateral symptoms. The proximity of the crus cerebri, third and other cranial nerves, leads to other complications in the pathological picture (p. 349). The association of hemianopia with contralateral third nerve paralysis and ipsilateral hemiplegia suggests a tract lesion. As a rule the fixation point does not escape in tract hemianopia. Partial atrophy of both optic nerves manifests itself by pallor of the discs in these cases, preceded in cases of raised intracranial pressure by papilloedema. The lesion is usually syphilitic meningitis or a gumma, tuberculosis or tumour of the optic thalamus or temporo-sphenoidal lobe; softening and haemorrhage are rare. It is important that the patient is subjectively unaware of his visual defect in lesions above the geniculate body, but is conscious of a hemianopic defect from geniculate or infra-geniculate causes. Primary lesions of the optic tract are very rare and the tract is usually disturbed by compression. Chordomas, pituitary adenomas, tentorial meningiomas, temporal lobe gliomas or aneurysms of the upper basilar distribution or on the superior cerebeller arteries or posterior cerebral arteries are the common causes. Tract hemianopias are incongruous with a variation in density.

Lesions of the optic chiasma. Bitemporal hemianopia is usually caused by tumours in the region of the sella turcica, pressure by a suprasellar aneurysm or by chronic arachnoiditis; these press upon the chiasma, so that the fibres going to the nasal halves of each retina are destroyed (Fig. 24.1:3). Tumours of the pituitary body are most common; but suprasellar tumours, particularly cranio-pharyngiomata derived from Rathke's pharyngeal pouch and suprasellar meningiomata must be considered. Other lesions are gliomas of the third ventricle, ectopic pinealomas, dermoid tumours and third ventricular dilatation due to obstructive hydrocephalus.

Enlargement of the pituitary body, whether from functional hyperplasia, adenoma, or malignant growth, leads to visual defects in about 80% of cases, due to pressure upon the chiasma which lies immediately above it and upon the inner sides of the optic tracts. The earliest visual symptoms may be a unilateral central scotoma simulating retrobulbar neuritis for one side is usually compressed before the other. This may be followed by homonymous hemianopia from pressure on one tract, or rarely by *altitudinal hemianopia*, i.e., loss of the upper or more rarely the lower halves of the fields from pressure upon the chiasma; early loss in the upper half of the field may be caused by intra- or extrasellar tumours, early loss in the lower half suggests a suprasellar tumour. More commonly bitemporal hemiachromatopsia, passing into a complete hemianopia, supervenes. The field does not show the accurate delimitation characteristic of homonymous hemianopia, but gradually contracts from the temporal side inwards and from above downwards, finally involving the nasal field from below upwards and leading to complete blindness. Then, or at a much earlier stage, the vision of the other eye becomes affected in a similar manner. If the second eye becomes involved before vision is lost in the first, the fields show bitemporal hemianopia. Complete temporal hemianopia in one eye, for example, may be associated with temporal achromatopsia in the other; such a combination emphasizes the importance of charting the colour fields in all cases. Many patients have a homonymous hemianopia, due to pressure and traction on one optic tract. Variations in the type and progress of the visual defects are thus not uncommon.

A chronic *chiasmal arachnoiditis* of obscure origin may also cause bitemporal hemianopia due to compression of the chiasma by fibrous cicatricial bands. The same field defect has also resulted from antero-posterior injury to the chiasma in fracture of the base of the skull.

Binasal hemianopia is very rare. It necessitates two lesions, one on each side of the chiasma, destroying the fibres to the temporal halves of each retina while leaving the nasal fibres intact. It may be due to distension of the third ventricle, causing the optic nerves to be pressed downwards and outwards against the internal carotids, or to atheroma of the carotids or posterior communicating arteries.

Cases have been described in which there has been loss of half of the field in one eye and depression of vision progressing to blindness in the other. These are due to a lesion at the point where one optic nerve meets the chiasma so that the crossed fibres from the opposite side are involved as they loop forward into the nerve (Fig. 24.1:2).

In all cases of chiasmal damage a careful survey of the central nervous system must be made as well as an enquiry into the function of the pituitary. X-rays may provide valuable information, showing, for example, erosion of the sella, enlargement of the pituitary fossa or vascular calcification; simple radiography should be supplemented, by computerized tomography. If, as frequently occurs, vision progressively deteriorates, transfrontal or naso-pharyngeal extirpation may be advisable in many cases, particularly of pituitary tumours; the prognosis of operative removal, if undertaken in time, is reasonably good.

Amblyopia (αμβλυς, blunt) and Amaurosis (αμαυρός, dark)

These are the terms used for partial and complete loss of sight, respectively in one or both eyes in the absence of ophthalmoscopic or other marked objective signs.

Unilateral amblyopia is usually either *congenital* or results from psychical suppression of the retinal image — *amblyopia ex anopsia*: these varieties are discussed elsewhere (p. 297). Unilateral amblyopia may be due to high refractive errors, a condition sometimes curable with suitable spectacles in early life if sufficient perseverance is exercised, but rarely in older people. Unilateral amblyopia is also a symptom of retrobulbar neuritis (*q.v.*).

Bilateral amblyopia is found in the various forms of toxic amblyopia (*q.v.*). Bilateral amaurosis occurs in uræmia and in meningitis. Both amblyopia and amaurosis occur in hysteria.

Uraemic amaurosis occurs particularly in acute nephritis, especially complicating pregnancy or after scarlet fever, but is also found with chronic renal disease. The onset of blindness is sudden or rapid (8–24 h); it is bilateral and complete. The fundi show no changes, unless, as in some cases, there is a coincident hypertensive retinopathy. Vision usually improves in 10–18 h, and is fully restored in about 48 h, especially if a lumbar puncture is done. In cases occurring during pregnancy there is usually eclampsia. In uræmic amaurosis the pupils are dilated, but generally react to light, showing that the lower centres are not affected. The condition is probably due to circulation of toxic material which acts upon the cells of the visual centres.

Amaurosis fugax is a term given to sudden temporary failure of sight in one eye which is usually the result of embolization of the retinal circulation. The onset is acute and the episode usually lasts for several minutes. The sudden loss may appear like a curtain falling from above or rising from below and vision may be completely absent at the height of the attack. Recovery occurs in the same pattern. Examination during or shortly after an attack may reveal retinal ischaemia in the form of retinal oedema, small haemorrhages and in some cases visible emboli in the retinal vessels. The emboli are fibrin-platelet aggregates originating on the irregular surfaces of an ulcerating atheroma within the carotid or the aorta or cholesterol crystals. Repeated attacks of amaurosis fugax indicate the need for arteriography especially if associated with transient cerebral symptoms.

Cardiovascular abnormalities such as valvular defects or arrythmias may cause similar visual phenomena. Prolapse of the mitral valve, a congenital cardiac abnormality, is associated with a similar history. Fibromuscular hyperplasia is a disease occurring in young females. In these patients proliferation of the medial muscular coats of medium-sized blood vessels occurs causing carotid artery, renal artery and vertebral artery stenosis. Arteriography shows a characteristic 'string of beads' sign. Migraine is an occasional cause of unilateral visual loss. Some patients with migraine have retinal manifestations presumed secondary to vaso-spasm in the retinal vessels and this may be substantiated by the presence of oedema in the retina.

Patients with optic nerve-head swelling experience brief obscurations of vision lasting 30–60 sec. It may occur unilaterally in patients with asymmetric disc oedema due to increased intracranial pressure or to giant-cell arteritis.

Venous stasis retinopathy (Fig. 24.2) consists of micro-aneurysms, small punctate haemorrhages and patches of neovasularisation. It originates from ischaemia and resultant anoxia and its presence indicates either occlusion or severe stenosis of the internal carotid artery. The retinal artery pressure is invariably low on the affected side. Ischaemic orbital pain may be produced by anoxia lessened by lying down.

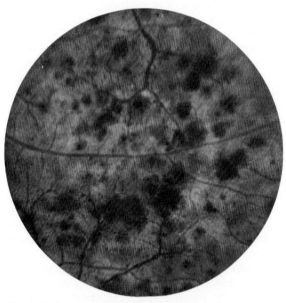

Fig. 24.2 Venous stasis retinopathy in left eye of patient with arteriographically shown occlusion of left internal carotid artery. Note dilated, dark and irregular veins. (By courtesy of T. P. Kearns.) Published with permission from the Am. J. Ophthalmol. 88: 714–722, 1979. Copyright by the Ophthalmic Publishing Company

Treatment with aspirin or persantin may alleviate symptoms due to platelet emboli. Disobliteration of the carotid is indicated for an isolated atheromatous plaque but often such plaques are multiple.

Hysterical amblyopia, as might be expected, exhibits protean manifestations. It may be unilateral, but is more commonly bilateral. There is usually concentric contraction of the fields, with or without colour defects; very characteristic is a spiral field which continually diminishes while it is being taken, so that it may be finally limited to the fixation point. The patients, however, get about perfectly well unaided, an impossibility in cases of genuine contracted fields (p. 212). Sometimes there are irritative symptoms — blepharospasm, blinking, lacrimation. The pupillary reactions are perfect, affording an invaluable objective diagnostic sign. Treatment must be directed to the psychogenic cause, but great care must be taken to eliminate organic disease before the diagnosis is finally accepted.

Scintillating scotomata

Scintillating scotomata of various kinds occur in *migraine*. In typical migraine the patient feels unusually well before the attack. A positive scotoma appears in the field of vision while obscuring sight it has a peculiar shimmering character. It gradually increases in size until ultimately one-half of the field is clouded, the fixation point remaining relatively clear. In the dark field bright spots and rays of various colours are often seen, frequently arranged in zig-zags when they are called 'fortification spectra' (*teichopsia*). Both half fields are usually affected, so that there is homonymous hemianopia. In other cases the whole field becomes clouded, but in spite of this the fixation point is usually seen momentarily, and then becomes obscured until the eyes are moved to a fresh spot. Vision usually clears in about a quarter of an hour, but the attack is soon followed by violent headache, generally intensified on the side of the head opposite the hemianopic field (*hemicrania*), and accompanied by nausea and even sickness ('bilious attack'). During the attack numbness in the mouth and tongue as well as slight aphasia are frequent as well as a copious secretion of urine of low specific gravity. Attacks occur periodically, but vary greatly in number and severity. In mild attacks, and especially as age advances, the scotoma may occur without the headache or the headache without scotoma.

Migraine is to be attributed to vasomotor changes in the brain. Vasodilatation, associated with a feeling of well-being, is followed by vasoconstriction, especially in the occipital lobes. Rest, warmth, and sleep are the best measures to combat the attacks; they can sometimes be warded off or alleviated by ergotamine tartrate.

Occasionally people who suffer from ordinary migraine have attacks in which, without any scotoma, the headache is followed by partial paralysis of the third nerve (*ophthalmoplegic migraine*) on the same side as the hemicrania. Slight ptosis, diplopia, and sluggishness of the pupillary reactions continue for some hours and gradually disappear. The paresis is worse and persists longer with succeeding attacks, and has sometimes eventually become permanent. Probably most of these cases are not migrainous, but due to some organic nerve lesion such as pressure on the optic nerve by a distended artery.

Night-blindness

This occurs *par exellence* in pigmentary retinal dystrophy (*q.v.*) and in xerophthalmia (*q.v.*), but in rare cases it is a familial congenital affection. It is also found after exposure to bright sunlight in hot countries amongst patients who are debilitated by malnutrition or prolonged fasting; the condition generally improves rapidly if the eyes are protected and the nutrition attended to. The affection is local, as is shown by the fact that covering one eye with a bandage during the day has been found to restore sight enough for the ensuing night, the unprotected eye remaining as bad as ever. Night-blindness is to be attributed to interference with the functions of the retinal rods, due to deficiency in visual purple. In xerophthalmia and the endemic cases the symptom is a manifestation of deficiency of fat-soluble vitamin A in the diet, and therefore cod-liver oil is specially indicated. It also occurs in diseases of the liver, especially cirrhosis, and may appear as a functional nervous disorder associated with other symptoms of neurosis or malingering.

Coloured vision (chromatopsia)

This is a rare symptom. *Erythropsia* (red vision) occurs particularly after cataract extraction if the eyes are exposed to bright light. Objects look red, but the visual acuity is not affected, and no permanent damage results. Patients should be warned of the possibility of erythropsia, as it is somewhat alarming and suggestive of hæmorrhage. It is met with also in snow-blindness. Chromatopsia also occurs in some cases during the resolution of optic neuritis when the ensuing atrophy is not complete. In normal people black print will sometimes suddenly turn deep red owing to strong lateral light entering the eye through the sclera.

Colour blindness or achromatopsia

This may be congenital or acquired. *Acquired colour blindness*, partial as in cases with relative scotomata or complete as in disease of the optic nerve, has been referred to incidentally in discussing the various disorders of the eye in which it occurs. In most diseases of the retina and choroid, changes in colour perception affect mostly the blue end of the spectrum. Slight diminution in acuity of perception of these rays is caused normally, owing to their physical absorption, by the increase of amber pigment in the nucleus of the lens (*blue blindness*), and this may be abnormally great in sclerosing lenses (*black cataract*); it has been said to affect the pictures of artists in their old age.

Congenital colour blindness occurs in two chief forms, total and partial. The former is very rare and is generally associated with nystagmus and a central scotoma. All colours appear grey, of different brightness. The spectrum appears as a grey band like the normal scotopic spectrum (p. 19), and like it with the maximum brightness at 510 mμ. It is probable that total colour blindness is caused by a central defect.

The partial form is seldom discovered unless special tests are made since the subjects compensate for their defect by attention to shade and texture, combined with experience. Gross cases occur in 3–4% of males, but are rare in females (0.4%); slighter cases are more common in males. It is an inherited condition, being transmitted through the female who is usually unaffected, and is probably due to the absence of one of the photopigments normally found in the foveal cones. In most cases reds and greens are confused, so that the defect is a source of danger in certain occupations, such as engine-drivers and sailors. The red-green cases fall into two chief groups, *protanopes* and *deuteranopes*. For the former the red end of the spectrum is much less bright than for normal people and is often actually shortened; in deuteranopes the green sensation is defective. These groups are said to have *dichromatic* vision. In both groups the defects may not be complete and these cases are called *protanomalous* and *deuteranomalous* respectively. It is clear that theoretically there might be other cases of colour blindness due to absence of the blue sensation, and such have been described, but are very rare (*tritanopes*).

There are two objects in testing for colour blindness: (1) the exact nature of the defect; (2) whether the subject is likely to be a source of danger to the community. The first is an exhaustive investigation involving stringent tests with a pure spectrum. In testing for danger, it is obvious that the names given to the colours are of value, for if a man repeatedly calls red green or *vice versa* he is unsuited to be an engine-driver or look-out man on a ship. Whatever the object in view, several tests should be employed; for the spectrum tests the student must be referred to special monographs on colour vision. The following are the other chief tests.

1. *The lantern test.* The subject names various colours shown by a lantern, and is judged by the mistakes he makes. Much here depends upon the size of the apertures of the lantern (i.e., the size of the retinal areas stimulated) and the nature and intensity of the light source. Many lanterns are worse than useless. Edridge–Green's lantern is efficient if used by an expert.

2. *Holmgren's wools.* These consist of a selection of skeins of coloured wools from which the candidate is required to make a series of colour-matches. This test has been much criticised, but if properly carried out

gross defects of colour vision are easily recognized and an expert will be put on his guard in almost every case of even minor defect.

Test I consists in presenting to the candidate a pale green sample and telling him to select from the heap of wools all those which seem to correspond in colour. If he is colour defective he will probably select several of the 'confusion colours' — greys, buffs, straw colour, etc. — as well as greens. He is next given a rose colour II: if he matches this with blues or violets he is red-blind; if with greys or greens he is green-blind. He is then given a bright red skein III: if he is red-blind he will choose dark greens and browns, if green-blind pale greens and browns. IV is a purple skein: if the candidate is colour defective he will probably select any shade of blue or green, also pinks and greys. V is a yellow skein: the colour-defective candidate will probably select greenish-yellows, light yellow-greens, fawns and pinks. In blue-blindness purples, red and orange are confused in test II.

3. *The Farnsworth–Munsell 100 hue test* represents hue discrimination by an error score, the greater the score the poorer the colour vision. Patients with toxic optic neuropathy display a characteristic pattern.

4. *Isochromatic charts.* These consist of coloured lithographic plates in which bold numerals are represented in dots of various tints set amid dots of the same size but of tints which are most readily confused with those of the figures by colour-defective people. Normal trichromats can easily read the numbers, some of which are indistinguishable to the various types of colour-defective while tests are included in which the numbers can be read by the colour-defective, but not by the normal sighted. Stilling's original tests have now been largely replaced by the Japanese test of Ishihara, while good alternatives are the Swedish Boström test or the American H-R-R test.

5. *Nagel's anomaloscope.* This is an instrument in which on looking down a telescope a bright disc is seen, divided into two halves by a horizontal line. One half is illuminated by light of the sodium line of the spectrum (yellow), and this has to be matched by a mixture of red (lithium line) and green (thallium line) in the other half. By turning screws the relative amounts of red and green in the mixture and the brightness can be varied.

Defects of colour vision have led to much acrimonious discussion. Their detection may be easy, but is often difficult and no single test is infallible.

Word-blindness

This occurs as a not very uncommon congenital anomaly, due to defects in the association areas of the brain, which often runs in families; it affects 0.1% of primary school children, being much commoner in boys than girls. Owing to backwardness in learning to read the children are often brought to the ophthalmic surgeon because a visual defect is suspected. In spite of normal fundi and often normal acuity of vision, the patients fail to recognize printed or written words. The auditory memory of words is unimpaired, and generally numerals and music can be read. Hence the patients learn well orally and are good at arithmetic. They are often quite intelligent and may be wrongly punished for inattention and stupidity. The defect is not necessarily complete, and much improvement can be obtained by careful individual tuition and perseverance. As an acquired condition (*aphasia*) it is commonly found after a cerebrovascular accident.

Malingering

Cases occasionally occur of people who hope to gain some advantage by pretending to be visually defective. It is rare for complete blindness to be assumed, and such cases can only be detected by constant watching of the person's behaviour. When one eye is said to be blind, in spite of absence of sufficient objective evidence to account for the condition, the demonstration of malingering resolves itself into a contest of wits between the surgeon and the individual. Many tests have been devised, and several should be employed in each case.

1. A low concave or convex glass (0.25 D) is placed before the 'blind' eye, and a high convex (+10 D) before the 'good' eye, and the examinee is told to read the distant types. If he succeeds malingering is proved.

2. A prism is placed base downwards before the 'good' eye and the examinee is told to look at a light. If he admits to seeing two lights malingering is proved.

3. The surgeon stands behind the patient and covers the 'blind' eye with his hand, at the same time holding a prism of 10 degrees base down before the 'good' eye in such a manner that the edge of the prism passes horizontally across the centre of the pupil; uniocular diplopia results. The surgeon then simultaneously removes his hand from the 'blind' eye and shifts the prism upwards so that the whole pupil is covered by it. If the examinee still admits to seeing two lights malingering is proved.

4. While the examinee looks at a light a prism of 10 degrees is placed base outwards before the 'blind' eye. If the eye moves inwards in order to eliminate diplopia it is not blind.

5. Snellen's coloured types may be employed. The letters are printed in green and red. If a red glass is placed before the 'good' eye, and the patient reads all the letters, the other eye is not blind, for the eye looking through the red glass can only see the red letters. Care must be taken in this test that the red glass cuts off all the rays from the green letters as tested by the surgeon's own vision.

25

Intra-ocular tumours

Intra-ocular tumours are rare, but of great importance, since they are usually malignant and endanger the life of the patient.

Tumours of the uveal tract
The common primary malignant tumour of the uveal tract is derived from the sheaths of Schwann and is thus ectodermal; it is best, therefore, to refer to these tumours as *malignant melanomata*.

Tumours of the iris
It is not uncommon to see irides with dark brown spots (melanomata), due to congenital aggregations of pigment cells. As a rule these are benign *nævi*, but occasionally they take on malignant proliferation. Any increase of size must be watched with suspicion.

Malignant melanoma is the only neoplasm of importance met with in the iris but is rare. Composed of pigmented or unpigmented spindle-shaped or round cells, it occurs as an isolated nodule which grows rapidly (Fig. 25.1), and if untreated it may penetrate the corneosclera and perforate the globe. Diagnosis from a granulomatous lesion depends on the absence of inflammation and the density of pigmentation, but the occasional absence of pigmentation may give rise to difficulties.

Treatment. The growth should be watched for a short time, preferably by repeated photography and if found to increase in size should be removed by iridectomy if this is feasible. If the tumour involves the root of the iris and the ciliary body it should be removed by iridocyclectomy. If completely removed the prognosis is excellent.

Malignant melanoma of the choroid
This arises from the outer layers of this tissue. It forms at first a lens-shaped mass, raising the retina over it. As it grows tension is thrown upon the elastic membrane of Bruch, which finally ruptures; the tumour then proliferates through the opening to form a globular mass in the subretinal space, separated from the part in the choroid by a narrow 'neck'. The retina remains in contact with the tumour at the summit, but is detached from the

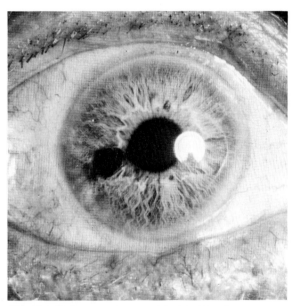

Fig. 25.1 Malignant melanoma of the iris. Note the deformation of the pupil

choroid at the sides, the intervening space being filled with exudative fluid. The growth may be in any situation, and the fluid may sink down to the lowest part of the eye, forming there a detachment isolated from that over the tumour, but with continuing growth the retina becomes more and more detached, until no part remains *in situ*; the nutrition of the lens then suffers, so that it becomes opaque. The tumour may fill the globe before perforating the sclera, or this may occur relatively early along the perivascular spaces of the vortex veins or ciliary vessels. The orbital tissues then become infiltrated. The lymph nodes are not affected, but metastases occur abundantly in the liver and elsewhere.

The growth is usually pigmented but is occasionally unpigmented, a distinction which is relatively unimportant; metastases from melanotic growths are often unpigmented. The pigment is chiefly melanin, but hæmatogenous pigmentation occurs after haemorrhages. The cells are usually spindle-shaped; they may be cylindrical or palisade-like, arranged in columns or around blood vessels, or even endothelial in appearance; most tumours are mixed-celled. Silver staining reveals a variable amount of argyrophil 'reticulin' fibres, generally more numerous in spindle-celled sarcomata. There is evidence that those with the most reticulin are the least malignant.

Flat malignant melanoma of the choroid. In rare cases the choroid becomes widely infiltrated so that a uniform thickening results, with a shallow 'detachment' of the retina.

The *clinical course* of malignant melanoma of the choroid is commonly divided into four stages: (1) the quiescent stage; (2) the glaucomatous stage: (3) the stage of extra-ocular extension; (4) the stage of metastasis. This is probably the typical chronological order of events, but secondary glaucoma may arise sometimes acutely, at an early stage or be delayed until after extra-ocular extension has taken place, and metastases may occur at any stage.

The cause of the glaucoma is obscure: in some cases it is due to the lens and iris being forced forwards, so that the angle of the anterior chamber becomes blocked and a sudden rise in tension is precipitated or it may be infiltrated with neoplastic cells. In other cases, particularly those of early onset, obstruction to the venous outflow from the eye is a possible explanation, the tumour being in some instances so situated as to press upon a vortex vein.

The tumour usually occurs in adults between 40 and 60. It is always primary, single, and unilateral. The earliest patients to seek advice are those in whom the tumour is near the macula, since vision is then most strikingly affected. In the periphery the tumour has usually attained a considerable size, and the patient may apply for treatment for relief of the pain of glaucoma.

It is of the utmost importance that the cause of the detachment of the retina should be diagnosed in these cases. If the tension is raised, a growth may be diagnosed almost with certainty. A simple detachment shows numerous more or less parallel folds, and undulations can be seen to travel over the surface when the eye moves. The detachment at the summit of a tumour is usually rounded and fixed, though in the surrounding parts it may show all the signs of a 'simple' detachment. Patches of pigment upon the rounded part support the diagnosis of a tumour, but pigmentary disturbance, more particularly at the periphery, is not uncommon in simple detachment. A simple detachment of the non-exudative type probably always has a hole or tear in the retina somewhere; if it can be found it is the most positive evidence that a growth is probably not present. Rarely a system of blood vessels having an entirely different mode of distribution from the retinal vessels can be made out between the latter; this is the most positive

evidence of a growth, but it is only occasionally seen. A very small, round detachment in the macular region or upper part of the globe is almost certain to be due to a tumour of the choroid. If the detachment is anterior, transillumination (p. 78) will afford assistance in diagnosis; a simple detachment is transparent, a choroidal growth opaque.

Diagnosis may be extremely difficult if the patient is first seen when glaucoma has already supervened. Dependence must then be placed largely upon the history. Defective vision may have been noticed months previously, and deteriorated without remissions. One eye only is involved; the other may be normal, or at least not of the glaucomatous type with a narrow angle, and the field of vision in this eye will show no typical glaucomatous defects. The affected eye will probably have no perception of light. Ultrasonography (B-scan) is a valuable investigation when the media are opaque.

Radio-active tracers. Neoplastic tissue has an increased rate of phosphate uptake and retains the isotope longer than non-neoplastic tissue. P32 emits beta-rays and is relatively safe because 20% of the dose administered is excreted in the first 24 h. The range of beta rays is small, averaging 2–3 mm with a maximum of 7–8 mm and this restriction makes the technique of the measurement of P32 uptake difficult. A solid state detector is capable of distinguishing clearly between the majority of benign and malignant intraocular lesions. Most malignant tumours show uptakes in excess of 80% of controlled values, a level which is not reached by benign tumours. The P32 uptake should be read 48 hours after the administration of the isotope.

In the diagnosis, two rare simple tumours must be kept in mind, particularly in the early stages. A *choroidal nævus* appears as a bluish patch with somewhat feathered edges, usually about the size of the optic disc and situated near the posterior pole of the eye. It is congenital and symptomless but, like nævi elsewhere, may occasionally assume malignant characteristics.

A *cavernous haemangioma* of the choroid, another rare tumour of congenital origin and of exceedingly slow growth, is also usually situated near the disc. It has a greyish hue and indefinite margins and often causes a retinal detachment.

Brawny scleritis may be difficult to differentiate from a malignant melanoma of the choroid if localised posteriorly.

Angiography in the diagnosis of choroidal malignant melanomata

There are no absolute criteria for angiographic differentiation of malignant melanomata from other choroidal lesions. However the angiographic picture taken in conjunction with the clinical examination may provide sufficient evidence for a correct diagnosis.

The fluorescence of lesions in the differential diagnosis depends on the same histopathological features but each of them may have certain distinguishing features.

1. Choroidal hæmangiomata: the vascular channels within these tumours fluoresce before the surrounding chorio-capillaris. This phenomenon may be masked by overlying pathology in the retina.

2. Naevi of the choroid obscure choroidal fluorescence and are associated with drusen and absence of late staining.

3. Metastatic tumours tend to produce poor fluorescence in the early phase but are probably indistinguishable from malignant melanomata in the late phase.

4. Disciform degenerations usually have a confluent intense late phase fluorescence.

5. Choroidal hæmartomata are non-fluorescent.

6. Retinal cysts are non-fluorescent.

Treatment. Evidence is accummulating to suggest that the trauma of enucleation leads to vascular spread of the tumour by embolization. Thus deaths from secondaries are rare before surgery and their incidence rises dramatically in the period immediately following surgery. While the patient can see well with the affected eye and there is no evidence of scleral involvement conservative management is therefore recommended.

The occasional long interval between enucleation of the involved eye and the appearance of secondaries elsewhere suggests an immunological mechanism at work. Furthermore spontaneous necrosis is a prominent feature of some choroidal melanomata associated with lymphocytic infiltration. If the growth has already burst through the globe, the orbit should be exenterated and, in addition, irradiated with X-rays or radium. When the tumour is small and the affected eye is the only seeing eye, destruction by light-coagulation or suturing cobalt discs to the sclera over the site of the neoplasm may be considered.

The disease is invariably fatal, usually within five years, if not eradicated by operation, but metastases may be delayed for 10 years or more. Prognosis is fair if the tumour is small (under 10 mm in size) and entirely intra-ocular especially if it contains much reticulin.

Malignant melanoma of the ciliary body

This is fundamentally of the same nature and gives rise to the same symptoms as the corresponding neoplasm of the choroid, the differences being only those dependent upon the anatomical disposition of the parts (Fig. 25.2). Thus the retina, being here more adherent to the underlying uvea and being reduced to a double layer of epithelial cells, is not detached until the growth has spread to the choroid. The tumour may attain a considerable size before it causes symptoms, which are then referable to displacement or distortion of the lens and interference with the ciliary muscle. The ciliary circulation is impeded, and conspicuous dilatation of one or two anterior perforating ciliary vessels should always arouse suspicion. The growth may invade the angle of the anterior chamber when it then has the appearance of an iridodialysis, a dark crescent showing at the root of the iris; that it is not an iridodialysis is shown by the fact that no reflex can be obtained through it on illuminating with the ophthalmoscope and from the absence of a history of a blow. In an unpigmented tumour the crescent may be yellowish, but vessels will usually be visible upon the surface and these render the diagnosis easy. The growth may be visible by oblique illumination with a widely dilated pupil and by gonioscopy, and is opaque to transillumination. Occasionally it takes on a *ring* or

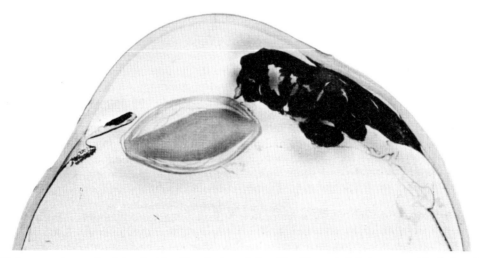

Fig. 25.2 Malignant melanoma involving the iris, ciliary body, and choroid, with a metastatic tumour on iris of other side. (By courtesy of Doherty.)

annular distribution, extensively infiltrating the ciliary region.

Malignant melanoma of the ciliary body is less common than that of the choroid; the treatment and prognosis are the same.

Epithelial hyperplasia of the ciliary processes is not uncommon in old eyes. Rarely *malignant epitheliomata* occur; also growths resembling embryonic retina (*diktyoma*). They cause the same clinical signs as malignant melanoma.

Secondary carcinoma of the choroid

This occurs as a metastatic growth in cases of cancer, particularly of the breast and alimentary tract. There is obscuration of vision, and ophthalmoscopic examination reveals a widespread shallow elevation of the retina, usually at the posterior pole. The disease is nearly always bilateral, and as it is usually only one of many metastatic deposits and the patient is generally in the stage of general carcinomatosis, excision of the eye is not usually indicated. These metastases, however, are radiosensitive and treatment by radiation will often effect sufficient improvement to maintain some vision and prevent the occurrence of pain until death supervenes. They may be hormone dependent and respond to ovarectomy or cytotoxic drugs.

Reticulum cell sarcoma

The malignant cell of reticulum cell sarcoma resembles a histiocyte. It originates usually within the reticuloendothelial system, but less commonly in the central nervous system where the neoplasm is referred to as a microglioma. When a reticulum cell sarcoma affects the eye it may do so as a primary ocular affection. When it is associated with a similar lesion elsewhere, the site is usually the CNS.

Patients are typically in their sixth or seventh decade at the time of presentation. They complain of decreased visual acuity with floaters or photopsia. The principal finding is vitreous involvement with 'inflammatory' cells which are refractory to topical steroid therapy. There may be a mild anterior segment reaction resembling a non-granulomatous iritis with or without keratic precipitates.

In some cases fundus lesions resemble retinal or subretinal infiltrates. The lesions are patchy with yellow-white fluffy outlines and quickly become confluent. If the macula is affected diminished visual acuity rapidly results. The vitreous may be so involved as to obscure retinal details.

Vitrectomy may provide the only available source for tissue diagnosis in ocular reticulum cell sarcoma. The tumour cells are large and pleomorphic with scant cytoplasm and prominent nuclear membranes. Nuclei are round or oval, occasionally multiple and with frequent mitoses, clumped chromatin and prominent nucleoli.

The differential diagnosis is from leukaemic infiltrates, retinitis secondary to bacterial or fungal sepsis, toxoplasmosis and cytomegalovirus infection.

The diagnosis is of some importance because radiation therapy has proved efficacious in affected eyes leading to permanent improvement in visual acuity.

Tumours of the retina

Retinoblastoma

Retinoblastoma used to be commonly known as 'glioma' retinae; malignant proliferations of neuroglia such as occur in the brain and optic nerve, are very rare in the retina. The usual malignant growth of the retina is due to proliferation of neural cells which have failed to evolve normally, and is better termed retinoblastoma.

The tumour is confined to infants and is probably always congenital, although it may remain quiescent or pass unnoticed until the fifth or sixth year or even later. The disease is rare; the second eye is affected, independently and not by metastasis or continuity *via* the chiasma, in about one-fourth of the cases, but frequently the growth cannot be recognised even on careful examination until after months or even years. Several children of the same family are sometimes affected as it presents dominant inheritance with variable gene penetrance.

The child is brought to the surgeon on account of a peculiar yellow reflex from the pupil, sometimes called 'amaurotic cat's eye'. If left untreated retinoblastoma runs through the same stages as melanoma of the choroid: (1) the quiescent stage, lasting from six months to a year; (2) the glaucomatous stage; (3) the stage of extraocular extension; (4) the stage of metastasis. The second stage results in enlargement of the globe, with apparent or real proptosis. Pain is severe during this stage, but is relieved when the tumour bursts through the sclera, an event which usually occurs at the limbus and is followed by rapid fungation. Metastasis first occurs in the preauricular and neighbouring lymph nodes, later in the cranial and other bones. Direct extension by continuity to the optic nerve (which is early affected) and brain is more common, and metastases in other organs, usually the liver, are relatively rare.

The growth consists chiefly of small round cells with large nuclei resembling the cells of the nuclear layers of the retina; many of these stain badly, showing that they are undergoing necrosis (Fig. 25.3). Among them may be found rosette-like formations of cells resembling the rods and cones.

Retinoblastoma is invariably multiple. When noticed very early, as may occur in the second eye, a larger mass is seen surrounded by numerous punctate satellites. Microscopically, minute deposits are seen scattered in various situations throughout the globe. It may grow

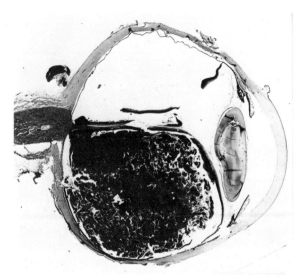

Fig. 25.3 Exophytic retinoblastoma. The neoplasm is entirely external to the detached retina. (By courtesy of Wolter.)

principally outwards, separating the retina from the choroid ('*glioma exophytum*'), or inwards towards the vitreous ('*glioma endophytum*'); between the two there is no fundamental distinction, but the ophthalmoscopic appearances differ. In the former the condition resembles a detachment of the retina; in the latter polypoid masses, sometimes with hæmorrhages on the surface, may be seen spreading into the vitreous. Hypopyon with esotropia is sometimes the presenting clinical picture.

Several conditions occurring in children may give rise to similar signs, and cause great difficulty in diagnosis. These have been grouped together under the term '*pseudo-glioma.*' The chief are: (1) inflammatory deposits in the vitreous, with or without detachment of the retina following a plastic cyclitis or choroiditis; (2) tuberculosis of the choroid, especially the confluent type; (3) toxocara infestation; (4) congenital defects, due to persistent hyperplastic vitreous at the back of the lens; and (5) retrolental fibroplasia. In all cases atropine should be instilled and both eyes should be thoroughly examined ophthalmoscopically, under general anæthesia if necessary. The tension may then be satisfactorily tested and may afford useful information which cannot be obtained without an anæsthetic. Raised tension is in favour of

retinoblastoma, lowered of pseudo-glioma. Even when every precaution is taken, in some cases it is impossible to be certain of the diagnosis; considering that the life of the patient is at stake and that the eye is in any case useless as an organ of sight, these should be treated as malignant. Lactic dehydrogenase activity if raised in the aqueous relative to the serum level is suggestive of retinoblastoma. Calcification occurs in 75% of cases and is pathognomonic of retinoblastoma.

Treatment. The treatment of large tumours is excision of the eye. The optic nerve should be cut long, and the cut end invariably submitted to microscopical examination. If there is any doubt of extension of the disease to the conjunctiva or orbital tissues exenteration of the orbit is indicated. When the diagnosis is doubtful the eye should be removed, for in inflammatory pseudo-glioma the eye is destined to shrink and become unsightly.

In treatment by radiation the sources used are, radio-active cobalt discs stitched to the sclera over the site of the nodule; the object is to deliver a dose of 4000 r to the summit of the tumour in one week. Late sequelæ of irradiation are thin greyish exudates at the macula appearing eighteen months after treatment, and posterior cortical lens opacities becoming evident after a period varying from nine months to eight years. Alternatively, X-rays may be used with an apparatus to confine the radiation to the posterior segment of the globe and thus avoid damage to the lens.

The prognosis of retinoblastoma, if untreated, is always bad; the patient invariably dies. The prognosis is fair if the eye is removed before extra-ocular extension has occurred. In the absence of disease of the second eye the patient may be regarded as out of danger if there is no recurrence in the orbit within three years, but the remaining eye should be carefully examined under atropine at frequent intervals for a much longer period. There are several cases on record of survival after removal of both eyes. Owing to its familial tendency the eyes of subsequent siblings or descendants should be carefully watched during infancy and childhood.

Spontaneous regression of retinoblastomata due to massive necrosis followed by calcification has been reported many times. Evidence is accumulating to suggest an immunological mechanism at work in some patients.

26

Injuries to the eye

The eye is protected from direct injury by the lids and the projecting margins of the orbit. Nevertheless, it is not exempt from foreign bodies, the action of caustics, contusions and wounds.

Extra-ocular foreign bodies

Foreign bodies

Foreign bodies which are usually small — particles of coal dust, emery, steel, etc. — may pitch upon the conjunctiva or upon the cornea. In the former case they cause sudden discomfort and reflex blinking. The foreign body sticks to the palpebral conjunctiva and is liable to be dragged across the cornea, which it excoriates. It may be washed by tears towards the inner canthus, and so into the nasal duct; more frequently it becomes lodged at about the middle of the upper sulcus subtarsalis where it is most likely to irritate the cornea, or in the upper fornix, or it may occasionally become embedded in the bulbar conjunctiva. Quite large foreign bodies, such as a grain of corn, may be retained for a long time in the upper fornix and give rise to much irritation and some discharge; they may be overlooked unless the upper lid is everted. They are generally embedded in a mass of granulation tissue, which may simulate the cockscomb type of tuberculosis (p. 123). The wing-cases of insects and the husks of seeds may adhere by their concave surfaces to the cornea, usually at the limbus, for several weeks.

Particles of steel and emery are very liable to fly straight onto the cornea and penetrate into the epithelium or substantia propria. Larger particles of steel, or less commonly stone, glass, etc., may perforate the globe (p. 247). When situated in the cornea they cause great pain and irritation. The pupil is often constricted. If allowed to remain they expose the cornea to the dangers of infection by organisms in the conjunctival sac with resultant ulceration which may lead to the extrusion of the foreign body in the slough. The ulcer thus formed may heal, but if virulent organisms are present a spreading ulcer, with or without hypopyon, may develop.

It is not always easy to discover a foreign body upon the cornea. In case of doubt the eye should be anæsthetised and the cornea thoroughly examined under oblique illumination with a slit-lamp. The use of fluorescein will nearly always, reveal the position. The slit-lamp is of great assistance in determining the nature and position of the foreign body, for by its use the depth of an embedded foreign body can be estimated by the length of the shadow which it casts.

Treatment. Foreign bodies must be removed as soon as possible. If lying loosely in the lower fornix they are easily removed with a clean swab or handkerchief after everting the lower lid. If not found in this position the upper lid should be everted (p. 71); the particle will generally be found in the sulcus subtarsalis and can be removed in the same manner. If it is still not seen the upper fornix should be brought into view (p. 71) and the particle removed. In case of difficulty, the previous anæsthetisation of the conjunctival sac will materially assist.

If the foreign body is embedded in the bulbar conjunctiva it should be picked out by a needle after topical anæsthesia. If a discission needle is not at hand a disposable sterile hypodermic needle may be used.

Removal of foreign bodies from the cornea is effected as follows:

The eye is anaesthetised and the patient seated in a chair. The surgeon holds the lids apart with the first and second fingers of his left hand, pressing slightly backwards so as to steady the globe. A light is focused upon the cornea, the patient being told to look in the direction which affords the best view of the particle. An attempt may first be made to remove the foreign body by touching it with a slip of clean blotting-paper which exercises a capillary attraction. If this fails a sterilised spud is used. Only if this also fails after repeated efforts should a needle be used, preferably a discission needle. The greatest care should be exercised not to scrape the epithelium more than is absolutely necessary. Emery and steel particles leave behind them a little ring of brown stain which should be scraped off if this can be done without too much trauma.

If there is any sign of ulceration or a greyish infiltration around the abrasion, and if the probability of acute (closed-angle) glaucoma can be excluded, a drop of 1%. Cyclopentolate should be instilled. In every case an antibiotic ointment should be inserted and the eye kept bandaged for a day. If ulceration occurs it is treated in the appropriate manner (p. 133). Special attention should be given to particles of stone which show a greater tendency than metal to cause ulceration, probably because metallic particles are often hot and therefore sterile when they enter the eye.

Occasionally sharp steel and other particles penetrate deeply into the cornea, without, however, perforating. The efforts made to remove them may push them in still deeper or even into the anterior chamber. When such an accident is feared, special precautions must be adopted. If the particle is magnetisable and a large magnet is available, magnetic removal should be tried (p. 250), but it is usually necessary to incise the cornea overlying the foreign body. This method may fail, particularly if the particle is small. If the foreign body escapes into the anterior chamber it must be removed by other methods (p. 251).

Fragments of aniline pencil in the eye cause much irritation and a very unsightly staining and may lead to ulceration and necrosis. The eye should be treated with glycerin drops (p. 365), since this substance is a solvent of aniline violet.

Prophylactic measures. Foreign bodies in the eye are extremely common in industrial workers, especially in grinding tools, lathe work, or hammering on a chisel with a mushroomed head. Apart from the danger to the sight of the worker, they are a source of great economic loss from expenditure of time and compensation. In addition to the banning of tools with overhanging edges, the fitting of guards on machines for grinding and other available preventive measures, such accidents could in most cases be entirely prevented by the use of goggles, but it is often impracticable to enforce this measure among workmen. Every attempt should be made by the provision of comfortable goggles and by educative means, such as 'Safety First' notices and lectures by welfare officials, to point out the dangers of failure to protect the eyes in this way.

Burns and chemical injuries

Burns by hot water or steam, hot ashes, exploding powder or molten metal, and injuries by caustics such as lime usually from fresh mortar or whitewash, or strong acids and alkalis may involve considerable damage either by injuring the cornea or by producing symblepharon. Strong ammonia is particularly harmful, causing necrosis of the cornea; acids (hydrochloric, sulphuric) much less so. Immediately after the accident there is intense conjunctivitis and chemosis, but the cornea often looks clear; in this state it is difficult to be certain of the severity of the injury. A drop of fluorescein solution will reveal the extent of the area denuded of epithelium. Prognosis should therefore be guarded, care being taken to impress upon the patient the gravity of the injury and the necessity of supervision. In the worst cases the cornea is dull or opaque. In the succeeding days an eschar forms and is thrown off; this is followed by granulation of the injured conjunctiva and frequently by ulceration of the cornea. The corneal condition should be treated as an ulcer (p. 133). In severe lime burns the whole cornea may be destroyed; perforation takes place, and the eye shrinks. In less severe cases a dense leucoma forms, porcelain-like in lime burns, and sight is lost. The chief danger derived from the condition of the conjunctiva is that of adhesion of the lid to the globe. It is most likely to occur with the lower lid where the lower fornix is obliterated by organisation of the granulation tissue. The symblepharon thus produced impedes the movements of the globe and may even interfere with its nutrition. Every precaution must be adopted to prevent its occurrence.

Treatment. In injury by caustics the excess of deleterious material must be removed at the earliest possible moment. Acids may be neutralised by dilute alkalis (lotio sodii bicarbonatis, 3%) and alkalis by weak acids (lotio acidi borici) or milk. In no case, however, should there be any delay in obtaining these solutions and if they are not immediately at hand, the eye should be copiously irrigated at once with water. Particles of lime must be perseveringly picked out with forceps, after the previous instillation of amethocaine: irrigation with 10% neutral ammonium tartrate or preferably a solution of the sodium salt of ethylene-diamine tetra-acetic acid (Appendix p. 369) diminishes scarring in lime burns. An antibiotic ointment should be instilled. A potent agent in reducing the inflammatory reaction and preventing the excess of granulation tissue which determines the development of symblepharon, is a corticosteroid applied topically as drops or ointment (Chap. 14).

Symblepharon may occasionally be prevented by sweeping a glass rod well coated with a lubricant round the upper and lower fornices, so that they are well packed with ointment, a procedure which should be repeated several times each day according to the severity of the case. The fitting of a contact lens separates the two mucosal surfaces and prevents their adhesion.

Poison gases

Poison gases used in warfare include lacrimatory gases, phosgene, mustard gas, arsenicals, and other agents.

The *treatment* of conjunctivitis caused by lacrimatory gases is irrigation with bland lotions — normal saline or sodium bicarbonate (3%). The eyes should not be bandaged, but dark glasses used.

Arsenical vesicants are neutralised by the local application of BAL ointment (British Anti-lewisite) which, however, is only effective if it is applied within a few minutes of the injury.

Contusions

Injuries by blunt instruments vary in severity from a simple corneal abrasion to rupture of the globe. A great number of lesions may result; indeed, every part of the eye may be so injured by a contusion as seriously to diminish vision. Moreover, in some cases the changes are delayed or progressive so that *in all cases a guarded prognosis should be given.*

As a general rule either the anterior segment of the eye in front of the iris-lens diaphragm, or the posterior half, is preferentially affected. The mechanism is as follows. When a force impinges upon the cornea this tissue is thrust inwards and may even be forced against the lens and iris; the wave of aqueous pushes these structures backwards and as the compression wave rebounds from the back of the eye, they are thrust forwards again. In this way they may be severely traumatised; and at the same time the wave of pressure, striking the retina and choroid as well as the angle of the anterior chamber, may do considerable damage. Delayed complications such as secondary glaucoma, hæmophthalmitis or traumatic iridocyclitis may follow.

The various conditions resulting therefrom will now be briefly enumerated.

The cornea

The cornea may suffer an abrasion, deep opacities may develop, or partial or complete rupture may occur.

A simple *abrasion* may be caused. It is recognised by distortion of the corneal reflex and by the use of fluorescein (p. 72).

Recurrent erosion (recurrent traumatic keratalgia). This may occur spontaneously but is particularly liable to happen after scratches especially with babies' finger-nails; in many cases, however, it is indicative of a degenerative condition of the cornea. The abrasion, however produced, usually heals quickly, but is followed some days, weeks, or even months later, by acute pain and lacrimation, generally on first opening the eyes in the morning. If the cornea is then stained with fluorescein an abrasion will be found, usually at the original site but sometimes elsewhere, or there may be one or a group of vesicles. The attack rapidly passes off with appropriate treatment, but often recurs again and again, particularly on awakening in the morning. There is no doubt that in these cases the epithelium is abnormally loosely attached to Bowman's membrane, and is liable to be torn off by the lid on waking. Early attacks should be treated in the same manner as a simple abrasion, but if the attacks are repeated debridement is indicated where-by the epithelium which is loose is removed and the eye padded for 48 h so that firm healing is established.

A *deep opacity* in the substance of the cornea may result from a contusion, usually in the form of delicate grey striæ interlacing in different directions, due to œdema of the corneal stroma or occasionally to wrinkling of Descemet's membrane (p .146). It generally clears up without leaving a permanent opacity. There may be ruptures in Descemet's membrane followed by acute oedema of the stroma.

Blood-staining of the cornea. This occasionally results from a contusion which has caused haemorrhage into the anterior chamber usually accompanied by a rise of tension of the eye and endothelial damage. The whole cornea is at first stained, the colour varying according to the duration of the condition. It may be reddish-brown, or greenish; in the latter case the condition simulates dislocation of the clear lens into the anterior chamber (p. 246). The cornea gradually and very slowly clears from the periphery towards the centre, the whole process taking two years or more. Microscopically there are myriads of minute, highly refractile rods packed in the lamellæ of the stroma, and sometimes round granules of pigment in the corneal corpuscles. These are derivatives of hæmoglobin which may or may not contain iron and are removed by phagocytic action — a slow process. In the absence of other causes of defective vision, sight may eventually be completely restored but is usually permanently impaired.

Sclera

Rupture of the globe. This is generally due to its being suddenly and violently forced against the orbital walls. It is often caused by a fall upon some projecting object, such as a knob or a key in a door. The force usually comes from the direction down and out, where the eyeball is least protected by the orbital margin and the globe is pushed against the pulley of the superior oblique muscle; the sclera gives way up and in at its weakest part, in the neighbourhood of the canal of Schlemm. The wound runs obliquely from the canal outwards and backwards through the sclera to appear more or less concentric with the corneal margin and about 3 mm behind it. The conjunctiva is often intact, but there are always severe injuries to other parts of the eye. The iris is generally prolapsed or torn away (iridodialysis) or retroflexed (*vide infra*). The lens may be expelled from the eye or escape under the conjunctiva (subconjunctival dislocation of the lens) or be forced back into the vitreous, in which case the anterior chamber becomes deep. Intra-ocular bleeding may be profuse, filling the anterior chamber and vitreous, and the condition may be complicated by a detachment of the retina with or without subretinal or subchoroidal haemorrhage. Ultimately, the eye usually shrinks and is lost.

Treatment. The eye must be carefully examined, using lid retractors, under an anæsthetic if necessary. In severe cases nothing remains but to excise the collapsed globe. In less severe cases without extrusion of the intra-ocular contents, the wound should be sutured, atropine instilled and the patient kept in bed.

In subconjunctival dislocation of the lens there is always escape of vitreous. Attempts should be made to remove the vitreous by a vitrector and close the wound so that it is free of vitreous strands.

The iris and ciliary body

This may suffer functional defects or may be actually torn.

A *traumatic miosis* due to irritation of the nerves occurs initially in every severe contusion.

In *traumatic mydriasis* following a contusion, the pupil is large and immobile and usually remains moderately dilated permanently.

The substance of the iris is often torn. The most common lesions are minute *ruptures in the pupillary margin* which are of little significance; *radiating lacerations* of the iris, sometimes extending to the ciliary margin, are rare. *Iridodialysis*, wherein the iris is torn away from its ciliary attachment for a variable distance, occurs more frequently (Fig. 26.1). A black biconvex area is seen at the periphery, and the pupillary edge bulges slightly inwards. With the ophthalmoscopic mirror a reflex can be obtained through the peripheral gap, and the fibres of the suspensory ligament and the edge of the lens may be visible. Uniocular diplopia may be produced by this injury. In extensive iridodialysis the detached portion of the iris may be completely rotated so that the pigmented back of the iris faces forwards (*anti-flexion of the iris*). The iris becomes re-attached only in exceptional cases, but, apart from other injury, the lesion rarely causes se-

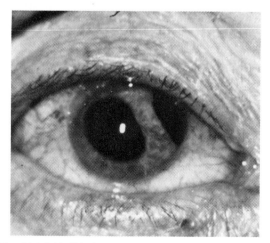

Fig. 26.1 Iridodialysis

rious results. In *traumatic aniridia* or *irideremia* the iris is completely torn away from its ciliary attachment, contracts into a minute ball, and sinks to the bottom of the anterior chamber, where it may be invisible. Rarely the same appearance is caused by *total inversion* or *retroflexion* of the iris, the whole iris being doubled back into the ciliary region out of sight. More commonly inversion is partial so that the appearance of a coloboma (*q.v.*) is obtained, but the fibres of the suspensory ligament cannot be seen. The ciliary body may also be torn or ruptured near its anterior attachment resulting in its subsequent retraction with a deepened anterior chamber and a tendency to glaucoma. Histologically there are longitudinal tears in the face of the ciliary body which split the circular from the radial fibres and result in angle recession. In all these cases there is usually a hyphaema and other injuries may be present.

The *treatment* consists of rest. Atropine should be instilled in iridodialysis, but not in ruptures of the iris or if the lens is subluxated. When the eye has settled, if the iridodialysis is gross and causes symptoms such as diplopia, the torn peripheral edge of the iris may be anchored with a silk suture into a scleral incision just behind the limbus.

The lens

The lens may show cataractous changes or be dislocated. In some cases a circular ring of faint or stippled opacity is seen on the anterior surface of the lens due to multitudes of brown amorphous granules of pigment lying on the capsule (*Vossius's ring*). It usually has about the same diameter as the contracted pupil, and is due to the impress of the iris on the lens, produced by the force of the blow driving the cornea and iris backwards. Minute discrete subcapsular opacities may be seen after resorption of the pigment.

Concussion cataract. This may assume many varied forms. It is due partly to the mechanical effects of the injury on the lens fibres and largely to the entrance of aqueous due to damage to the capsule, either impairment of its semi-permeability or often the result of actual tears which, particularly if they are small and peripheral, may not be clinically visible. They frequently occur at the thin portion of the capsule covering the posterior pole of the lens. Sometimes, especially if they are covered by the iris, such tears are rapidly sealed, at first with fibrin and later by the proliferation of the subcapsular epithelium which secretes a new capsule; in these cases the entrance of aqueous is stopped and the opacity in the lens may remain stationary or even regress. Alternatively, the tear may remain open and opacification progress to involve the entire lens.

The most typical appearance is that of a *rosette-shaped cataract*, usually in the posterior cortex, sometimes in the anterior or both. In this condition an accumulation of fluid marks out the architectural arrangement of the lens (p. 11). The star-shaped cortical sutures are therefore delineated and from them radiate feathery lines of opacities outlining the lens fibres. Occasionally the rosette disappears; sometimes it remains stationary and sometimes it progresses to total opacification of the lens, a complication which may appear rapidly within a few hours after the injury or may be delayed for many months.

A *late rosette-shaped cataract* may develop in the posterior cortex one or two years after a concussion. It is smaller and more compact than the early type and its sutural extensions are short.

The treatment of such cataracts is on general lines (p. 260) but, unless the rapid intumescence of the lens leads to a secondary glaucoma which may then require immediate measures for its relief (p. 178), any surgical interference should be delayed for some months until the final outcome is apparent. If possible, the eye should be left until all signs of inflammation have subsided, where-after it should be treated as indicated for unilateral cataract (p. 178).

Dislocation of the lens. This may occur when the relatively fragile suspensory ligament is torn by the to-and-fro wave of pressure set up by the contusion. If the tear is partial the lens may be *subluxated* so that it is displaced laterally and sometimes slightly rotated. This leads to a variation in the depth of the anterior chamber which is deeper in the part unsupported by the lens. With the pupil dilated, the edge of the lens may be seen as a grey convex line by oblique illumination, but more readily and unmistakably as a black line with the ophthalmoscope (p. 84). The lack of support to the iris causes tremulousness when the eye is moved.

If the rupture to the suspensory ligament is complete the lens is *dislocated*, usually into the vitreous. Sometimes it remains clear and can be seen only with difficulty; at other times it turns opaque and appears as a yellow mass. Alternatively, particularly if the blow has been slanting, the lens is dislocated into the anterior chamber, an accident which may follow a trivial injury if the lens is shrunken. A clear lens in the anterior chamber is not always easily recognised, but it does not long remain clear and diagnosis is then easy. It is more globular than normal owing to its freedom from the restraint of the suspensory ligament. When still clear it looks like a globule of oil in the anterior chamber. With oblique illumination it has a golden rim, due to total reflection of the light; this is the exact opposite of the total reflection when the edge of the lens is seen with the ophthalmoscope, the light being then totally reflected away from the observer's eye. The lens in the anterior chamber causes spasm of the sphincter pupillæ, which may occur at the moment when it is passing through the pupil. An iridocyclitis or an intractable secondary glaucoma is then set up so that the eye is usually lost if the anteriorly dislocated lens is allowed to remain.

Dislocation of the lens always causes a considerable disturbance of vision. In subluxation there is astigmatism which is much increased by tilting of the lens. The slackening of the suspensory ligament causes increased curvature and myopia which, however, may be more than compensated by backward displacement.

If the lens is displaced so much laterally that the edge crosses the pupil, uniocular diplopia is present. Through the aphakic area of the pupil the eye is highly hypermetropic, through the phakic portion it may be myopic, in addition to which the periphery of the lens acts as a prism. Ophthalmoscopic examination by the indirect method in these conditions shows two images of the disc differing considerably in size, and by the direct method the fundus may be observed through the phakic or through the aphakic portion of the pupil. In total dislocation into the vitreous the effect is that of the old cataract operation of couching; the pupillary area is aphakic and the refraction is highly hypermetropic, requiring cataract spectacles for its correction. In these cases the vision may be retained for many years.

Treatment. In dislocation forwards the lens should be extracted by a cryoprobe combined with vitrectomy. Vision may be improved by suitable glasses in cases of total luxation into the vitreous and subluxation. In the latter case it is usually impossible to correct the astigmatism so that a correction for the aphakic part of the pupil may give better visual results. A dislocated lens into the vitreous should be left there. If the capsule leaks phakolytic glaucoma will supervene and this may demand its extraction.

The vitreous

The vitreous is usually disorganised to some extent by detachment either anterior or posterior or by a combination of both. The most common occurrence is the appearance of clouds of fine *pigmentary opacities*, the vitreous frame-work when examined with the slit-lamp being bespangled with innumerable golden-brown dots derived from the uvea (p. 181).

Haemorrhage into the vitreous is also common. The whole vitreous chamber may be filled with blood so that no reflex will be obtained with the ophthalmoscope, but with oblique illumination a dull red hue may be seen, especially if the pupil is dilated (p. 183).

The choroid

The choroid may be torn or haemorrhages may occur.

Rupture of the choroid. This follows a severe contusion by a blunt body striking the front of the eye. Immediately after the injury the view is obscured by extravasation of blood. When it has become absorbed the rupture, usually not far from the disc, concentric with it and on its temporal side, is seen as a curved white streak over which the retinal vessels pass and which rapidly becomes pigmented along its edge (Plate 5, Fig. C); the white appearance is due to the sclera shining through. Sometimes multiple ruptures occur more or less concentric with each other. If the choroid is ruptured near the macula, loss of central vision results, but simple ruptures of the choroid in which the macula is not involved cause little impairment of vision. The treatment consists of the instillation of atropine and rest in the upright position with head erect until the extravasated blood is absorbed.

A contusion may cause a *choroidal haemorrhage.*

The retina

The retina may suffer oedematous changes, be torn, or degenerative changes or hæmorrhages may occur.

Commotio retinae (Berlin's oedema). This is a common result of a blow on the eye. A milky-white cloudiness due to oedema appears over a considerable area at the posterior pole. Sometimes it disappears after some days when vision is usually restored. In other cases, although vision may be good at first, central vision gradually diminishes, the loss of function being associated with the development of pigmentary deposits at the macula.

Traumatic macular degeneration. This may often appear slight and the fine pigmentary changes are easily overlooked immediately after the accident. The pigmentation, however, which mainly aggregates at the fovea, has a tendency to increase progressively and has a serious and permanent effect on central vision. Alternatively, the oedematous changes may lead to the formation of cystic changes at the macula, and on the rupture of a cyst a *macular hole* may be formed. Either appears clinically as a round or oval, deeply red patch just as if a hole has been punched out. In cystic formation some central vision may remain; in the case of a hole central vision is lost.

Tears in the retina. These may follow a contusion, particularly in the peripheral region in eyes already suffering from myopic or senile degeneration. It has already been pointed out that these are frequently the precursors of *retinal detachments (q.v.).*

Occasionally, particularly in the concussion injuries associated with gunshot wounds, a rupture of the retina is associated with a similar rupture of the choroid. Such cases present a characteristic picture of *traumatic proliferating chorioretinopathy* secondary to haemorrhage into the vitreous, leading to traction bands.

Prognosis should be guarded in *all* cases of serious blows upon the eye.

Optic nerve

The optic nerve is not infrequently injured in fractures of the base of the skull (p. 350). Injuries by sticks, knives or other penetrating instruments are rare. Avulsion of the optic nerve is very rare in civilian life but occurs in gunshot wounds of the orbit (p. 340).

The tension

This may be seriously disturbed following concussion injuries, particularly if they are severe. A condition of *hypotony* or, alternatively, of *traumatic glaucoma* may supervene. Angle-recession is associated with traumatic effects on the outflow channels leading to an insidious glaucoma resembling glaucoma simplex in its course Ghost-cell obstruction of the trabeculae may also induce a secondary glaucoma. Such a glaucoma may be controlled by miotics, but sometimes, particularly when complicated by haemorrhages, it is intractable even to operative treatment so that the permanent visual loss may be profound or complete.

A violent and intractable *post-traumatic iridocyclitis* is not uncommon.

Perforating injuries

Perforating injuries caused by sharp instruments or foreign bodies are all potentially serious and should be treated as emergencies. Their seriousness arises from four causes.

1. The *immediate trauma.* This will be considered in the following sections.

2. The introduction of *infection.* Occasionally in a corneal wound caused by a dirty implement, pyogenic organisms are carried into the eye, multiply there and cause rapid necrosis of the whole cornea. In these cases a ring of deep infiltration appears 2 or 3 mm internal to and concentric with the corneo-scleral margin — so-called *ring abscess.* If the organism is the *Ps. aeruginosa* (an anaerobic gram-negative rod), there is much chemosis of the conjunctiva sometimes with a greenish discharge. Enzymes released by the organism cause liquifaction of the cornea. Usually panophthalmitis is set up and the whole of the central part of the cornea is cast off. The only chance of saving such an eye is by a paracentesis directly the infiltration is observed and the institution of intensive treatment with polymyxin B and gentisin (p. 158).

If it finds access into the anterior chamber, pyogenic infection leads to a purulent iridocyclitis with hypopyon (p. 152) and usually panophthalmitis (p. 157).

Two special infections should be noted. *Gas-forming organisms,* such as *Cl. welchii,* are occasional contaminants. They excite a virulent panophthalmitis with a brownish discharge and gas bubbles in the anterior chamber. Although they are sensitive to penicillin destruction of vision has always followed. *Tetanus* is a rare complication; if this infection is introduced into the eye, the localised cephalic type of tetanus often results. Whenever such a complication may be suspected, as in agricultural or road accidents, if the patient is not already immunised, prophylactic treatment should be instituted.

3. *Post-traumatic iridocyclitis* is a common sequel to a perforating wound.

4. *Sympathetic ophthalmitis*, one of the most dreaded complications of perforating wounds, will be discussed subsequently (p. 252).

Wounds of the conjunctiva

Wounds of the conjunctiva are common and should be stitched.

Wounds of the cornea

These may be linear or lacerated. The margins swell up soon after the accident and become cloudy through imbibition of fluid thus facilitating closure of the wound and restoration of the anterior chamber. If small and limited to the centre, corneal wounds heal well unless they become infected; atropine is instilled, an antibiotic ointment inserted, and a pad and bandage applied. If the wound becomes infected it must be treated like a perforating ulcer.

If the wound is large an adhesion of the iris or its prolapse is almost certain to occur. The prolapsed iris should never be replaced, even if this is possible, since it may carry infection into the eye. It must be abscised (p. 258); the technique of this operation will be discussed subsequently (p. 258). In large wounds, which are often corneo-scleral in type, healing is facilitated by direct suturing.

If the wound is large, events may be more turbulent. The lens rapidly opacifies and flocculent grey masses protrude through the opening in the capsule; sometimes the whole chamber is full of white flocculi.

A traumatic cataract of this type is liable to set up serious complications if not aspirated at once. Traumatic iridocyclitis is invariable and may be severe. The swelling of the lens, keeps the iris in contact with the cornea.

The *treatment* of traumatic cataract in association with perforating wounds especially if complicated by vitreous loss is by the use of a vitrectomy instrument. The aim of surgery is to remove the cataract, perform an anterior vitrectomy, suture the globe and take adequate steps to ensure control of infection by intra-ocular antibiotics as a *primary procedure* including the insertion of an intra-ocular lens implant in suitable cases.

Treatment. If the injury is so severe that there is no likelihood of the recovery of useful vision, the eye should be excised. If there is a chance of useful vision

the sclera may be sutured and the sutures tied after vitrectomy. Seriously injured eyes usually shrink.

Wounds of the lens

Such wounds cause traumatic cataract and are always a serious complication. If the wound in the capsule is small, the entry of aqueous causes a localised cloudiness in its vicinity and, irrespective of the site of the wound, opacities in the form of feathery lines appear in the posterior cortex, which later develop into a rosette-shaped cataract resembling that of early concussion cataract (Fig. 26.2). Occasionally the wound in the capsule becomes sealed, particularly if a posterior synechia develops, in which case these changes may be stationary; usually they are progressive until a complete cataract is formed.

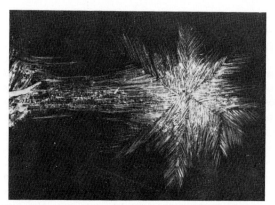

Fig. 26.2 Rosette-shaped cataract at the posterior pole following perforation of the lens by a foreign body. A disturbance in the lens along the track of the foreign body is seen

Perforating wounds with the retention of foreign bodies

The retention of a foreign body adds considerably to the danger and anxieties of a perforating injury. The foreign bodies most likely to penetrate the eye and be retained are minute chips of iron or steel (accounting for 90% of the foreign bodies in industry), stone, and particles of glass, lead pellets, copper percussion caps, less frequently spicules of wood. In chipping stone with an iron chisel, it is a chip of the chisel and not of the stone which enters the eye.

The *size and velocity* of the missile are of importance. If the foreign body is large so much damage is usually caused that the eye has to be removed. Very minute particles can, however, penetrate the cornea or sclera and lodge in the deeper parts of the eye.

The entrance of a foreign body into the eye may cause damage in one of three ways — by mechanical effects, by the introduction of infection, and sometimes by specific action (chemical and otherwise) on the intra-ocular tissues. We will first consider the mechanical effects.

The foreign body may enter the eye either through the cornea or sclera. Having penetrated the cornea it may be retained in the anterior chamber where it may fall to the bottom and, if very small, lie deeply in the angle hidden by the scleral ledge where it can only be seen gonioscopically. It is generally, however, caught in the iris, and can be recognised with the slit-lamp. A piece of glass in the anterior chamber is exceptionally difficult to see because its refractive index differs so little from that of the surrounding media.

The foreign body may pass into or through the lens, either by way of the iris or of the pupil. In each case a traumatic cataract is produced, which undergoes the usual changes (p. 248). If the particle has passed through the iris there will be a hole in this structure; this looks black by oblique illumination, but shows a red reflex when illuminated by the ophthalmoscope, unless the lens behind the hole is cataractous. A hole in the iris is of great diagnostic significance, since it rarely occurs except as the result of perforation by a foreign body. The foreign body may be visible in the lens, either before or after dilatation of the pupil, but it is possible for it to pass through the iris and through the circumlental space without wounding the lens.

The foreign body may be retained in the vitreous to which it may obtain access by various routes: through the cornea, iris and lens; through the cornea, pupil and lens; through the cornea, iris and zonule; or directly through the sclera. If it comes to rest in the vitreous it may remain suspended for some time but eventually sinks to the bottom of the vitreous chamber owing to degenerative changes in the gel which lead to liquefaction, partial or complete. If the particle is small, the lens clear, and there has been little hæmorrhage, the body may be seen ophthalmoscopically in the vitreous or retina; the track through the vitreous often looks like a grey line. Most commonly the particle has enough energy to carry it directly onto the retina where it may ricochet once or even twice before it comes to rest; occasionally it pierces the coats of the eye and comes to rest in the orbital tissues (*double perforation*).

If it lies in the retina, the foreign body, generally black and often with a metallic lustre, is surrounded by white exudate and red blood-clot, but eventually fibrous tissue usually encapsulates it and the retina in the neighbourhood becomes heavily pigmented.

The lodgement of a foreign body in the posterior segment frequently leads to degenerative changes, apart altogether from its chemical nature, which may considerably damage the sight. These may entail a widespread degeneration, but most frequently fine pigmentary disturbances at the macula, often the result of concussion (*q.v*), diminish or destroy central vision. The vitreous usually turns fluid, bands of fibrous tissue

may traverse it along the path of the foreign body, hæmorrhage may be extensive, and retinal detachment may follow. Particles greater than 2 mm in size usually lead to destruction of the eye.

Infection. As with other perforating wounds, the introduction of infection is an ever-present danger when a foreign body enters the eye. Some types of foreign body are more likely to be associated with infection than others. Fortunately, owing to the heat generated partly on their emission and partly by their rapid transit through the air small flying metallic particles are frequently sterile, and it is notorious that infections are more likely to follow the introduction of pieces of stone or wood than anything else. The infection should be treated prophylactically as in perforating wounds; despite treatment, the prognosis in terms of vision is seldom good.

The *reaction of the ocular tissues to a foreign body* varies with its chemical nature. Non-organised materials are either (1) inert, or (2) excite a local irritative response which leads to the formation of fibrous tissue, often resulting in encapsulation, or (3) produce a suppurative reaction, or (4) cause specific degenerative effects. Organised material, on the other hand, tends to produce a proliferative reaction characterised by the formation of granulation tissue. Although the inert materials cause little or no reaction at the time, iridocyclitis and disorganisation may eventually develop.

Glass, *plastics* and *porcelain* are inert. *Stone* may occasionally give rise to chemical changes depending on its composition. Of the metals, *gold*, *silver*, *platinum* and *tantalum* are inert. *Lead*, usually occurring as shot-gun pellets, becomes coated with the carbonate and excites little reaction. *Aluminium* frequently becomes powdered and excites a local reaction; so also does *zinc* which may excite suppuration — a reaction often associated with *nickel* and constantly with *mercury*. Iron and copper, the two most common materials found, undergo electrolytic dissociation and are widely deposited throughout the eye causing important degenerative changes.

Iron. This causes the condition of siderosis; so also does steel in proportion to its ferrous content. The condition is probably due to the electrolytic dissociation of the metal by the 'current of rest' in the eye, which disseminates the metal throughout the tissues and enables it to combine with the cellular proteins, thus killing the cells and causing atrophy. The tissues are not uniformly affected. The earliest clinical manifestation is the deposit of iron in the anterior capsular cells of the lens where oval patches of the rusty deposit are arranged radially in a ring corresponding with the edge of the dilated pupil. This appearance is pathognomonic and leads eventually to the development of cataract. The iris also becomes characteristically stained, first greenish and later reddish-brown. The vision of these eyes, however little affected by the primary injury, gradually fails owing to degenerative changes in the retina and lens. The retinal degeneration, associated with great attenuation of the blood vessels, eventually becomes generalised, taking the form of pigmentation resembling that of pigmentary retinal dystrophy. Secondary glaucoma of the chronic type is a common late complication; and, unless the foreign body becomes encapsulated or is removed in time, most of these eyes go blind.

Pathologically the deposits of iron are revealed by the Prussian blue reaction with Perls's micro-chemical stain. The characteristic blue pigmentation is found particularly in the corneal corpuscles, in the meshes of the trabeculæ, on the inner surface of the ciliary body, and in the retina where the whole retinal vascular system is clearly marked out. The anterior layers of the iris are impregnated, and in addition to subcapsular deposits in the lens, the fibres are also stained. There is always intense blue coloration immediately around the foreign body.

The reaction of *copper* or *brass* (as from percussion caps) varies with the content of pure copper. If the metal is relatively pure, a violent reaction ensues. Occasionally this results in the profuse formation of fibrous tissues so that the particle becomes encapsulated; more usually a suppurative reaction follows, which eventually retrogresses so that it results in shrinkage of the globe.

If, however, the metal is heavily alloyed, a much milder reaction ensues — *chalcosis*. It becomes electrolytically dissociated and is deposited particularly where resistance to its migration is offered by continuous membranes. The typical sites for deposition are in the deeper parts of the cornea where it accumulates mostly at the periphery causing the appearance of a golden-brown Kayser-Fleischer ring (p. 146), under the capsule of the lens where it is deposited to form a brilliant golden-green sheen aggregated in radiating formations like the petals of a flower (*sun-flower cataract*), and occasionally on the retina at the posterior pole where lustrous golden plaques reflect the light with a metallic sheen. Not entering into chemical combination with the proteins of the cells as does iron, however, degenerative changes do not appear and the vision may remain indefinitely good.

Organised materials. Wood and other vegetable matter, produce a proliferative reaction characterised by the formation of giant cells. Eyelashes may be carried into the anterior chamber in perforating wounds of the cornea, whether accidental or operative; proliferation of the epithelium of the root hairs frequently leads to the formation of intra-ocular cysts. *Caterpillar hairs* may penetrate the eye (p. 124) exciting a severe iridocyclitis characterised by the formation of granulomatous nodules (*ophthalmia nodosa*).

The *diagnosis* of an intra-ocular foreign body is a matter of extreme importance, particularly as the patient is often unaware that a particle has entered the eye. In all suspicious cases particularly with a history of the use of a hammer and chisel, a careful search must be made for a wound of entry; and it may be very minute and difficult to find. If the particle has passed through the cornea, however, the most minute scar can always be seen on careful examination with the slit-lamp; its detection in the sclera may be much more difficult or sometimes even impossible.

The anterior segment of the eye must be thoroughly explored with the slit-lamp and the angle of the anterior chamber with the gonioscope. A hole in the iris or an opaque track through the lens is pathognomonic. These tracks, together with the position of the wound of entrance, often give a valuable clue in localising the foreign body. If the media are clear, the entire fundus must be similarly searched under full mydriasis.

Radiography is indispensable for the discovery and location of such foreign bodies as are radio-opaque. Fortunately these particles are usually metallic and many — although by no means all — can thus be demonstrated. Many methods of localisation are available. One of the most useful — that exploited in the techniques of Mackenzie Davidson and the Bromley localiser in Britain, and Sweet and Dixon in America — depends on taking two stereoscopic pictures at two fixed angles, and calculating the position of the foreign body from the displacement of its shadow with reference to a known opaque marker. This method is capable of great accuracy.

A second method, involves the suturing of a metal ring at the limbus and taking X-ray photographs in the antero-posterior and lateral axes. The foreign body can then be located in terms of the meridian and the number of millimetres behind the limbus or corneal apex.

A third method consists of the use of the CAT scan which is capable of localising a foreign body with great accuracy.

A useful method of detection and localisation in the operating theatre is to exploit the alterations in a secondary induced current produced by a metallic particle in its vicinity. This principle has been incorporated in instruments (*locators*) wherein the searching element is a pointed probe and alterations in the current in the neighbourhood of the particle are revealed by the deflections of a dial or changes in the pitch of a loud speaker. Ultrasound in the form of an A scan may localise a foreign body in line with a probe.

Treatment. A foreign body should be removed unless (1) it is inert and was probably sterile; (2) little damage has been done to vision; and (3) the process of removal will almost inevitably destroy sight. These conditions are most often fulfilled in the case of minute foreign bodies in the retina. Magnetisable foreign bodies are more easily removed than others since the use of the magnet considerably facilitates the technique.

Electro-magnets such as are used in ophthalmology utilise the principle of the solenoid wherein a coil wound around a central core renders the latter magnetic: this is fitted with suitably shaped terminals. The power of such a magnet depends on the electric current available (which is limited), the length and diameter of the wire in the coil and the mass of the core. The latter two are limited by the requirments of weight and manœuvrability. The effectiveness of any magnet depends on the magnetisability of the particle, its size which determines the number of lines of force which traverse it, and its distance away: the effectivity of a magnet diminishes as the cube of the distance from the particles to be attracted.

Intra-ocular foreign bodies are often lightly magnetisable and always small. *Hand magnets* (Fig. 26.3) which can readily be manipulated by hand, are employed.

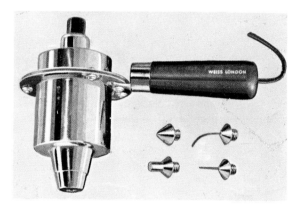

Fig. 26.3 Hand electro-magnet. Four small terminals are seen which screw into the point of the magnet. (By courtesy of Hamblin.)

The time over which a magnet can be applied is limited by the amount of heat generated; prolonged applications can therefore only be made by repeated short exposures which are effective by gradually loosening a foreign body from an encapsulated bed or slowly drawing it through the tissues of the eye.

If the foreign body lies within the lens, magnet-extraction is usually difficult; it is better to treat such particles as if they were non-magnetic (*vide infra*).

If a magnetic foreign body is in the vitreous or retina, a magnet is necessary for its removal. Extraction is undertaken by the posterior route whereby the particle is extracted directly through a scleral incision into the posterior segment of the globe. Accurate localisation of the foreign body is essential so that it is removed by the shortest possible path.

Extraction by the posterior route. This is done through an incision as close to the foreign body as is practicable, as determined by previous localisation; if the particle

lies in the vitreous the incision is best made 5 mm behind the limbus — the so-called 'safe zone' in that it traverses the pars plana of the ciliary body, largely obviating any danger of immediate hæmorrhage or subsequent retinal detachment. The conjunctiva is reflected, the area around the incision is touched with the cryo-probe as in the operation for retinal detachment (*q.v.*), the sclera carefully incised down to the ciliary body, and the point of the terminal of the magnet inserted into the lips of the wound but not into the cavity of the eye. The current is then turned on; if the operation is successful the particle approaches and adheres to the terminal which is at once withdrawn, and after the terminal is free from the eye, the current is switched off. The scleral wound is then closed by previously placed sutures.

The immediate effect of extraction of foreign bodies with the large magnet is often good, but prognosis should be guarded. The tracks through the vitreous may become filled with fibrous tissue; as this organises and contracts, the retina may be pulled up and total detachment destroy vision. Victrectomy instruments have helped the management of cases of perforating wounds with intra-ocular foreign bodies. Lens opacities and vitreous haemorrhage, bands and membranes can be removed at the time of initial surgery. The extent of retinal damage can be accurately assessed and treated thus minimising late post-operative complication.

The extraction of a non-magnetic foreign body from the anterior segment of the eye is often easy; from the posterior segment it presents great difficulties.

If the foreign body lies upon the iris it can usually be picked out by iris forceps through a suitably placed keratome incision. If it is entangled in this tissue, it is removed in the course of an iridectomy in the manner already described.

If it lies in the angle of the anterior chamber it is impossible to get at it with forceps by an ordinary keratome incision immediately over it (Fig. 26.4A). The incision should be made at 3 mm inside the limbus in the quadrant of the cornea lying over the foreign body, the point of the keratome being directed straight at it (Fig. 26.4B). The foreign body can then be lifted out with

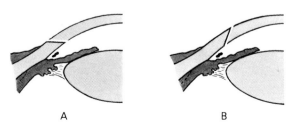

A   B

Fig. 26.4 The removal of a non-magnetic foreign body from the anterior chamber: A, the wrong incision; B, the correct incision to allow access to the foreign body

toothless forceps, and the risk of prolapse of iris is also minimised.

If the foreign body is in the lens, a few days should be allowed to elapse for the aqueous to act upon the lens fibres. An aspiration (p. 261) is then performed and the foreign body will probably be evacuated with the lens matter. In elderly patients it may be necessary to extract the lens by the operation for extraction of senile cataract (p. 263).

If a non-magnetisable foreign body lies in the posterior segment of the globe its removal is difficult. If it lies on the retina, and *if accurate localisation has been attained*, preferably verified at the time of operation by bone-free radiography, it may sometimes be directly removed by forceps through an incision, preceded, as already described, by cryo application to the sclera immediately over the site. If it is in the vitreous and the media are clear, successful instances have been recorded of its removal by special forceps introduced through a pars plana incision and manipulated under microscopic control.

The prognosis of the retention of a foreign body in the eye is always serious, even if little mechanical damage has been done at the time of injury. It varies with the site and the chemical nature of the particle. If the foreign body is allowed to remain and is inert, it may be retained indefinitely without affecting vision, although an iridocyclitis, sometimes appearing after many years, may be anticipated. If it is not inert and allowed to remain, the visual prognosis is bad. If the foreign body has been removed from the anterior chamber, the prognosis is usually good provided the lens was not wounded. A wound of the lens, however, gravely aggravates the position owing to the immediate difficulties of its evacuation, the subsequent irritative reaction, and the tendency for the development of secondary glaucoma. Even if the particle has been successfully extracted from the posterior segment of the globe, the subsequent history over a five- or ten-year period shows that many such eyes eventually lose useful vision from degenerative changes or retinal detachment, no matter how dramatically successful the operation had been.

Sympathetic ophthalmitis

Sympathetic ophthalmitis
This is the condition in which serious inflammation attacks the sound eye after injury of the other. In recent years sympathetic ophthalmitis has become a rare disease.

Sympathetic ophthalmitis almost always results from a perforating wound. Wounds in the ciliary region — the so-called 'dangerous zone' — involving the ciliary body and leading to its incarceration in the scar, have always been considered especially dangerous; it is

doubtful if, *per se*, they are more dangerous than others. On the other hand, it is certain that wounds in which iris, ciliary body or lens capsule is incarcerated are more likely to set up sympathetic ophthalmitis than others. It very rarely occurs if actual suppuration has taken place in the exciting eye. It is also extremely rare without perforation, if indeed it ever occurs in these circumstances.

Children are particularly susceptible, but it occurs at any age. It usually begins four to eight weeks after the injury to the first eye (the exciting eye) has taken place, rarely earlier, but the onset has been reported as occurring nine days after the accident and may be delayed for many months or even years.

There is always iridocyclitis in the exciting eye. Usually it is a plastic iridocyclitis which has been set up by injury and has not subsided in the course of three or four weeks. Instead of quietening down the ciliary injection remains, there is lacrimation and the eye is tender: special attention should be directed to the presence or absence of precipitates ('k.p.') on the back of the cornea. In the rarer cases of delayed sympathetic ophthalmitis the exciting eye has passed into a quiescent state and may have shrunk completely. The onset of sympathetic ophthalmitis in the second eye is then ushered in by return of irritation — ciliary injection, tenderness, etc. — in the shrunken globe. The exciting eye, while showing evident traces of old iridocyclitis, may yet possess useful vision.

Sympathetic ophthalmitis — the disease in the second or sympathising eye — is almost always a plastic iridocyclitis differing clinically in no respect from this form of iridocyclitis due to other causes. In rare cases it manifests itself as a neuro-retinitis or choroiditis. In cases which the surgeon knows to be liable to the condition the first sign may be the presence of precipitates ('k.p.') on the back of the cornea, noticed at this early stage because they have been anticipated. In other cases the patient first seeks advice for photophobia and lacrimation, or defective vision in the uninjured eye (sympathetic irritation).

Prodromal symptoms are sensitivity to light and transient indistinctness of near objects due to weakness of accommodation. On examination at this stage there may be lacrimation, slight ciliary injection, tenderness of the eyeball, as shown by the patient shrinking from an attempt at examination, precipitates on the back of the cornea, and vitreous opacities; occasionally there is some œdema of the optic disc. The prodromal symptoms may occur in intermittent attacks, spread over a considerable period.

When fully developed all the signs and symptoms of iridocyclitis are present, varying in degree according to the severity of the case. The prognosis as to vision is always doubtful, but if there is much deposition of plastic exudates in the pupillary area it becomes extremely grave. Cases showing little exudation ('serous iritis') but a deep anterior chamber and 'k.p.' have a more favourable prognosis, but they may at any moment develop into the severe plastic type. Sympathetic ophthalmitis sometimes takes two or more years to run its course but the disease is self-limiting.

Pathologically the microscopic features in both the exciting and the sympathising eye are the same. In the earliest stages, examination shows nodular aggregations of lymphocytes and plasma cells scattered throughout the uveal tract. The pigment epithelium of the iris and ciliary body proliferates to form nodular aggregations (Dalén–Fuchs nodules) and the tissues become invaded by lymphocytes and epithelioid cells. The retina also becomes heavily infiltrated especially in the neighbourhood of the vessels. In the later stages the infiltrate becomes diffuse and giant cells appear; in fact, the condition is scarcely distinguishable from tuberculosis of the uveal tract, although caseation is never present. These are merely the signs of reaction to a relatively mild form of irritation.

The aetiology of the condition is unknown but two theories usually receive preference — that it is infective or allergic in nature. Since no organismal invader has been demonstrated, a hypothetical virus infection is often inculpated which, like many other viruses, may have the habit of remaining long quiescent.

On the other hand, a purely allergic origin to uveal pigment has been postulated. Uveal pigment can act as an allergen and sufferers from sympathetic diseases show a skin sensitivity to it. Viral infection may be the initiating factor by modifying uveal proteins to the extent that they become unusually antigenic or, by damaging the cells directly, uncover intracellular antigens.

The *treatment* of sympathetic ophthalmitis demands the exercise of great judgment.

It is, in the first place, prophylactic. In every case of perforating wound, with or without the retention of a foreign body, the question of excision of the eye on account of danger to its fellow arises. It may be assumed as an axiom that *sympathetic ophthalmitis never occurs after the excision of an injured eye unless it has already commenced at the time of operation.* Hence, early excision is a positive safeguard against the disease. The rule should be to excise any eye which is so injured that it is im-

probable that useful vision will be regained. In cases wherein this is doubtful, expectant treatment, including the topical administration of steroids, may be adopted for a time. If the eye quietens down quickly it is unlikely to set up sympathetic inflammation. The chief causes which keep up irritation are entanglement of the iris or ciliary body or lens capsule in the wound; every effort must therefore be made to obviate this.

During this expectant period if, despite treatment, the eye continues to be irritable, with ciliary injection, photophobia, and lacrimation, and above all if 'k.p.' appear, the eye should be excised. It is seldom wise to wait longer than a fortnight unless there are undoubted signs of amelioration. It must be remembered that children are more susceptible to the disease than adults.

Even more difficult to decide is the course to adopt in those cases in which sympathetic ophthalmitis has already supervened. If the case is seen early, shortly after the onset of inflammation in the sympathising eye, and if the injured or exciting eye has no useful vision, this useless eye should be excised at once. There is no question that the excision of the exciting eye has a good effect upon the process in the sympathising eye if performed early. At a later stage there is no evidence to show that it exerts any influence.

The treatment of sympathetic iridocyclitis is that of iridocyclitis in general (p. 156) with the proviso that steroid preparations have a more dramatic effect than in most other ocular inflammations. At the earliest suggestion of inflammation, steroids should be given systemically in large doses of 100 mg of Prednisone (p. 369); subconjunctival injections reinforced by the topical use of dexamethasone 0.1% drops are the most effective method. In all cases the treatment should be continued for many months lest relapses follow its cessation, and the eye should be watched over a period of years. Daily doses of steroid are employed initially but later it should be possible to change to alternate day steroid therapy. If the immediate crisis can be tided over in this way and recurrences prevented, comfort may be derived from the fact that the disease is self-limiting. The use of steroids has completely altered the prognosis of this disease *if such treatment is commenced early.* If, however, the inflammation has taken a firm hold and the uvea is heavily infiltrated, the outlook is much less bright.

27

Operations upon the eyeball

In this chapter the more important operations only will be noted. Of these the commoner classical procedures will be described in some detail; only the general principles of more specialised techniques will be indicated.

PRELIMINARY MEASURES

Before intra-ocular operations, particularly major operations such as cataract extraction, *a general survey* of the patient is advisable which should include an investigation of the blood-pressure the haemoglobin level and the general cardio-vascular condition and of the urine to exclude the presence of sugar, albumin and bacteria (particularly in the presence of overflow incontinence in the male). Few general diseases are a complete contraindication to an ocular operation; but it is well to be forewarned of possible complications.

Local bacteriological precautions should also be taken by clinical inspection and a preliminary swab if there are signs of conjunctivitis. Suitable antibiotic treatment is given if any infection is present in the conjunctival sac based on sensitivity studies of the bacteria cultured. Prophylactic gentisin drops are always employed preoperatively. Dacryocystitis should be eliminated and a nasal-drainage operation should be performed if necessary.

ANAESTHESIA FOR EYE OPERATIONS

Most ophthalmic operations can be conducted under local analgesia, preferably with premedication. While the co-operation of the patient is always desirable, it is not always given, and it is unfair in the trying circumstances of an operation to expect that it should be; but it is easy by adequate basal sedation, analgesia and akinesia to ensure that events will not get out of hand. General anaesthesia is the standard procedure in the U.K. for ophthalmic surgery.

Local analgesia
1. *Surface analgesia.* Amethocaine 1% drops are readily absorbed by the conjunctiva and cornea, and produce complete analgesia after the instillation of 4 drops at intervals of 3 min. The iris, however, is not rendered completely analgesic by this method

2. *Infiltration and regional analgesia.* Infiltration analgesia with procaine or a suitable substitute is employed to effect analgesia of the iris. A retro-ocular injection may be used to infiltrate the ciliary ganglion and the surrounding tissues: 1 ml of procaine (4%) with 1 in 100 000 adrenaline is injected with a fine needle, 5 cm long, passed through the skin of the lower lid at the outer and lower angle of the orbit and directed towards the apex of the orbit for a distance of 3.5 cm. Occasionally a large vein is punctured giving rise to a proptosis sufficient to delay an intra-ocular operation for a few days. An alternative is to make a similar injection into Tenon's capsule just behind the equator about half-way between the temporal border of the superior rectus and the upper edge of the lateral rectus. A fine needle is used, and care is taken to insert it very obliquely through the conjunctiva, to avoid the site of a vortex vein, and to keep close to the sclera.

Pre-medication
It is usually wise to administer sedatives before operation to allay the natural fear and apprehension of the patient. For this purpose droperidol, a neuroleptic tranquillizer and anti-emetic is given with diazepam in a dose of 10 mg of each in the average adult by mouth 2 h before operation. Children over 1 year of age are premedicated with trimeprazine syrup (Vallergan Forte) at a dose of 4 mg/kg body weight 2 h before surgery, followed by an injection of atropine 0.2–0.6 mg 30 min before surgery.

General anaesthesia
Basal anaesthesia by the intravenous administration of drugs is peculiarly suited to ophthalmic surgery. A useful drug for this purpose is thiopentone a rapidly acting barbiturate which produces a fall of blood pressure and intra-ocular pressure, good relaxation and moderately quick recovery of consciousness. A single injection

suffices for an operation of 10–20 min duration. For longer operations more of the solution is periodically injected. Conjunctival and corneal reflexes are abolished, but it is wise to use local analgesia and akinesia in addition.

AKINESIA FOR EYE OPERATIONS

In intra-ocular operations involving a wide opening of the globe (e.g., cataract) temporary paralysis of the orbicularis muscle is advisable in order to prevent squeezing together of the lids.

For this purpose a *facial block* may be employed. Four to 5 ml of procaine are injected down to the periosteum covering the neck of the mandible where the upper branches of the facial nerve pass forwards and upwards. The patient should be instructed to open his mouth, and the position of the condyle and temporo-mandibular joint is located by the operator's left forefinger. After closing the jaw the needle is inserted at a point half an inch below the position of the condyle and passed straight down to the periosteum where the solution is injected, and firm pressure and local massage are applied. Paralysis of the orbicularis rapidly follows. The main trunk of the facial nerve may be reached before its bifurcation by a 5/8 inch needle injected its whole length just below the external auditory meatus between the mastoid process and the posterior border of the mandibular ramus.

Alternatively the branches of the facial nerve may be blocked as they run over the malar bone. A needle is inserted down to the periosteum of the malar bone at a point about 1 cm below and behind the outer canthus and passed upwards towards the temporal fossa, forwards and downwards towards the infra-orbital foramen, and downwards and backwards towards the tragus for an inch or so.

When the lids have been paralysed in this way, postoperative closure should be ensured either by filling the conjunctival sac with an antibiotic ointment and carefully closing the lids or by inserting a stitch into the skin of the upper lid 3 mm above its margin. This is fixed to the cheek by adhesive plaster after the operation and removed at the first dressing.

Fixation of the globe by a stitch passed through the tendon of the superior rectus muscle is necessary in intra-ocular operations conducted under general anaesthesia and is advisable in all intra-ocular operations. It is more effective after the injection of 0.5 ml procaine into the belly of the muscle. During the operation the stitch is clamped without tension to the head-towels by artery forceps.

Akinesia affecting particularly the extra-ocular muscles can be attained by the systemic injection of curare-like preparations such as *d*-tubocurarine chloride (5–9 mg intravenously). Small doses only are required since these muscles are the most susceptible in the body to the action of these relaxants, but they should be used with care and only by an expert. The use of long-acting muscle relaxants to produce akinesia of the ocular muscles without controlled respiration is potentially dangerous. The use of hyperventilation by a mechanical ventilator with tubocurarine moreover lowers intra-ocular pressure by reducing alveolar carbon dioxide concentration.

The speculum. In most operations a simple speculum of Barraquer is adequate. Many others are available which are supported on the orbit but the simplest and safest method is to employ lid-stitches. The upper lid stitch (*vide supra*) instead of being inserted in the middle is passed through the skin twice at the junctions of the middle third with the outer and inner thirds, and it, as well as the central superior rectus stitch, is clamped on the head-towels to keep the upper lid back. A skin stitch in the lower lid depresses it by the weight of a bull-dog clip hanging down over the cheek.

General routine

The preparation of the eye immediately before the operation is the same in all cases. The skin of the lids is dried and painted with Betadine (povidone-iodine 10%, alcoholic solution). Two or three drops of an antibiotic are instilled. Five drops of Amethocaine are instilled at 3 min intervals and one drop into the other eye to diminish the risk of closure of the lids. The orbicularis oculi is paralysed; an injection of procaine is made into Tenon's capsule or the ciliary ganglion if necessary. Sterile towels are draped round the head, neck and chest and the face covered with a mask of steri-drape in which an aperture has been cut to give access to the eye. The lid stitching is inserted after local injection of procaine into the skin. The speculum (if employed) is inserted and the eye is ready for operation.

In most operations *fixation of the eye* is required. This is usually attained by fixation forceps which should take a deep grip of the conjunctiva so as to include the episcleral tissue or an insertion of one of the muscles; otherwise they are liable to tear the conjunctiva if much traction is exerted, as by an involuntary movement of the patient. The eye is then pulled gently forwards; the forceps should never be pressed backwards, particularly in operations wherein the globe is opened, lest the pressure expel some of the intra-ocular contents. As an alternative in some operations a fixation suture may be inserted into each of the rectus muscles and immobility in a particular direction attained by gentle but firm traction thereon.

The routine *post-operative treatment* is the insertion of

antibiotic ointment, the application of a light gauze pad and bandage. When the globe has been widely opened, protection against accidental injury may be obtained by a rigid cover shaped to the orbital rim; a cartella shield of stiff plastic is suitable (Fig. 27.1). This and the pad can be secured in place by adhesive micropore. Both eyes are never covered and the patient is allowed out of bed on the day following surgery.

Most ophthalmic operations are performed with surgical cutting instruments; two techniques, however, should be noted which have special indications.

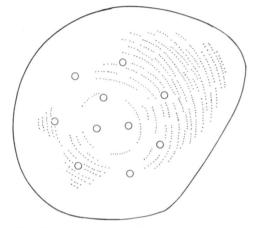

Fig. 27.1 'Cartella' shield for right eye

Operations with cryotherapy

Cryotherapy has replaced surface diathermy which has a necrotic effect on the sclera. It is employed: (1) to excite a plastic choroiditis to cause adhesions between the retina and choroid and close a retinal hole in retinal detachment, or as a prophylactic measure to prevent its occurrence in cases in which thin and degenerate areas occur in the retina, and before opening the posterior segment of the globe as for the removal of a foreign body; (2) in glaucoma to cause an atrophy of the ciliary body; (3) to destroy intra-ocular inflammatory lesions (retinal periphlebitis) or neoplasms, either simple (as an angioma) or malignant, as an alternative to radiation when excision of the eye is contra-indicated.

Cryosurgery is a technique used to injure tissues by the application of intense cold. This is achieved by a cryoprobe, a pencil-like instrument held by the surgeon, cooled to a temperature varying from $-40°C$ to $-100°C$ by solid carbon dioxide or liquid nitrogen (Fig. 27.2). The method is useful in such procedures as the surgery of cataract and particularly retinal detachment because of its slight effect on scleral integrity.

Light-coagulation

This is a useful technique wherein a chorioretinal burn is caused by a brilliant beam of light derived from a

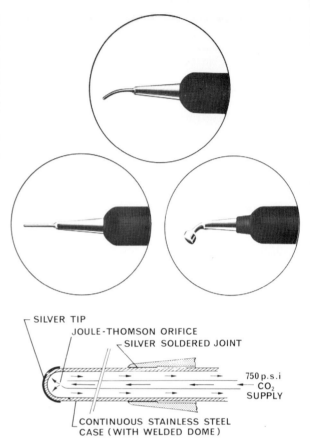

SILVER TIP
JOULE-THOMSON ORIFICE
SILVER SOLDERED JOINT
750 p.s.i
CO_2
SUPPLY
CONTINUOUS STAINLESS STEEL
CASE (WITH WELDED DOME)

Fig. 27.2 Cryoprobes

specially designed Xenon arc-lamp. The apparatus is elaborate and allows an ophthalmoscopic view of the retinal lesion. It may be used in cases of retinal detachment to coagulate the region of the tear in the central area of the fundus, provided the retina is not far removed from the underlying choroid. It may also be used to destroy a small neoplasm or inflammatory lesion in this region of the fundus or on the iris. A smaller lesion of the same type can be made by an argon or krypton laser applied under direct view of a slit-lamp microscope and contact lens.

OPERATIONS ON THE CORNEA

Paracentesis

This may be employed for hypopyon ulcers, hyphaema with raised tension or occasionally for hypertensive cyclitis. As a rule the paracentesis is performed near the periphery of the cornea using a keratome.

The eye is steadied with fixation forceps and an incision made approximately 2 mm within the limbus at the point selected. Generally the temporal limbus is most convenient; for the evacuation of a hypopyon the lower limbus is used. A keratome, a broad needle or a paracentesis needle may be employed. This is inserted in the plane of the iris to make a valvular opening, and directly the point traverses the cornea the plane of the blade is altered so that it lies close to the inner surface of this tissue to avoid wounding the iris or lens. It is then pushed inwards until the incision is sufficiently long, and carefully withdrawn so that little or no aqueous escapes. A sudden withdrawal with loss of much aqueous may lead to hæmorrhage or a prolapse of the iris; the means to deal with this should therefore be at hand. An iris repositor is then inserted and the peripheral lip of the wound slightly depressed so that the aqueous escapes slowly with a minimum of disturbance. Such an incision can be repeatedly re-opened on successive days by the iris repositor.

Keratoplasty

The general principles of corneal grafting are as follows. In perforating keratoplasty a disc in the centre of the cornea is involved. From the donor eye, usually a cadaver eye preserved by refrigeration, the cornea is removed and a disc of the required diameter is punched out with the larger of two paired trephines and transferred to a watch-glass containing saline or glutothione Ringer's solution. A corresponding disc is then marked on the recipient cornea with the smaller trephine and double-armed sutures inserted at the limbus so that they cross over the proposed site of the graft in order that the graft may later be secured by direct suturing. The trephining is then continued through the thickness of the cornea until aqueous begins to escape; the host disc, including any tags of Descemet's membrane, is then completely removed by a specially designed scissors or knife. The donor graft is then carefully laid upon its bed and the cross sutures tied. Air is placed in the anterior chamber to protect the corneal endothelium during the insertion of a continuous perlon suture. Miosis is induced by miochol which reforms the anterior chamber. Miochol is acetylcholine 1%, mannitol 5% powder in vial made up to a solution of 2 ml with diluent immediately before use. The continuous suture is removed some months later.

In *lamellar keratoplasty* a trephine is used fitted with a guard so that the cut reaches only a desired depth. A disc of the required depth (usually about 0.4 mm) is cut in the donor's cornea with the trephine and the lamella removed with a special corneal knife. A similar procedure is performed on the recipient's eye and sutures inserted as for penetrating keratoplasty. The graft is then inserted into its bed and the sutures tied.

Allograft rejection caused by histo-incompatibility depends successively on recognition of the foreign antigen by thymus-dependent host lymphocytes, stimulation of lymphoid cells in draining lymph nodes and destruction of donor tissue by sensitised lymphocytes and their products.

Within the first few weeks corneal graft failure is more likely to be due to defective donor endothelium resulting from surgical trauma, autolysis or degenerative change related to the age of the donor. Other causes are defective wound closure, secondary infection or secondary glaucoma.

Usually there is a period of three weeks during which the graft appears technically successful and clear and this is followed by oedema and cellular precipitates on the back of the graft. There is also a line of opacity corresponding to the interface between the rejected endothelium and the advancing inflammatory infiltrate. A favourable response to corticosteroids is usual. Graft survival is greatest in corneae which are avascular prior to surgery and immunological rejection is almost always heralded by ingrowth of vessels from the limbus. Good correspondence between donor and host transplantation antigens is a possible explanation for the occasional survival of grafts in heavily vascularised recipients.

Tarsorrhaphy

Although not strictly a corneal operation tarsorrhaphy, is performed for corneal conditions, particularly neuro-paralytic or exposure keratitis. The operation may aim at more or less total closure of the lids or alternatively be confined to one half, usually the external, so that the palpebral aperture is narrowed rather than closed. Apart from the placement of the sutures both operations follow the same technique.

The mucous membrane is dissected up from the margin of the lower lid just posterior to the grey line (p. 258) over rectangular areas about 6 mm long on each side of the middle of the lid. The edge of the upper lid is similarly treated at the corresponding positions. Two mattress sutures are then passed through rubber sheet-

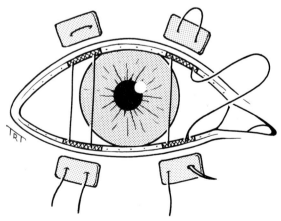

Fig. 27.3 Tarsorrhaphy

ing and the skin so that they come out at the posterior edge of the bare surface (Fig. 27.3) – not on the posterior surface of the lid where they would rub against the cornea. After being similarly carried through the skin of the other lid and the rubber they are tied, the freshened surfaces being brought into contact. In a few days the lids will be firmly adherent.

OPERATIONS UPON THE IRIS

Iridectomy

Iridectomy, which consists of the abscission of a portion of the iris, is performed for the following conditions: (1) prolapsed iris; (2) closed-angle glaucoma; (3) as part of cataract extraction; (4) threatening ring synechia; (5) foreign bodies in, or small cysts or tumours of the iris.

Iridectomy for prolapsed iris. The prolapse is seized with iris forceps held in the right hand, as close to the cornea as possible, and drawn well out from the wound. A second pair of iris forceps, held in the left hand, is then applied again as near the cornea as possible, and the iris drawn still further out. De Wecker's scissors are then taken in the right hand and the iris is cut off close to the cornea (Fig. 27.5). If the operation has been successfully performed the stumps of iris retract into the anterior chamber and are free from the wound. Atropine is instilled and a pad and bandage applied.

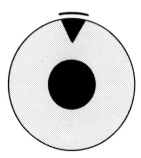

Fig. 27.4 Diagram of wound and coloboma in peripheral iridectomy at the site of election

Iridectomy for iritis. This should be performed in the upper part of the iris, and in this operation the coloboma should be wide as in

Iridectomy in combined extraction of cataract.

Iridectomy for closed-angle glaucoma. This is usually peripheral ('button-hole') or occasionally total. In the first case, the operation is designed to re-establish communication between the posterior and anterior chambers; the second is rarely required.

An easy and safe procedure is the *ab externo incision* as an approach to the classical broad iridectomy (Fig. 27.5). A conjunctival flap is cut 3 mm from the limbus from 2

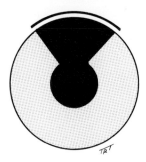

Fig. 27.5 Diagram of wound and coloboma in a sector iridectomy

to 10 o'clock. An incision is then made at the conjunctival reflection from 12.30 to 1.30 o'clock by a few strokes of the blade of a Bard–Parker knife to open the anterior chamber. The lens cannot be wounded since this opening is peripheral to its equator. When the incision enters the anterior chamber the iris presents in the wound or will do so on slight pressure on the cornea.

In a peripheral iridectomy the eye is gently rotated downwards by the superior rectus stitch, a conjunctival flap is turned down at 11 or 1 o'clock meridian with a sterile swab and the surgeon opens the globe by a small *ab externo* incision. A knuckle of iris is induced by pressure on the posterior lip of the wound to prolapse and a portion of the iris near its base is abscised leaving the sphincter intact. It should be possible to retain the anterior chamber during this manœuvre (Fig. 27.4).

Iridotomy

Consists of section of the iris without the abscission of any portion. It is employed for making a new pupil when the normal pupil is closed or has been drawn up to the wound of a faulty cataract extraction with incarceration of the pillars of the coloboma. A more effective method of reforming a pupil when the iris is drawn up to the wound is by a central iridectomy performed as shown in Figure 27.6.

Iridotomy in the treatment of primary closed-angle glaucoma may be carried out by a pulsed argon laser or by the Coherent 900 continuous-wave argon laser adapted to the Zeiss slit-lamp.

Division of anterior synechiae. This is a form of iridotomy. It is most easily done by the use of Lang's twin knives, two tiny but similar knives, one with a sharp point and blunt edges, the other with a blunt point and a sharp edge. The first is introduced through the cornea near the limbus some distance from the synechia at a point which provides a good fulcrum and then withdrawn. The second is introduced through the same puncture, with the sharp edge facing the synechia. These manœuvres should be done without losing aqueous. The second knife is then swept across the

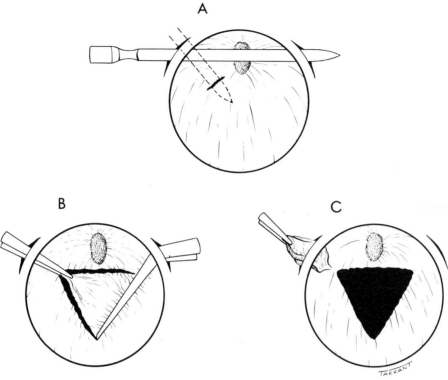

Fig. 27.6

synechia cutting it close to the cornea and then withdrawn. If the synechia is extensive, two or even more operations may be required, a portion of the adherent iris being severed each time.

OPERATIONS FOR SIMPLE GLAUCOMA

Sclerotomy

If puncture of the posterior segment of the globe is required it is usually most safely performed through the pars plana of the ciliary body 5–6 mm behind the limbus to avoid the risk of a retinal detachment.

Anterior sclerectomy

This is the name given to various operations for simple glaucoma in which a piece of sclera is excised to form a filtering scar. It will be convenient to note all the operations for simple glaucoma at this point although strictly speaking they are not all sclerectomies.

In *Elliot's trephining* a large flap of conjunctiva and Tenon's capsule is made, almost concentric with the margin of the cornea. The trephine (1.5–2 mm diam.) is applied, so that half the aperture lies on the cornea, the other half on the sclera. The corneo-scleral disc is cut by a few rotatory movements. When the anterior chamber is entered aqueous escapes, and the pupil is

displaced upwards. The trephine is removed, a knuckle of iris protrudes from the wound and the disc is forced out. The root of the iris is picked up with iris forceps, drawn slightly outwards and a small piece excised to form a peripheral iridectomy. The disc is then seized with Elliot's disc forceps and excised with spring scissors.

There is some tendency for iritis to develop immediately after trephining. Hence atropine and topical steroids should always be used daily for at least a week.

A contact lens placed on the eye with a haptic may prevent the development of an avascular bleb.

Owing to the prominence and thinness of the overlying conjunctiva *late infection* may occur long after the operation.

Other filtration operations, have been devised. In *Lagrange's operation* an ordinary iridectomy is performed with a Graefe Knife but before closing the wound a small piece of its anterior lip is snipped off without wounding the conjunctival flap. In *Scheie's operation* of cauterisation of the sclera with a peripheral iridectomy, more permanent drainage is usually ensured. The sclera is lightly cauterised along a line 1 mm behind the limbus underneath a reflected conjunctival flap, an incision is made with a knife along this line, the posterior lip of the wound thus made is again cauterised, the incision is completed to enter the anterior chamber, a peripheral iridectomy is performed and finally the conjunctival flap is sutured in place.

In *iridencleisis* a tongue of iris is incarcerated in a scleral incision near the limbus and partially severed from the main body of the iris to prevent the progressive bulging which tends to follow an iris prolapse.

In trabeculectomy (Fig. 27.7) a conjunctival flap is lowered and a trap-door of two third's thickness of sclera is fashioned so that it is 5 mm square and hinged at the limbus. A deeper trap-door measuring 4 mm square is fashioned to expose the ciliary body, the attachment of the ciliary body to the scleral spur and the root of the iris. This deep scleral flap is excised and peripheral iridectomy performed. The superficial flap is then sutured with two fine silk sutures and the conjunctiva closed by a key-pattern collagen running suture. Trabeculectomy probably acts by subconjunctival filtration helped by some drainage through the opened Canal of Schlemm.

In *cyclodialysis*, which is useful in aphakic eyes, a channel is opened up between the anterior chamber and the supra-choroidal space. Under a conjunctival flap an incision about 3 mm long is made in the sclera 4 mm behind and concentric with the corneo-scleral junction in the lower temporal quadrant. A spatula specially curved to fit the inner aspect of the sclera is inserted and passed forwards between the scleral spur and the ciliary body into the filtration angle, the point being tilted towards the sclera during the manoeuvre. Here it is swept transversely through a small arc, breaking down the adhesions between the root of the iris and the cornea. The conjunctival flap is sutured over the wound. Alternatively a small radial incision is made at 12 o'clock over the limbus and the ciliary body separated from the scleral spur by a spatula passed into the eye circumferentially. A basal iridectomy may be performed after separating two fifths of the circumference.

Partial destruction of the ciliary body. This is a further method of dealing with a recalcitrant case of glaucoma. This used to be done with diathermy (*cyclodiathermy*) whereby a partially penetrating or a surface electrode is used to make a ring of applications 3–6 mm behind the sclera. The entire ciliary body may be induced to undergo some degree of atrophy in this way, but an operation involving the whole ciliary body is best done in two or three stages. The first type of electrode is more safely

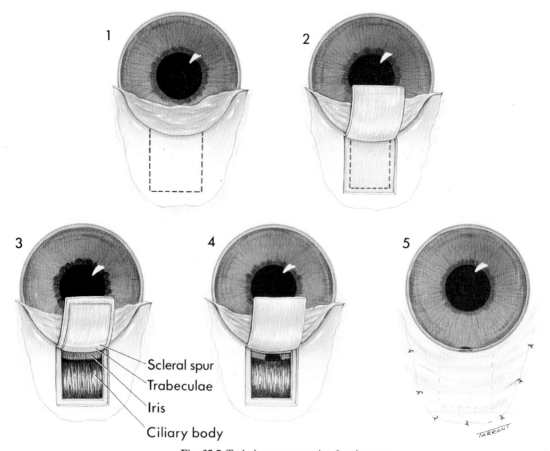

Scleral spur
Trabeculae
Iris
Ciliary body

Fig. 27.7 Trabulectomy operation for glaucoma

employed under a conjunctival flap; the second can be applied to the conjunctiva. An alternative procedure is to induce ciliary atrophy by *cryosurgery* through the conjunctiva placing a retinal probe over the ciliary body applying it for 60 seconds at a temperature of −70°C in six equidistant positions.

OPERATIONS FOR CATARACT

Aspiration

Aspiration by a microsurgical technique is the most suitable operation for cataract before the age of 15; it may be employed up to the age of 30, before the nucleus of the lens has become hard.

Aspiration of the soft lens in young patients requires a general anaesthetic; the pupil must be fully dilated with atropine and phenylephrine.

The globe is fixed by a silk stitch in the superior and inferior rectus muscle. A butterfly needle is attached to a container of saline by tubing and enters the anterior chamber by a horizontal track through the lower cornea. It is guarded by an assistant whose job is to maintain an anterior chamber of saline by raising or lowering the container. Continuous infusion with a 2-way Cannula and two syringes is an alternative method (Fig. 27.8).

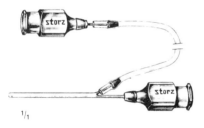

Fig. 27.8 Jensen–Thomas anterior capsule suction-irrigating cannula

A small limbal-based conjunctival flap is made above and an ab externo approach made with a Bard–Parker knife. A broad needle completes the incision and a silk suture passed through the anterior lip. A basal or peripheral iridectomy is performed and the anterior capsule incised just in front of the equator of the lens by an incision large enough to accommodate an 18-gauge bevelled needle. Lens matter is hydrated and then sucked out in the presence of an intact anterior chamber. The wound is closed and a sub-conjunctival injection of Gentisin and Betnesol is given. The pupil is kept dilated for 3 weeks and topical Predsol N drops applied three times each day.

Capsulotomy

This may be required if the capsule membrane thickens. This is best carried out by a Ziegler knife through an infused anterior chamber which keeps the vitreous in place. The knife is inserted through the capsule, run along for a very short distance and then cut in a forward direction until an effective gap has been achieved.

Lensectomy

Cataracts secondary to chronic anterior uveitis as occur in Still's disease present a particular problem. *Lensectomy*, by which lens material is cut and aspirated through a fine-bore needle is a simple and atraumatic technique applicable to this problem. A small limbal incision, which does not require suturing, has the advantage of reducing the risk of vitreous loss and the amount of surgically-induced astigmatism to a minimum. It is a technique also applicable to the treatment of traumatic, presenile and congenital or juvenile cataract. It is not suitable for the removal of calcified lenses or those with hard nuclei because of the danger of endothelial damage, loss of lens matter into the vitreous and possibly retinal detachment.

An oblique incision is made with a von Graefe knife at 10 o'clock just inside the limbus (Fig. 27.9). If the cataract is soft and suitable for lensectomy the corneal incision is enlarged to allow the introduction of the vitrectomy instrument (Fig. 27.10). As much of the lens matter as possible is removed keeping the tip of the instrument within the capsular bag to minimise excessive irrigation of the corneal endothelium by the infusion stream. Aspiration should be forceful so as to engage the lens material into the aspiration port. After the greater part of the lens has been aspirated the anterior capsule is removed (Fig. 27.11). Finally the posterior capsule is removed and a shallow anterior vitrectomy performed (Fig. 27.12). In eyes with congenital cataract uncomplicated by uveitis it is possible to leave the posterior capsule behind. Air is inserted into the anterior chamber and

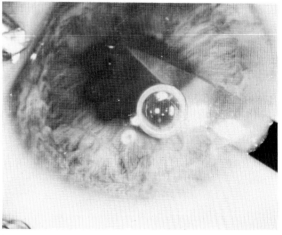

Fig. 27.9 Oblique incision with a Graefe knife. (By courtesy of J. J. Kanski.)

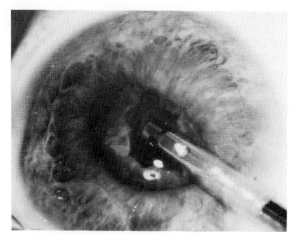

Fig. 27.10 Introduction of SITE vitrector. (By courtesy of J. J. Kanski.)

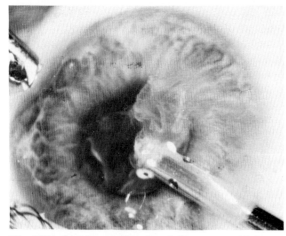

Fig. 27.11 Anterior capsule removed. (By courtesy of J. J. Kanski.)

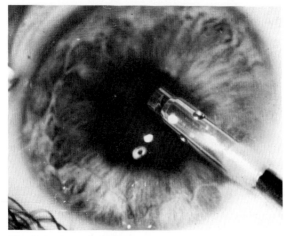

Fig. 27.12 Posterior capsule removed with anterior vitrectomy. (By courtesy of J. J. Kanski.)

no sutures are required for the corneal wound. The instruments employed in this technique are either the Klöti vitreous stripper or the Keeler–Federman S.I.T.E. – Suction Infusion Time Extractor.

These instruments are particularly useful when patients have small pupils with extensive posterior synechiae making access to the lens difficult. With the vitrectomy instruments it is possible to enlarge the pupil and remove all adhesions before the lens is aspirated.

Curette evacuation or linear extraction

This is the operation whereby after discission, whether accidental (traumatic cataract) or intentional, the softened lens matter is aspirated through a corneal or limbal incision.

Extraction of senile cataract

This may be performed by several methods. In extracapsular extraction the anterior capsule is opened the lens nucleus is expressed and the posterior capsule left behind so a subsequent needling may be required (p. 263). In intracapsular extraction the lens is removed in its capsule at one surgical intervention.

In the various types of operation the two common factors will be discussed first — the section and the use of sutures.

The section can be made in the classical way with the Graefe knife. A good section is an important factor in determining the success of the operation and more precise methods have been developed.

In the *ab externo* section a conjunctival flap 3 mm in breadth is dissected down to the limbus around the upper half of the cornea above the horizontal meridian and deflected downwards. While the eye is steadied by forceps a Bard–Parker knife with a D-blade incises the sclera 1 mm from the reflection of the conjunctiva through two-thirds of the depth of the sclera. A narrow flap of sclera is then fashioned by under-mining the anterior lip of the incision. When this has been done the anterior chamber is entered usually on the temporal side of the right and the nasal side of the left eye. Curved corneal scissors are inserted with one blade in the anterior chamber and the incision completed.

This technique provides great accuracy in the location of the section, a matter often of importance when pre-placed sutures are employed, and ensures protection by a broad and complete conjunctival flap.

Alternatively an *ab externo* incision may be made which is entirely corneal. A razor blade or diamond knife is used to cut through the anterior two-thirds of clear cornea just in front of the limbus. The incision is then completed by curved corneal scissors.

Sutures should always be used in cataract surgery. With efficient corneo-scleral suturing the patient can get up out of bed on the next day. A multitude of suturing techniques has been devised, many of them unnecessarily elaborate. For the *ab externo* approach three to five preplaced interrupted sutures of monofilament silk are necessary, while the conjunctival flap can be secured after the operation by a few post-placed conjunctival sutures. The corneo-scleral sutures are most safely inserted before the section is completed; they are left slack and tied after the lens is removed; if silk sutures are employed they are buried under the conjunctival flap.

Corneal incisions are best closed by a continuous 10.0 perlon suture whereby the deep bites are radial. The knot is buried in the wound so as to avoid irritation and the encouragement of vascularisation. The first bite of the incision is passed through the posterior lip of the wound and the last bite on the return half of the continuous suture passes through the anterior lip only. The suture is cut short and the knot slips into the depths of the corneal wound.

The injection of balanced salt solution into the anterior chamber through a fine-angled needle insinuated under the conjunctival flap at the end of the operation after the sutures have been tied, has some advantages. The chamber is re-formed immediately, the iris and vitreous pushed back to their original positions and the danger of prolapse of the iris lessened. A water-tight wound is desirable.

Extracapsular extraction. After the corneo-scleral sutures have been inserted and the section made, a peripheral iridectomy is performed.

The cystitome is introduced, the blade flat and the blunt curved edge leading, until the point is near the lowest part of the pupillary margin. The cutting edge is then directed backwards, the handle is slightly raised, and the lens capsule is incised vertically and horizontally. Alternatively the cystitome may make a series of serrated incisions in the anterior capsule in the form of a ring. During this manoeuvre the endothelium may be protected by a cushion of air or by the use of a cystitome which is hollowed to permit simultaneous perfusion of balanced salt solution. When the ring has been completed non-toothed iris forceps pick up the anterior layer of the capsule and remove it from the globe.

The cystitome is then taken in one hand, and the curette or the lens expressor in the hand corresponding to the eye being operated upon. The back of the curette or the lens expressor is placed horizontally upon the lower part of the limbus and gentle but firm pressure is made in a direction backwards and slightly upwards. This causes the nucleus of the lens to be tilted so that the upper edge appears presenting in the wound. The lens nucleus is coaxed out of the wound by continuing the pressure with the curette, but more and more in an upward direction. Meanwhile the lens may be gently helped out by the cystitome in the other hand. If there is much clear soft lens matter, this is coaxed out of the

wound by irrigation of the anterior chamber with balanced salt solution at body heat through a cannula inserted into the anterior chamber and attached to a syringe. More sophisticated instruments are now available to combine suction and irrigation such as the Cavitron Extraction–Irrigation System.

This instrument provides control of irrigation and aspiration by a vacuum control system whereby a sterile irrigating fluid is introduced into the anterior chamber to replace aspirated fluids and materials. The system allows an extracapsular procedure to be performed with an intact posterior capsule and a clean posterior chamber. All cortical matter should be removed. It is particularly liable to lie behind the iris in the 12 o'clock meridian. The iris repositor is now again used to free the iris from the angles of the wound and push back into the anterior chamber any tags of capsule which may be presenting. These are so transparent as to be invisible, and it is extremely important that they should not become incarcerated in the wound. Finally, the posterior capsule is cleared of adherent cells by a suffusing iris repositer with a roughened tip. Thus Elschnig's pearls are unlikely to develop. The corneo-scleral suture should then be tied, the conjunctival flap sutured to its normal position, atropine instilled and appropriate dressing applied.

Intracapsular extraction. After the section is made, two small peripheral iridectomies are performed. α-Chysmotrypsin is introduced by a cannula through the iridectomies so that the zonule may be lysed. Capsule forceps are introduced and the lens capsule grasped above just in front of the equator. Alternatively the cornea is lifted by an assistant, the anterior chamber dried by a triangle of spontex and the cryo-probe applied to the lens with the help of an iris retractor so as to form an iceball within the lens substance. The lens is then lifted slightly, rotated and is removed through the wound. As it is delivered isotonic sterile pilocarpine or miochol (acetyl-choline) is introduced from a syringe so as to ensure pupillary contraction. The sutures are then tied, the iris replaced and the conjunctival flap adjusted and sutured.

A complication which may occur during cataract extraction is prolapse of vitreous. In high myopes in whom vitreous may be lost care should be taken to prevent this occurence by the use of preoperative acetazoleamide 500 mg intravenously, an intravenous drip of 200 ml, Mannitol (20% solution) to deturgese the vitreous, a Fleiringa ring sewn onto the globe to avoid its collapse, the use of relaxants by the anaesthetist to prevent muscle spasm and a mechanical ventilator to avoid a rise in pCo_2. Digital pressure to soften an eye may also be employed.

If vitreous is lost the aim of the surgeon must be to perform a vitrectomy so that eventually the vitreous lies

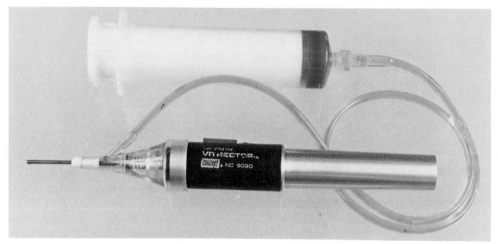

Fig. 27.13 Kaufman vitrector vitreous suction cutter

entirely behind the plane of the iris and well away from the wound. This is best achieved by the Kaufman Vitrector (Fig. 27.13). The cutting tip is inserted into the pupil just behind the iris with the cutting port posterior. The sterile disposable cutting head is attached to a syringe which is operated by an assistant, who sucks out enough vitreous to enable the remaining gel to lie behind the iris. The anterior chamber is reformed by B.S.S. after closure of the wound.

After-treatment. The patient lies quietly upon his back with his head and shoulders raised, in the semi-sitting (Fowler's) position, and is directed to avoid all straining. The slight amount of post-operative aching is readily controlled by sedatives. It is a wise precaution with restless patients to tie their hands loosely to the bed at night lest they knock or rub their eyes when they are half asleep.

On the day following the operation the eye is dressed using swabs with warm lotion and, in an extracapsular extraction, a drop of sterile 1% cyclopentolate solution instilled; this is not necessary in an intracapsular extraction in which the eye remains white. The wound is inspected, but should not be disturbed more than is absolutely necessary.

The cornea should be bright, and the pupil round. Faint greyness in the cornea above (striate opacity, p. 146) need cause no alarm.

It is wise to keep healthy patients who have had a general anaesthetic in bed for one day with the operated eye covered. If they show any signs of early mental disturbance or wandering in speech and the unoperated eye is blind, the operated eye should be uncovered and dark glasses substituted; this is safe in the presence of efficient suturing. Normally however, a light dressing is kept on for 1 day; afterwards tinted glasses are worn; temporary cataract glasses can be ordered at once and permanent spectacles in about 3 weeks.

The *post-operative complications* of cataract extraction are striate keratopathy (p. 146), incarceration of the iris in the angles of the wound, prolapse of the iris, iridocyclitis, secondary glaucoma, intra-ocular haemorrhage, infection of the wound and panophthalmitis.

Prolapse of the iris is most effectively prevented by iridectomy, the use of sutures and the injection of B.S.S. into the anterior chamber. It usually occurs in the first day or two, but may result later from injury to the eye by rubbing or knocking it, straining or coughing. It must be treated *at once* by abscission of the prolapse. As the iris is irritable the operation is painful, and general anaesthesia or retrobulbar local anaesthesia is generally necessary. The wound is reopened by insinuating the tip of an iris repositor under the conjunctival flap and gently uncovering the prolapse. The flap is turned down over the cornea, the iris pulled out with iris forceps and snipped off with de Wecker's scissors. The iris is then replaced with a clean repositor and the conjunctival flap brought back into position. A small subconjunctival knuckle of iris can sometimes be replaced by an iris repositor.

Delayed re-formation of the anterior chamber may be due to a leaking section, or be associated with choroidal and possibly ciliary body detachment with hyptonia. It is much less common in cataract extraction than after iridectomy or trephining for glaucoma. In these cases a leaking wound should be repaired. The administration of Diamox may be helpful and the injection of air into the anterior chamber with release of choroidal fluid is occasionally necessary in unresponding cases.

Expulsive haemorrhage is fortunately rare. It occurs during or soon after operation in old people with arteriosclerosis. There is sudden severe pain, and on removal of the dressings the wound is found to be gaping and filled with blood clot, vitreous, etc. The eye is always lost and should be excised. This may be necessary in order to stop the bleeding, the socket being then packed and firmly bandaged.

Septic infection may occasionally occur, especially in diabetic patients, from the twelfth to thirty-sixth hour after operation. There is severe aching pain, due to the accompanying acute iridocyclitis. On removing the dressing the upper lid is oedematous. When the lids are separated tears gush out and there is muco-pus in the conjunctival sac. The lids should be separated gently, if necessary with retractors. The cornea is then seen to be dull and hazy, especially in the upper part, the lip of the wound being yellow, intense iritis is present, the pupil and coloboma become filled with exudate, a hypopyon appears and, finally, the vitreous becomes infected and panophthalmitis leads to the destruction of the eye. Treatment as for panophthalmitis (p. 158) should be applied quickly and energetically and in severe cases vitrectomy should be considered. Iritis in mild degree probably occurs in all cases of extra-capsular cataract extraction. In its more pronounced form it is especially associated with retained lens matter (p. 263). The worst cases occur with acute septic infection or fungus infection.

Detachment of the choroid. See p. 168.

Secondary glaucoma may occur after cataract extraction usually due to pupillary blockage (relieved by a peripheral iridectomy at 6 o'clock), or peripheral anterior synechiae. Sometimes it is due to the anterior chamber's being lined with epithelium when there has been delay in healing and the corneal epithelium has grown down into the wound and spread over the surface of the iris, lens capsule and posterior cornea. Ingrowing epithelium is best treated by application of laser light to destroy the epithelium on the iris followed by cryotherapy to the epithelium on the back of the cornea over a bubble of air and wide removal of the dead epithelium on the iris by a vitrectomy instrument introduced by a pars plana approach. Glaucoma due to peripheral anterior synechiae is best treated by cyclodialysis. If it fails, repeated cryopexy may be tried.

Cystoid macular oedema (Fig. 27.14) is a common complication following cataract extraction. Typically visual acuity is initially good and then declines 4–12 weeks after extraction. A significant percentage of eyes presenting this complication have vitreous attached to the posterior surface of the wound. Perifoveal capillary leakage of fluorescein is present in 60% of patients who have had cataract extraction. In those eyes presenting vitreous attachment to the wound an anterior vitrectomy is worth considering. Indomethacin, a potent inhibitor of prostaglandin synthesis may be given as a prophylactic in doses of 25 mg orally four times daily for 4 weeks starting the day after surgery. Gastro-intestinal irritation is a common side-effect.

Intra-ocular lenses Implant surgery of an anterior

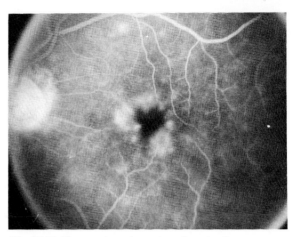

Fig. 27.14 Fluorescein angiography at 2 weeks after uncomplicated intracapsular extraction. Moderate perifoveal leakage is apparent 7 min after fluorescein injection. (By courtesy of Meredith.)

chamber lens, an iris clip lens or a posterior chamber lens is performed with the help of an operating microscope and a watertight closure of the wound is all important. Post-operative flat anterior chambers with plastic-endothelial contact give rise to corneal endothelial decompensation. Patients who suffer from uncontrolled glaucoma, overt corneal dystrophy, diabetes particularly in the young, retinal detachment in either eye, or if they possess only one eye are unsuitable for implantation.

Primary implantation may be carried out after intracapsular extraction providing a rapid return of visual function, although there may be a higher incidence of cystoid macular oedema by this method, a more noticeable endophthalmodonesis and a higher incidence of post-operative retinal detachment.

Planned extracapsular surgery offers capsular fixation by a two loop lens with a deep anterior chamber, a normal pupillary function, less prosthetic movement and a lower incidence of endothelial corneal dystrophy, cystoid maculopathy and retinal detachment. Some 20–30% of such operations require a subsequent capsulotomy.

An intraocular lens may be inserted secondarily sometime after cataract extraction using an anterior chamber lens.

Anterior chamber implants are inserted under general anaesthesia preceded by intravenous Acetazolamide 500 mg and 2% Pilocarpine drops. They are inserted diagonally or horizontally. A barrage of cautery is laid down about 1 mm behind the limbus to catch the limbal capillary plexus and avoid bleeding. The temporal section is made at the limbus large enough to accommodate the width of the lens. After insertion there may be some bulging of the iris between the feet of the inserted implant in which case a small peripheral iridectomy should be performed at that site. The wound is closed by interrupted 7–0 chromic catgut sutures. Air is injected to re-establish the anterior chamber and push the iris behind the plane of the implant.

The Choyce Mark VIII anterior chamber lens (Fig. 27.15a) can be used either as a primary or secondary implant. It is simple to insert and rests on the iris root posterior to the scleral spur. The Epstein–Copeland Maltese cross iris plane lens (Fig. 27.15c) is simple to insert but is prone to pupillary block glaucoma. The Binkhorst and Federov four-loop iris-supported lenses (Fig. 27.15d and e) can be used after intracapsular or

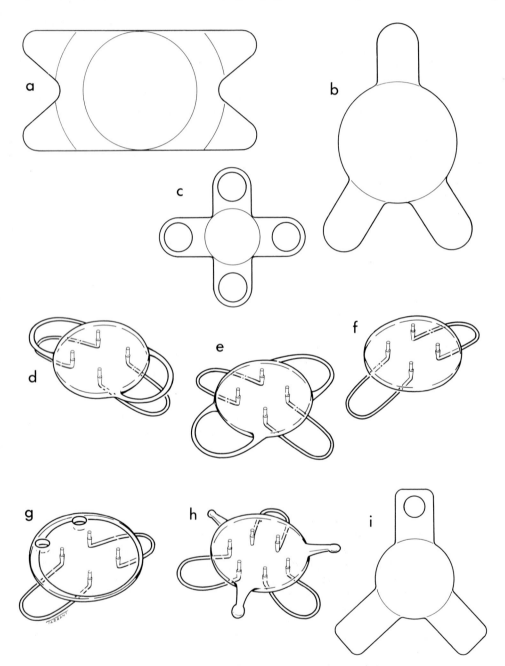

Fig. 27.15 a, Choyce lens (mark VIII); b, Ridley's tripod lens; c, Epstein–Copeland Maltese lens; d, Binkhorst 4-loop iris-clip lens; e, Federov iris-supported lens; f, Binkhorst 2-loop lens; g, Worst medallion lens; h, Federov sputnic lens; i, Pearce tripod posterior chamber lens

extracapsular extraction. Adequate peripheral iridectomies are essential to avoid pupillary block glaucoma. A
Binkhorst two-loop iridocapsular lens (Fig. 27.15f) is
used after extracapsular extraction. The Worst medallion lens (Fig. 27.15g) is also suitable for intracapsular
or extracapsular extraction and is sutured to the iris.
Posterior chamber lenses include the Pearce tripod and
bipod posterior chamber lens, used after extracapsular
extraction with or without direct iris suture fixation
(Fig. 27.15i), and the J-loop Sinsky posterior chamber
lens which lies in the capsular bag and is uniplaned.

Development of a safe permanent-wear soft contact
lens giving the same optical qualities as an intraocular
lens may make implantation an unnecessary risk. A conservative approach to intraocular lens implantation consists of a selection of suitable patients over the age of 65,
and the avoidance of monocular patients.

Results of intraocular lens implantation are excellent.
A corneal incision with a diamond knife, discission of the
anterior capsule with a suffusing cystitome, using the
'can opener' method, and removal of the anterior layer
with non-toothed forceps leads to easy removal of the
nucleus through an enlarged corneal incision. All the remaining lens matter can then be removed by irrigation
with suction and all cells adherent to the posterior capsule may be evacuated by mild friction. A posterior
chamber implant made entirely of methyl methacrylate
can be put into the capsular bag through a protective
layer of Healonid, which leaves the corneal epithelium
untouched. The lower loop of the lens is placed behind
the iris and the upper loop wheeled into a horizontal position by gentle rotation. A peripheral iridectomy is usually
required. Miochol contracts the pupil and washes out the
Healonid. The wound is brought together by a continuous nylon suture with a buried knot. A subconjunctival injection of Genticin 20 mg is given. Pilocarpine 2% drops are placed in the conjunctival sac before the eye is padded.

The patient, after recovery, returns to the ward: the
pad is removed next day and the patient discharged
home. The stitch is only removed if it disturbs the patient after a 6 weeks' period or if it induces above average
astigmatism. Even the most enthusiastic contact lens
practitioner would find it difficult to compete with the
results of such a method and it will be remembered that
the implanted lens lies in exactly the same position as the
normal crystalline lens which has been removed. The
presence of a small peripheral iridectomy makes the eye
look cosmetically attractive as well as thoroughly
efficient.

Phako emulsification performed through a small limbal incision offers a safe method of performing extracapsular extraction in young people with a soft nucleus
and in high myopes. In the average patient with cataract,
however, it has nothing more to offer.

OPERATIONS FOR RETINAL DETACHMENT

Operations for retinal detachment can only be performed after accurate localisation of the retinal hole
(p. 218). Anaesthetic drops should not be used to
attain analgesia since they cloud the cornea and preclude
accurate ophthalmoscopic examination. General anæsthesia is the method of choice.

In the operation using surgery a flap of conjunctiva
and Tenon's capsule is reflected over the site of the
retinal hole. Owing to the fact that the cryoprobe can, if
required, be slipped under an extra-ocular muscle, it is
rarely necessary to reflect these unless a posterior position of the retinal hole makes it necessary to rotate the
eye to an extreme degree to gain access to the site. An
application of the probe is then made at the presumptive
site of the retinal lesion and the intensity and location of
the reaction checked by indirect ophthalmoscopic examination. Its relationshiop to the retinal lesion determines
the sites of further applications of the probe. After satisfactory circumvallation of the hole or holes an ophthalmoscopic examination should show apposition of the
retina to the choroid; if it is not so apposed a scleral
plomb should be applied and apposition ensured if
necessary by the use of air introduced through a separa-
ate perforation in the region of the pars plana to force
the retina against the choroid mounted on the plomb.
Both eyes are bandaged, and the head is immobilised in
a position such that the torn portion of the retina tends
to fall gravitationally on the underlying choroid. In
favourable cases adhesion between retina and choroid is
fairly firm in two days but for some time care must be
taken not to jeopardise its security by undue physical
exertion.

A third technique is to cause a choroidal burn by
light-coagulation in the region of the retinal hole. Since
the light is absorbed by the pigmentary epithelium, this
is only effective if the detachment is shallow and the
hole is not too peripheral.

A fourth technique involves a scleral buckling operation, wherein the sclera is indented over the retinal hole
by stitching onto it an implant of silicone rubber. In
such cases subretinal fluid does not need to be released
if the hole is well mounted and the central retinal artery
circulation is not compromised. If the central retinal
artery is pulsating or reduced in calibre indicating functional obstruction of flow, the intra-ocular pressure may
be reduced by paracentesis and diamox intravenously. In
addition, when there are many holes, an encircling
operation may be tried; a band of silicone rubber is passed round the eye beneath the rectus muscles and tied
after release of some subretinal fluid so as to produce a
circumferential buckle. In these cases also further adhesions between the retina and the choroid can be ensured
by light-coagulation or cryosurgery. This encircling pro-

cedure may be used prophylactically in the second eye if the first presents with a non-traumatic giant tear. The complications of retinal surgery are macular pucker, massive vitreous retraction (p. 185) and anterior segment ischaemia.

A fifth technique is applicable when vitreous traction is the cause of a persistent detachment. In such cases vitrectomy is required to break the pulling force on the retina combined with vitreous replacement with liquid silicone to act as an internal support.

EXCISION OF THE EYEBALL

It is mandatory to mark the forehead above the eye to be removed before the anaesthetic is administered, and to reexamine the fundus immediately before surgery.

A general anaesthetic is always given. The technique is as follows:-

After the speculum is inserted, the surgeon seizes the conjunctiva just outside the limbus at the upper part of the cornea with fixation forceps and incises it here with blunt-pointed scissors, one blade being passed under the conjunctiva as far as possible round the cornea. By carrying the point out under the looser bulbar conjunctiva it may be taken a third of the distance round the circumference; the edge is then brought close up to the limbus before the conjunctiva is divided. The manoeuvre is repeated on the other side of the cornea. Finally, the portion below the cornea is divided. The conjunctiva should be divided completely round the cornea, and close to it, in three or four cuts. The peripheral edge of the cut conjunctiva is then taken up by the forceps, and the bulbar conjunctiva is separated from the globe as far back as the equator in all directions by a series of small snips, the blades of the scissors being kept flat in close contact with the eyeball. In this manner the capsule of Tenon is simultaneously opened.

The tenotomy hook is then taken in the left hand, the scissors being retained in the right. The rectus muscles are taken up one by one and divided close to the globe. It is well to begin with the superior rectus, since it is the most difficult to reach. The tendon of the lateral rectus of the right eye or the medial rectus of the left eye should be left long. The obliques are found by passing the hook farther back and carrying it round close to the globe.

The speculum is then taken and held widely open and pressed back into the orbit. If the muscles have been properly divided the globe springs forwards between the blades of the speculum. If it does not do so the speculum is removed and the eye dislocated by pushing the lids behind it with the fingers; in children, in whom the orbit is small in relation to the size of the globe, it may

be necessary to lever it out with the points of the excision scissors. The heavy excision scissors are taken in the right hand, the appropriate long tendon stump seized with toothed forceps and the globe pulled forward and rotated towards the left side of the patient so that the optic nerve is easily reached. The points of the closed scissors are passed into the orbit — to the outer side of the eye on the right side, to the inner on the left. The optic nerve is felt with the closed scissors: it is easily recognised. The scissors are withdrawn a short distance, opened, and the blades pushed down, one on each side of the nerve, which is then divided; the sensation of dividing the nerve is unmistakable. The eyeball can then be freely drawn forwards so that any remnants of the obliques still attached to the globe can be divided close to the eye. To control bleeding, the inside of the muscle cone is packed with gauze wrung out in hot saline and pressure kept up for two or three minutes. The edges of the conjunctiva are then drawn together by a continuous silk suture, antibiotic ointment inserted, the lids closed, and the dressing applied with firm pressure. This should consist of a small spherical pad of gauze, then a round flat pad of sterilised or cyanide gauze, then a thick round pad of sterilised wool. The bandage is applied also with firm pressure. The patient is kept in bed for one or two days. The suture is removed after forty-eight hours. Subsequently there is always some mucoid secretion which necessitates washing out the orbit twice a day with an astringent lotion.

If the globe is perforated and collapsed the rupture should be closed by sutures before proceeding to excise the eye.

It is easy to cut the sclera instead of the nerve, especially with curved excision scissors. Particularly when the nerve has to be cut long, as in excision for neoplasms, it is preferable to use straight scissors and to pass them along the inner wall of the orbit; indeed, straight instruments should always be used in preference to curved when possible, because it is easier to judge the position of the point.

Evisceration of the eyeball. This is recommended only in some cases of panophthalmitis (*q.v.*) in order to prevent the extension of the infection up the optic nerve sheaths.

In this operation an opening is made into the cornea which is then removed with scissors and all the intraocular contents are scooped out, the inner surface of the sclera being thoroughly cleansed with a swab. If the entire sclera is left there is considerable reaction and delayed healing. These disadvantages may be obviated by cutting the insertions of the extra-ocular muscles and excising the greater part of the sclera, leaving only a small collar of it around the optic nerve so as to leave the nerve sheaths unopened (*frill excision*).

Excision with the introduction of an implant. This has

the advantage that it provides support for the artificial eye, making it look less sunken and endowing it with some mobility so that the simulation of a real eye is closer. All implants, however, unless firmly fixed and buried, have a tendency subsequently to be expelled.

The simplest technique is to bury a plastic implant in Tenon's capsule and to it the extra-ocular muscles are sutured. Cat-gut sutures are pre-placed in the muscle tendons before these are cut and the implant secured by suturing Tenon's capsule and the conjunctiva over it.

The Allen implant makes use of a magnet to keep the extra-conjunctival part of the prosthesis in close approximation to the implant.

An *artificial eye* of plastic should not be worn less than 2 weeks after excision. A small eye may be worn for an hour or two a day until the conjunctiva becomes used to the foreign body. Eight or nine weeks after the operation a full-sized eye may be worn; a plastic eye need be taken out and washed only once a week.

Contracted socket is the result of injury, faulty excision, cellulitis in the orbital tissues, or the continued wearing of a rough artificial eye. The first three causes lead to the formation of dense cicatricial bands across the socket, rendering the wearing of a prosthesis impossible. The last cause usually results in obliteration of the lower fornix, so that the eye cannot be kept in place.

Contracted sockets are difficult to remedy. It is easy to divide the bands and make a new groove to hold the eye in position, but unless the wounds become covered with epithelium the edges heal together and no improvement is produced. A thorough dissection of all fibrous bands should be made, and the raw surface covered by a Stent mould. The Stent is cooled *in situ* by drops of cold saline and removed. A clamp is applied to the lower lip, which is then everted to expose its inner aspect. The Stent mould is placed over this, and a graft of buccal mucous tissue nearly twice the size is cut. The submucous tissue is dissected off and the graft sutured in position in the orbit. The Stent is secured in place over this by mattress sutures; the eyelids are closed and covered with a dressing of tulle-gras gauze wrung out in saline, and a pad and bandage are applied. This grafting procedure, however, is not by any means invariably successful.

In bad cases of contracted socket restoration can only be obtained by dissecting away all the remaining conjunctiva and fibrous tissue and grafting an ample split-skin graft with the aid of a Stent mould. In skin-grafted sockets, however, there is always an unpleasant discharge and smell from desquamating epithelium, and it is usually preferable in such cases to close the lids with a permanent tarsorrhaphy or wear a prosthesis attached to a pair of spectacles, leaving the socket alone.

EXENTERATION OF THE ORBIT

See p. 338.

Disorders of motility of the eyes

28

Anatomy and physiology of the motor mechanism

If each eye is to be rapidly and accurately fixed upon any object so that its image is thrown upon the fovea, and if the two eyes in their every movement are to move in unison so that binocular vision is to be attained, it is obvious that their motility and co-ordination must be subserved by an unusually accurate and responsive neuromuscular apparatus. We shall first study the extra-ocular muscles and then their central nervous control.

The extra-ocular muscles
A team of six muscles controls the movements of each eye. Four of them, the *rectus muscles*, have the general action of rotating the eye in the four cardinal directions — up, down, out and in (Fig. 28.1A). They arise in a fibrous ring around the optic foramen to the nasal side of the axis of the eye and run to be inserted in the sclera by flat tendinous insertions about 10 mm broad. The medial rectus is inserted into the sclera about 5.5 mm to the nasal side of the corneo-scleral margin, the inferior rectus 6.6 mm below, the lateral rectus 7 mm to the temporal side, and the superior rectus 7.75 mm above (Fig. 28.2). The *oblique muscles*, the primary function of which is rotation of the globe, are differently arranged (Fig. 28.1B). The superior oblique arises from the common origin at the apex of the orbit, runs forwards to the trochlea, a cartilaginous ring at the upper and inner angle of the orbit and, having threaded through this, becomes tendinous; the tendon changes its direction completely and runs over the globe under the superior rectus to attach itself above and lateral to the posterior pole (Fig. 28.3). The action of the muscle is thus determined by the oblique direction of its tendon after it has left the trochlea. The inferior oblique maintains a similar direction throughout its course and is the only muscle not rising from the apex of the orbit. It arises anteriorly from the lower and inner orbital walls near the lacrimal fossa and, running below the inferior rectus, finds an insertion in the sclera below and lateral to the posterior pole of the globe.

In order to control their movements all these mucles are provided with fascial *check ligaments* intimately connected with Tenon's capsule and the periosteum.

The action of the extra-ocular muscles
These rotate the eye around a *centre of rotation*, which lies in the horizontal plane some 12 or 13 mm behind the cornea, and in every movement of the globe every muscle is involved in some degree, either by contraction or inhibition. Three types of rotation or 'degrees of freedom' are possible around the centre of rotation:

1. Rotation around the vertical axis whereby the globe is turned from side to side.
2. Rotation around the horizontal axis whereby the globe is turned upwards and downwards.
3. Rotation around the antero-posterior axis — an involuntary movement of *torsion:* intorsion when the upper pole of the cornea rotates nasally, extorsion when temporally.

When the medial or lateral rectus acts it rotates the eye horizontally inwards or outwards. Owing to the obliquity of their course, however, contraction of the superior and inferior recti must involve torsion (Fig. 28. 4A and B). Thus, when the superior rectus acts upon the globe in the primary position, it not only pulls the eye upwards, but also inwards and intorts it. Similarly when the inferior rectus acts the eye is pulled down and in and extorted. Since the obliques are inserted behind the centre of rotation, their direction of action is from behind forwards and inwards. When the superior oblique contracts, therefore, if the globe is in the primary position the main effect is intorsion, but it also rotates the eye downwards and outwards; the inferior oblique causes primarily extorsion but rotates the globe upwards and outwards. The mechanism is so arranged that when the superior rectus and inferior oblique act simultaneously the eye moves directly upwards, the upward movement caused by each muscle being summated, while the inward movement and torsion of the superior rectus are exactly compensated by the outward movement and contrary torsion of the inferior oblique. Similarly when the inferior rectus and superior oblique act simultaneously the eye moves directly downwards.

Every movement of the eyeball is thus a synkinesis.

Not only is there uniocular synkinesis: in normal circumstances there is always also binocular synkinesis.

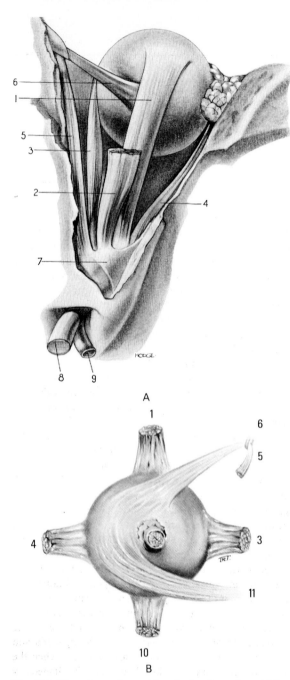

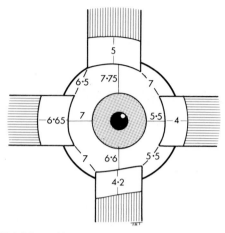

Fig. 28.2 Lines of insertion of the rectus muscles of right eye seen from the front

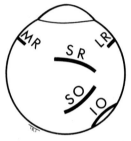

Fig. 28.3 Lines of insertion of the superior and inferior oblique muscles and of the superior, medial and lateral recti of right eye, seen from above

Fig. 28.1 The extra-ocular muscles: A, view from above (right eye); B, view from behind (left eye). 1, superior rectus; 2, levator palpebræ superioris; 3, medial rectus; 4, lateral rectus; 5, superior oblique; 6, reflected tendon of superior oblique; 7, annulus of Zinn; 8, optic nerve; 9, ophthalmic artery; 10, inferior rectus; 11, inferior oblique

Abduction of one eye is accompanied by adduction of the other — conjugate deviation; elevation or depression of one eye is always accompanied by elevation or depression respectively of the other. The only exception to this rule is the bilateral adduction of the eyes in convergence. Elevation of both eyes is accompanied by slight abduction (divergence), depression by slight adduction (convergence).

In these movements the muscles which contract together are called *synergists*; those which suffer inhibition, *antagonists*. The correlation may be summarised thus:

In rotation to the right — synergists: R. lat. rectus, L. med. rectus. Antagonists: R. med. rectus, L. lat. rectus.

In rotation to the left — synergists: L. lat. rectus, R. med. rectus. Antagonists: L. med. rectus, R. lat. rectus.

In rotation upwards — synergists: R. and L. superior recti primarily, R. and L. inf. obliques secondarily. Antagonists: R. and L. inf. recti, R. and L. sup. obliques.

In rotation downwards — synergists: R. and L. inf. recti primarily, R. and L. sup. obliques secondarily. Antagonists: R. and L. superior recti primarily, R. and L. inf. obliques secondarily.

The *nervous control of the ocular movements* is complicated. The muscles are supplied by nerves arising from nuclei in the mid-brain. Their action is co-ordinated by

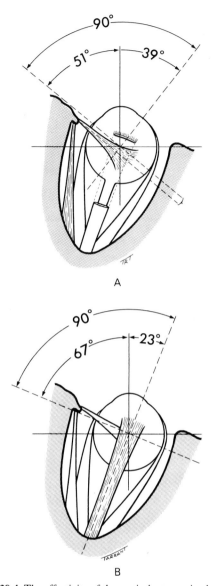

Fig. 28.4 The effectivity of the vertical rotators in elevation. When the visual axis lies in the muscle plane, rotation upwards will be maximal; in this position there is one direction of movement only — upwards and downwards; the further the visual axis is removed from this position, the more effective the muscle becomes in torsion. A, The superior (or inferior) oblique is 100% effective in depression (or elevation) when the eye is adducted 51°. It is ineffective when the eye is abducted 39°. B, The superior (or inferior) rectus is 100% effective in elevation (or depression) when the eye is abducted 23°. It is ineffective when the eye is adducted 67°. In the primary position three-quarters of its efficiency is devoted to vertical rotation and one-quarter to torsion

intermediate 'centres' situated in this region by which reflex activities are governed. Finally these intermediate centres are linked with the vestibular apparatus whereby they become associated with the equilibration reflexes,

and also with the cerebral cortex so that voluntary movements and participation in the higher reflexes involving perception become possible (Fig. 28.7).

The oculomotor, or third cranial nerve, supplies all the extrinsic muscles except the lateral rectus and superior oblique: it also supplies the sphincter pupillæ and ciliary muscle. The superior oblique is supplied by the fourth (trochlear) nerve, and the lateral rectus by the sixth (abducens) nerve.

The third and fourth nuclei form a large continous mass of nerve cells situated near the middle line in the floor of the aqueduct of Sylvius beneath the superior colliculus (Fig. 28.5). The cells nearest the middle line towards the anterior part of the third nucleus are smaller than the others: they form the Edinger–Westphal (and Perlia's) nucleus which probably supplies fibres to the ciliary muscle (accommodation) and sphincter pupillæ (constriction of the pupil). The main mass of the large-celled nucleus is composite, divided into cell-masses subserving the individual extrinsic ocular muscles as is seen in Fig. 28.5. The levator palpebrae is represented most caudally, while abduction is relegated to the sixth nucleus, situated much farther caudally in the brain-stem. There is little decussation of the fibres from the third nuclei of the two sides in their anterior parts, but a considerable amount in the posterior part.

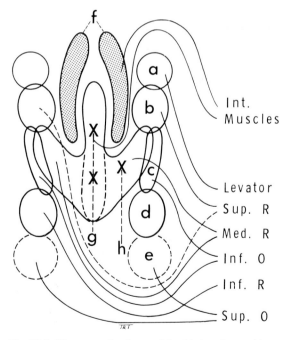

Fig. 28.5 Diagrammatic scheme of the third nucleus and its associated cell groups (after Brouwer): a, levator palpebrae; b, superior rectus; c, inferior oblique; d, inferior rectus; e, superior oblique–nerve IV; f, intrinsic ocular muscles (sphincter of iris and ciliary muscles); g, medial rectus–convergence; h, medial rectus–inward movement

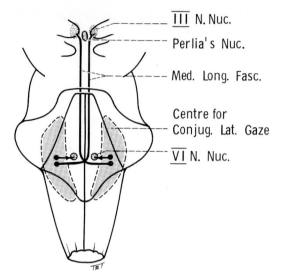

III N. Nuc.

Perlia's Nuc.

Med. Long. Fasc.

Centre for Conjug. Lat. Gaze

VI N. Nuc.

Fig. 28.6 Diagrammatic representation of dorsal surface of the brain stem showing the connection of the pointine centers for conjugate lateral gaze with the abducens nuclei and with the oculomotor nuclei by way of the medial longitudinal fasciculus

The fourth nerve is unique among motor nerves in having a dorsal decussation. Nearly, if not quite all the fibres decussate in the superior medullary velum and are distributed to the superior oblique muscle of the opposite side.

The sixth nucleus is in the immediate vicinity of the facial (seventh) nucleus (Fig. 28.6), the fibres from which make a large bend around it. Hence vascular and other lesions of the sixth nucleus are very liable to be accompanied by facial paralysis on the same side. All the fibres of the sixth nerve are distributed to the ipsilateral lateral rectus.

The peculiarities of distribution of the fibres from the third, fourth and sixth nuclei to muscles partly on one side and partly on the opposite side of the body show that the nervous mechanism of co-ordination of these muscles is extremely complex.

The *intermediary mechanism* co-ordinating the activities of these nuclei is also complex. The nuclei are interconnected to a considerable extent by fibres participating in the *posterior longitudinal bundle* (Fig. 28.8), a large and important tract of nerve fibres derived in part from the anterior columns of the spinal cord, lying in close relation to the third, fourth and sixth nuclei. These fibres have important functions in the co-ordination of movements and equilibration, which are so intimately related with vision. The nuclei are also inter-related through this bundle so that co-ordination of the two eyes is maintained. One of the most important of such connections is the fibres which link up the sixth nucleus of one side with the third nucleus of the other.

In this region there are 'centres' which control conjugate movements.

There is a centre controlling horizontal conjugate movements in the neighbourhood of the sixth nucleus; an area controlling vertical movements lies just above the two third nerve nuclei and is involved in the early development of a pinealoma; the centre for convergence

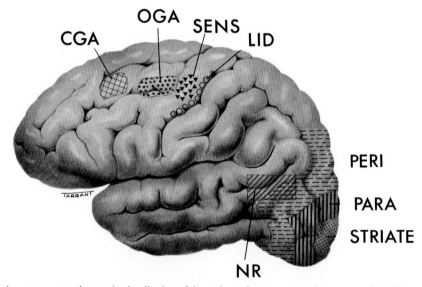

CGA OGA SENS LID

PERI

PARA

STRIATE

NR

Fig. 28.7 The ocular motor areas. A tentative localisation of the main ocular motor areas in part transferred from the brain of primates to that of man. It is to be noted that the apparently accurate localisation of certain areas is by no means factual or constant. CGA, cephalogyric area, OGA, oculogyric area. LID, lid movement area. PARA, parastriate area (area 18). NR, approximate area for convergence and the near reflexes (in the macaque) (areas 19 and 22), PERI, peristriate area (area 19). STRIATE, striate area (area 17). SENS oculo-sensory area

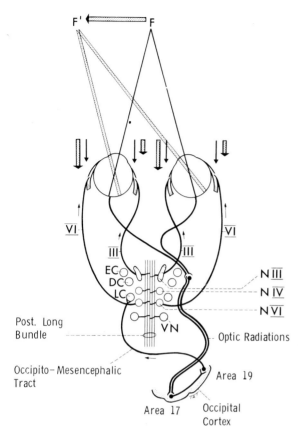

F' F

VI   VI

III   III

EC
DC
LC

N III
N IV
N VI

Post. Long
Bundle

VN

Optic Radiations

Occipito–Mesencephalic
Tract

Area 19

Area 17   Occipital
Cortex

Fig. 28.8 The organisation of the psycho-optical reflexes
(fixation, refixation, fusional, etc.). So long as the fixation point
(F) is imaged on each macula, the fixation reflex maintains the
posture of the eyes steady by an equality of muscular tone
(black arrows). If, however, F is moved to F', the retina on the
right of the macula is stimulated and sets up a refixation reflex.
The afferent path is: (a) retinæ — optic nerves — chiasma —
right optic tract; (b) lateral geniculate body — right optic
radiations — striate area of occipital cortex; (c) peristriate
occipital cortex. The efferent path is conjectural, but traverses
the posterior part of the optic radiations and reaches the
opposite cerebral peduncle where connection is made with the
vestibular nucleus (VN), the mid-brain ocular motor centres
governing conjugate elevation, depression and lateral
movements (EC, DC, LC), whence impulses are relayed
through the posterior longitudinal bundle to the ocular motor
nuclei (III, IV, VI). In the present case, acting essentially
through the left VIth and the branch of the right IIIrd to the
medial rectus, the muscular tone is altered (broken arrows) to
orientate the eyes so that F' again falls on each macula

is associated with the third nerve nucleus and almost
certainly lies in the Edinger-Westphal complex; and an
area co-ordinating divergence possibly exists.

This elaborate mechanism in the mid-brain is controlled from three sources, one voluntary and three
reflex.

1. *Voluntary ocular movements* are initiated in the
pyramidal cells of the motor area of the frontal cortex in
the second and third frontal convolutions of both sides

(Fig. 28.7). The fibres enter the knee of the internal
capsule as part of the pyramidal tract close to the fibres
governing facial movements and break off in the mid-
brain, first the fibres for vertical movements (and movements of the upper lid) and then those for lateral movements. These fibres control conjugate movements, vertical and horizontal, of both eyes; movements of individual muscles are not represented in the cortex. Stimulation of the cortex or the tracts therefore produces
conjugate movements of the eyes to the opposite side;
destruction, paralysis of voluntary conjugate movements
away from the side injured, in either case without involving disalignment of the eyes or diplopia. These pathways
are tested clinically by asking the patient to look to the
right, left, up or down. A destructive lesion in the right
prefrontal lobe would lead to an inability to look con-
jugately to the left. When the patient is asleep the eyes
would be found in the position of right conjugate gaze
(the eyes are looking towards the lesion).

2. The involuntary reflexes which depend on vision
(fixation, fusional movements, convergence, etc.) — the
psycho-optical reflexes — are centred in the visual cortex
of the occipital lobe (Fig. 28.7). The afferent path for
these reflexes is the visual pathway; the efferent runs
down the optic radiations to the posterior longitudinal
bundle (Fig. 28.8) and thence to the ocular motor nuclei. These pathways are tested by asking the patient to
follow an object which is passed horizontally and vertically so that the conjugate following movements of the
eyes may be elicited.

3. An elaborate system of *stato-kinetic reflexes* of great
phylogenetic antiquity co-ordinates the position of the
eyes when the head is moved in space; their afferent
path runs from the semicircular canals of the inner ear
to the mid-brain centres. They induce conjugate movements of both eyes, a slow tonic movement in the direction of equilibration and a quick return (nystagmus).
This pathway is tested by passive movements of the
head. If the chin is depressed the eyes normally elevate
if fixation is maintained and if the head is rotated on a
vertical axis the eyes maintain fixation as a result of the
stato-kinetic reflexes. These movements are often referred to as 'doll's-head' movements and they may be selectively maintained when voluntary conjugate gaze and
following conjugate gaze are disturbed as in the Silvian
aqueduct syndrome.

4. A similar system of *static reflexes* co-ordinates
movements of the eyes in respect of movements of the
head upon the body. They are mediated mainly by
proprioceptive impulses from the neck muscles which
are linked with the ocular motor centres through the
posterior longitudinal bundle. A unilateral lesion of
the posterior longitudinal fasciculus produces a characteristic clinical picture known as *internuclear ophthalmoplegia* consisting of paresis of the ipsilateral medial

rectus on attempted conjugate lateral gaze. One medial rectus only is involved unless the lesion is bilateral. The medial rectus however is still capable of acting on convergence. On gazing to each side there is a relative lag of the adducting eye and a monocular nystagmus of the abducting eye (ataxic nystagmus). Multiple sclerosis is the common cause of bilateral internuclear ophthalmoplegia and a vascular occlusion often associated with diabetes is the commonest cause of a unilateral internuclear ophthalmoplegia.

Skew deviation is a hypertropia that is referrable to neither a peripheral neuromuscular lesion nor to a local mechanical factor in the orbit. Lesions within the central nervous system cause skew deviation but evidence is scanty for localisation, other than in the general region of the posterior fossa.

Skew deviation is characterised by a maintained deviation of one eye above the other, frequently fixed for all directions of gaze but equally often variable for different directions of gaze. It may simulate palsies of individual vertically-acting muscles and be differentiated from these only through the absence of mid-brain or peripheral nerve disease.

Skew deviation may occur with any lesion of the brain stem or cerebellum but is more common with unilateral than with bilateral lesions. It is characteristically present with unilateral internuclear ophthalmoplegia. The eye on the side of the lesion is usually hypotropic. The fact that a vertical divergence occurs on stimulating the labyrinth or with unilateral labyrinthine disease suggests that the pathogenesis of skew deviation is linked with the vestibulo-ocular pathways. It is found with cerebellar tumours, acoustic neuromas, compressive lesions, platybasia and vascular accidents of the pons and cerebellum (especially thrombosis of the cerebellar and pontine arteries). It is infrequent with demyelinating lesions.

Fixation and binocular vision

We have already seen that the image of an external object on the retina is determined by a line passing from the object through the nodal point of the eye. Conversely an object is *projected* in space along the line passing through the retinal image and the nodal point. When a distant object is looked at the visual axes are practically parallel; the object forms an image upon each fovea centralis. Any other object to one side forms its retinal images upon the temporal side of one retina and upon the nasal side of the other; these retinal areas are co-ordinated visually in the occipital cortex so that such an object is seen with both eyes as a single object. These are known as *corresponding points*, the most important pair of which, of course, is the foveae. Points on the two retinae which are not corresponding points in this sense of the term are called *disparate points*, and if an object forms its retinal images thereon it will be seen double (binocular diplopia). If the disparity is slight there is a tendency to move the eyes so that the images may be fused by means of the fusion reflexes from the occipital cortex.

Since the most accurate vision is attained by the foveae it is necessary that the eyes be rapidly orientated so that the image of an object of interest falls upon them or that of a moving object be retained on them. This ascendancy of the foveae is maintained by the *fixation reflex* (Fig. 28.8) and whenever the image leaves the foveae, the eyes are at once reorientated so that it falls upon them. The activity of this reflex is demonstrated by the rapid to-and-fro movements of the eyes of a person looking out of the window of a moving train, and can be demonstrated clinically by regarding a revolving drum or a moving tape on which black and white stripes are painted (*optokinetic nystagmus*). The latter phenomenon can be used as a test to demonstrate the integrity of the reflex paths.

The same reflex produces *involuntary fusional movements* of the eyes to maintain single binocular vision. They may be demonstrated clinically by placing a small prism in front of one eye while the patient regards a distant light. The eye will at once turn out of the primary position to allow the deflected rays to fall again upon the fovea. The strongest deviation which can thus be overcome is a measure of the *reflex fusional capacity* (Fig. 28.12A and B). A prism bar consists of a battery of prisms of increasing strength and is a convenient instrument in clinical testing (Fig. 28.9).

Binocular vision

In view of the distance between the two eyes it is obvious that the retinal images of both eyes cannot be identical since each eye regards a slightly different aspect of any object observed. If the object is a solid body the right eye sees a little more of the right side of the object, and *vice versa*. The two images are fused psychological, and this fusion of the slightly diverse images, combined with other facts derived from experience, enables the person to appreciate the solidity of objects.

Moreover, it is obvious from Fig. 28.10 that if an object is regarded, the images of other objects nearer or further away cannot fall upon corresponding points. If their projection through the nodal point is continued to the retina, it is seen that the images of objects nearer than the object of fixation fall on the temporal side, those farther away to the nasal side of the fovea. This can be easily demonstrated by holding a pencil in front of the eyes: if the pencil is fixated, more distant objects appear doubled; if a distant object is fixated, the pencil appears doubled. It will be found in this way that near objects suffer a *crossed (heteronymous) diplopia*; distant

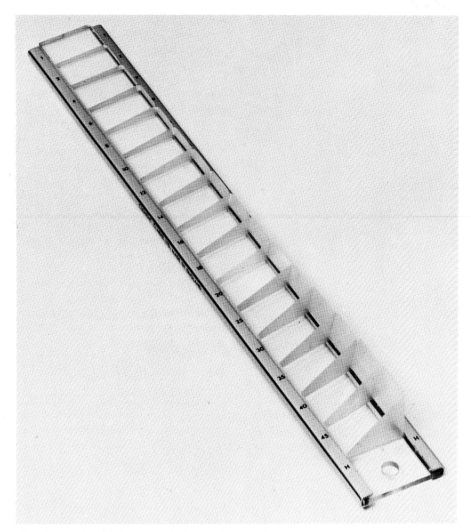

Fig. 28.9 Prism bar, (By courtesy of Clement Clarke International Ltd.)

objects an *uncrossed (homonymous) diplopia*. This diplopia is physiological and is perceptually suppressed in actual vision, but it produces a psychological impression

which is translated into appreciation of distance. It follows that accuracy of stereoscopic vision depends upon good sight with both eyes simultaneously.

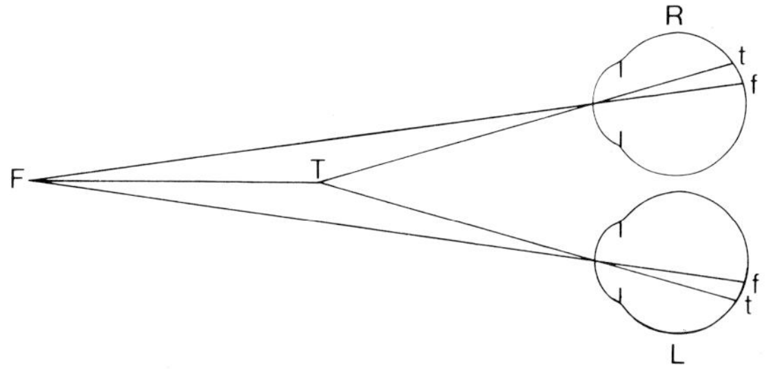

Fig. 28.10 To illustrate physiological binocular double vision. For the sake of clarity the distances are out of proportion. The images of the fixation point (F) fall on each fovea (*f*); those of an object near the eye (T) will fall on *t*, giving rise to crossed diplopia

Convergence and accommodation

When a distant object is observed by an emmetropic person the visual axes are parallel and no effort of accommodation is made. If, however, a near object is regarded, the eyes converge upon it and an effort of accommodation corresponding to the distance of the object is made. These movements are reflex and are controlled, as we have seen, by a centre in the occipital cortex (Fig. 28.7), the afferent path being the visual pathways, the efferent path running to the Edinger–Westphal nucleus. The associated pupillary contraction is a purely low-level reflex arc, the afferent path running from the medial recti to the Edinger–Westphal nucleus

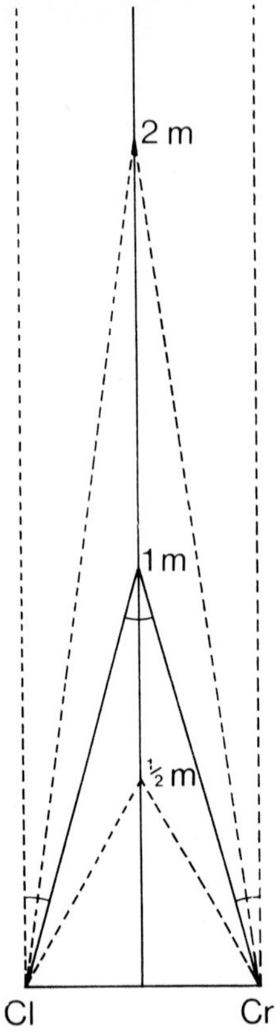

Fig. 28.11 Diagram of the metre angle. *Cr., Cl.,* centres of rotation of the right and left eyes

and the efferent by the parasympathetic fibres in the third nerve (Fig. 4.8).

Convergence is usually measured by employing the *metre angle* as a unit. Suppose an object to be situated in the median line between the two eyes at a distance of one metre from them. Then the angle which the line joining the object with the centre of rotation of either eye makes with the median line is called one metre angle (Fig. 28.11). With an interpupillary distance of 60 mm this angle is about 2°. If the object is two metres away the angle is approximately half as great, or ½ m.a. If the object is 50 cm away the angle will be 2 m.a. Now, the amount of accommodation which an emmetropic eye exercises in order to see clearly an object 1 m away is 1 D, 2 m away 0.5 D, 50 cm away 2 D, etc. Hence with an emmetropic person the amount of convergence, reckoned in metre angles, is the same as the amount of accommodation reckoned in dioptres. Just as the difference in the amount of accommodation between the far point and the near point is called the amplitude of accommodation, so the difference in convergence between the far point and the near point is called the *amplitude of convergence..*

Clinically, convergence can be tested roughly by making the patient fix a finger or pencil which is gradually brought nearer to the eyes in the middle line. The eyes should be able to maintain convergence when the object is 8 cm (3½ inches) from the eyes. If outward deviation of one eye occurs before this point is reached the power of convergence is deficient.

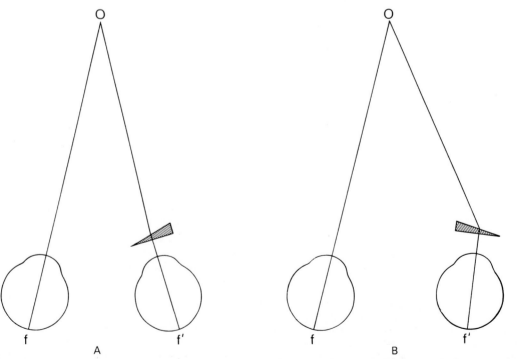

Fig. 28.12 Diagrams of the action of adducting and abducting prisms. O, object of fixation; *f, f′*, left and right foveæ centrales

More accurate measurements can be made by instruments held in front of the eyes wherein a vertical pointer slides along a scale. The amount of convergence can also be measured by prisms, as an extension of the method described to measure fusional capacity (Fig. 28.12A and B). In this case the prism is directed base outwards; the strongest prism which can thus be used without inducing diplopia when a *distant* object is regarded is a measure of the amplitude of convergence.

Although related, it is obvious that the association between convergence and accommodation must be elastic — otherwise a hypermetrope whose accommodation is always used in excess would always have diplopia, or a presbyope who could not accommodate would be unable to converge. If a person fixates (and accommodates for) a *near* object, the amount of *positive convergence* is measured by the strongest prism, base out, which can be borne without causing diplopia (Fig. 28.12A); the amount of *negative convergence* (or relative divergence) by the strongest prism, base in (Fig. 28.12B). The amplitude of convergence therefore consists of a negative portion and a positive portion which vary with each distance of the object fixated.

The convergence synkinesis is so co-ordinated that the energy exerted is accurately divided between the two medial recti. Hence it is found that the effect is the same in the above experiments whether the prism is placed before only one eye, or a prism of half the strength is placed before each eye.

29

Paralytic and kinetic strabismus: synkineses: nystagmus

Strabismus (στραβός, *crooked*) *or squint*)

This is a generic term applied to all those conditions in which the visual axes assume a position relative to each other different from that conforming to physiological conditions. We have seen that the motility of the eyes is controlled by voluntary and reflex mechanisms centred in the cerebral cortex. Lesions at this level or in the supranuclear pathways produce *conjugate deviations* or *pareses* which affect both eyes equally; although their movements or positions are abnormal, they maintain their relative co-ordination and diplopia is not produced. Simple ptosis, however, may result from such a lesion. The clinical incidence of these deviations will be discussed in Chapter 34 as well as the mixed palsies resulting from lesions in the mid-brain. If, however, the lesion is situated at the level of the lower neurons, affecting the nuclei, the nerves or the muscles, the relative co-ordination of the eyes is disturbed and diplopia and other symptoms appear. The usual result of such a lesion is paralysis (*paralytic squint*); sometimes it is due to irregular or spasmodic activity of individual muscles or groups of muscles (*kinetic squint*); We shall see presently that a further type of squint exists when the visual axes, although abnormally directed, retain their relative position in all movements of the eyes; this is therefore termed *concomitant squint*.

Paralytic strabismus

Signs and symptoms

The signs and symptoms of paralytic squint comprise limitation of ocular movements, diplopia, false orientation, abnormal position of the head and vertigo.

1. *Limitation of movement*. In paralysis of an ocular muscle the ability to turn the eye in the direction of the normal action of the muscle is diminished or lost. In slight paresis the defect in mobility may be so small as to escape observation without special tests. In all positions in which the affected muscle is not brought actively into play the visual axes assume their normal relationship.

Limitation of movement is tested roughly by fixing

the patient's head and telling him to follow the movements of the surgeon's finger. The finger should be held vertically in testing horizontal movements, horizontally in testing vertical movements. An accurate record of the movements of each eye can be obtained by taking the *field of fixation* with the perimeter as for recording the field of vision. With the head immobile and the other eye screened the patient looks as far as possible along the arc of the perimeter, test types being moved in from the periphery until he is just able to read them. The normal field of fixation is about 50° downwards and 45° in all other directions.

The relative movements of the two eyes when each is used for fixation are of importance. This is most readily explored by the *screen test*. When the eyes are turned in the direction of the normal action of the paralysed muscle movements of the affected eye are impeded. It therefore deviates relatively to the other eye; this position is called the *primary deviation* (Fig. 29.1A). The angle of deviation is the angle which the line joining the object of fixation and the nodal point makes with the visual line.

If, on the other hand, the paralysed eye is used for fixation it will have difficulty in moving in this direction; since the nervous energy required for movement is equally distributed between the two, the normal eye will share in this abnormal effort. If, therefore, the sound eye is covered by a screen, and an attempt is made to fix an object so situated that the paralysed muscle is brought into play, it will be found that the normal eye behind the screen deviates more than the primary deviation of the paralysed eye. For example, if the right lateral rectus is paralysed and the left eye is covered, then on attempting to fix an object situated to the right with the right eye, the left eye will deviate very much to the right, so much in fact that its line of vision is well to the right of the object fixed. Hence, if the screen is removed suddenly the left eye will spring back to the left so as to take up fixation. This deviation of the sound eye is called the *secondary deviaiton* (Fig. 29.1B) and is due to over-action of the contra-lateral synergist of the palsied muscle. This feature is of great importance because when well marked it distinguishes paralytic squint from

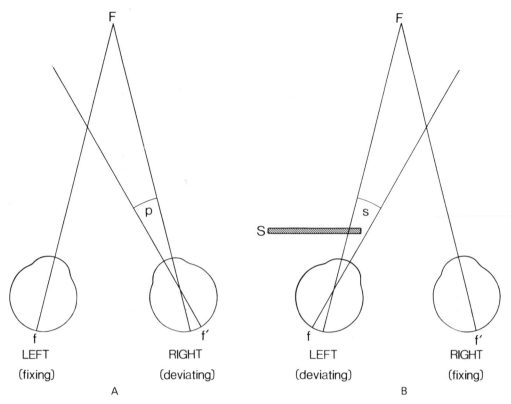

Fig. 29.1 Primary and secondary deviations. In concomitant squint (affecting the right eye) the primary deviation (p, A) is equal to the secondary deviation (s, B) obtained when the non-squinting eye is occluded by a screen, S. F, fixation point. In paralytic squint the secondary deviation is greater than the primary

the concomitant type in which the secondary deviation is equal to the primary.

2. *Diplopia.* The chief complaint of patients with paralysis of an extrinsic muscle is usually that they see double. Diplopia occurs only over that part of the field of fixation towards which the affected muscle or muscles move the eye. If both eyes are functional and one deviates, *binocular diplopia* results.

The image seen by the squinting eye (*false or apparent image*) is usually less distinct than that seen by the fixing eye (*true image*), because only in the latter case does the image fall upon the fovea centralis. The angular displacement of the false image is equal to the angle of deviation of the eye.

Suppose the left eye fixes accurately while the right deviates inwards, a bright, sharply defined foveal image is seen with the left eye. The image formed by the object on the right retina, falling as it does upon the line joining the nodal point with the object, lies to the nasal side of the retina. The patient, being unconscious of the malposition of his eye, orientates the object subjectively as if the eye were straight. He knows from experience that objects which form their images upon the nasal side of the retina are situated to the temporal side. He therefore projects the object with this eye to the right of its

actual position. This is called *homonymous diplopia*, because the object as seen by the right eye is to the right of the object as seen by the left eye (Fig. 29.2A). If the right eye deviates outwards, *heteronymous* or *crossed diplopia* results, because the object as seen by the left eye lies apparently to the right of the object as seen by the right eye (Fig. 29.2B).

3. *False orientation.* It will be seen from what has already been said that false orientation is a necessary accompaniment of binocular diplopia. Suppose that a patient whose right lateral rectus is paralysed shuts his left eye and attempts to fix an object situated towards the right. Let him now quickly point at the object with his extended index finger; the finger will pass considerably to the right of the object. This is called *false projection*. It depends upon the same principle as the increase of the secondary deviation, for the object is projected according to the amount of nervous energy exerted; as this is greater than that exerted in normal circumstances, the object is projected too far in the direction of action of the paralysed muscle. It is essential that the finger should be directed at the object quickly, otherwise the error is noticed and compensation is made. For example, if in the same circumstances the patient is told to walk towards an object situated at some distance to

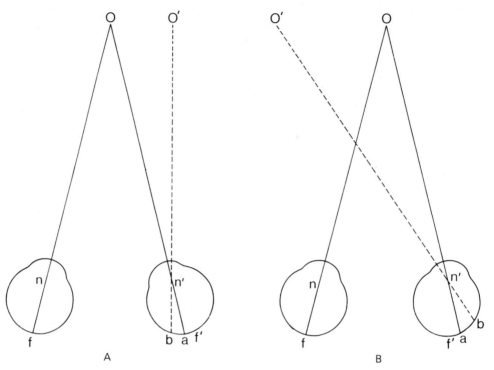

Fig. 29.2 A, Diagram of homonymous diplopia; B, diagram of heteronymous (crossed) diplopia: f, f', left and right foveæ; n, n', left and right nodal points. The image of O formed at a is projected as if a were the fovea, i.e., to O' from b

the right, he first steps too far to the right, then recognises his mistake and corrects it. In long-standing paralysis the patient may learn by experience to compensate for the error.

4. *Position of the head.* The patient holds his head so that his face is turned in the direction of action of the paralysed muscle. For example, in paralysis of the right lateral rectus the patient keeps his head turned to the right. The object of this manœuvre is to lessen the diplopia and its attendant unpleasant consequences as much as possible. In complex paralysis the position of the head is still such as to relieve the diplopia to the maximum extent, the position being unconsciously adopted.

'Ocular torticollis' is a term sometimes applied to tilting of the head to compensate for defective vertical movements of one eye. It is distinguished from true torticollis due to contraction of the sternomastoid muscle in that there is a simple tilting of the head without rotation of the chin towards the opposite shoulder; moreover, the sterno-mastoid is not unduly contracted. It occurs chiefly in cases of congenital origin but it follows traumatic palsies if binocular single vision can be obtained by adjusting head posture. The vertical squint is made manifest by placing the head straight, when diplopia is also elicited.

5. *Vertigo.* Vertigo, leading to nausea and even vomiting, is due partly to diplopia, partly to false projection.

It occurs chiefly when the paralysed muscle is called upon to exert itself. When the gaze is turned from the region of correct to that of false localisation, objects appear to move with increasing velocity in the direction in which the eye is moving. The unpleasant symptoms are counteracted partially by altering the position of the head, or completely by shutting or covering the affected eye.

In congenital strabismus these symptoms are not obtrusive since the vision of one eye is suppressed or false retinal correspondences develop; in these cases contraction of the antagonistic muscles does not occur. In acquired cases they are at first very distressing and incapacitating. In paralyses of long standing, however, relief is gradually obtained: false orientation and diplopia tend to disappear or become less troublesome, for the patient learns to ignore the impressions derived from the affected eye. Moreover, contracture of the antagonists of the paralysed muscle gradually sets in, which has the effect of increasing the deviation. Since the retinal image is thus thrown farther to the periphery of the retina where the senstivity is less, its suppression is facilitated.

Investigation of a case of ocular paralysis
The patient usually seeks advice on account of diplopia. In some cases the nature of the case is obvious immediately from the strabismus or from the manner in which the head is held. In most cases these features are

too slight to decide the diagnosis and special tests must be made.

1. The first procedure should be to cover one eye in order to determine whether the diplopia is uniocular or binocular.

2. If it is decided that the diplopia is binocular, the patient should fix the surgeon's finger, and the field of fixation of each eye should be carefully investigated. In cases of complete paralysis of one or more muscles it may be possible to make an accurate diagnosis from the observation of the defective movements. In cases of paresis the limitation of movement of the eye may be so slight as to be unidentifiable.

3. In such cases the diplopia must be investigated by more delicate tests. In a dark room a red glass is placed before one eye and a green before the other in order to distinguish their images. A bar of light through a steno-pæic slit in a hand-torch is then moved about in the field of binocular fixation at a distance of at least four feet from the patient, the patient's head being kept stationary. The positions of the images are accurately recorded upon a chart with nine squares marked upon it (Fig. 29.6). The examination may be carried out by the surgeon turning the patient's head in various directions while the light is kept stationary. The following data are derived from this examination:

(a) the areas of single vision and diplopia;
(b) the distance between the two images in the areas of diplopia;
(c) whether the images are on the same level or not;
(d) whether one image is inclined or both are erect;
(e) where the diplopia is homonymous or crossed.

These data, if concordant, are sufficient to diagnose the paralysis. The false image, which is frequently tilted and the fainter of the two, is determined by the direction in which the images are most separated from each other, in which case it is displaced farthest in the direction of the normal action of the paralysed muscle. By covering one eye it can be shown to which eye this image belongs.

The deviation of the false image is most easily determined when the eye is turned in the *cardinal positions*. For lateral palsies where only two muscles are involved, the test is easy; greatest diplopia occurs in the horizontal line to the right in paralysis of the right lateral or left medial rectus, to the left for the left lateral or right medial rectus.

For vertical movements the action of four muscles must be analysed. They are most easily differentiated thus.

In view of the obliquity of their course (p. 275) the recti are most effective as vertical rotators as the eyes are abducted from the primary position, the obliques when adducted. On looking up to the right the right superior rectus and the left inferior oblique are therefore primari-

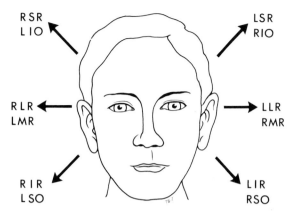

Fig. 29.3 The fields of action of the ocular muscles in binocular movements. The maximum effectivity as elevators is attained by the RSR and the LIO when acting as right-hand elevators

ly involved, the false image being higher than the true and tilted. The corresponding displacements in the four cardinal positions are seen in Figure 29.3.

It must be remembered that these tests are purely subjective. In many cases the patients are uncooperative or their intelligence is obscured by intracranial disease; or contracture of the antagonistic muscles may have set in. Consequently the answers are not infrequently discordant, and accurate diagnosis may be extremely difficult or impossible. As additional complications, the paresis may unmask a latent squint (p. 293) or the patient may fix with the paralysed eye, especially if this eye has the greater acuity of vision.

Considerable ingenuity has been used to devise mnemonics for determining the position of the false image. One of the most satisfactory is that of Maddox shown in the accompanying diagram (Fig. 29.3); if the field is divided into areas as shown, in vertical palsies the paresis is due to failure of the 'same-named' rectus muscle (in the left superior area, the left superior rectus) or the most 'crossed-named' oblique muscle (right inferior oblique). In all cases the most peripheral image belongs to the palsied eye.

In clinical practice these principles are applied thus:
1. First decide whether the diplopia is horizontal or vertical from the history of the patient and by testing with red and green goggles, red in front of the right eye.
2. If horizontal:
  a. Find the position of gaze where the separation of the images is maximal — right or left by moving a light in the horizontal plane.
  b. In that position the furthest displaced image belongs to the eye with the muscle palsy.
  c. Application of the mnemonic of Maddox will identify the palsied muscle.
3. If vertical:
  a. Find the position of gaze where the separation of

the images is maximal, moving the light vertically in the median plane. If the separation is greatest above there is an elevator palsy, if greatest below there is depressor palsy.

b. Find out if the separation is maximal to the right (above or below) or to the left (above or below).

c. The furthest displaced image belongs to the eye with muscle palsy.

d. The application of the mnemonic of Maddox will identify the palsy muscle.

It may be pointed out that all the signs, with the exception of the deviation of the eye — defective movement, false projection, increase of diplopia secondary deviation, and position of the head — are towards the side of the paralysed muscle.

To measure the degree of deviation, especially if torsional, and particularly to measure any progressive in-crease, the *Hess screen* (Fig. 29.4) is useful. It consists of a tangent screen marked in red lines on a black cloth with red spots at the intersection of the 15° and 30° lines with themselves and with the horizontal and vertical lines; over it three green threads are suspended in such a way that they can be moved over the screen in any direction by a pointer. The patient, wearing red-and-green glasses, is asked to place the junction of the three threads over the red spots in turn. Through the red glass he can only see the red markers and through the green, the green threads, so that he indicates the point at which one eye is looking when the other fixes a spot. The position on which the indicator appears to coincide with the spot gives a permanent record of the primary and secondary deviation. The test also provides an accurate measure of comitance. In a concomitant squint the fields of each eye, although relatively displaced, are

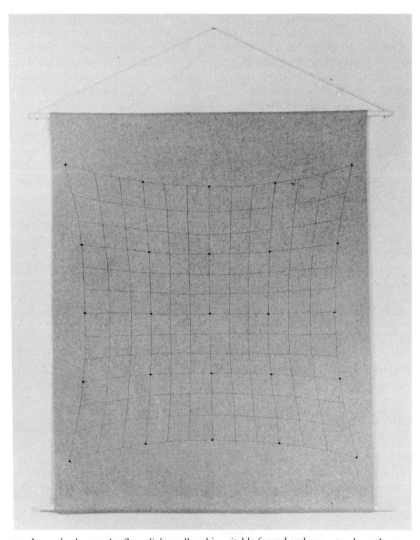

Fig. 29.4 Hess screen. A grey background reflects light well and is suitable for red and green torch markers

equal in area and undistorted; in paretic squint the area on the affected side is diminished away from the affected muscle and in spastic squint it is increased towards the affected muscle.

Varieties of ocular paralysis

If one muscle alone is affected it is generally the lateral rectus or the superior oblique, since each of these is supplied by an independent nerve. Affection of several muscles simultaneously is usually due to paralysis of the third nerve. All the extrinsic and intrinsic muscles of one or both eyes may be paralysed — *total ophthalmoplegia*. If only the extrinsic muscles are affected the condition is called *external ophthalmoplegia*; if only the intrinsic (sphincter pupillæ and ciliary muscle) *internal ophthalmoplegia*.

Paralysis of the lateral rectus. There is limitation of movement outwards, and the face is turned towards the paralysed side. Homonymous diplopia occurs on looking to the paralysed side; the images are on the same level and erect, becoming more separated on looking more towards the paralysed side. The false image is slightly tilted on looking up or down as well as towards the paralysed side (Figs 29.5–6).

Paralysis of the superior oblique. There is limitation of movement downwards and towards the sound side; the face is turned downwards and towards the *sound* side. Homonymous diplopia occurs on looking down (Fig.29 8); the false image is lower and its upper end is tilted towards the true image. The distance between the images increases on looking down and towards the sound side and the inclination of the false image increases on looking down to the *paralysed* side. The patient has great difficulty in going downstairs, and vertigo is usually a particularly prominent symptom.

Paralysis of the third nerve. In complete paralysis of the third nerve there is ptosis, which prevents diplopia.

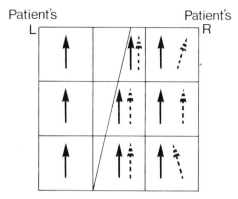

Fig. 29.6 Diplopia chart for the right lateral rectus. The oblique line through the chart shows the limit of the fields of single vision and of diplopia. The dotted arrows show the positions of the false image in different parts of the field of diplopia

On raising the lid with the finger the eye is seen to be deflected outwards and rotated internally, owing to the tone of the two unparalysed muscles. The pupil is semi-dilated and immobile, and accommodation is paralysed. There is a slight degree of proptosis, owing to loss of tone of the paralysed muscles. There is limitation of movements upwards and inwards, to a less degree downwards. With the lid raised there is diplopia, which is crossed, the false image being higher, with its upper end tilted towards the paralysed side (Figs 29.7, 29.9).

Paralysis of the third nerve is often incomplete, and individual muscles may occasionally be affected alone.

The ætiology of paretic strabismus

This is composite. The central nervous diseases which may entail *a lesion of the ocular motor nuclei* are discussed in Chapter 34. The most common cause is a small haemorrhagic or thrombotic lesion in the mid-brain associated with arteriosclerosis or diabetes; syphilis used

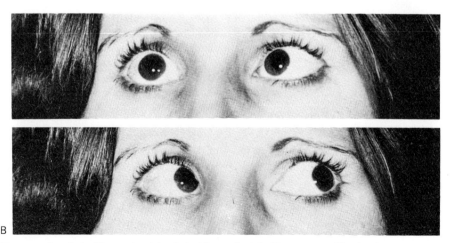

B

Fig. 29.5 R VI nerve palsy: A, looking to the right; B, looking to the left. (By courtesy of Sanders.)

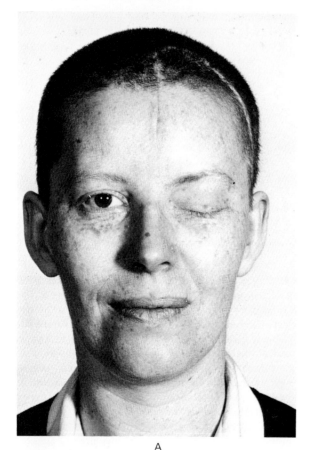

A

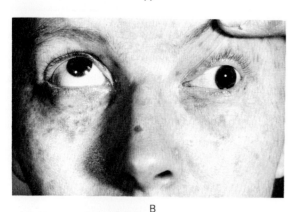

B

Fig. 29.7 A, L Complete III Nerve Paralysis due to a posterior communicating aneurysm to show left ptosis and the craniotomy scar. B, Complete L III Nerve Paralysis with the lid elevated and the patient attempting upward gaze to show the L dilated and fixed pupil with failure of L adduction and elevation. (By courtesy of Sanders.)

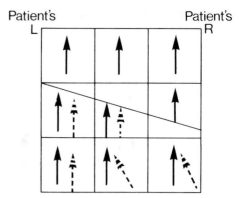

Fig. 29.8 Diplopia chart for paralysis of the right superior oblique

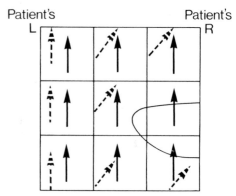

Fig. 29.9 Diplopia chart for the right third nerve paralysis. The area enclosed by the curved line is the area of single vision

(diphtheria) or exogenous (lead, botulism) origin, and thiamine deficiency.

Lesions of the nerve trunks are similarly common. They may be involved in infections of the meninges, cavernous sinus or orbit, by pressure from tumours, or trauma involving a fracture of the base of the skull. Among tumours, secondary invasion of the orbit or skull by malignant nasopharyngeal tumours (p. 337) should be remembered; of these, ocular palsies are a common early symptom. In pressure paralysis the nerve most frequently involved is the sixth; paralysis of the lateral recti is thus common in cases of intracranial tumours with high intracranial pressure, and generally has no localising value. It may be due to traction on the nerves as they bend over the apex of the petrous portion of the temporal bone, or to pressure by the anterior inferior cerebellar and internal auditory arteries, which cross them at right angles and often lie ventral to them; the nerves are strangulated between the vessels and the œdematous and swollen pons. The paralysis, generally of the lateral rectus, following spinal anæsthesia may be due to the same cause; the onset is rapid, and recovery usually takes many weeks. Since the third nerve passes

to be the most frequent ætiological factor. Other causes are infections of the central nervous system (encephalitis lethargica, polioencephalitis, etc.), toxins of endogenous

between the superior cerebellar and the posterior cerebral arteries, the same mechanism may account for ophthalmoplegic migraine (*q.v.*).

Misdirection in the regeneration of the third cranial nerve is common after total interruption of function usually by head trauma. The ocular signs of misdirection are:

1. Pseudo-Graefe lid sign. As the eye attempts to move downwards the upper lid retracts.
2. Pseudo-Argyll–Robertson pupil. There is a slow light reflex and a better constriction of the pupil to the near synkinesis.
3. Horizontal gaze lid dyskinesis. The upper lid retracts as the eye is adducted and falls as the eye is abducted.
4. Difficulty in vertical gaze.
5. Adduction on attempted vertical gaze.
6. Monocular optico-kinetic responses. As vertical optical targets are presented to the patient the normal eye develops good vertical optico-kinetic nystagmus whereas the affected eye does not.

Lesions of the muscles as well as of the branches of the nerves may occur with orbital disease or injury; the latter is relatively common. A palsy due to inefficiency of the superior oblique owing to dislocation of the trochlea is one of the more common lesions of this type.

Treatment. Aetiological treatment should be directed to the cause of the palsy.

The diplopia, if minor, may sometimes be relieved by suitable prisms, but this treatment is rarely of much use owing to the variation in the amount of the deviation in different positions of the eyes. Surgery is indicated when the deviation has become stabilised — usually recession of the contra-lateral synergist muscle, followed, if necessary, by recession of the antagonistic muscle in the same eye, thus putting the affected muscle under better mechanical conditions. Those operations should always be done in stages to assess the effects of each; the techniques are described in Chapter 30.

Congenital strabismus

This is not uncommon. It is usually due to ineffectivity of a muscle owing to its mal-insertion, sometimes to a defect or absence of the nervous motor mechanism, sometimes to fibrosis of the muscle, and occasionally to absence of the muscle itself. Sometimes the defects are extensive and movements irregular or grossly deficient. More often one or a few muscles are involved, most commonly the lateral rectus, the superior rectus and oblique. If the defect is slight the squint eventually takes on the characteristics of a concomitant strabismus from which it is frequently difficult to differentiate in later life.

One of the common congenital defects is *Duane's retraction syndrome*. It is due to a fibrosis of the lateral rec-

tus or a co-contraction of the lateral and medial rectus; in the primary position the eyes are straight or show some latent convergence, but a restriction or absence of abduction. On adduction there is a retraction of the globe and a narrowing of the palpebral fissure while on attempted abduction there is a slight exophthalmos. A second anomaly is the *superior oblique sheath syndrome* wherein there is a marked defect of elevation in the adducted position somewhat resembling the effects of a paresis of the inferior oblique muscle. The taut superior oblique tendon may be treated by a 3 mm tenectomy within the intermuscular septum. If post-operative palsy of the operated muscle occurs it can be managed by recession of the ipsilateral inferior oblique or the contralateral inferior rectus.

Kinetic strabismus

Aberrant forms of strabismus occur as the result of irritative intracranial lesions, and are due, not to paralysis, but to irregular action or over-action of certain muscles, caused by unequal stimulation of the nerve centres or nerves. Such squints may occur in meningitis and lesions of the mid-brain or cerebellum, such as tumours (glioma, tubercle, gumma, etc.). The occurrence of the squint only during epileptiform fits or its irregularity of type may render the diagnosis from paralytic squint easy, especially when there are other prominent symptoms of cerebral irritation. In other cases, especially in the early stages of the disease, the diagnosis from paralytic or concomitant squint may be extremely difficult.

A second, more common, cause of such a squint is the spasmodic contracture which develops in the antagonist of a paretic muscle. The muscle usually affected is the inferior oblique following a paresis of the superior rectus or superior oblique, frequently congenital in origin. The deviation is typical. On looking away from the affected side, as the eye is adducted and the inferior oblique comes into play, it is suddenly jerked up and in (Figs. 29.10). Treatment is by myectomy or recession of the muscle (p. 302).

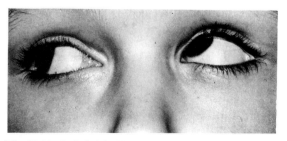

Fig. 29.10 L Inferior oblique overaction. (By courtesy of Fells.)

Synkineses

The extrinsic muscles take part in many normal and pathological synkineses. When the eyes look up, the levatores palpebrarum raise the lids and in extreme upward movements the frontales also contract. In congenital ptosis (q.v.) upward movement of the eyes is often defective. On looking down the lid follows the globe; in exophthalmic goitre the lid follows tardily or not at all (von Graefe's sign); in total facial paralysis the lid follows the globe on looking down, although the eye cannot be closed voluntarily. On closing the lids, as in sleep, the eyes generally turn upwards and outwards (Bell's phenomenon). The same movement of the eyes occurs on attempted closure in total facial paralysis.

Other pathological synkineses are probably due to congenitally abnormal associations between two nerves or to aberrant regeneration of nerve fibres along the wrong nerve sheath after disease or injury. The 'jaw-winking' synkinesis (of Marcus Gunn) is particularly striking. In these rare cases one levator palpebræ is thrown into spasm during eating, and sometimes on reading aloud. The upward lid movement is especially associated with lateral movements of the jaw, due to action of the pterygoid muscles which are innervated by the fifth nerve. In most cases, but not all, there is slight ptosis of the affected lid, and in cases with congenital ptosis the synkinesis occurs on sucking. Allied to the jaw-winking cases are others in which spasmodic lid movements occur on lateral deviation of the eyes.

The convergence pupillary synkinesis has already been mentioned: to it may be added the contraction of the pupil on forced closure of the lids. In rare cases spontaneous rhythmical variations in the size of the pupil are accompanied by ocular or lid movements. They are usually associated with congenital or early infantile paresis of the third nerve. Of these, a rhythmic cyclic oculomotor spasm is one of the most dramatic. In the mydriatic phase there is total ophthalmoplegia with ptosis, and at intervals of a minute or less a miotic phase develops in which the upper lid retracts, the eyes converge, the pupil contracts and the accommodation undergoes spasm.

Nystagmus

Nystagmus (νυσταξειν, to nod) is the term applied to rapid oscillatory movements of the eyes, independent of the normal movements which are not affected. The oscillations are involuntary, although in rare cases normal persons can imitate them. They are usually lateral, but vertical, rotatory, and mixed rotatory and lateral or vertical nystagmus occur. The condition is almost always bilateral, although the movements may be much more marked in one eye than the other. In such cases it may be necessary to examine the eye very carefully with the ophthalmoscope before the presence of nystagmus

can be demonstrated in the magnified ophthalmoscopic image. Unilateral nystagmus does occur, but it is probable that many of the cases described are really bilateral. In latent nystagmus no movement is present when both eyes are open but nystagmus is elicited when either eye is covered. Latent nystagmus is often associated with alternating sursum-duction or dissociated vertical divergence characterised by either eye slowly elevating with an excyclorotation when the eyes are dissociated. This may occur spontaneously when the patient is tired or day-dreaming or on occlusion of one eye. The deviation is usually bilateral but may be asymmetrical.

Diplopia is rarely a problem because of the ability to suppress but there may be a disturbing cosmetic problem. If the disfigurement is due to the upward deviation of one eye then attempts should be made to make the patient fix with the affected eye.

Surgical correction is first aimed at correcting the horizontal deviation and eliminating oblique muscle overactions. If this fails to solve the problem then recession of the superior rectus by 6–9 mm is required. The procedure consists of passing a suture through the muscle, whip-locking it and then disinserting the muscle. The suture is then passed through the old insertion site, the muscle is allowed to fall back a predetermined distance and the suture is tied at the original insertion. Limitation of elevation may occur but there is little change in the primary position other than the elimination of the sursum-duction.

Nystagmoid jerks — larger rhythmic jerking movements, most pronounced at the extreme limits of the normal movements of the eyes — should be distinguished from true nystagmus. They are not uncommon in normal people in certain conditions such as fatigue. It is a jerk-type nystagmus which is slightly more pronounced in the abducting eye and is poorly sustained. The rapid component is in the direction of gaze. The fundamental cause is probably quite different from that of true nystagmus, although both may occur together. Opticokinetic nystagmus has already been noted (p. 278).

Nystagmus may be congenital or early infantile, or it may be acquired. These two groups of cases should be carefully distinguished on account of their different pathological foundations. Congenital and early infantile nystagmus dating from birth or within a few weeks of birth, occurs in congenitally malformed eyes, in albinism, and in eyes with congenital or early acquired opacities of the media (such as leucoma or anterior polar cataract due to ophthalmia neonatorum) or macular disease. The cause in these cases is inability to develop normal fixation. Fixation is normally developed during the first few weeks of life, the eyes being moved aimlessly and independently before it is acquired. Any cause operative at this period seriously diminishing the acuity of macular vision is liable to give rise to nystagmus; if the eye is blind, nystagmus does not develop but vague 'searching movements' are seen. Nystagmus is present in most cases of total colour blindness (*q.v.*) in which vision is carried out by the rods alone, and there is therefore a central scotoma. In some congenital cases it is impossible to discover any cause. In a few such cases ancestors or relations have been albinos.

Nystagmus in infancy may be acquired after the period at which fixation is developed. This form occurs in the first year of life as *spasmus nutans*, in which it is associated with nodding movements of the head. The nodding of the head may be antero-posterior (affirmation), lateral (negation), or rotatory. It develops some weeks before the nystagmus, ceases during sleep, and disappears before the nystagmus. The nystagmus is very fine and rapid, and may be vertical, rotatory, or lateral and is generally more marked in one eye. The whole symptom-complex disappears in time — one of the few cases in which nystagmus spontaneously resolves. The nystagmus may disappear in one eye before the other; such cases may be mistaken for true unilateral nystagmus. In rare cases head nodding with nystagmus is congenital and hereditary, a condition which persists throughout life.

Congenital jerky nystagmus is not associated with any recognisable pathological lesion in the eyes. The causative lesion probably lies in the complex nervous mechanisms in the brain stem which are concerned in the centring and in the 'steady fixation' of the eyes. Nystagmus may be regarded as an exaggeration of the fine persistent movements of the eyes (micro-saccades, slow motion random drifts, and rapid impulsive saccades which correct the random drifts) which are essential in the maintenance of a clear foveal perception of the retinal image.

The basic aim of surgical treatment is to transfer the 'neutral point' (where the nystagmus is least apparent) from an eccentric position to a straight-ahead position so that there is an eliminaiton of the compensatory head posture. Prismotherapy may be applied to achieve the same effect. The Fadenoperation is based on the idea that the necessary muscle force for any given ocular movement steadily increases after leaving the arc of contact of the globe. The operation consists of creating a second insertion of certain extrinsic ocular muscles (usually both medial recti) at least 10 mm behind the physiological insertion. Attempts have been made to convert the movements of a nystagmus into audible stimuli which can be heard by the subject who uses this feedback signal to control the nystagmus by maintaining a constant tone.

There are a number of ocular motility disorders which occur in childhood and resemble nystagmus. This group includes ocular bobbing, flutter-like oscillations of the eyes, ocular dysmetria, opsoclonus, ataxic conjugate movements of the eyes and ocular myoclonus.

In ocular bobbing the eyes remain motionless in the primary position and then suddenly the eyes deviate downwards or less commonly upwards after which they slowly return to the primary position. Children with this affliction characteristically have loss of coloric responses on cold water irrigation of the ears with total horizontal conjugate gaze palsies. They usually have a massive neoplastic lesion involving the pontine brain stem and the prognosis is extremely poor.

Flutter-like oscillations of the eyes and ocular dysmetria are ocular signs of interruption of cerebellar connections into the brain stem. They represent the dysmetric overshoots of the eyes and inability to fixate a target accurately when gaze is shifted from one point in space to another. The eyes may either overshoot (or undershoot) the target.

Opsoclonus consists of wild, chaotic, apparently conjugate movements of the eyes. There are frequent myoclonic movements of the face, arms and legs. Patients have a clear sensorium; the disorder often follows an episode of benign encephalitis and usually has a good prognosis.

Oculopalatal myoclonus is an unusual disorder in which the patient develops associated movements of the eyes, palate, face, platysma, larynx, eustachian tube orifice, tongue and occasionally the extremities. It follows severe brain stem damage in the myoclonic triangle which has as its boundaries the red nucleus above, inferior olive below and dentate nucleus of the cerebellum posteriorly. It occurs most commonly in association with vascular disease.

Nystagmus in adults occurs in diseases of the midbrain, cerebellum and vestibular tracts, and of the semicircular canals. It is common in multiple sclerosis wherein the movements are generally horizontal and are elicited in the early stages only in extreme lateral position of the eyes. Cerebellar irritative lesions cause coarse nystagmus towards the side of the lesion and fine nystagmus to the opposite side. Nystagmus may also occur in adults as an 'occupation neurosis', the commonest form being coal-miners' nystagmus (*vide infra*).

In congenital and early infantile nystagmus the patient is wholly unconscious of the movements, since objects do not appear to move. Vision is usually defective in spite of correction of errors of refraction which generally accompany the defect. In some cases of acquired nystagmus in adults, objects appear to move.

Labyrinthine nystagmus

This occurs in disease of the internal ear in which the semicircular canals are involved, and can be produced in normal subjects by rotation in a specially designed chair or by syringing the ears. Conjugate movement to the opposite side may be induced by syringing one ear with cold water. Vertical gaze upwards may be induced by syringing both ears with cold water and vertical conjugate gaze downwards induced by syringing both ears with warm water. The nystagmus is rhythmic, with a rapid and a slow component, is bilateral, and horizontal or rotatory, but varies according to the semicircular canal stimulated. Any pair of semicircular canals can be stimulated by rotation with the head in a suitable position. Destruction of one labyrinth causes rhythmic nystagmus towards the opposite side, which ceases if the other labyrinth is destroyed.

Miners' nystagmus
This occurs chiefly in those who have worked long at the coal face. The patient complains of defective vision which is worse at night, headache, giddiness, photophobia, the dancing of lights and movements of objects. The nystagmus is essentially rotatory and very rapid; in latent cases it is elicited by fixing the head and making the patient look up. In severe cases the lids are nearly closed and the head is held backwards; there is tremor of the head and eyebrows. The frequency of the disease varies inversely with the illumination in the mine suggesting that fixation difficulties in the dim illumination may be an ætiological factor; it will be remembered that vision in a dull light is carried out almost entirely by the rods. In these circumstances visual acuity is greatest 10–15% outside the fovea, and there is a physiological central scotoma making fixation difficult. There is, however, a large psychoneurotic factor in all cases. Improvement in miners' lamps and in the lighting of mines eliminates the disease which was a cause of considerable economic loss in time and compensation.

See-saw nystagmus of Maddox is a disjunctive pendular type of nystagmus in which the patient's eyes move in opposite directions with an associated torsional component. As the right eye moves up, the left eye moves downwards and there is a distinct torsional movement, the right eye intorting and the left eye extorting. The reverse is then seen. It is classically considered as a sign of parachiasmal disease.

Retraction nystagmus and convergence nystagmus are two special forms found with neurological damage localised to the upper mesencephalon. They are a part of the Silvian aqueduct syndrome. In young patients retraction nystagmus should suggest the diagnosis of mid-brain glioma or pinealoma. The ocular features of the Silvian aqueduct syndrome consist of:
1. Retraction (convergence) nystagmus.
2. Vertical nystagmus.
3. Difficult voluntary vertical gaze (especially up gaze).
4. Vertical gaze is better to following or doll's head movements than on command with an intact Bell's phenomenon.
5. Adduction movements with attempted vertical gaze.
6. Defective convergence.
7. Retraction nystagmus with downgoing opticokinetic targets.
8. Pupillary abnormalities (light-near dissociation).
9. Pathological lid retraction.

Gaze related nystagmus
In gaze direction nystagmus there is no movement of the eyes in the primary position but as the patients gaze is gradually diverted in any direction, particularly horizontally, a rather course, jerk-like nystagmus develops with its rapid phase in the direction of gaze. This builds to a maximum intensity in the extremes of conjugate gaze and is well sustained.

This type of nystagmus suggests drug intoxication, especially with barbiturates. Gaze direction nystagmus shows a frequency of 3–8 beats per second on an electronystagmogram.

Gaze paretic nystagmus has a frequency of 1–2 beats per sec and the eye tends to return to the primary position with the slow phase of the nystagmus. This nystagmus disappears completely when total gaze paralysis occurs. It is always seen in association with some degree of conjugate gaze weakness. It is common in brain stem disorders at the pontine level.

Down-beating vertical nystagmus indicates posterior fossa dysfunction often at the foramen magnum level.

30

Concomitant strabismus: heterophoria

We have already seen that in concomitant squint, as opposed to the paralytic type, although the eyes are misaligned, they retain their abnormal relation to each other in all movements. In paralytic squint the afferent pathways and centres are intact, but the efferent, effector mechanism breaks down. In concomitant squint the efferent pathways are normal and can still maintain coordination of the eyes, but either the afferent path is defective (usually due to poor visual acuity owing to a defect in the eye) or the central mechanism mediating the fixation and fusional reflexes is undeveloped or has broken down. The break-down may be due to peripheral causes, such as the excessive effort of convergence required with the sustained accommodation necessary in hypermetropes or a slight weakness in an extra-ocular muscle such as is not sufficient to cause a paralytic squint.

If the fusion mechanism is well-developed and the defect slight, visual alignment may be maintained in normal circumstances by a continued effort of fusion: the squint is then *latent* and can only be made manifest when fusion is made impossible (as by covering up one eye). This condition is called *heterophoria* or *latent squint*. If, on the other hand, the maintenance of alignment becomes impossible, a true or *apparent concomitant squint* develops and remains constant.

Heterophoria or latent strabismuts
We have just defined heterophoria as a condition wherein there is a tendency to misalignment of the visual axes which is corrected by the fusional capacity. As with all deviations the tendency is equally shared between the two eyes. Since the position of rest is usually one of slight divergence, few people are *orthophoric* and some degree of heterophoria is almost universal. If the latent deviation is one of convergence the condition is called *esophoria*, of divergence, *exophoria*, if vertical, *hyperphoria*: it is impossible to be sure whether there is absolute hyperphoria of one eye or hypophoria of the other, the condition being relative. If the deviation is torsional the term *cyclophoria* is applied. Lateral deviations are the most common, due often to over-stimulation of convergence with accommodation in hypermetropia (*esophoria*) or under-stimulation in myopia (*exophoria*). Hyperphoria is also common and is probably often due to abnormal insertions or slight weakness of one or other of the vertically rotating muscles. Cyclophoria is rare.

The *symptoms* of heterophoria may be considerable since parallelism of the visual axes is only maintained by tonic contraction of the appropriate muscles. Symptoms of eyestrain are therefore encountered in the higher degrees; but the smaller degrees give rise to little or to trouble. This particularly applies to eso- and exophoria since the muscles involved are accustomed to act unequally in convergence; only when the deviation is great — 5 to 10° or more — is asthenopia generally present. Slight degrees of hyperphoria, however, may cause discomfort, for in these cases more complicated adjustments are necessary involving the non-physiological action of muscles which are not accustomed to work together in order to keep the visual axes in the same plane. For the same reason cyclophoria gives the greatest discomfort of all.

As might be expected the deviation is liable to become manifest in conditions of bodily fatigue and to vary in amount from time to time. Some periodic squints are due to this cause, and the periodicity may be rhythmic. Thus a child may squint in the evening when he is tired; after a good night's rest the squint may disappear and may not return until the second or third day, the sequence being accurately repeated. Often latent squints give no trouble until school age arrives or adult life is reached when the demands of near vision increase the strain. No symptoms arise perhaps until after reading or writing for an hour or two when 'the letters seem to run together'. This is due to relaxation of the overstrained muscles; the eyes momentarily assume the position of rest, and diplopia, which is not appreciated as actual double vision, causes blurring of the print. With an effort the blurring is overcome, but eventually this becomes impossible, headache supervenes, and the work has to be abandoned.

The *diagnosis* of heterophoria simply depends on abolishing fusion so that, without its control, the eyes assume their position of rest. Several tests for this are available.

The most simple is the *cover test*. When a distant object is regarded and both eyes are uncovered there is no deviation. One eye is then screened the eyes dissociate and the latent deviation appears; when the screen is removed this eye moves at once to regain the position of binocular fixation. The other eye reacts similarly, the deviation in both being the same.

Other tests depend on altering the appearance of the retinal image in one eye so that no stimulus is given to fusion.

Of these the simplest is the *Maddox Rod Test*. The patient is placed 6 m from a bright spot of light in a dark room. A Maddox rod, which consists of four or five cylinders of red glass side by side in a supporting disc, is placed in the trial frame before one eye: the same effect is given by a disc of deeply grooved red glass (the Maddox groove, Fig. 30.1). The spot of light seen through the red cylinders appears as a long red line. If the cylinders are placed with their axes horizontal the red line will be vertical. If there is orthophoria the bright spot will appear to be in the centre of the vertical red line; if there is eso- or exophoria the red line will be to one side of the spot. The angle of the deviation is measured by the strength of the prism which it is necess-

ary to place in front of the Maddox rod (or the other eye) in order to bring the red line and the spot together. The nature of the deviation is indicated by the position of the base of the prism, whether out or in. The Maddox rod is then rotated so that the cylinders are vertical; the red line will now be horizontal. If there is no hyperphoria the line will pass through the bright spot. If there is hyperphoria the red line will be below or above the spot according to whether the relative hyperphoria is associated with the eye with the rod in front of it or with the other. In each case the amount of deviation is measured either on a graduated tangent scale set on the wall or by the strength of the prism required to correct it.

The deviation in latent squint is often different in near vision from that in distant vision. An exophoria appearing when near objects are regarded is in fact an *insufficiency of convergence*, a condition which may give rise to symptoms when much near work is undertaken.

The deviation in near vision is conveniently tested by the *Maddox wing test* (Fig. 30.2) in which, when the patient looks through the two slit-holes in the eyepieces of the instrument, the fields which are exposed to each eye are separated by a diaphragm in such a way that they glide tangentially into each other. The right eye sees a white arrow pointing vertically upwards and a red arrow pointing horizontally to the left. The left eye sees a horizontal row of figures in white and a vertical row in red. These are calibrated to read in degrees of deviation. The arrow pointing to the horizontal row of figures and the arrow pointing to the vertical row should both be at zero; any deviation indicates an eso- or exophoria or a hyperphoria, the amount of which can be read off on the scale. There are several *diaphragm tests* on somewhat similar principles.

Besides the actual measurement of the deviation in latent strabismus the strength of the muscles involved should also be tested by forcing them to a maximum effort against prisms (*prism vergence tests*). With the patient seated 6 m from a light the highest prism which

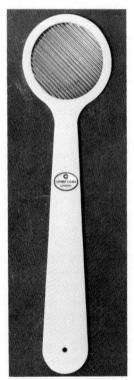

Fig. 30.1 Maddox groove. (By courtesy of Clement Clarke international Ltd.)

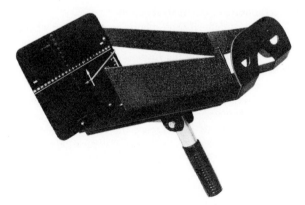

Fig. 30.2 The Maddox wing test

can permit single vision gives the *verging power* for the particular direction involved. The converging power varies very much and with practice can be raised to the neighbourhood of 50 degrees (25° d) or more; if it falls below 20 degrees, it may be taken to be definitely insufficient. The diverging power should be 4–5 degrees, and normal limits of super- and subduction are from 1.5 to 2.5 degrees.

Treatment. The lower degrees of esophoria, and to a less extent of exophoria, cause no symptoms and need no special treatment. If symptoms are apparent after any error of refraction has been corrected with spectacles, a rational treatment of eso- or exophoria consists in exercising the weak muscles against prisms, or by the use of the stereoscope. Unfortunately this is usually not or only temporarily beneficial, but relief may be maintained by repeating the exercises at intervals, an activity which the patient can practise himself. If this is ineffective the symptoms may be relieved by ordering prisms in spectacles to correct the defect, i.e., prisms with their bases directed in the opposite sense to those used for exercise. This should be avoided if possible since it generally tends to increase the defect, so that stronger prisms have to be ordered from time to time. The total prismatic error should be divided equally between the two eyes in ordering the correction. Hyperphoria in its less degrees should unhesitatingly be treated in this way; in this condition exercises are useless.

In all cases when the deviation is large and is unaffected by such treatment, operation may be considered, one or other muscle being recessed or resected, the case being treated as if it were a manifest squint (*q.v.*). Even if not curative, the deviation may thus be reduced to such a degree as to abolish asthenopia.

Insufficiency of convergence may be treated by prism exercises. The following simple exercise is often sufficient without having recourse to prisms. A pencil is held in the hand and slowly approximated to the nose until, despite an effort of convergence, it appears double; this is repeated until the distance at which diplopia occurs is gradually shortened. At about every tenth time the patient looks into the distance, so as to relax his accommodation and convergence. The exercise should be repeated three or four times a day for several weeks but never at night when tired.

Concomitant strabismus

We have already seen that in concomitant strabismus, the visual axes, although abnormally directed, retain their abnormal relation to each other in all movements of the eyes. The final lower pathway in the efferent tracts controlling ocular movements is undisturbed, but either the visual impressions arriving at the cortex from one eye are defective or the fusional reflexes have not developed or have been weakly developed and have

broken down so that an ocular deviation results. The cause or causes of this failure are unknown and many theories have been stated and restated so frequently that they are often accepted as proved. The fact remains, however, that no theory of the fundamental causation has yet been advanced which satisfactorily explains the condition.

Many important factors in the ætiology of concomitant strabismus are known, and a proper appreciation of them is essential to rational treatment. In the first place, defective vision in one eye, such as high ametropia, opacities in the media or ocular disease, makes it easy for the affected eye to lose fixation. If the defect exists from birth or early life, the cortical cells normally subserving both eyes may never develop binocular connections so that fusion is impossible. Disturbances in muscular equilibrium usually due to a congenital malinsertion or defective development of one or more of the extrinsic muscles, may act in the same way, the squint being perhaps preceded by a period of heterophoria during which fusion was maintained. The forced dissociation between accommodation and convergence, a matter early pointed out by Donders, is also of importance; the continuous effort of accommodation in the hypermetrope in order to see clearly even in the distance stimulates convergence to a greater degree than is compatible with binocular fixation; faced with the dilemma of either relaxing his accommodation and not seeing clearly or converging too much, he chooses the latter and squints inwards. Conversely, the myope squints outwards. These relationships between the refractive condition and the direction of squint, however, are by no means invariable.

Concomitant strabismus may be either convergent or divergent.

Convergent strabismus is the more common and is most frequent in hypermetropes. It always commences in childhood. It may become manifest after a fright, an attack of whooping cough, measles or other debilitating illness, and is often popularly attributed to some such cause. The deviation is not always quite horizontal: in many cases the eye deviates upwards as well as inwards. In most of these cases there is a vertical element, and the deviation may have been primarily paretic.

Divergent strabismus, on the other hand, is most common in myopes, often commencing at a later age; it may, indeed, arise late in life when one eye loses most or all of its vision. The better eye is then used and the other is allowed to take up the position of rest, which is usually one of divergence. There is an undoubted tendency for the deviation in all cases of convergent strabismus to diminish with the diminution of accommodation in age. Spontaneous cure rarely if ever occurs in divergent strabismus, which tends to increase with time.

If one eye habitually fixes and the other squints the case is usually termed one of *unilateral strabismus*. Sometimes fixation is retained by either eye in which case the squint is said to be *alternating*. Usually in a divergent squint an object towards the right in the field of vision will be fixed with the right eye, in the left of the field by the left eye; the converse may occur in convergent squint. (cross-fixation) Occasionally patients with alternating strabismus can fix with either eye voluntarily, but usually they are unconscious of which eye is fixing. Concomitant squint may be *constant*, or occur only at intervals — *periodic*.

The investigation of strabismus

The first step is to ensure that any apparent deviation is indeed real. An *apparent squint* may be due to the configuration of the palpebral aperture. If, for example, as commonly occurs in children, epicanthus (*q.v.*) is present and the medial canthi approach the cornea eccentrically, the appearance of an internal squint results. More commonly such an appearance is due to a divergence beween the visual axis and the optic axis, a divergence which gives the appearance of convergent squint to myopic eyes, of divergent squint to hypermetropic eyes — the opposite relation to a real squint.

The optic axis upon which the cornea and lens are centred passes through the centre of rotation of the eye and approximately through the centre of the pupil. The visual axis passes through the nodal point and the fovea centralis, thus crossing the optic axis and making a small angle with it. This angle (although the convention is slightly inaccurate) is commonly spoken of clinically as the angle γ (gamma) (Fig. 30.3). In the emmetropic eye the angle γ is said to be positive, since the optic axis usually cuts the retina internal to the fovea centralis. In hypermetropic eyes the angle γ is also positive but greater than in emmetropia. In myopia the angle γ is absent or negative for the visual axis and the optic axis coincide or the latter cuts the retina external to the fovea centralis

Neither of these lines can be seen, and the direction of the line of vision is judged by the position of the pupil. Hence the greater the size of a positive angle γ the more the eye will appear to look outwards. If the angle γ is negative the eye will appear to look inwards. In high hypermetropia, therefore, there will be an apparent divergent squint, in high myopia an apparent convergent squint. The latter is the more striking because the emmetropic eye usually has a positive angle γ of 5°, thus producing an apparent divergence of 10°, which, however, we are accustomed to regard as the normal position of the eyes.

The next step is to differentiate a concomitant from a paralytic squint. Both these conditions are analysed by the *screen test*. In an apparent squint there is no devi-

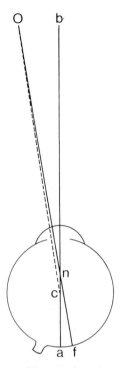

Fig. 30.3 Apparent strabismus. *a b*, optic axis upon which the refractive surfaces are centred; *f*, fovea centralis; *n*, nodal point; *c*, centre of rotation; O, point of fixation; O *c*, line of fixation; O *n f*, line of vision; O *c b*, angle γ. It is practically equal to O *n b*, which can be measured. In actual practice the guide to *a b* is taken from the centre of the pupil; *a b* does not usually pass accurately through the centre of the pupil, so that the result is always only approximate. The angle γ is to the nasal side in hypermetropia and emmetropia

ation when either eye is covered up and then is uncovered to resume fixation. In paralytic squint we have already seen that the secondary deviation is greater than the primary; in concomitant squint, both deviations are equal. No extra effort is required to look in any direction, so that when either eye is covered and then uncovered, the deviation suffered by each is the same. If, moreover, the movements of the eye are found to be full in all directions, and there is no complaint of diplopia, it may be concluded that there is no paralysis. It must be remembered, however, in performing this test in a marked squint, that the eyes do not move as much as usual in the direction opposite to that of the deviation. Thus, in convergent squint it may be very difficult to get the eyes to move outwards to the full extent so that the margin of the cornea lies inside the lateral canthus. This defective movement may be due to muscular contracture.

When the fixing eye is covered with the screen the deviating eye usually moves so as to take up fixation. In unilateral squints of long standing this eye may remain motionless or move only slightly, a condition which is called *eccentric fixation*. Since it occurs only with marked deviation of long standing there is generally no difficulty in distinguishing it from apparent squint.

Apart from the loss of binocular vision, concomitant squint is asymptomatic: diplopia may be present in the initial stages, but it rapidly disappears due to psychological suppression of the macular image of the squinting eye. In most cases suppression is aided by an actual visual defect in this eye, but it also occurs in alternating squint, in which both eyes are frequently normal or have the same degree of ametropia. Suppression is doubtless aided in all cases by the peripheral situation of the image in the squinting eye, but the essential seat of suppression is the brain. Since the image of any object falls on disparate points diplopia results, and since the brain finds this intolerable, it actively inhibits the image of the squinting eye. This prolonged active suppression results in a permanent lowering of the vision of the squinting eye — *amblyopia ex anopsia*. In contrast, it is noteworthy that, because this purposeful and active inhibition is not involved, an eye which has been blind for many years from cataract, immediately attains good vision after a successful operation.

The suppression affects mainly the fovea; indeed, the acuity of vision may become greater at the eccentric point of the retina where the new fixation axis falls habitually in the squinting position, a result which leads to the development of a 'false macula' with abnormal retinal correspondence and abnormal projection. This abnormal relationship is maintained only when both eyes are in use; when the squinting eye only is used, the fovea is usually (but not invariably) used again for fixation. So fixed may this abnormal system become that if the eyes are straightened, diplopia may result, to overcome which the eyes naturally tend to return to their old squinting position. The elimination of false correspondences is therefore of importance before operation is attempted. Eventually all power of fixation may be lost by the amblyopic eye.

Measurement of the angle of the deviation is important in all cases of concomitant squint as a guide to treatment. Many methods are available, but much the most useful and accurate is by a calibrated *amblyoscope* (*the synoptophore* or *orthoptoscope*, an instrument based on the principle of a simple amblyoscope) (Figs. 30.4–5). The patient looks down two adjustable tubes at two easily fixated small objects, and the angle between the tubes is altered until each eye attains fixation when they are used separately, one rapidly after the other. This gives the position of the visual axes. The corneal reflexes are then centred on the pupil; this gives the position of the optic axes. The difference between the two gives the angle of deviation. An attempt is then made to make both eyes fixate the objects simultaneously so that they appear superimposed; if the deviation is different from that

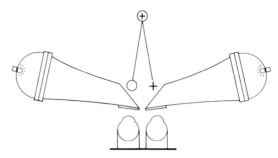

Fig. 30.4 The Amblyoscope

obtained with each eye separately, the presence of abnormal correspondence is shown, and the difference gives the angle of false projection. Other less accurate methods are available.

A rough indication of the angle of the squint can be obtained from the position of the corneal reflex when light is thrown into the eye with the ophthalmoscope, from a distance of about two feet (Fig. 30.6). The patient is told to look at the light; an infant does this reflexly. In the fixing eye the corneal reflex will be in the centre of the pupil, or slightly to the inner side if there is a large angle γ, to the outer side if there is a negative angly γ. The light is then turned onto the squinting eye. If the reflex is about half-way between the centre of the pupil and the corneal margin there is a deviation of about about 20°; if it is at the corneal margin, about 45°. This test gives only an approximate estimation.

The angle of deviation of the squinting eye can also be measured on the perimeter or the tangent scale; in either case the patient fixes the central point with the good eye, and the surgeon carries a light along the arc of the perimeter or the arm of the tangent scale until the corneal reflex thus obtained is centred on the pupil of the squinting eye. The angle at which this occurs is the angle of squint (Fig. 30.7A and B).

Treatment. The routine treatment of a case of concomitant convergent strabismus in a child is as follows:

1. *Preliminary.* Record the distant vision of each eye if the child is not too young (by the E Test, p. 133, or by the Sheridan Gardner test types), the angle of deviation, and any false projection. Order ung. atropinæ, 1%, three times a day for at least four days. At the end of this period estimate the error of refraction by retinoscopy and confirm the result subjectively if possible; reliance should be placed on the retinoscopy rather than on subjective tests. Again measure the angle of the squint, which is likely to be less under atropine than without a mydriatic. Order the full spectacle correction for constant use. A smaller deduction for the effect of atropine should be made than in hypermetropia without squint; indeed, if the refractive error is small no deduction may be made. Great care must be taken to correct all astigmatism, especially in the squinting eye.

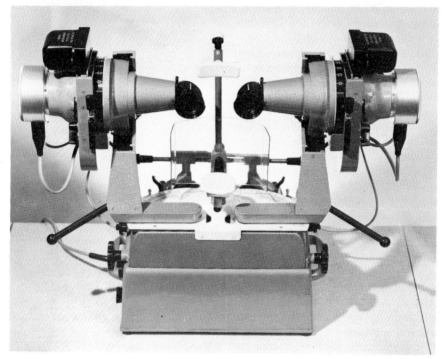

Fig. 30.5 A modern synoptophore for examination of binocular vision, the capacity for fusion and the muscle balance. (By courtesy of Clement Clarke.)

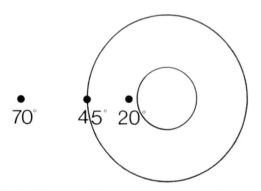

Fig. 30.6 Diagram of the position of the corneal reflex as a guide to the angle of the squint

The patient should be re-examined in a month's time.

If the child is less than two years old, is a hypermetrope and has an internal squint, it is easier to eliminate accommodation by keeping both eyes under the influence of atropine; the 1% ointment need be applied only once every second day. The child should be examined at regular intervals until it is considered advisable to order spectacles.

2. Occlusion of the fixing eye. If, when the vision is tested, the squinting eye is amblyopic, as is usually the case, an effort should be made to improve the vision in it by continual exercise. In order that this eye may be used, the other must be prevented from seeing, or at any rate from seeing clearly. The only satisfactory method of ensuring this is by complete occlusion, effected by a patch covering the better eye; to prevent the child removing it, it is well to fix it to the skin by adhesive material. The patch is changed when it becomes dirty or loose. *Occlusion should be absolute* since if both eyes are used together active inhibition of the squinting eye rapidly undoes any good result achieved; it may have to be continued for six to twelve weeks, but if there is little improvement after this interval the practice may be discontinued. In cases of eccentric fixation the good eye should be occluded for a time in the hope that foveal fixation will develop in the other. In some cases the deviation becomes transferred to the occluded eye: this is a good sign, as it indicates that the vision with the originally squinting eye is only slightly worse than that of the fixing eye.

An alternative method is to activate the entire population of visual neurones in the visual cortex by a range of spatial frequency gratings covering all orientations. This is accomplished by slowly rotating a disc with black and white lines of varying widths before the amblyopic eye and in this way the vision may improve in the amblyopic eye faster and more completely than with other techniques. Patients observe the gratings with the amblyopic eye for seven minutes and play drawing

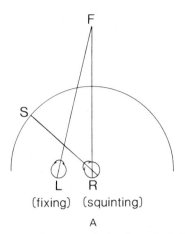

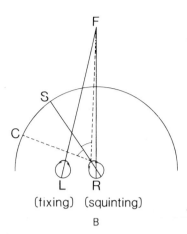

Fig. 30.7 Angular strabismometry. A, Javal's method. The R.E. (squinting) is central in the perimeter. The L.E. fixes F. The surgeon carries a light (S) along the arc of the perimeter until the corneal reflex in R is central. Angle SRF (less the angle γ) is the angle of squint. B, Charpentier's method. The R.E. (squinting) is central in the perimeter. The L.E. fixes F. A light is placed on the perimetric arc on the line FR and the surgeon moves round the arc (to C) until he sees the corneal reflex in R central. Half the angle FRC (i.e., FRS) (less the angle γ) is the angle of squint

games on a Perspex plate over the rotating grating. Children are treated at weekly intervals and the non-amblyopic eye is not occluded.

In very young children or in recent squinters in whom the habit of suppression has not become fixed, the less drastic procedure of instilling atropine into the *fixing* eye every two days may be sufficient; in this event the squinting eye must be used for seeing near objects.

3. *Orthopic training.* The further treatment depends upon the size of the angle of deviation, the condition of vision in the squinting eye, and a variety of other factors which differ in each case. An attempt is made to cultivate binocular vision and stereoscopic fusion by *orthoptic training.* This consists essentially in specially designed exercises undertaken mainly on a synoptophore devised, not to increase the power of the muscles (which is unimpaired) but to encourage the development of binocular vision and the capacity for fusion. It is obvious that only a small and recently acquired squint can be cured in this way and in the majority of cases such training must be combined with surgery. As a rule in this way only can a complete 'cure' be attained since the patient is placed in the same condition as a normal person; his eyes are straight and he has binocular vision. The eyes can be put straight surgically, but this cures only the deviation and leaves the fundamental disability unaltered. If eccentric fixation is well established, it is often well to occlude the affected eye for some weeks and then to stimulate the macula by special *pleoptic methods* (flashing devices, the production of after-images, etc.); but such treatment is time-consuming and exacting and not always successful.

There are three stages in orthoptic treatment: (a) the production of simultaneous vision with the two eyes; (b) the production of binocular vision and the elimination of false projection; and (c) the production of stereoscopic vision, i.e., the fusion of two images of the same object seen in perspective, resulting in the perception of solidity and relief.

Although orthoptic treatment is of great value in inculcating correct visual habits such as the training of binocular vision and the abolition of false projection, it rarely if ever by itself cures a squint of over 10° deviation or one of long standing. In many cases it is useless to attempt it, and in all cases it is useless unless carried out systematically and thoroughly, and it is rarely worth while to persist with it as a sole method of treatment if the deviation is not corrected within three months. For the details of the treatment monographs on the subject must be consulted. Its most valuable function is as an adjunct to operative treatment — to develop binocular vision and reduce the intensity of abnormal projection before operation, to consolidate results and correct any residual deviation after surgery.

4. *Surgical treatment* of concomitant unilateral convergent squint is indicated when the angle of squint is 10° or more when wearing correcting lenses, and in children when orthoptic training has failed to correct the deviation within a reasonable time. As a general rule it should be undertaken early and certainly as soon as the child is old enough to co-operate in post-operative orthoptic treatment, usually between four and five years of age. Postponement until the child is ten or more usually results in the permanence of amblyopia and failure to establish binocular vision. The operation is then purely cosmetic.

The safest operations for general use are a resection or a recession of the appropriate muscle. Free tenotomy of the medial rectus tendon and its expansions into Tenon's capsule is usually followed by divergence and retraction of the caruncle and plica semilunaris, owing to failure of reattachment to the globe. A tenotomy of the lateral rectus muscle, however, is sometimes permissible. The medial rectus should not be recessed more than 5 mm. lest weak convergence occur, leading to discomfort in reading and near work and to headaches. An approximate guide to expected results is given in the Table 30.1.

The treatment of alternating concomitant convergent squint without appreciable error of refraction is purely cosmetic. These patients have no binocular vision, and it is useless to attempt to develop it unless the case is seen when the patient is very young or immediately after the squint has been first noticed. There is often a considerable deviation so that surgery may be required on both eyes.

The treatment of concomitant divergent strabismus is similar to that of the convergent type. The refraction must be first carefully corrected, and it is advisable to order a full correction for constant use unless the myopia is very high. Recession of the lateral rectus is seldom indicated in these cases because the benefit derived is too slight; it will not correct much more than 5° deviation. Hence resection of the medial rectus is usually necessary, reinforced, if required, by recession of the lateral muscle. In divergent strabismus slight over-correction is indicated, for these eyes show a great tendency to revert to their former position.

Sometimes the patients develop diplopia after the eyes have been straightened. This may be due to false projection (p. 283), but also occurs with alternating squints. It is a troublesome complication, usually persisting for some weeks or months, and is distressing to the patient; but it usually eventually disappears.

'A' and 'V' phenomena

A tendency for the eyes to diverge on elevation is physiological. The 'A' and 'V' phenomenon should be assessed by the cover test in 25° upward and downward gaze. The cover test should be carried out for near distance and also in the far distance beyond 6 m, particularly in cases of divergent strabismus. Glasses should

Table 30.1 An approximate guide to expected results

	Surgery (in mm)	Correction (in degrees)	(in prism dioptres)
Esotropia			
Minimum MR recessions each eye	3	12°–15°	20–25Δ
Maximum MR recessions each eye	5	up to 25°	up to 40Δ
Minimum (MR recession) same (LR resection) eye	3 / 5	12°–15°	20–25Δ
Maximum (MR recession) same (LR resection) eye	5 / 8	30°	50Δ
Exotropia			
Minimum LR recessions each eye	5	15°	25Δ
Maximum LR recessions each eye	7	up to 30°	up to 50Δ
Minimum (LR recession) same (MR resection) eye	5 / 4	12°	20Δ
Maximum (LR recession) same (MR resection) eye	7 / 8	30°	50Δ
Vertical rectus surgery			
Minimum SR or IR recession	2.5	up to 5°	up to 8Δ
Minimum SR or IR resection	3	up to 5°	up to 8Δ
Maximum SR or IR recession (or resection)	4.5	up to 8°	up to 15Δ
Combined maximum vertical recti recession/resection of same eye	4.5	15°	25Δ

Key: MR = medial rectus; LR = lateral rectus; SR = superior rectus; IR = inferior rectus. (By courtesy of Fells.)

be worn if necessary and in assessing the cover test for near a small target to stimulate accommodation is necessary.

If no binocular vision is achievable and therapy is desired only for cosmetic purposes the grosser amounts of 'A' and 'V' phenomenon may require surgical adjustment.

If useful binocular vision is present, and this is only maintained by a compensatory chin elevation (in 'A' esophoria or 'V' exophoria) or chin depression (in 'V' esophoria or 'A' exophoria) then surgical adjustment is indicated. Binocular vision in the primary position and in downward gaze is more important than binocular vision on upward gaze and surgery should be planned accordingly.

In general it is found that the oblique muscles are of more importance in the production of 'A' and 'V' phenomena than are the vertical recti muscles. Weakening or strengthening of the obliques, therefore, are well-recognized methods of influencing 'A' and 'V' phenomena.

'A' estropia

In the absence of vertical muscle anomaly, resection of the lateral recti with displacement of the insertions downwards should be effective in patients with a greater deviation for distance than for near. In those with A esotropia associated with convergence excess, recession of the medial recti with elevation of the insertions is effective.

Large degrees in small children, with gross overaction of the superior obliques, may respond to bilateral weakening of the muscle.

'A' exotropia

Smaller degrees may be helped by bilateral resection of the inferior recti, or resection of the medial recti with elevation of the insertions but the results are disappointing.

Large degrees in small children with overaction of the superior obliques respond to bilateral weakening of this muscle.

'V' esotropia

In the the absence of vertical muscle anomaly, recession of the medial recti with displacement of the insertions downwards is effective. If overation of the inferior obliques is present this responds to bilateral antero-position of this muscle with recession of the medial rectus muscles. If the overaction is gross, the antero-position should be combined with recession of the inferior oblique.

'V' exotropia

In the absence of significant vertical muscle anomaly,

recessions of the lateral recti with displacement of the insertions upwards is effective. If overaction of the inferior obliques is present, bilateral anteroposition of the muscle is effective, with or without recession of the muscle, depending on the degree of overaction. Recession of the lateral recti may be performed at the same time.

Microtropia

The features of microtropia are a small esotropia of less than 10Δ with a minor degree of amblyopia. There is eccentric fixation and harmonious ARC. Cover test is not reliable in demonstrating a microtropia and its detection is facilitated by the use of a 4Δ prism test which demonstrates a small scotoma in one eye. If a 4Δ prism is placed base-out before the sound eye then this eye adducts to resume fixation, and the fellow eye abducts without showing a fusional recovery movement. When the prism is placed base-out before the squinting eye then the image is moved onto the foveal scotoma so that no movement of either eye results.

The aetiology of microtropia is uncertain although anisometropia is a common finding. Patients are usually referred because of the discoverry of a slight amblyopia in one eye on routine testing. Some patients may complain of reading difficulties because they experience the crowding phenomenon or become aware of their scotoma on reading with one eye. There is nothing to offer in the way of treatment.

Operations on the extrinsic muscles

In operating for squint with a general anæsthetic it is important to remember that the position of the eyes varies in different stages of anæsthesia so that it gives no criterion of the final position after the anæsthetic has passed off; in squint surgery the deviation as previously measured should be remembered and the position actually present under the anæsthetic ignored. With local anaesthesia discomfort results when tension is put upon a muscle — which is almost impossible to avoid. In the case of children a general anæsthetic should be used. In all cases the preparation of the eye for operation should follow the lines already indicated.
Post-operative padding is unnecessary.

Recession of the medial rectus

A vertical incision is made with scissors in the conjunctiva over the medial rectus and a flap undermined towards the inner canthus exposing the muscle covered by Tenon's capsule; alternatively a limbal conjunctival incision may be employed. Tenon's capsule is then button-holed with scissors and slit for 7 mm along the upper and lower edges of the muscle: the part of the capsule covering the muscle should be preserved. The point of a strabismus hook is passed into Tenon's capsule at the posterior limits of the incisions and retracted. Dividers measuring the amount desired to set the muscle back are placed along the upper and lower borders of the muscle, the distance measured off from the tendon insertion, and marked on the sclera. Catgut sutures are passed through the upper and lower edges of the muscle 2 mm behind its insertion in the so-called 'whip stitch' fashion. The tendon is divided, and the stitches are passed through the superficial layers of the sclera at right angles to the long axis of the muscle at the points already marked. They are tied, and the conjunctival incision is then closed with a continuous suture.

Resection of the lateral rectus
An incision is made 2 mm behind and concentric with the corneo-scleral junction in front of the insertion of the muscle, and the conjunctiva undermined. The muscle is exposed in the same manner as in recession. A strabismus hook is passed between the muscle and sclera, and the length of muscle and tendon for resection determined and marked with gentian violet. Whip-stitch sutures are passed through the upper and lower edges of the muscle 2 mm behind the mark and ensnaring a breadth of about 2 mm of the muscle fibres. The muscle is divided at the mark, the distal part being held in fixation forceps so as to steady the globe whilst the scleral sutures are inserted. The needles are passed through half the thickness of the sclera at the level of the insertion. The tendon is then divided at its insertion, the shortened muscle drawn forwards, the sutures tied, and the conjunctival incision closed.

The superior and inferior recti are resected and recessed in the same way.

In antero-positioning of the inferior oblique
The muscle is approached through conjunctiva and separated at its insertion. It is reattached closer to the inferior rectus muscle on an arc which joins the insertions of the medial and inferior rectus muscles. In recession of the inferior oblique the posterior end of the muscle is reattached 7 mm behind the lower end of the lateral rectus attachment and 7 mm downwards along a line concentric with the limbus. The anterior corner of the oblique muscle is attached 3 mm posterior to and 2 mm lateral to the lateral end of the inferior rectus insertion.

The superior oblique tendon weakening procedure
This procedure is carried out in two different clinical conditions:
  1. An A-pattern horizontal strabismus with overacting superior oblique muscles.
  2. *Brown's Syndrome*, secondary to a taut superior oblique tendon. Tenon's capsule is opened 10 mm posterior to the limbus. While the globe is depressed

maximally with a muscle hook introduced temporally under the superior rectus muscle, and Tenon's capsule is retracted superiorly with a Desmarre's lid speculum the superior oblique is visualised 8 mm posterior to the nasal border of the superior rectus muscle insertion lying in its bed of intermuscular septum. A 1 mm hole in the intermuscular septum is made either just anterior or just posterior to the tendon border so that a small hook may be introduced just nasal to the superior rectus muscle to isolate and pick up the superior oblique tendon. All surgery is performed on the insertional sub-Tenon's half of the tendon. The tendon is never-exposed in the extra-Tenon's space between the trochlea and the site of penetration of Tenon's capsule.

In Brown's Syndrome, there is an inability to elevate the adducted eye above the mid-horizontal plane. Less restriction of elevation is apparent in the mid-line and an even smaller elevation deficiency is detectable in abduction. Slight down-shoot of the adducting involved eye is often present. A widening of the palpebral fissure on adduction is associated with this restriction of elevation. Ten per cent of cases are bilateral.

Brown's Syndrome is caused by a tight or short relatively inelastic superior oblique muscle and/or tendon and this is present in varying degrees.

When operating on A-pattern patients with overacting superior oblique muscles a 6 mm tenectomy is advised. The intermuscular septum is left in tact, 6 mm of tendon are excised at the nasal border of the superior rectus muscle and the tendon remains attached to all the tissues it is normally attached to — the sleeve of elastic tissue at the site of its penetration through Tenon's capsule, its normal scleral insertion and the intermuscular septum which invests it between Tenon's capsule penetration and the insertion. The pulling power of the proximal end of the severed tendon is transmitted through the contiguous intact intermuscular septum to the distal end of the severed tendon reducing the possibility of muscle palsy after tenectomy.

For Brown's Syndrome a similar procedure is carried out whereby 3 mm of tendon is tenectomised.

Enhancing superior oblique action
This operation is performed on the lateral side of the superior rectus through a conjunctival incision running horizontally from the lateral edge of the superior rectus. A squint hook picks up the whole of the superior oblique insertion which is then split half way along with a second hook. Two 6 0 collagen sutures are placed in the anterior half of the superior oblique insertion before it is cut from the sclera. The anterior half of the superior oblique tendon is then swung anteriorly and this moves the line of muscle pull forwards ensuring improved intorsion. It is a valuable operation when patients suffer from excyclophoria following closed head injury.

Marginal myotomy

Marginal myotomy weakens a muscle without altering its attachment to the sclera and is usually applied to a medial rectus muscle which has already been fully recessed. Up to four-fifths of the muscle is clamped from opposite sides in two places and the crushed muscle is then cut with scissors.

Muscle transposition procedures

(For total lateral rectus palsy.) In Jensen's operation the medial rectus is detached and recessed. The superior and inferior recti are split along their lengths and joined to the adjacent halves of the similarly split lateral rectus. A 5 1 1 0 Mersilene suture ties the half muscles together at the level of the equator.

Fadenoperation

The Fadenoperation is a procedure designed to change the anatomical and thereby the functional arc of contact of a muscle by suturing the muscle to the sclera 12– 18 mm posterior to its insertion. The effect is to alter the deviation in the field of maximum deviation with no effect in the primary position thus the dynamic angle is increased whereas the static angle of strabismus remains unaffected.

When mechanical factors are important in the pathogenesis of a squint resulting from orbital trauma or poor surgery simple recession-resection procedures do not usually suffice. The conjunctiva need not be closed at the end of an operation if by its closure the eye would be drawn back into its previous condition. Provided that it is sutured to the sclera a bare crescent of sclera may be left between the conjunctival edge and the limbus. A muscle, usually a medial rectus can be recessed much further back than the maximum 5 mm by two whip stitches which are sewn through the insertion of the medial rectus and the muscle tendon itself allowed to slip back as far as necessary into the orbit. This may produce a straight eye in the primary position and still allow for adequate adduction.

SECTION 6

Diseases of the adnexa of the eye

31

Diseases of the lids

Anatomy

The lids are covered anteriorly by skin and posteriorly by mucous membrane – conjunctiva tarsi. They contain muscle, glands, blood vessels and nerves, all bound together by connective tissue which is particularly dense at the posterior part where it forms a stiff plate – the tarsus (Fig. 31.1).

The skin of the lids is peculiar in its thinness, its loose attachment, and the absence of fat in its corium. It is covered with fine downy hairs, which are provided with small sebaceous glands, and there are also small sweat glands. At the margins these structures are specially differentiated. The cilia or eyelashes are strong, short, curved hairs, arranged in two or more closely set rows. Their sebaceous follicles, like the cilia themselves, are specially differentiated, and are called *Zeis's glands* which, apart from being larger, are identical with other sebaceous glands. The sweat glands near the edge are also unusually large and are known as *Moll's glands*; they are situated immediately behind the hair follicles, and their ducts open into the ducts of Zeis's glands or into the hair follicles, not directly onto the surface of the skin as elsewhere.

The margin or free edge of the lid is called the *intermarginal strip* (Fig. 31.2). It is covered with stratified epithelium which forms a transition between the skin and the conjunctiva. The anterior border is rounded; the posterior, which lies in contact with the globe, is sharp. The capillarity induced by this sharp angle of contact is of importance in the proper moistening of the surface of the eye. Immediately anterior to the posterior border the orifices of the ducts of the meibomian glands form a single row of minute orifices, just visible to the naked eye. Between them and the anterior border is a fine grey line, which is important in operations in which the lid is split since it indicates the position of the loose fibrous tissue between the orbicularis palpebrarum and the tarsus.

The tarsus consists of dense fibrous tissue; it contains no cartilage. Embedded in it are some enormously developed sebaceous glands, the *meibomian (tarsal) glands*, consisting of nearly straight tubes, directed vertically,

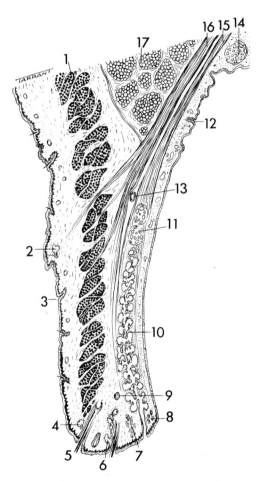

Fig. 31.1 Section through the upper lid. 1, orbicularis muscle; 2, sweat gland; 3, hair follicle; 4, gland of Zeis; 5, cilium; 6, gland of Moll; 7, pars marginalis of orbicularis muscle; 8, pars sub-tarsalis of orbicularis muscle; 9, inferior arterial arcade; 10, meibomian gland; 11, gland of Wolfring; 12, conjunctival crypts; 13, superior arterial arcade; 14, gland of Krause; 15, Müller's muscle; 16, levator palpebræ superioris; 17, fat

twenty to thirty in number in each lid, each opening by a single duct on the margin of the lid.

The orbicularis palpebrarum occupies the space be-

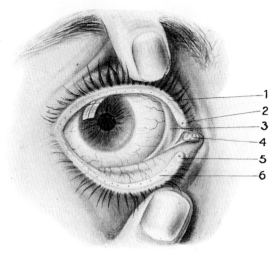

Fig. 31.2 The surface anatomy of the lid margins and the conjunctival sac. The lids have been pulled aside to display their margins and expose the structures at the inner canthus. 1, intermarginal strip; 2, upper punctum; 3, plica semilunaris; 4, caruncle; 5, lower punctum; 6, openings of tarsal glands

tween the tarsus and the skin. The main central band of the levator palpebræ superioris is inserted into the upper border of the tarsus; an anterior slip passes between the bundles of the orbicularis to be inserted into the skin of the middle of the lid; a posterior slip is inserted into the conjunctiva at the fornix. The inferior rectus and oblique muscles send fibrous strands forwards into the lower lid to be attached to the tarsus and palpebral ligament.

Besides these striped muscles there are layers of unstriped muscle in each lid, constituting the superior and inferior tarsal muscles of Müller. The fibres of the former arise among the striped fibres of the levator, pass down behind it, and are inserted into the upper border of the tarsus; the inferior tarsal muscle lies below the inferior rectus and is inserted into the lower tarsus.

The arteries of the upper lid form two main arches, the superior lying between the upper border of the tarsus and the orbicularis, the inferior, in a similar position just above the hair follicles. In the lower lid there is one arch near the free edge. There are two venous plexuses in each lid: a post-tarsal passing into the ophthalmic veins, and a pre-tarsal opening into subcutaneous veins.

The sensory nerve supply is derived from the trigeminal. The third nerve supplies the levator palpebræ, the seventh the orbicularis, and the sympathetic Müller's muscles.

Oedema of the lids

This is common and, owing to the looseness of the tissue, may be so great as to close the eye (Fig. 31.3). It may be inflammatory or passive. *Inflammatory oedema* may be caused by an inflammation of the lid itself (dermatitis, stye, insect bite, etc.), of the conjunctiva (when it may be associated with chemosis), of the lacrimal sac, or by purulent inflammation in the eye, Tenon's capsule, the orbit or the underlying nasal sinuses. Chronic thickening of the lids, resembling œdema but harder in consistency, may follow recurrent attacks of erysipelas – so-called *solid œdema*.

Passive oedema, due to circulatory obstruction, is seen in general disease (renal disease, cardiac failure) or local conditions such as cavernous sinus thrombosis. An intermittent and acute oedematous condition due to a general anaphylaxis is accompanied by swollen lids. (angio-neurotic œdema).

Inflammation of the lids

Almost any of the inflammatory conditions which affect the *skin* in general may attack the lids. In this region dermatitis is common and frequently marked, particularly allergic manifestations due to sensitization to innumerable allergens — cosmetics, dyes, drugs, etc. (Fig. 31.3). Atropine irritation is a typical example. An

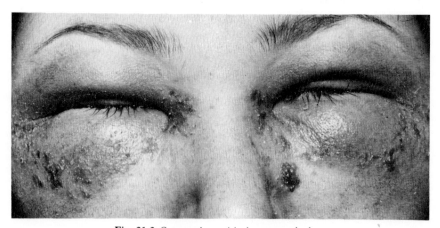

Fig. 31.3 Contact dermatitis due to eye-shadow

eczema may occur in association with a discharging conjunctivitis or where there is much lacrimination. The ordinary coccal infections cause boils and abscesses; specific infections may occur such as anthrax or zoster (*q.v.*). Erysipelas is dangerous in that it may spread to the orbit, leading to cellulitis, thrombosis of the cavernous sinus, or meningitis.

Blepharitis

This is a chronic inflammation of the margins of the lids, appearing as a simple hyperæmia or as a true inflammation which may occur in two forms. In *squamous blepharitis* small white scales accumulate among the lashes which fall out readily, but are replaced without distortion. If the scales are removed the underlying surface is found to be hyperæmic, but not ulcerated. The condition is often essentially metabolic and of the nature of seborrhœa associated frequently with dandruff of the scalp. Such ætiological factors require treatment.

Ulcerative blepharitis is an infective condition. Yellow crusts glue the lashes together and on removing them small ulcers which bleed easily are seen around the bases of the lashes. This distinguishes the condition from matting together of the lashes by conjunctival discharge; removal of these crusts reveals normal lid margins. The symptoms are redness of the edges of the lids, itching, soreness, lacrimation, and photophobia.

The sequelae of the ulcerative form are serious. If not treated energetically and with perseverance the disease is extremely chronic, causing or being accompanied by chronic conjunctivitis. The ulceration is liable to extend deeply, destroying the hair follicles so that the lashes fall out and either are not replaced or only by a few small, scattered, distorted cilia (*madarosis*). When the ulcers heal the cicatricial tissue contracts. Neighbouring hair follicles are drawn out of place and a false direction is given to the remaining cilia so that they may rub against the cornea (*trichiasis*). Occasionally the development of cicatricial tissue may be extreme so that the edge of the lid becomes hypertrophied and droops in consequence of its weight (*tylosis*).

The lower lid is particularly liable to be displaced by prolonged ulcerative blepharitis. The contraction of the scar tissue drags the conjunctiva over the margin; the posterior lip of the intermarginal strip, instead of being acute-angled, becomes rounded, so that its capillarity is impaired. Tears then tend to spill over (*epiphora*), a condition which is accentuated if the punctum becomes everted so that it ceases to lie in accurate contact with the bulbar conjunctiva. The continual wetting of the skin with tears leads to eczema, which is followed by contraction. The condition is made worse by perpetually wiping the eyes, so that eventually *ectropion* develops; this causes still more epiphora and a vicious circle is set up.

The causes of blepharitis are very varied. The condition may follow chronic conjunctivitis due to staphylococci carried to the lid margins by infected fingers. Occasionally parasites cause blepharitis — *blepharitis acarica*, due to demodex folliculorum, and *phthiriasis palpebrarum*, due to the crab-louse, very rarely to the head-louse.

Treatment. The local treatment of blepharitis must be energetic in the ulcerative form. The crusts must first be removed and loose, diseased lashes epilated. This is effected most easily by thorough bathing with warm bicarbonate of soda lotion, 3%. The application softens the deposits, so that they can be picked or rubbed off with a pledget of cotton-wool. When the crusts have been entirely removed an antibiotic drop depending on the sensitivity of the organism is prescribed. When the infection has been eliminated simple daily swabbing of the lid margins with a warm bland lotion must be established as a daily habit. Rubbing of the eyes or fingering the lids with unwashed hands must be barred completely. In most case, if the treatment is carried out properly, there is a speedy cure.

Syphilis

A *primary chancre* near the lid-margin is a rarity. There is generally a small ulcer covered with scanty greyish secretion, much indurated about the base, considerable oedema and involvement of the regional lymph nodes. The swelling of the lymph nodes is always suggestive of syphilis or tuberculosis, but in all doubtful cases scrapings should be examined for treponemata. Systemic penicillin treatment should at once be undertaken.

Vaccinia

The margin of the lid is occasionally inoculated from the recently vaccinated arm of a baby, and one lid may infect the opposing margin of the other. Usually the pustule is at the outer canthus, and the pre-auricular lymph node is swollen and painful. The history generally serves to elucidate the case. Sometimes the cornea becomes affected. *Treatment* is outlined on p. 140 (Fig. 31.4).

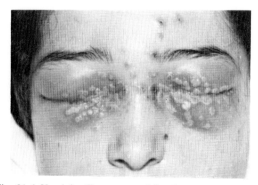

Fig. 31.4 Vaccinia. (By courtesy of Ogg.)

Molluscum contagiosum is a small white umbilicated swelling, generally multiple, due to a large poxvirus from which a substance resembling sebum can be expressed. Histologically large intracytoplasmic inclusion bodies occur within acanthotic epidermis. It produces a severe conjunctivitis and occasionally a keratitis which are intractable to treatment unless the primary nodules on the lid margin are dealt with. Each should be incised and expressed and the interior touched with tincture of iodine or pure carbolic acid by (Fig. 31.5).

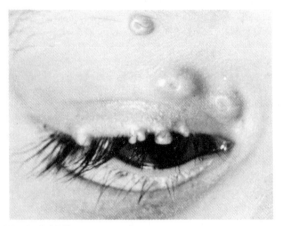

Fig. 31.5 Molluscum contagiosum

Inflammation of the glands of the lids

Hordeolum or stye

This is a suppurative inflammation of one of Zeis's glands (Fig. 31.6). In the early stages the gland becomes swollen, hard and painful, and usually the whole edge of the lid is œdematous. An abscess forms which generally points near the base of one of the cilia.

The pain is considerable until the pus is evacuated. Styes often occur in crops, or may alternate with boils on the neck, carbuncles, or acne, usually indicating a deficient resistance to staphylococci. It is commonest in young adults, but may occur at all ages, especially in debilitated persons.

Treatment. Hot compresses should be used in the early stages. When the abscess points it may often be evacuated by pulling out the affected cilium; alternatively, it is incised with a small knife, which may be momentarily painful. Thereafter a hot compress is applied. Antibiotic ointments may prevent recurrences.

If crops of styes occur, conditions such as diabetes must be excluded and rubbing the eyes must stop. A general course of tetracycline may stop recurrences.

Hordeolum internum.

This is a suppurative inflammation of a meibomian gland, is less common; it may be due to secondary infection of a chalazion. The inflammatory symptoms are more violent than in an external stye, for the gland is larger and is embedded in dense fibrous tissue. The pus appears as a yellow spot shining through the conjunctiva when the lid is everted. It may burst through the duct or the conjunctiva, rarely through the skin. *Treatment* is the same as for the external type, except that the incision should be made exactly as for a chalazion (*vide infra*).

Chalazion (tarsal 'cyst', meibomian 'cyst')

Figure 31.7 is not a cyst but a chronic inflammatory granuloma of a meibomian gland. Chalazia are often multiple, occurring in crops, a condition commoner in adults than in children. The glandular tissue becomes replaced by granulations containing giant cells, probably as a result of chronic irritation by an organism of low virulence. The gland becomes swollen, increasing in size very gradually and without inflammatory symptoms so that patients usually seek advice on account of the disfigurement. The smaller chalazia are difficult to see, but are readily appreciated by passing the finger over the skin. If the lid is everted the conjunctiva is red or purple over the nodule, in later stages often grey, or rarely, if

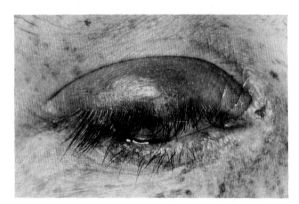

Fig. 31.6 Stye

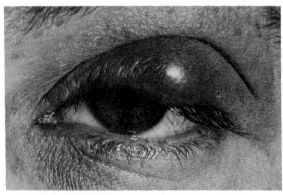

Fig. 31.7 Chalazion of the upper lid

infection has occurred, yellow (hordeolum internum). The grey appearance is due to alteration in the granulation tissue which becomes converted into a jelly-like mass. Complete spontaneous resolution rarely occurs. The contents may be extruded through the conjunctiva, and in these cases a fungating mass of granulation tissue often sprouts through the opening, keeping up conjunctival discharge and irritation. Sometimes the granulation tissue is formed in the duct of the gland, from which it projects as a reddish-grey nodule on the intermarginal strip (*marginal chalazion*).

Treatment. Chalazia should be incised and thoroughly scraped.

The conjunctival sac is well anæsthetised, and the lid with a regional injection of Procaine, the lid everted and at the point of greatest discoloration a vertical incision is made through the palpebral conjunctiva with a sharp scalpel Any semi-fluid contents which may be present escape and the walls of the cavity are thoroughly scraped with a small sharp spoon. Bleeding soon stops and no dressing is usually necessary. A clamp is a useful adjunct in the manipulations.

The patient should be warned that the swelling will remain for some time since the cavity becomes filled with blood. Sometimes, especially if the scraping has not been sufficient, granulation tissue sprouts from the wound. This must be snipped off with scissors and the cavity again scraped out.

Very hard chalazia are occasionally met with, particularly near the canthi; these may be adenomata of the glands and require excision. Malignant changes occur but are rare; in all cases wherein recurrences persist, however, a histological section should be examined.

Anomalies in the position of the lashes and lids

Blepharospasm

This consists of involuntary sustained and forcible eyelid closure which may occur spontaneously — *essential blepharospasm* or be precipitated by sensory stimuli — *reflex blepharospasm*. Essential blepharospasm has an insidious onset between the ages of 45 and 65 of brief involuntary eye closure affecting one or both eyes and leading to an inability to open the lids. It is less apparent during periods of heightened attention. Treatment consists of facial denervation. All temporal–zygomatic and buccal branches of the VIIth nerve which cause contraction of the upper facial muscles are avulsed. The mandibular branch of the VIIth nerve is identified and the function of its branches are assessed by electrical stimulation.

Trichiasis (θριξ; τριχός, *a hair*)

This is the condition of distortion of the cilia, so that they are directed backwards and rub against the cornea.

Any condition causing entropion (*q.v.*) will cause trichiasis, trachoma and spastic entropion being among the most common; other causes are blepharitis, and the scars resulting from injuries, burns, operations, or destructive inflammations such as diphtheria. A few of the lashes may be effected, or the condition may be due to entropion involving the whole margin of the lid. It may also be caused by congenital distichiasis (*q.v.*).

The symptoms are those of a foreign body continually present in the eye — irritation, pain, conjunctival congestion, reflex blepharospasm and lacrimation. Recurrent erosions, superficial opacities and vascularisation of the cornea are eventually produced; recurrent corneal ulcers are not infrequently due to this cause.

Treatment. Isolated misdirected cilia may be removed by epilation but this must be repeated every few weeks. Destruction of the hair follicle by diathermy or electrolysis is preferable.

With the former, a fine needle is inserted into the hair follicle and a current of 30 mA is applied for 10 sec. With the latter, the flat positive pole is applied to the temple; the negative, a fine steel needle, is introduced into the hair follicle: a current of 2 mA is used. The negative pole is determined by placing the terminals in saline, when bubbles of hydrogen are given off by it. The strength of current can be gauged by the rate of evolution of gas. It should be remembered that electrolysis is both painful and tedious; the pain may be avoided by injecting Procaine into the margin of the lid. If the current is of the proper strength, the bubbles produced at the site of puncture cause the formation of a slight foam, and the lash with its bulbous root can be easily lifted out.

If many cilia are displaced, resort must be had to operative procedures as for entropion (*vide infra*).

Entropion (εν; *in*, τρεπειν, *to turn*)

Rolling in of the lid, occurs in two forms, spastic and cicatricial. The symptoms are those of the trichiasis (*q.v.*) which is induced.

Spastic entropion. This is due to spasm of the orbicularis in the presence of degeneration of the palpebral connective tissue separating the orbicularis muscle fibres thus allowing them to ride up in front of the tarsal plate towards the lid margin. Degeneration of the tarsal muscle of Müller (a lower lid retractor) plays a part in failing to anchor the lower margin of the tarsal plate to the bony orbit. The inferior lid aponeurosis maintains the orbicularis muscle in such a position that it presses against the lower tarsus and prevents an entropion by contraction of the capsule-palpebral head of the inferior rectus. If the aponeurosis degenerates then strong contraction of the circularly arranged fibres tends not only to approximate the lid margins, but also to turn them inwards. If the support is insufficient, entropion is pro-

duced. This is well seen when the eyeball has been removed, but it also occurs when the globe is deeply set
owing to absence of orbital fat, especially if the skin of
the lids is also redundant. These conditions are found
particularly in old people who are therefore liable to
spastic entropion. It is also caused by tight bandaging as
after a surgical operation and is favoured by narrowness
of the palpebral aperture (blepharophimosis). Spastic
entropion is almost invariably restricted to the lower lid
(Fig. 31.8).

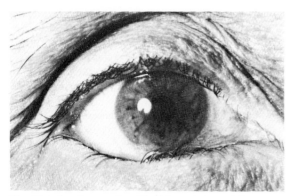

Fig. 31.8 Spastic entropion. The lid margin is partially curled
in and the lashes sweep the cornea

Cicatricial entropion. This is caused by cicatricial contraction of the palpebral conjunctiva; in the worst
forms, found in trachoma, the tarsal plate is also bent
and distorted, sometimes by atrophic, sometimes by
hyperplastic changes. It is an exaggeration of the effect
produced by the various causes of trichiasis (*q.v.*).

Treatment of spastic entropion. If due to bandaging, the
condition is often cured by simply leaving off the bandage. In the spastic entropion of old people temporary
relief may be obtained by everting the lid, by painting
collodion on the skin, by pulling it out with a strip of
adhesive plaster or by a subcutaneous stitch. Injection of
1 ml of 80% alcohol subcutaneously along the edge of
the lid, with or without canthoplasty, has been advocated. Permanent relief can be obtained only by
operation.

Attempts may be made to produce a ridge of tarsal
tissue in the orbicularis muscle and thus prevent fibres
from sliding in a vertical direction. A horizontal incision
is made 4 mm below the lid margin through all the lid
structures. Two double-armed sutures are placed
through the tarsal plate in the inferior lip of the wound,
entering from the conjunctival surface. These sutures
are inserted under the skin of the upper lip of the
wound to exit just below the lid margin. The skin incision is closed, the clamp released and the deep sutures
tied.

In congenital epiblepharon and in senile entropion

affecting bed-ridden patients a simple suturing of the
lower lid with double-arm 5–0 chromic catgut may
prove efficacious. The needle is passed through the lid
from conjunctiva to skin adjacent to but not through the
inferior border of the tarsus. Slight downward traction
is applied to the skin when the needle is passed through
the muscle and skin. The second needle is placed 3 mm
horizontally from it. The suture is tied firmly and left to
fall out spontaneously in three weeks.

Bick procedure modified by Reeh. In patients with particularly lax lower lids and entropion it is necessary to
remove some of the excessive lid tissue next to the lateral canthus. An inverted house-shaped lid shortening is
performed as shown in the diagram. (Fig. 31.9 (1)) One
4.0 silk suture is brought through the skin of the medial
edge 2 mm from the wound margin. The suture is carried through two-thirds of the thickness of the tarsus
and does not penetrate the conjunctiva. The needle is
then carried through the equivalent tissue of the lateral
margin prior to piercing the lateral canthal tendon. A
similar 4.0 silk suture is carried through the skin and
lower tarsus on the medial wound margin and through
the orbicularis laterally prior to being fixed to the
periosteum of the lateral orbital rim. (Fig. 31.9 (2))
These sutures are left *in situ* and 6.0 chromic gut sutures
close the tarsus and the equivalent tissue laterally.
(Fig. 31.9 (3)) A marginal 6.0 silk suture is passed
through the grey line of the two wound margins; it is
tied and left long for subsequent fixation to the forehead
where it remains in place for two or three days.
(Fig. 31.9 (4)) The skin margin is closed with interrupted 6.0 silk sutures. (Fig. 31.9 (5)) At the end of the
procedure the two 4.0 silk sutures are tied firmly to fix
the tarsal edge to the lateral canthal tissue. The skin
sutures are removed in four or five days and the 4.0 silk
fixation sutures are allowed to remain in position for
10–12 days.

Tucking of inferior lid retractors (Jones, Reeh and Wobig).
In cases of severe entropion tucking of the inferior
lid retractors is advised (Fig. 31.10). The lower lid is
placed in an entropion clamp and an incision made
5 mm beneath the lid margin from the lateral canthus to
the junction of the inner and middle third. The pretarsal
part of the obicularis is severed from the pre-septal part
and the lower border of the tarsus is identified.

The orbital septum is stripped from the tarsus at its
point of attachment to the lower border to open the
preaponeurotic space. Detachment of the preseptal muscle to the fascia is freed by blunt dissection over an area
of about 10 mm when excessive preseptal skin and orbicularis muscle may be resected.

A 4.0 silk suture is then brought through through the
preseptal skin at the level of the middle and the lateral
third of the lower lid. The suture is carried through the
inferior lid aponeurosis about 8 mm inferior to the tar-

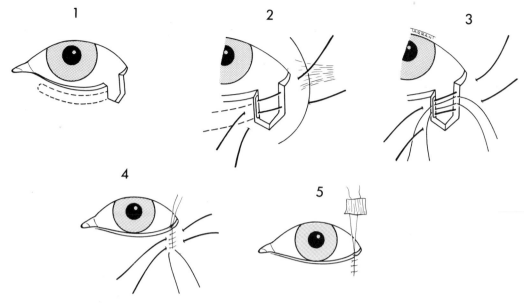

Fig. 31.9 Bick procedure modified by Reeh

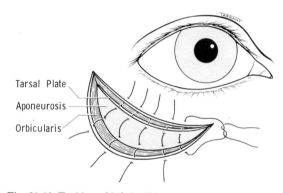

Fig. 31.10 Tucking of inferior lid retractors (Jones, Reeh and Wobig)

sus with a small bite. Then the needle is affixed to the aponeurosis at the level of the lower border of the tarsus prior to penetrating the inferior tarsal margin. The needle then penetrates the upper skin margin and is tied in a slip knot.

Ideally the lower lid should move down 3 mm when the patient gazes downwards. This may require a modification of the placing of the lower bite through the aponeurosis. When the central stitch is satisfactory then 3 or 4 similar sutures are applied. The sutures are kept in place for 6–10 days.

Treatment of cicatricial entropion. Many plastic operations have been devised for the relief of cicatricial entropion: only the more simple will be described here. The principles governing the various operations are: (1) altering the direction of the lashes, (2) transplanting the lashes, (3) straightening the distorted tarsus. Sub-

cutaneous injection of Procaine or a general anaesthetic is indicated; the former method does not obviate all pain, especially if the tarsus is cut.

The simplest procedure is some modification of *Burow's operation.* The lid is everted over the end of a metal lid spatula. A horizontal incision through the conjunctiva and passing completely through the tarsal plate, but not through the skin, is made along the whole length of the lid in the sulcus subtarsalis, about 2–3 mm above the posterior border of the inter-marginal strip. The temporal end of the strip may then be divided by a vertical incision through the free edge of the lid, including the whole thickness. In this manner the edge of the lid is left attached only by skin, and when cicatrisation has occurred the edge is turned slightly outwards, so that the lashes are directed away from the eye. The edge of the lid may be kept everted during the process of healing by means of a spindle-shaped pad of oiled silk kept in position by sutures suitably applied.

There is an alternative operation. The incision is made as before. The tarsal plate is pared down to a chisel-edge along the whole length and mattress sutures are passed through the plate and lid margin, emerging through the grey line (p. 307); they are tied over rubber tubing, thus bending the lid margin forwards and upwards.

In the *Jaesche-Arlt operation* the zone of hair follicles is transplanted to a slightly higher position. The globe is protected by the spatula inserted between it and the lid, or held by a lid clamp. The lid is split from the outer canthus to just outside the punctum along the grey line. The incision extends between the tarsus and the orbicularis for a depth of 3–4 mm, so that the zone containing the hair follicles is loosened. A crescentic piece of skin is then removed from the lid. The lower incision extends through the skin down to the tarsus at a distance of 3–4 mm from the edge of the lid and parallel with it for its whole length. The middle part of the upper incision is 6–8 mm from the edge of the lid. The crescentic piece of skin thus marked out is removed, without taking any orbicularis. The two skin incisions are then sutured. In this manner the zone of lashes is transplanted to a higher level. The gaping wound in the intermarginal strip may be filled in with a graft of mucous membrane from the lip; this tends to prevent the follicles from being drawn down again when the wound cicatrises. Care should be taken not to produce ectropion by removing too much skin.

Ectropion

Rolling out of the lid, occurs in several forms, the chief being senile, cicatricial, and paralytic. The symptoms are due to the epiphora induced and to the chronic conjunctivitis caused by exposure. In long-standing cases the exposed conjunctiva becomes dry and thickened, red and very unsightly and in severe cases the cornea may suffer from imperfect closure of the lids.

Senile ectropion. If the ectropion is most pronounced in the mid section of the lower lid full-thickness lid shortening is recommended in that area. Full-thickness shortening should not be done closer than 5 mm to the punctum. An inverted house-shaped incision of tissue is made and is then repaired as described on p. 312.

If the degree of ectropion is severe and marked over the lateral half of the lower lid a Kuhnt–Szymanowski procedure as modified by Byron Smith is recommended. A line is drawn with gentian violet dye 3 mm inferior to the lid margin following the contour of the lower lid (Fig. 31.11 (1)). The line is drawn slightly past the lateral canthus in an upward manner at which point it is sloped downwards. A skin flap is prepared and a full-thickness lid shortening is then performed at the lateral canthus as previously described (Fig. 31.11 (2 & 3)) Excess skin is then pulled gently upwards and outward (Fig. 31.11 (4)). The excess skin is removed and the skin margins are sutured with 7.0 silk (Fig. 31.11 (5)). Traction sutures are kept at the point of the lid margin meeting and are taped to the forehead at the end of the procedure.

In paralytic ectropion *lateral tarsorrhaphy* may be indicated. In this operation the palpebral aperture is shortened by uniting the lids at the outer canthus. The edges of the upper and lower lids are freshened for the requisite distance, the lashes being excised. The lids are then sutured together as in central tarsorrhaphy (p. 258).

Cicatricial ectropion requires some form of *blepharoplasty*, employing whole or split-skin grafts or flaps of skin taken from the upper lid, behind the ear or the inner upper arm, or strips of fascia lata. Each case must be treated on its own merits and will often exercise the ingenuity of the surgeon.

Symblepharon (συν, *with, together,* βλεφαρόν, *eyelid*)

This is the condition of adhesion of the lid to the globe (Fig. 31.12) Any cause which produces raw surfaces upon two opposed spots of the palpebral and bulbar conjunctiva will lead to adhesion if the areas are allowed to remain in contact during the process of healing — burns from heat or caustics, ulcers, diphtheria, operations, etc. Bands of fibrous tissue are thus formed, stretching between the lid and the globe, involving the

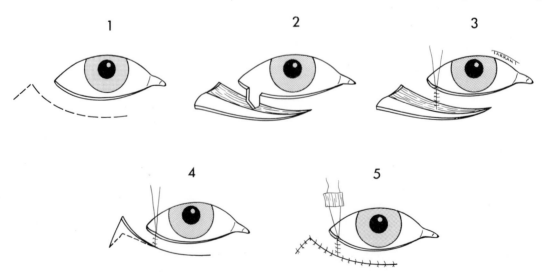

Fig. 31.11 Byron Smith modification of a Kuhnt–Szymanowski procedure

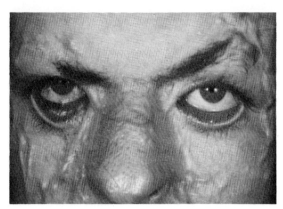

Fig. 31.12 Symblepharon

cornea if this has also been injured. The bands may be narrow, but are more frequently broad, and may extend into the fornix so that the lid is completely adherent to the eyeball over a considerable area (*symblepharon posterior*). Bands limited to the anterior parts and not involving the fornix are called *symblepharon anterior*. *Total symblepharon*, in which the lids are completely adherent to the globe, is rare.

Pronounced adhesions cause impairment of mobility of the eye resulting in diplopia. The adhesion may be so intimate that it is impossible to close the lids efficiently, lagophthalmos with its baneful consequences resulting (*vide infra*). There is often much disfigurement.

Treatment. The prevention of symblepharon is of the utmost importance (p. 243). When it is already established operation is necessary and this may be difficult especially when the bands are broad or if there is symblepharon posterior. There may be no guide to the limitations of sclera and tarsus, and great care has to be exercised lest the globe be punctured. The prevention of the re-formation of adhesions is much more difficult, and is successful only if the raw surfaces are covered with conjunctival or buccal mucous membrane grafts. A therapeutic contact lens may be helpful.

Ankyloblepharon (αγκυλη, *a thong*, βλεφαρον, *eyelid*)
This is adhesion of the margins of the two lids. It may be either a congenital condition or due to burns, etc. It may be partial or complete, and is often combined with symblepharon. The treatment depends upon the amount of symblepharon. If it is very extensive operation may be contra-indicated. In other cases the lids are separated and kept apart during the healing process. If the adhesion extends to the angle of the lids, the latter must be covered with an epithelial graft, otherwise the condition will recur.

Blepharophimosis (βλεφαρον, *eyelid*, φιμος, *a muzzle*)
This is the condition in which the palpebral fissure

appears to be contracted at the outer canthus. The outer angle is often normal, but is obscured by a vertical fold of skin formed by eczematous contraction of the skin following prolonged epiphora and blepharospasm (*epicanthus lateralis*). Mere narrowing of the palpebral aperture is often called blepharophimosis, and may be a congenital condition: it is really a form of ankyloblepharon. The condition may require no treatment, disappearing spontaneously after the inflammation has subsided. In other cases canthoplasty is indicated.

Lagophthalmos (λαγως, *a hare*)
This is the condition of incomplete closure of the palpebral aperture when an attempt is made to shut the eyes. It may be due to contraction of the lids from cicatrisation or a congenital deformity, ectropion, paralysis of the orbicularis, proptosis due to exophthalmic goitre, orbital tumour, etc., or to laxity of the tissues and absence of reflex blinking in people who are extremely ill or moribund. Owing to exposure the cornea becomes epidermoid (xerosis corneæ) or keratitis sets in. The treatment is that of keratitis e lagophthalmo (*q.v.*).

Ptosis (πτωσις, *falling*)
This is the term given to drooping of the upper lid, usually due to paralysis or defective development of the levator palpebræ superioris. It may also occur as a purely mechanical ptosis due to deformity and increased weight of the lid brought about by trachoma or tumours, or from lack of support in phthisis bulbi or anophthalmos.

The condition may be unilateral or bilateral, partial or complete. In the higher degrees the lid hangs down, covering the pupil more or less completely and interfering with vision. An attempt is made to counteract the effect by overaction of the frontalis and by throwing back the head, the eyes being rotated downwards at the same time. A very characteristic attitude is thus adopted; forced contraction of the frontalis causes the eyebrows to be raised and throws the skin of the forehead into wrinkles (Fig. 31.13). Partial ptosis may be

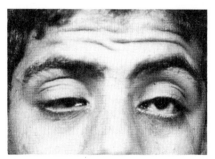

Fig. 31.13 Congenital ptosis, more marked on the right side. Note the wrinkling of the forehead in the attempt to open the eyes. (By courtesy of Kamel.)

masked by this means, but becomes manifest if the patient is asked to look up while the eyebrows are fixed by firm pressure with the fingers against the frontal bone.

Ptosis may be congenital or acquired. The congenital form is usually, but not invariably, bilateral, and is due in most cases to defective development of the muscles. The condition is not infrequently hereditary. There is often an associated defect in the upward movement of the eyes, due sometimes to absence of the posterior insertion of the levator into the fornix, sometimes to coincident maldevelopment or defective innervation of the superior rectus. Defective upward movement of the eyes is the commonest congenital defect of the bilaterally associated extrinsic muscles. A *periodic ptosis* may be present in association with abnormal synkineses (p. 290).

Congenital ptosis is the commonest form of this affliction. In congenital ptosis the history is all important and the presence of congenital ptosis should be confirmed by photographs taken during childhood. Other causes of ptosis must be eliminated, such as trauma a systemic disease or a neurological disorder.

In the normal eye the upper lid margin rests midway between the upper border of the pupil and the limbus. A simple diagram in the notes is sufficient for record purposes (Fig. 31.14).

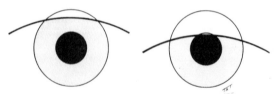

Fig. 31.14 How to record the position of the upper lid

The amount of levator function must be assessed. The examiner places the thumb of one hand horizontally over the patient's brow. The patient is directed to look down without moving his head. With his other hand, the examiner places a millimeter rule just in front of the upper lid and notes the reading on the ruler opposite the lid margin. The thumb is now pressed firmly on the brow fixing the frontalis. The patient is asked to look up as far as possible without moving his head. The difference in the two readings is a practical measurement of levator function. Infants respond better to this test if an assistant provides a fixation light.

In tiny children if the eyelid is everted and the infant encouraged to look up the lids may remain in that position while the eyes are elevated indicating an extreme weakness of levator function.

It is important to examine young people with ptosis for congenital anomalies, disturbances of binocular vision and motility, refractive error and for corneal insensitivity.

Paresis of the elevators of one eye may lead to downward deviation of the globe and a pseudo ptosis.

It is mandatory to investigate Bell's phenomenon particularly if a frontalis sling procedure is being considered. A defective closure combined with the loss of Bell's phenomenon leads to exposure of the cornea during sleep.

One of the objects of surgery on unilateral ptosis is to produce a close match of the contra-lateral upper lid fold. In order to do this it is important to record whether there is a fold in the unoperated lid with a sketch and description of its contour, its depth and any change in depth produced on elevation of the lid; the presence of more than one fold and the distance of the fold from the lid margin must also be registered and copied.

Acquired ptosis is usually unilateral. It may be part of the symptom-complex of paresis or paralysis of the whole of the third nerve, or may be due to paresis or paralysis of the branch supplying the levator. Isolated ptosis without other signs of oculomotor paralysis may result from disease of the supranuclear pathways (p. 349). It may also be due to direct injury of the muscle or its nerve supply, as by wounds or fractures. Bilateral ptosis may occur in the acquired form, notably as part of the syndrome of myasthenia gravis or occasionally in myotonic dystrophy.

Myasthenia gravis is a disease characterised by generalized muscular weakness and rapidly developing fatigue of the muscles due to an auto-immune disorder in which damage of acetylcholine receptors takes place at the post-synaptic membrane. Anti-acetylcholine receptor antibodies are found in approximately 80% of patients with myasthenia with levels correlating with the severity of the disease. Attempts can be made to modify the defective immune mechanism with corticosteroids, immunosuppressives, plasmapheresis and thymectomy. The symptoms fluctuate and after a short rest recovery follows rapidly in the early stages. Ptosis and failure of convergence are early and prominent features. The ptosis is nearly always bilateral and is increased by prolonged fixation or attempts to look upwards; effective compensation by overaction of the frontales is impossible. Ophthalmoplegia externa, partial or complete, occurs in 50% of the cases, but the intrinsic muscles are not affected. Nystagmoid jerks are not uncommon. Remarkable temporary improvement in the action of the muscles is obtained by injections of Prostigmin (Fig. 31.15) or Tensilon intravenously.

Tensilon is a rapidly acting and quickly hydrolised anticholinesterase. Thus acetylcholine briefly accumulates in greater than normal amounts in ganglia, post ganglionic sympathetic nerve endings and in neuromuscular junctions in all types of muscle.

Treatment In cases of paralysis of the third nerve

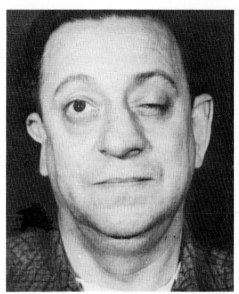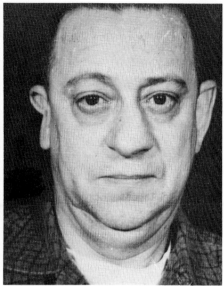

Fig. 31.15 A-B Myasthenia gravis, before and after edrophonium. (By courtesy of Cogan.)

treatment must be directed to removal of the cause. The fact that this nerve is frequently affected in syphilis must be borne in mind; these cases respond to treatment better than others. In cases of incurable paralysis and in congenital and mechanical ptosis the deformity can be relieved only by operation. In complete paralysis of the third nerve, operation is usually contra-indicated on account of the abduction of the eye since if the lid is raised in these cases the diplopia becomes manifest.

Operations for ptosis ameliorate the condition but seldom give perfect results. Three techniques may be applied: (1) if the levator is not completely paralysed this muscle may be shortened; (2) if the levator is paralysed but the superior rectus is active, the latter muscle used to be pressed into service to lift the lid often with disasterous complications; (3) if both levator and superior rectus are paralysed, the action of the frontalis muscle may be utilised in raising the lid.

The Fasanella-Servat operation is indicated for cases of minimal ptosis (1.5–2 mm) with adequate 8 mm function of the levator, showing a good lid fold. The lid is everted and two curved hæmostats are placed grasping conjunctiva, tarsus, levator and Müller's muscle. Pulling up the haemostats the upper tarsus is excised by small bites (4–5 mm). A running suture is carefully placed and the knot is buried by bringing both ends of the suture out through a skin wound made in the outer part of the lid fold.

In the Blaskowics' operation the upper lid is doubly everted over a Desmarres' lid retractor. The conjuctiva above the tarsus is ballooned with saline. An incision is made through the conjunctiva near the tarsal border and dissected back to the fornix (Fig. 31.16). A buttonhole

incision is made on the temporal side and scissors are passed across just above the aponeurosis to the nasal side. A ptosis clamp is inserted one blade being above and the other below the aponeurosis of the levator. The aponeurosis of the levator is cut free and drawn downwards, 1 or 2 mm of the upper border of the tarsus is excised. The levator horns are identified with traction and they are cut with scissors.

The amount of aponeurosis to be resected is measured with a caliper when three double-armed 5.0 chromic gut sutures are passed through the aponeurosis from the anterior surface at this point and tied with three knots. The excess aponeurosis is excised and these sutures are passed completely through the upper edge of the tarsus starting at the posterior edge. When they have passed through the upper edge of the tarsus they are carried along the anterior surface to emerge through the muscle and skin in a line which will produce the lid fold. The three mattress sutures are drawn up and tied over a wisp of cotton wool. The conjunctiva is closed with a continuous 6.0 chromic suture. A Frost suture is then inserted in the lower lid and a firm dressing applied.

In Everbusch's technique the line of incision is in the future lid fold. The skin should be drawn up before the markings are made. Excess skin to be removed later should be taken from the upper lip of the wound.

The skin of the lid is held taut and the incision is made with a razor blade. After the incision is completed the dissection is carried upward and downward under the obicularis muscle to expose the orbital septum. A vertical incision is made through the septum with a knife and spread open with a small scissors.

Pressure on the globe usually causes the preaponeur-

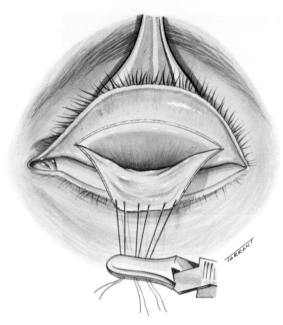

Fig. 31.16 Blaskovics' operation. The upper eyelid is maintained in a position of double eversion in order to expose the conjunctival surface of the lid and the region of the superior fornix, and this is achieved by the use of Desmarres' eyelid retractor which presses on the skin surface of the eyelid.

The palpebral conjunctiva is incised in the region of the upper border of the tarsal plate and three double-ended silk sutures with the loop of each suture on the inner surface of the conjunctiva are inserted into the upper edge of the incised conjunctiva so that this portion of the conjunctiva is retracted into the region of the superior fornix with exposure of the underlying superior palpebral muscle and levator tendon. (Reproduced from Miller S J H (ed) 1976 Eyes. In: Rob and Smith's Operative Surgery, 3rd edn, by courtesy of the publishers Butterworths, London

otic fat to appear in the wound. The glistening aponeurosis of the levator tendon lies directly beneath the fat. The aponeurosis should be carefully identified and when this has been done the lid is everted and the conjunctiva above the tarsal border is ballooned with saline. A small buttonhole incision is made through the conjunctiva on the temporal side and blunt scissors are passed across watching the blades through the thin conjunctiva. This separates the conjunctiva from Müller's muscle and the aponeurosis. A second buttonhole incision is made on the nasal side. A ptosis clamp is passed as the scissors are withdrawn with one blade under the conjunctiva and the other on top of the aponeurosis.

With the aponeurosis in the ptosis clamp and all tissues freed from both surfaces, the horns should be incised being careful not to damage the superior oblique tendon or the lacrimal gland. The amount of aponeurosis to be excised is measured with a caliper. Three 6.0 chromic gut double-armed sutures are passed through the aponeurosis from below upwards and tied securely

with three knots. The excess aponeurosis is removed. One needle from each of the double-armed sutures is passed through the outer layer of the tarsus parallel to the lid border and approximately 4 mm from the lid margin. These sutures are tied. Three or more additional interrupted 6.0 chromic gut sutures are added to ensure firm fixation of the entire aponeurosis. A good fold is produced with a 6.0 silk suture for adults and chromic catgut for children.

In order to produce a firm scar each suture should pass through the depth of the wound about 1.5 mm back and through the outer layer of the aponeurosis. When the suture is drawn up and tied the skin is firmly anchored to the aponeurosis producing a permanent fold. A 4.0 silk Frost type suture is inserted below the lash line for at least 10 mm and brought up to be passed through the skin just below the brow. A firm dressing is applied.

The anterior approach is recommended in patients who require larger sections. A 10 mm resection is minimal for congenital ptosis and maximal for senile ptosis. A mild congenital ptosis with 8 mm or more of levator function and an intact aponeurosis may be corrected with a 10–12 mm of resection; a patient with 4 or 5 mm of ptosis with 5 or 6 mm of levator function and a thin aponeurosis may need 18–24 mm of resection to produce an acceptable result if the levator function is feeble and the ptosis severe.

Frontalis suspension. When the levator muscle is intact but the function is poor (3 mm or less) strengthening by resection of the levator is not recommended.

Suture techniques (Fig. 31.17). A 4.0 Supramid extra suture with two swedged-on needles facilitates easy passage through the outer layers of the tarsus. After attachment to the tarsus, the needles are removed and the two sutures are carried upwards through the deeper layers of the lid with a one-half curved, cutting needle to emerge through the wound made above the brow. These sutures are deep enough to prevent visible suture marks.

The operation is useful for young children as a tem-

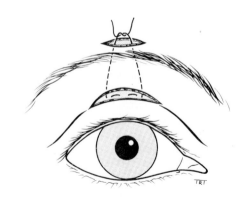

Fig. 31.17 Hildreth-Silver lid suspension

porary measure until they are able to co-operate better as they grow older. It is also useful in elderly and infirm patients. If a levator resection has produced a mild under-correction a Supramid suture may be used. The suture may be removed at any time.

Infection of the suture bed is one of the annoying complications and the suture should be guarded carefully during surgery keeping it way from the skin and lashes and the wound in the brow should be carefully closed. A broad spectrum antibiotic post-operatively for four or five days is important. To reduce the forehead scar, it is well to close the deeper parts of the wound. A deeply placed mattress suture, of 6.0 silk or Mersilene brings the muscle, fascia and skin together. This removes the strain on the fragile skin.

Fascia lata for frontalis suspension (Fig. 31.18). Three incisions are made in the upper lid about 4 mm from the lid margin. A short deep incision is made 5 mm above the medial and lateral portions of the brow. The third incision is made midway between the two, some 16 mm above them. The fascial strips are drawn through the openings in the lid and then upward emerging with two ends in each of the openings above the brow. One end of the fascia is cut off and the other emerges at the central incision. The fascia must lie deep in the lid tissue and be drawn up quite tightly because there is a tendency towards undercorrection.

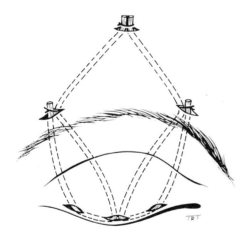

Fig. 31.18 Fascia lata lid suspension

The fascial strips are secured with 5.0 chromic catgut at each brow incision. The forehead wounds are closed with deep mattress sutures followed by a Frost-type 4.0 silk suture in the lower lid. A broad spectrum antibiotic should be given for five days.

If after these operations it is found that when the eyeball is raised, the skin of the upper lid falls in an unsightly fold over the lashes, a horizontal strip of skin of suitable width is removed from the upper lid, the pos-

ition of the lower skin incision corresponding roughly to that of the upper edge of the tarsal plate. The sutures which join the edges of the skin incision are carried through the deep tissues in such a way as to stretch the skin over the tarsus and to produce a fold in the skin of the eyelid in the normal position.

Tumours of the lids and allied conditions

Benign growths

These include xanthelasma, molluscum, warts, nævus, angioma, and other tumours common to the skin and cutaneous glands.

Small clear *cysts* frequently occur among the lashes in old people, due to the retention of secretion of Moll's glands. They disappear if the anterior wall is snipped off.

Xanthelasma (ξανθος, *yellow*, ελασμα, *a plate*) or *xanthoma*. This is a slightly raised yellow plaque, most commonly found in the upper and lower lids near the inner canthus, and often symmetrical in the two lids and on both sides. They are most common in elderly women, and are sometimes associated with diabetes and excessive formation of cholesterol. They grow slowly, and only require treatment on account of the disfigurement produced. They may be excised or destroyed by trichloracetic acid or carbon dioxide snow.

Naevus or mole. Usually pigmented, may occur on the lids, generally affecting the margin and involving both skin and conjunctiva. Two may be symmetrically situated on the lids of the same eye, indicating their origin at a time when the lids were still united. The microscopical appearance is characteristic, consisting of nævus cells, often arranged in an alveolar manner. They may grow at puberty but very rarely take on malignant proliferation. They may be removed by excision but this ought to be complete and extensive.

Haemangioma. Often also called naevus, occurs in two forms — telangiectases and cavernous hæmangiomata (Fig. 31.19). The former are bright red or portwine coloured spots composed of dilated capillaries. The latter consist of dilated and anastomosing vascular spaces lying in the subcutaneous tissue having all the characteristics of erectile tissue; they are not infrequently strictly localised as if partially encapsulated. They appear bluish when seen through the skin and form swellings which increase in size on venous congestion as on crying or lowering the head. Cavernous hæmangiomata are rarely seen in adults, partly owing to the fact that they are generally treated in early life, but possibly due to spontaneous atrophy of the growth and thickening of the skin.

Haemangioma often follows the distribution of the first and second divisions of the fifth nerve. In the *Sturge-Weber syndrome* it is associated with haemangioma

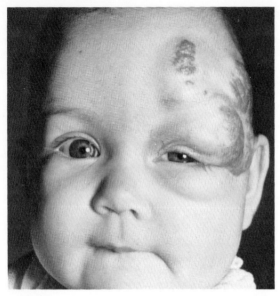

Fig. 31.19 Cavernous haemangioma of the lid and eyebrow. (By courtesy of Peeters.)

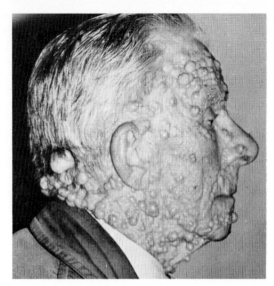

Fig. 31.20 Neurofibromatosis. (By courtesy of Jay.)

of the choroid and glaucoma, and also with haemangioma of the leptomeninges, causing homonymous hemianopia or epilepsy. The intracranial lesion may be diagnosed radiographically since there are often calcareous deposits underlying the cerebral cortex.

Telangiectases and small haemangiomata usually disappear and may well be left alone; if they increase in size, however, treatment is indicated, if the tumour is small by excision, if large they are best treated because of the danger of amblyopia or later strabismus. If the mass does not interfere with vision the child should be left until aged 3–5 years before cosmetic surgery is undertaken, but if vision is compromised an attempt may be made to tie off the feeder vessel from a branch of the internal carotid (upper lid) or external carotid artery (lower lid). Local injection of 40 mg triamcinolone and 6 mg betamethasone sodium phosphate into the tumour may lead to involution in some cases. Large diffuse tumours may be treated with alternate-day administration of large doses of steroids for several months under the direction of a paediatrician. Superficial radiotherapy (80–120 kv.) may be given in doses of 100–200 rad. monthly for six months with a total dose not exceeding 500–600 rad. Injection of sclerosing solutions is discouraged because of residual scarring.

Lymphangioma. Occurs rarely in the lids.

Neurofibromatosis (Elephantiasis neuromatodes, plexiform neuroma, von Recklinghausen's disease)

The lids and orbit may be affected. In typical cases the temporal region is also affected (Fig. 31.20). The swollen lid and temporal region form a characteristic picture.

The hypertrophied nerves can be felt through the skin as hard cords or knobs. The nerve fibres are little changed, the hyperplasia affecting the endo- and peri-neurium. In several cases the ciliary nerves have been found to be affected, both in the orbit, associated with a true glioma of the optic nerve, and inside the globe, which in many cases is buphthalmic. Operative measures are seldom satisfactory. The choroid and ciliary body may be much thickened by layers of dense fibrous-like tissue probably derived from the cells of the sheaths of Schwann. Laminated ovoid bodies resembling Pacchionian corpuscles also occur.

Symmetrical soft swellings above the inner canthus are sometimes seen in elderly people. They are due to prolapse of the orbital fat through an aperture in the orbital septum.

Malignant tumours

These include carcinomata, sarcomata and malignant melanomata, the first being much the more common. *Epitheliomata* (squamous-celled carcinomata) show a preference for sites where the character of the epithelium changes; they therefore commence generally at the edges of the lids. The patients are elderly; the preauricular lymph nodes may be enlarged, or if the growth is near the inner canthus, the submaxillary nodes. Any of the glands of the lid may in rare instances undergo carcinomatous proliferation.

The commonest malignant epithelial growth is the basal-celled carcinoma (rodent ulcer), which shows a predilection for the inner canthus (Fig. 31.21). It commences as a small pimple which ulcerates and if the scab is removed it is found that the edges are raised and indurated. The ulcer spreads very slowly, the epithelial

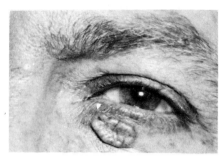

Fig. 31.21 Rodent ulcer. (By courtesy of Smithers.)

growth extending under the skin in all directions and penetrating deeply. The surrounding structures are gradually destroyed; lids, orbit, and bones are invaded. The growth is only locally malignant and probably originates in the accessory eptithelial structures of the skin — hair follicles and glands — but the lymphatic nodes are not affected. Rodent ulcer rarely occurs before forty year of age, and the rate of growth is usually measured in years.

Sarcoma is rare; it may be round- or spindle-celled. *Reticular tumours*, round-celled growths variously described as lymphoma, lymphosarcoma, pseudoleucæmic tumours, etc., sometimes affect both orbits and all four lids causing symmetrical proptosis; occasionally the patients show blood changes as in leukæmia. The growth is slow but continuous and the eyes may be endangered by lagophthalmos. Malignant melanomata are rare, as also is a more generalised pigmentation developing in adult life which may become cancerous (*melanosis*) (p. 129).

Treatment. Epitheliomata and sarcomata must be thoroughly extirpated by surgery even if it involves excision of the globe or exenteration of the orbit. Rodent ulcer is sensitive to radiation; if small, however, it is probably best excised; if so large as not to be amenable to operative treatment without sacrificing a good eye, it may be satisfactorily treated with radium or X-rays provided there is no involvement of the bones. Occasionally, however, the results of radiational treatment may be misleading, for the skin surface may show a firm scar while the growth continues to spread beneath the surface; in every case it is wise to keep a careful watch for any recurrence. In the later stages extensive plastic operations may have to be performed to protect the eyeball and when this becomes impossible the eye must be excised and the morbid tissues freely removed. Most reticular tumours are radio-sensitive as is melanosis in its pre-cancerous phase, although by no means always in its cancerous phase.

Injuries of the lids

Injuries of the lids of various kinds — contusions, wounds, burns, etc. — are very common. They must be treated upon general principles but special attention must be directed to associated injuries of the bones of the orbit (p. 339) and the eyeball.

Contusions

These are often more alarming in appearance than in reality (the 'black eye'). There is great swelling and ecchymosis both in the lids and conjunctiva. In all cases a guarded prognosis should be given, for it may be impossible to determine the full extent of the injury to the orbit or the eye.

Wounds

Wounds in the direction of the fibres of the orbicularis gape little and heal without conspicuous scarring; hence surgical wounds should be made in this direction as often as possible. Vertical wounds gape causing disfiguring cicatrices, and often lead to ectropion or other distortion, especially if there is adhesion to the subjacent bone. The worst wounds are those which sever the lid vertically in its whole thickness. If they do not unite by first intention, a notch (traumatic coloboma) is left in the lid margin, and disfigurement, lagophthalmos and epiphora result.

Treatment. Simple contusions with ecchymosis require only conservative treatment with cold compresses. Wounds must be thoroughly cleansed and brought together by sutures. On account of the rich blood-supply it is not necessary to make a wide excision of the edges: only obviously contused and devitalised tissue should be excised. As a prophylactic against infection the wound should be dusted with sulphonamide and penicillin powder. Lacerated wounds are likely to leave ugly scars and deformities: these must be treated by plastic operation. If suppuration occurs the abscess must be opened and treated on general surgical principles. Vertical wounds severing the canaliculus require special care (Chapt. 32).

Burns

It is important to diagnose the degree of a burn. First degree burns require cleansing and the application of sterile saline and penicillin packs every three hours during the day. Second degree burns should be cleansed, any vesicles opened and dead epithelium removed; subsequent treatment is similar. Third degree burns should be cleaned and immediately covered by whole or split-skin grafts, a temporary tarsorrhaphy being performed and allowed to remain until all risk of cicatricial ectropion has passed. This is the great danger from burns of the lids that they easily lead to a severe exposure keratitis with permanent impairment or even loss of vision. For this reason coagulants (tannic acid, etc.) should never be applied to burns of the lids. The best prophylactic is grafting before scar tissue has formed; if the initial graft does not take well it can be repeated at leisure. If scarring has developed cicatricial deformities resulting from burns are corrected by plastic operation.

Congenital abnormalities of the lids

Symblepharon, ankyloblepharon, ectropion, entropion and trichiasis occur occasionally as congenital malformations. Ptosis is a fairly common congenital defect.

Distichiasis (δις, double, στιχος, a row)

This is a rare condition in which there is an extra posterior row of cilia, occasionally in all four lids. The posterior row occupies the position of the meibomian glands which are reduced to ordinary sebaceous glands performing the normal function of lubricating the hairs; these lashes may irritate the cornea.

Coloboma of the lid

This is a notch in the edge of the lid (Fig. 31.22). The gap is usually situated to the inner side of the midline, generally affecting the upper lid but two or more defects may occur in the same lid. Sometimes a bridge of skin links the coloboma to the globe, or there is a dermoid astride the limbus at the site of the coloboma. There are often other congenital defects of the eye or other parts of the body such as coloboma of the iris or accessory auricles. Some cases are due to incomplete closure of the embryonic facial cleft, others probably to the pressure of amniotic bands. Occasionally there is a notch at the outer part of the lower lid, associated with maldevelopment of the first visceral arch (*mandibulofacial dysostosis*).

Cryptophthalmos (κρυπτος, hidden)

This is a very rare condition in which skin passes continuously from the brow over the eye to the cheek, associated with abnormalities of the eye and often of the orbit.

Microblepharon

This is the condition in which the lids are abnormally small; they may be absent or virtually so — *ablepharon*. These conditions usually occur only in cases of microphthalmos or congenitally small eyes. Microphthalmos may be associated with a congenital *orbito-palpebral cyst*, causing a swelling of the lower lid. The cyst is connected with the eyeball, contains retinal tissue in its lining, and is due to defective closure of the embryonic fissure — an extreme case of ectatic coloboma of the choroid (*q.v.*). The eyeball may be apparently absent (*congenital anophthalmos*), but there are always microscopic vestiges of ocular tissues.

Epicanthus

This is a semilunar fold of skin, situated above and sometimes covering the inner canthus (Fig. 31.23). It is usually bilateral and gives the appearance that the eyes are far apart and have a convergent squint and the bridge of the nose is flat. It may disappear as the nose develops. It is normal in Mongolian races. The deformity can be remedied by plastic surgery.

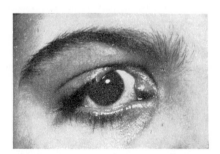

Fig. 31.22 Coloboma of the upper lid. (By courtesy of Reese.)

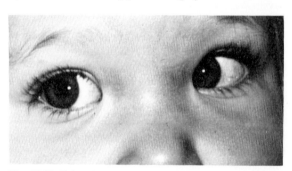

Fig. 31.23 Epicanthus

32

Diseases of the lacrimal apparatus

Anatomy and physiology

The lacrimal apparatus consists of the lacrimal glands and the lacrimal passages.

The *lacrimal glands* of each eye consist of the superior or orbital gland, the inferior or palpebral gland, and the accessory lacrimal glands or Krause's glands. All are serous acinous glands, scarcely distinguishable microscopically from serous salivary glands with which they are morphologically identical. The orbital gland, about the size of a small almond, is situated in the lacrimal fossa at the outer part of the orbital plate of the frontal bone; ten or twelve *lacrimal ducts* pass from it to open upon the surface of the conjunctiva at the outer part of the upper fornix. The palpebral gland consists of only one or two lobules situated upon the course of the ducts of the superior portion. It can be seen when the eye looks down and in after the upper lid has been everted. The accessory or Krause's glands are microscopic groups of acini, lying below the surface of the conjunctiva between the fornix and the edge of the tarsus (Fig. 31.1). There are about forty-two in the upper, six to eight in the lower fornix. The ducts of numerous acini unite to form a larger duct which opens into the fornix.

The *lacrimal passages* consist of the lacrimal puncta, the canaliculi, the lacrimal sac, and the nasal duct. The *lacrimal puncta* lie near the posterior border of the free margin of the lid about 6 mm from the inner canthus. Each lid has one punctum and one canaliculus. The punctum is situated upon a slight elevation, larger in elderly people, the *lacrimal papilla* (Fig. 31.2). As already mentioned, this is visible in normal circumstances only when the lid is slightly everted (p. 71). The *canaliculus* passes from the punctum to the lacrimal sac; it is first directed vertically for about 1–2 mm, then horizontally for 6–7 mm. The canaliculi usually open separately through the outer wall of the lacrimal sac. The *lacrimal sac* lies in the lacrimal fossa formed by the lacrimal bone; when distended it is about 15 mm long vertically, and 5–6 mm wide. The upper portion or *fundus* extends slightly above the level of the inner tarsal ligament and the sac itself is surrounded by fibres of the orbicularis muscle. The lower end narrows as it opens into the *nasal duct*, a tube varying much in size (12–24 mm long, 3–6 mm in diameter) passing downwards and slightly outwards and backwards, bounded by the superior maxilla and inferior turbinate, to open at the anterior part of the outer wall of the inferior meatus of the nose. The line of the duct is given by a point just outside the inner canthus and the groove between the ala of the nose and the cheek. The upper end of the nasal duct is the narrowest part. The canaliculi are lined by stratified epithelium, the lacrimal sac and nasal duct by columnar epithelium lying upon a corium which contains a venous plexus. The mucous lining forms an imperfect valve at the orifice into the nose.

The *lacrimal secretion* is a slightly alkaline fluid containing sodium chloride as its chief constituent. The ordinary amount secreted is just sufficient to moisten the eyeball, and is lost by evaporation. Only under reflex irritation, psychical or peripheral, is an excess secreted, and this is sucked into the lacrimal sac and forced through the nasal duct into the nose during the act of blinking, when the fibres of the orbicularis contract around the sac. It must be remembered that xerosis or dryness of the conjunctiva does not result from extirpation of the superior and inferior lacrimal glands, the moistening of the conjunctiva by Krause's glands and its own mucous cells being sufficient to prevent it. On the other hand, epiphora does not usually result from extirpation of the lacrimal sac, except in the presence of psychical or peripheral stimuli to increased secretion. The tears have some slight bacteriostatic properties owing to the presence of an enzyme, lysozyme.

Diseases of the lacrimal gland

Diseases of the lacrimal gland are rare. *Dacryo-adenitis* occurs occasionally in general infections (mumps, influenza etc;) sometimes leading to suppuration. Infectious mononucleosis may produce a red painful swelling with redness of the outer third of the upper eyelid. This may be associated with a follicular conjunctivitis, periorbital oedema, uveitis and sometimes optic neuritis. Occasionally the central nervous system is involved, but fortunately the disease is usually self-limited. A permanent *fistula* may result from the bursting of an abscess in the gland.

Dacryops is a cystic swelling in the upper fornix due to retention of secretion owing to blockage of one of the lacrimal ducts. It can only be distinguished from retention cysts of Krause's glands by its position.

Mikulicz's syndrome is characterised by symmetrical enlargement of the lacrimal and salivary glands. The ætiology varies but the swelling is usually of a lymphomatous nature. Both parotid and lacrimal glands are enlarged in uveoparotid inflammation (p. 161).

Tumours of the lacrimal gland show a very marked resemblance to those of the parotid. Much the commonest is a *pleomorphic adenocarcinoma*, frequently characterised histologically by myxomatous material (the so called 'mixed tumour'). Benign mixed lacrimal gland tumours present in middle life as slowly progressive painless swellings in the upper lid. Bone is not usually invaded. Malignant tumours present with a short history and pain. Benign tumours should be removed in their capsule. A painful tumour or one with bone invasion or calcification should have a biopsy through a trans-septal incision. If malignant radical surgical removal is necessary.

All conditions which cause swelling of the gland may lead to impairment of movement of the eye. The globe is pushed downwards and inwards; movement outwards, and especially outwards and upwards, is limited. There may be some proptosis.

Kerato-conjunctivitis sicca (Sjögren's syndrome)

A general systemic and auto-immune disturbance usually occurring in women after the menopause and often associated with rheumatoid arthritis, is characterised by deficiency of the lacrimal secretion leading to dryness of the eyes. This usually gives rise to chronic irritative symptoms and may be associated with epithelial erosions or filaments on the corneal surface; damage to the epithelium of the cornea and conjunctiva may be demonstrated clinically by staining with rose bengal. Pathologically, the lacrimal gland is found to be fibrotic and infiltrated with lymphocytes; similar changes in the salivary glands may lead to a dryness of the mouth, while desiccation may occur in other mucous membranes. A tear lysozyme ration of 0.1 is typical of keratoconjunctivitis sicca.

A dry eye

A dry eye produces discomfort and reduced vision when the tear film becomes chronically unstable and repeatedly breaks up into dry spots between blinks, exposing the corneal and conjunctival epithelium to evaporation. Tear film instability may be the result of (1) Deficiency of tears — Sjögren's syndrome (2) Deficiency of conjunctival mucus. Mucus from goblet cells of the con-

junctiva is necessary to keep the tear film stable. Lack of mucus causes premature tear film break-up even in the presence of abundant tear fluid. Mucus deficiency occurs in Stevens-Johnson's syndrome, ocular pemphigoid, avitaminosis A, old trachoma or secondary to practolol: (3) Altered corneal surface — changes and irregularities from past disease result in poor wetting with subsequent risk of further damage. (4) Insufficient resurfacing of the corneal surface by the lid as in decreased blink rate, lid paralysis or the formation of a dellen. Symptoms arising from a dry eye may be mimicked by chronic blepharo-conjunctivitis due to the staphylococcus, rosacea kerato-conjunctivitis or allegic conjunctivitis. These diagnoses should first be eliminated. Features which help in the diagnosis of a moderately dry eye are the presence of particulate matter in the tear film due to mucus which is stainable with alcian blue. A tear lysozyme ratio between 0.9 and 0.6 or a Schirmer test producing wetting less than 6 mm support the diagnosis.

The Schirmer test is performed by folding the 5 mm top end of the paper strip 90° and placing it in the lower conjunctival sac of the open eye. It is left in place for five minutes or until 30 mm of the strip is wetted. If tear fluid fails to diffuse over the lid margin along the strip within two minutes, it is removed to another site within the sac and timing is recommenced. Such a method obviates false positive results. The strip is removed from the eye after five minutes and the wetted portion is measured. The concentration of tear lysozme is measured in units per microlitre. The result is divided by the value of the critical lower limit to express the concentration as the tear lysozyme ratio.

G. Hypromellose B.P.C. 1968 and B.J.6 drops are effective artificial tears. The slow-release artifical tear is a pellet of a cellulose compound without preservative that is inserted below the tarsus of the lower lid where it dissolves slowly providing a continous source of tears. If obstruction of the canaliculi with gelatin plugs gives relief it is worth considering permanent obstruction of the lower puncta. Excess mucus may be treated by Acetyl Cysteine 5% drops buffered to pH 8.4 with sodium bicarbonate.

Diseases of the lacrimal passages

Eversion of the lower punctum

This occurs from laxity of the lids in old age, from chronic conjunctivitis or blepharitis or any cause leading to ectropion (q.v.) (Fig. 32.1). If on clinical examination the punctum is visible when the lower lid apposes the globe it may be considered to be everted. This causes epiphora, which in turn aggravates the condition.

Treatment In slight cases, especially in old people, the eversion may be sufficiently counteracted by burning a

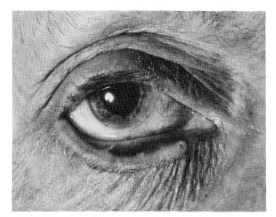

Fig. 32.1 Eversion of the punctum in a case of senile ectropion

row of deep punctures along the whole length of the lower tarsus preferably towards its lower border with the cautery. The maximum effect is expected in six weeks. As the cicatricial tissue contracts the punctum is pulled inwards towards the eye.

If this fails an incision of a tarso-conjunctival segment 2 mm below the punctum is made. It must be spindle-shaped and 8 mm in length. It is closed with 6.0 catgut burying the knots to avoid abrading the cornea.

The simplest method is the so-called 'three-snip' operation. The conjunctival sac is anæsthetised and Procaine injected into the tissues around the canaliculus. The punctum is dilated with Nettleship's dilator which is introduced vertically and then pushed inwards along the canaliculus. A canaliculus knife is then taken and the probe-point is passed into the punctum in the same manner, first downwards, then inwards, the back of the knife being directed forwards and slightly downwards. In this manner, as the knife is pushed inward, the posterior wall of the canaliculus is incised. While this manœuvre is being performed the lid is kept stretched outwards, so that the wall of the duct is kept taut against the edge of the knife. The triangular flap of the posterior wall formed between the vertical and horizontal parts of the canaliculus is then snipped off with scissors. A probe should be passed on the day following the operation, and occasionally on succeeding days, so as to prevent closure of the incision.

In cases of marked eversion of the lower punctum a radical operation for ectropion may be necessary.

Occlusion of the puncta

This may be congenital, which is extremely rare, or cicatricial. In either case epiphora is caused which is very difficult to treat. Before treatment is commenced the patency of the lacrimal passages should be ensured by syringing through the other (upper) punctum.

An endeavour should be made to slit up the occluded punctum — not the whole canaliculus. On inspection no trace of the punctum may be visible, but it is rare if some evidence of its presence cannot be seen on minute examination of the normal site with the slit lamp. The point of the dilator is inserted at this site, and may succeed in opening up the punctum sufficiently to admit the probe-point of the canaliculus knife.

Occlusion of the canaliculus

This may be due to a scar or a foreign body. It may follow the prolonged use of IDU drops. An eyelash is the commonest obstructive foreign body, a 'concretion' less frequent. An eyelash usually projects somewhat from the punctum and is easily removed with forceps. Concretions are masses of the mycelium of a fungus, usually actinomyces. They are removed by dilating the canaliculus, slitting it, curetting it and injecting a solution of penicillin.

Congenital anomalies of the puncta and canaliculi

These are occasionally seen. The puncta may be absent or constricted; there may be two puncta in a lid, both generally opening into the same canaliculus. Sometimes a groove is found instead of a canaliculus.

Lacrimal obstruction

Epiphora may be classified according to whether or not it is accompanied by a mucocoele. Mucocoeles can be divided into two groups according to whether or not there is regurgitation on pressure over the sac. Those with regurgitation on pressure are either patent or blocked on attempting to syringe down to the sac; if blocked a probe will enter the sac without difficulty and the condition is due to obstruction low in the sac or naso-lacrimal duct and dacryocystorhinostomy will act as a cure; on the other hand if patent on syringing and the probe enters the sac a space occupying mass within the sac is likely either fungal or neoplastic. If epiphora is accompanied by a mucocoele, but does not regurgitate on pressure there is a block both at the bottom of the sac and also at the entry of the common canaliculus in the sac wall: if there is a block on syringing with reflux from the upper punctum and increase in size of the mucocoele, a probe can usually enter the sac and the common canalicular obstruction is a flap valve on the sac wall, a condition which will respond to a D.C.R. with excision of the flap; on the other hand if syringing is blocked and does not distend the sac and the probe does not enter the sac the canalicular block is a mucosal stenosis in the sac wall which can be dealt with effectively by incision and temporary canalicular intubation combined with D.C.R.

Epiphora without a mucocele generally does not give regurgitation on pressure over the sac. Such cases may be divided into those in which there is a block to syringing with reflux through the upper punctum, those in which there is a block with no flow of fluid except reflux around the cannula and those in which syringing is patent down to the nose. Those that are blocked on syringing with reflux through the upper punctum may be divided into those in which a gently passed probe readily enters the sac, these have an obstruction low in the sac or in the naso-lacrimal duct and are cured by a D.C.R. Those in which a gently passed probe is held up in the common canaliculus, that is beyond the medial commisure at a distance of 8 mm or more from the punctum are due to a stenosis at the site and require a canaliculo-dacryocystorhinostomy with anastomosis of the common canaliculus to the sac. Epiphora with no mucocoele, and no regurgitation on pressure, blocked to syringing with no flow except some reflux around the punctum, whichever canaliculus is syringed, presents a difficult problem: if the gently passed probe stops in each canaliculus after entering 5–8 mm or more, then the patent canaliculus reaches the medial commisure and the canalicular obstruction at that site can be dealt with by canaliculo-dacryocystorhinostomy anastomosing each canaliculus separately to the sac but the success rate is only 50%. If however, the probe enters less than 5 mm and meets an obstruction then canaliculus to sac anastomosis is not practical and this condition is best dealt with by a Lester-Jones tube. Epiphora with no mucocoele, no regurgitation and no blockage on syringing to the nose may be due to a tight canaliculus or an everted punctum.

Epiphora with pain, nasal discharge, especially with intermittent nasal bleeding must always raise the suspicion of a neoplasm of the antrum or ethmoid.

The use of a Lester-Jones tube follows the operation of dacryocystorhinostomy. When the posterior mucosal flaps have been sutured attention is directed to the caruncle which is excised. A needle is then inserted in a slightly downward direction from a point some 2 mm behind the medial commisure to emerge just behind the anterior mucosal flap. It should lie anterior to the body of the ethmoid and middle turbinate. This track is then enlarged using a Graefe knife and a polythene tube is inserted. This tube is about 18 mm long and its medial end is trimmed short of the nasal septum and its expanded lateral end sutured at the inner canthus. The dacryocystorhinostomy is then completed and a few days later this tube is replaced by a 2 mm glass capillary tube some 10–16 mm in length. The lateral end of this tube has a cuff 3–4 mm in diameter and its medial end is expanded to 2.25 mm. The indication for the operation is the presence of persistent epiphora in a patient with less than 8 mm of the lateral part of the canaliculus remaining. Six months after the tube is inserted it may become blocked with inspissated mucus and its removal is necessary for adequate cleaning. Replacement of the tube is sometimes difficult and has to be carried out

under local anaesthesia. Lester–Jones tubes are not recommended for children.

The operation of canaliculo-dacryocystorhinostomy consists of dissecting out the common canaliculus, and a little of both upper and lower canaliculi removing any strangulating fibrosis in the region of the medial palpebral ligament, anastomosing the common canaliculus with the sac and completing the procedure with a dacryocystorhinostomy.

Dacryocystitis

Otherwise known as inflammation of the lacrimal sac is not uncommon. It may occur in an acute or chronic form.

Chronic dacryocystitis is the more common. The essential symptom is epiphora, aggravated by such conditions as exposure to wind. There may be a swelling at the site of the sac (a *mucocele*) and the caruncle and neighbouring parts of the conjunctiva are frequently inflamed. On pressure over the sac, muco-pus or pus regurgitates through the puncta, or more rarely passes down into the nose. Bacteriological examination of the fluid demonstrates the presence of an extraordinary number of bacteria — staphylococci, pneumococci, streptococci, etc.; of these the pneumococcus is sometimes present in virulent form. This fact is of considerable importance since it explains the frequency with which hypopyon ulcer arises in these cases and the danger of panophthalmitis if any intra-ocular operation is undertaken. Dacryocystitis is a constant menace to the eye since minute abrasions of the cornea are of almost daily occurrence and such an abrasion is liable at any moment to become infected and give rise to an ulcer.

Chronic dacryocystitis is commonly attributed to the effects of stricture of the nasal duct arising from chronic inflammation, usually of nasal origin. Obstruction to the lower end of the nasal duct may be caused by the pressure of nasal polypi, a hypertrophied inferior turbinate bone, extreme deviation of the septum, and so on.

Untreated chronic dacryocystitis never undergoes spontaneous resolution. The condition tends to progress and the walls of the sac ultimately become atonic, the contents never being evacuated except by external pressure. At any time an acute inflammation may arise leading to the formation of a lacrimal abscess. This sequel may be caused by injudicious treatment by probing which may result in an abrasion of the epithelial lining through which the pericystic tissues may become infected.

Treatment In the new-born, penicillin drops should be ordered and minute directions should be given for expressing the contents of the sac, a manœuvre which should be done very frequently. Most cases will be cured by this treatment. If, however, three months elapse without marked improvement, an anæsthetic should be given and *probing of the naso-lacrimal duct* performed through the upper canaliculus the greatest care being exercised to avoid injuring the walls of the duct; it is unnecessary to slit the canaliculus.

The punctum and canaliculus are dilated with a Nettleship's dilator and a small probe (No. 1 or 2) is inserted vertically downwards into the canaliculus, then passed gently but firmly inwards until the point is felt against the lacrimal bone. The probe is then rotated upwards and towards the middle line, and pushed down the nasal duct until it touches the floor of the nose; it should be remembered that the duct is short in the newborn. Little force is required if rightly applied in the line of the duct (p. 323). The passage of a probe *once* will cure most congenital cases.

In adults, repeated *syringing of the naso-lacrimal duct* may first be attempted particularly in recent cases with a view to reducing the swelling of the inflamed mucosa and restoring patency. The conjunctival sac is anaesthetised, the punctum dilated and the sac syringed out with a lacrimal syringe. The point of the cannula being inserted into the canaliculus, two or three syringefuls of penicillin solution (10 000 units per ml.) are passed; probably the whole of the fluid will regurgitate through the upper canaliculus. The operation should be repeated daily and in many cases the fluid will pass freely down into the nose in a few days; when this occurs the syringing should be repeated at increasing intervals. A number of cases can be cured in this manner particularly if the patient is told to squeeze out the contents of the sac frequently in the intervals between syringing.

The condition of the lacrimal passages may also be visualised radiologically after injecting lipiodol with a lacrimal syringe into the puncta and the upper part of the sac; in this way the site of an obstruction may be located. Anatomical assessment of the lacrimal drainage apparatus is more precise using subtraction macro-dacryo-cystography with canalicular catheterisation (Fig. 32.2). The functional efficiency of lacrimal drainage may be assessed by a technique using a radio-active tracer instilled into the conjunctival sac and visualised with an Anger gamma camera. The tracer employed is usually a sulphur colloid, Technetium (Figs 32.3 and 32.4).

If the case is still recalcitrant, the establishment of permanent drainage into the nose by dacryocystorhinostomy must be undertaken. This operation, properly performed, removes the obstruction and retains the function of drainage.

Dacryocystorhinostomy. The operation can be undertaken under general anaesthesia. The ipsilateral nasal fossa is sprayed with cocaine and adrenaline, and may be packed with ribbon gauze soaked in an oily solution of the same drugs. The canaliculi are then dilated, and the lacrimal sac irrigated with warm saline. The lids are

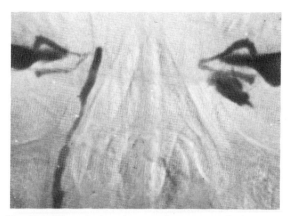

Fig. 32.2 *Bilateral subtraction macrodacryocystography.* Normal right lacrimal duct system. On the left side there is a block at the proximal end of the common canaliculus. (By courtesy of Glyn Lloyd.)

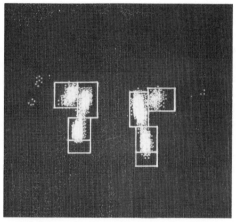

Fig. 32.3 Regions of interest within lacrimal excretory system: inner canthus, lacrimal sac, lacrimal duct and inferior meatal entrance of lacrimal duct. (By courtesy of Hurtwitz.)

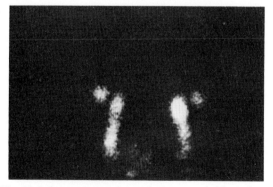

Fig. 32.4 Gamma camera image demonstrates hold-up of tracer in left lacrimal sac.(By courtesy of Hurtwitz.)

temporarily closed with mattress sutures passed through the skin of the lid margins in order to avoid the danger of an infected abrasion.

With the skin stretched by moderate traction at the outer canthus, a curved incision is made, beginning 2 mm above the medial palpebral ligament and 3 mm to the nasal side of the inner canthus; it is carried vertically downwards for 4 mm, and then outwards along the line of the anterior lacrimal crest to a spot 2 mm below the inferior orbital margin. The skin of the temporal edge of the incision is undermined for 2 or 3 mm, but not that of the nasal edge owing to risk of wounding the angular vein or its branches. The orbicularis is split in the line of the incision, and a lacrimal retractor inserted so as to retract it with the skin. The periosteum over the lacrimal crest is incised and separated from the lacrimal fossa to expose the lacrimal bone. The bony crest is removed with a gouge and hammer and when the nasal mucosa is reached the gap in the bone is enlarged so as to make the anastomosis of sac and nasal mucosa possible. The sac is opened through the periosteum and its nasal wall and the entrance of the common canaliculus inspected and tested for patency.

Acute dacryocystitis. Lacrimal abscess may be due to acute inflammation of the sac or to suppuration starting in the peri-cystic tissues. The skin over the sac becomes red and swollen. The redness and swelling rapidly extend to the lower lid and upper part of the cheek, so that the condition may be easily mistaken for erysipelas. There is severe pain, and often some fever. The abscess usually points below and to the outer side of the sac owing to gravitation of the pus to the margin of the orbit. If it opens spontaneously pus continues to be discharged for some time, and a permanent fistula is likely to result.

Treatment. General treatment by antibiotic drugs should be instituted at once (Chapt. 14). If seen at the beginning of the process an attempt may be made to draw the contents of the sac into the nose by cocainizing the ipsilateral nasal fossa and inserting a tampon soaked in adrenaline (1 in 100 000) over the opening of the nasolacrimal duct. An injection of penicillin into the sac may be helpful. In some early cases the mucopus can then be coaxed down the nasal duct.

Hot bathing should be persevered with and the abscess should not be opened unless it is pointing under the skin, in which case it should be opened by a small incision, the pus gently squeezed out, a piece of rubber-glove drain inserted, and a dressing of penicillin and sulphonamide powder applied.

If the discharge continues dacryo-cysto-rhinostomy is indicated.

Stricture of the nasal duct

This has already been referred to incidentally. It is probable that many intractable fibrous strictures are caused by probing; others arise spontaneously as the result of destruction of the epithelium by extension of inflammation from the nose or lacrimal sac. Occasionally bony strictures occur, usually caused by a fractured maxilla or inflammation of the antrum.

Treatment. A nasal drainage operation (p. 327) should be performed in these cases if probing fails.

33

Diseases of the orbit

It is unnecessary to describe the anatomy of the orbit and its contents here. The student is recommended to revise his knowledge of the subject, paying special attention to the relations of the nasal cavities and their accessory sinuses, and to the communications with the interior of the cranial cavity by way of the optic foramen and sphenoid fissure. The intimate adhesion of the dural sheath of the optic nerve to the walls of the optic foramen is of great pathological importance, and the relations of the intra-orbital to the intracranial circulation must be thoroughly appreciated. The eye is slung in position in the orbit by fascia, one sheet of which, Tenon's capsule, forms a socket in which the globe moves. This, with the sclera, forms a lymphatic space, lined completely with endothelium. The extrinsic muscles of the eye do not perforate this capsule, but invaginate it, the fascia being reflected from their surfaces.

From the surgical point of view there are thus four spaces which are relatively self-contained, within each of which inflammatory processes are contained for a considerable time, and each of which must, if necessary, be opened separately (Fig. 33.1): (1) The *sub-periosteal space* between the bones of the orbital wall and the peri-orbita; (2) The *peripheral orbital space* between the peri-orbita and the extra ocular muscles which are joined by fascial connections making a more or less continuous circular septum; (3) The *central space*, a cone-shaped area enclosed by the muscles (the 'muscle cone'); and (4) *Tenon's space* around the globe.

Computerised tomography in orbital lesions
Fat in the intraconal space, a tissue of low density, acts as a natural contrast medium. Its presence has made computerised tomography an accurate method of orbital

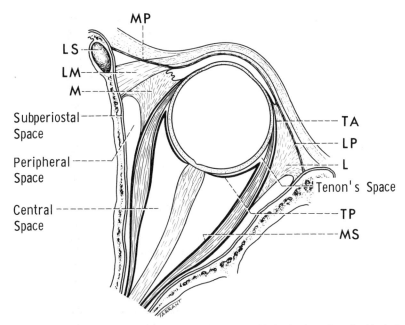

Fig. 33.1 Horizontal section through the orbit. L, lateral check ligament; LM, lacrimal portion of orbicularis muscle; LP, lateral palpebral ligament; LS, lacrimal sac; M, medial check ligament; MP, medial palpebral ligament dividing into a superficial and a deep band; MS, muscle sheaths; TA, anterior part of Tenon's capsule; TP, posterior part of Tenon's capsule

diagnosis when soft tissues are involved. After plain X-ray of the skull, it is the principal method of investigation of patients presenting with unilateral exophthalmos in suspected orbital disease. The advantage of using a body scanner for orbital diagnosis lies in the routine availability of making scans in planes other than the axial (CAT). Coronal (CCT), oblique and saggital sections of the orbit are feasible because of the large aperture of the body scanner. Whereas ultrasonic diagnosis is virtually confined to the eye and immediate retrobulbar space, computerised tomography may pinpoint the cause of proptosis whether intra- or extraorbital.

Orbital disease. The investigation of orbital disease may be considered in three stages: (1) is concerned with the imaging of bone structures by plain X-ray and conventional tomography; (2) is the imaging of soft tissues, principally by computerised tomography, aided in some patients by ultrasonography; and (3) is the demonstration of the vasculature by orbital venography or carotid angiography.

Plain X-ray examination in a patient presenting with proptosis should be backed by good conventional tomography, particularly axial hypocycloidal tomography which is most informative. After the second stage of investigation by computerised tomography the majority of the causes of unilateral exophthalmos will have been revealed. There remains, however, the third stage of investigation that of the demonstration of the vasculature by angiography. Such techniques are only required in a minority of patients, principally those with vascular anomalies in the orbit or within the cranium. Another indication for venography is in the diagnosis of inflammatory processes. In the rectus muscle cone and apex of the orbit, a high proportion of obstructions in the intraconal course of the superior ophthalmic vein is due to an inflammatory process. This applies to the Tolosa-Hunt syndrome wherein obstruction may be shown in the venous system due to granulation tissue.

The introduction of computerised tomography has made carotid arteriography less necessary for the routine investigation of proptosis. Arteriography should therefore only be carried out on selected patients particularly those who are clinically suspected of having an arterio-venous shunt or other vascular anomaly intracranially. Other patients requiring carotid angiography are those with a vascular tumour in the orbit where it is important to identify the feeding vessel prior to surgery.

The position of the eye in the orbit is important. The normal position of the eye is such that a straight-edge applied vertically to the middle of the upper and lower margins of the orbit just touches the closed lids over the apex of the cornea. There are individual variations which are of no pathological importance when symmetrical; in all cases of doubt the two sides should be compared. Accurate·estimates of the amount can be

obtained only by special mechanical devices (exophthalmometers); a simple one is illustrated in Fig. 33.2. A convenient test is the following: the patient is seated, the surgeon standing behind him. The surgeon holds the patient's head in such a manner that he looks straight down the nose. He then rotates the head backwards until he can just see the apex of one cornea. If he can see more of the other cornea, that eye is relatively proptosed.

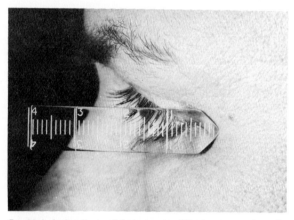

fig. 33.2 A simple exophthalmometer. The instrument is made of a transparent plastic with a groove which fits into the outer bony margin of the orbit. The scale is engraved on both sides of the solid bar of plastic and the observing eye is aligned to read off the level of the apex of the cornea so that the scales on either side of the bar and the apex of the cornea are in one straight line. In the illustration, the two scales at 3 cm are seen out of alignment, and at 4 cm this tendency is increased

Abnormal protrusion of the globe is called *exophthalmos* or *proptosis*. It is much commoner than abnormal retraction or *enophthalmos*. The former condition is due to many causes, among which increase in the orbital contents is the most important. Slight prominence of the eyes accompanies high myopia, paralysis of the extrinsic muscles, stimulation of Muller's muscle by cocaine, and occurs as an idiosyncrasy, especially in very obese people. Unilateral proptosis occurs in orbital cellulitis from any cause, thrombosis of the orbital veins with or without implication of the cavernous sinus, arterio-venous aneurysm, tumours of the orbit and its contents, and orbital haemorrhage or emphysema. Bilateral exophthalmos occurs in endocrine exophthalmos, bilateral proptosis in the later stages of thrombosis of the cavernous sinus, empyema of the accessory sinuses of the nose, symmetrical orbital tumours (lymphoma, pseudo-leukæmia), and as a result of diminished orbital volume in oxycephaly or 'tower-skull' and leontiasis ossea.

Enophthalmos is generally due to severe injury in which the bones of the floor of the orbit are fractured and soft tissues herniate, or to orbital cellulitis followed by mechanical retraction by fibrous tissue.

Orbital inflammation

Periostitis

This is rare but particularly affects the orbital margin. It is most often due to injuries, extension of inflammation from neighbouring parts, tuberculosis or syphilis. In traumatic cases the margin is naturally most affected, but a traumatic element is often an exciting cause in the other cases, so that in them also the margin most frequently suffers.

Periostitis of the deeper parts of the orbit causes less difinite signs. There is more pain of a deep-seated character. There may be proptosis with deviation of the direction of the eye. If the apex of the orbit is implicated, various ocular motor palsies may develop together with trigeminal anæsthesia and neuralgia, and occasionally amaurosis due to involvement of the optic nerve (the *syndrome of the apex of the orbit*). One of the lesions of the orbital apex is characterised by painful, acute ophthalmoplegia with or without involvement of the optic nerve and ophthalmic division of the trigeminal nerve and it responds promptly to steroid treatment. Tolosa described a case wherein a mass of granulation material was found around the carotid artery in the cavernous sinus and the syndrome is now referred to as The Tolosa – Hunt Syndrome. In this syndrome steroids usually relieve the pain within 24 – 48 h and the signs of compression. Other types of lesions may be responsive to steroids but the remission is not complete nor does it occur so rapidly after the onset of treatment. The Tolosa – Hunt Syndrome is not a pathological diagnosis and it should not be made without arteriography and venography and when there are atypical features — clinically, radiologically, or in response to treatment the patient should be fully investigated to eliminate such diagnoses as infraclinoid aneurysm, caratico-cavernous fistula, pituitary tumour, meningioma and orbital tumour.

Treatment In most cases general treatment by antibiotic drugs to which the infecting organism is susceptible has a dramatic effect. If suppuration supervenes, the abscess is opened and any carious bone removed.

In deep-seated periostitis an exploratory operation may be necessary and should not be too delayed.

Orbital cellulitis

This is purulent inflammation of the cellular tissue of the orbit. It is due most frequently to extension of inflammation from neighbouring parts, especially the nasal sinuses; other less common causes are deep injuries, especially those with a retained foreign body, septic operations, particularly evisceration, facial erysipelas, or metastases in pyæmia.

There is great swelling of the lids, with chemosis. The eye is proptosed, and its mobility impaired with result-

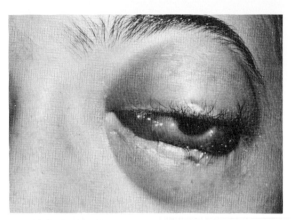

Fig. 33.3 Orbital cellulitis. (By courtesy of Jarrett.)

ing diplopia. Pain is severe, increased by movement of the eye or pressure. Fever is present, and cerebral symptoms may arise. Vision may not be affected, or it may be reduced owing to retrobulbar neuritis. The fundus is difficult to examine; it may be normal or show engorgement of the veins and optic neuritis, passing later into optic atrophy. An abscess is formed which usually points somewhere in the skin of the lids near the orbital margin, or it may empty into the conjunctival fornix. Panophthalmitis may supervene and there is grave danger of extension to the meninges and brain as purulent meningitis, cerebral abscess or thrombosis of the cavernous sinus.

Treatment. General treatment with antibiotic drugs should be instituted at once (Chap. 14), and if instituted reasonably early, resolution may rapidly follow.

Pseudotumour

Pseudotumour is of uncertain aetiology. It produces exophthalmos due to a non-neoplastic mass in the orbit. It is a diagnosis made by exclusion when all other causes of inflammatory masses have been discounted. It can occur at any age but is commonest between 40 and 60 years and slightly commoner in men. The symptoms are proptosis, pain, diplopia, lid swelling and redness. It is usually unilateral but occasionally bilateral. Radiography and ultrasonic scanning of the orbit show a diffuse infiltration of heterogeneous consistency.

A short course of steroids in high dosage is indicated and in most cases there is a rapid resolution although half the patients develop a recurrence on withdrawal of steroid therapy. In such cases radiotherapy is often effective in eliminating the disease permanently.

Thrombosis of the cavernous sinus

This may be due to extension of thrombosis from various sources.

The anatomy of the venous channels which communicate with the cavernous sinus is of great importance in

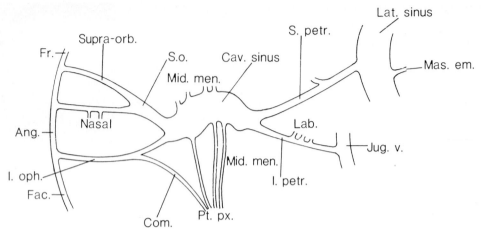

Fig. 33.4 Tributaries of the cavernous sinus (lateral view). (For explanation of lettering, see Figure 33.5.)

this connection (Figs 33.4, 33.5). The superior and inferior ophthalmic veins enter it in front and the superior and inferior petrosal sinuses leave it behind. It communicates directly with the pterygoid plexus through the middle meningeal veins and the veins of Vesalius, and indirectly through a communicating vein from the

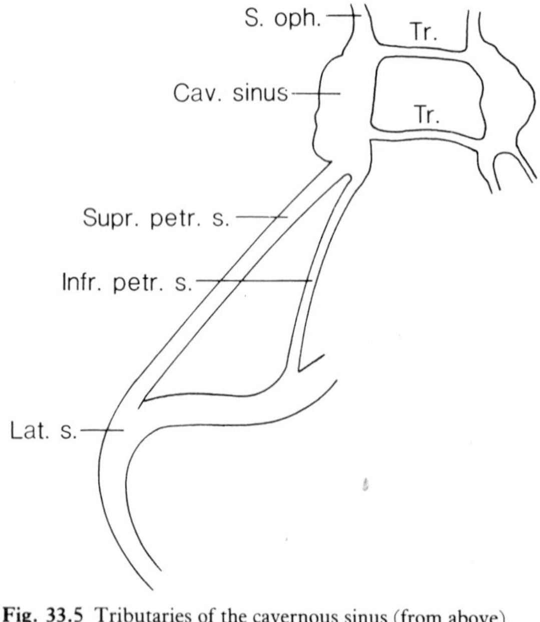

Fig. 33.5 Tributaries of the cavernous sinus (from above)
Explanation of Figure 33.4, 33.5: *Ang.*, angular vein. *Cav. Sinus*, cavernous sinus. *Com.*, communicating vein. *Fac.*, facial vein. *Fr.*, frontal vein. *I. oph.*, inferior ophthalmic vein. *I. petr.* (*Infr. petr.*S.), inferior petrosal sinus. *Jug. V.*, jugular vein. *Lab.*, labyrinthine veins. *Lat. Sinus.* (S.) lateral sinus. *Mas. Em.*, mastoid emissary vein. *Mid. Men.*, middle meningeal veins. *Nasal*, nasal veins. *Pt. px.*, pterygoid plexus. *S.o.* (*oph.*), superior ophthalmic vein. *Supra-orb.*, supra-orbital vein. *S.* (*Supr.*) *petr.*, superior petrosal sinus. *Tr.* transverse sinus

inferior ophthalmic to the pterygoid plexus. The anastomoses of the ophthalmic veins with the frontal and angular open up a communication with the face. Labyrinthine veins opening into the inferior petrosal sinus afford a communication with the middle ear. Numerous tributaries throw it into direct or indirect communication with most parts of the cerebrum. The mastoid emissary vein places the sinus in communication with the subcutaneous tissues behind the ear through the lateral sinus and superior petrosal sinus; it is this communication which is of great diagnostic importance, since swelling behind the ear may decide the question of thrombosis in each direction along these sinuses. The sinus of one side communicates with that of the other by two (or sometimes three) transverse sinuses which surround the pituitary body.

Infection may occur *via* the orbital veins, as in erysipelas, septic wounds of the face, orbital cellulitis, and infective conditions of the mouth, pharynx, ear, nose and accessory sinuses, or as a metastasis in infectious diseases or septic conditions. On more than one occasion the tragedy of bilateral blindness has resulted from an event so simple as the injudicious squeezing of a furuncle on the upper lip.

The patient presents almost the same symptoms and signs as in orbital cellulitis. If in addition there is œdema in the mastoid region behind the ear the diagnosis is certain, for this is due to thrombosis of the emissary vein. A further point of diagnostic importance is transference of the symptoms to the opposite eye, which occurs in 50 % of cases, whereas bilateral orbital cellulitis is very rare. The first sign is often paralysis of the opposite lateral rectus, and this should be carefully watched for in any suspicious case of inflammatory unilateral proptosis. It must be remembered, however, that thrombosis of the sinus may be a complication of cellulitis.

There is severe supra-orbital pain owing to implication of the branches of the ophthalmic division of the fifth nerve, and paresis of the ocular motor nerves. In the later stages the eye is immobile, the pupil dilated, and the cornea anæsthetic. Proptosis occurs in nearly all cases, but is of late onset in those of otitic origin.

It is commonly stated that the retinal veins are greatly engorged, but in many cases this is certainly not true. When this occurs it is usually accompanied by pronounced disc swelling, and both signs indicate extensive implication of the orbital veins and tissues. Simultaneous thrombosis of both cavernous sinuses, with proptosis and disc swelling, occurs in diseases of the sphenoid sinuses. Typical papillœdema is commonest in otitic cases and indicates meningitis or cerebral abscess: it is bilateral, but more pronounced on the side of the aural lesion.

Thrombosis of the cavernous sinus is accompanied by rigors, vomiting and severe cerebral symptoms. Before the advent of the modern antibiotic drugs the patient usually died, but their early use in massive (intravenous) doses together with anti-coagulants may bring about resolution.

Trichinosis

This is an infestation of striated muscles by the larva of the nematode Trichinella spiralis. The encysted larvae are ingested in undercooked pork and develop in the intestine into mature adults. Eggs develop and hatch in the female nematode and the larvae enter the general circulation. There may be muscle weakness and pain, remittent fever and oedema localised to the orbit, particularly the upper lid. There is pain on movement of the eyes.

The extra-ocular muscles themselves are tender and there is an associated eosinophilia. The inflammation may be suppressed with the use of corticosteroids.

Distension of the accessory sinuses of the nose

The accessory sinuses of the nose — the frontal, ethmoid and sphenoid sinuses, and the antrum of the superior maxilla — are separated from the orbit only by thin plates of bone. The orifices which form the communication between these cavities and the nose are liable to become occluded by catarrh, polypi or neoplasms, so that the normal sero-mucous discharge is unable to drain into the nose; the cavities therefore become distended with fluid, and if pyogenic organisms are present, pus may be formed. The treatment of the conditions thus set up cannot be considered part of the functions of the ophthalmic surgeon, but he must be prepared to diagnose them since they not infrequently appear for the first time in the ophthalmic clinic. This is particularly the case in distension of the frontal,

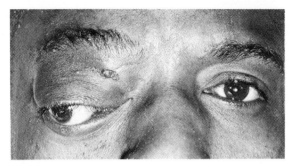

Fig. 33.6 Fronto-ethmoidocele. (By courtesy of M. M. Kulvin.)

ethmoid and sphenoid sinuses. Of these the frontal sinus suffers most often.

Distension or empyema of the frontal sinus causes bulging at the upper and inner part of the orbit (Fig. 33.6). There may be some proptosis and displacement of the eyeball downwards and outwards, œdema of the upper lid or slight ptosis. There is considerable pain and tenderness with severe headache.

Distension of the ethmoid cells by polypi, new growths or inflammatory products may also cause bulging into the orbit and displacement of the globe. Diplopia, chemosis, venous engorgement and ptosis may be caused.

In all cases there is often discharge from the nostril of the same side, or manifest disease of the nasal cavities. Owing to erosion of the walls of the sinus the fluid may extend under the periorbita causing bulging into the posterior part of the orbit or orbital cellulitis. Occasionally retrobulbar neuritis may occur, a complication most probable with inflammation and distension of the sphenoid cells which lie in close proximity to the optic nerve.

In doubtful cases help may be afforded by a skiagram. *Treatment*, apart from general antibiotic therapy, is essentially nasal, but an opening into the orbit may be necessary if cellulitis develops (*q.v.*)

Wegener's granulomatosis

This is a rare chronic disease affecting the upper respiratory tract, lungs and kidneys and characterised by widespread distribution of necrotising angiitis with surrounding granuloma formation. Ocular manifestations occur secondary to adjacent granulomatous sinusitis or as a result of focal vasculitis. The naso-lacrimal duct may be obstructed. There may be proptosis and extraocular muscle or optic nerve involvement.

Cytotoxic agents are required for the control of this systemic inflammatory disease. Cyclophosphamide is the preferred cytotoxic drug when used in low dosage with careful monitoring of the white blood count. A daily oral dose of 1–2 mg per kg of bodyweight should be administered. The treatment of conjunctivitis and episcleritis with topical corticosteroids is usually effective using 0.5% Prednisolone 3–4 times daily together with cycloplegics.

Tumours of the orbit

Orbital tumours are rare.

Benign growths

These include dermoid cyst, dermo-lipoma (p. 128), angioma, osteoma (Fig. 33.7), plexiform neuroma (p. 320), meningioma and meningo-encephalocele. *Dermoid cysts* appear as swellings under the lid, usually at the upper and outer angle; they contain sebaceous material derived from sebaceous glands in the walls, which are lined with epithelium and possess hair follicles; they sometimes contain fœtal remnants (teratoid cysts).

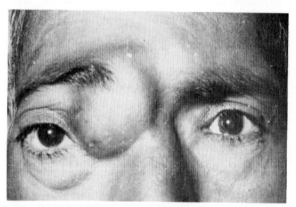

Fig. 33.7 Ethmoidal osteoma. (By courtesy of Mortada.)

Clinically they may be mistaken for *meningo-encephaloceles* protrusions of the cerebral contents, which usually occur at the upper and inner angle where there are most sutures between bones. In the latter: (1) the tumour is immovably attached to the bones; (2) the hole in the bone may be palpable; (3) pulsation, synchronous with respiration and the pulse, increasing in amplitude on straining, can be seen; (4) pressure may cause diminution in size due to fluid being pressed back into the cranium; (5) exploratory puncture (which should only be undertaken with full aseptic precautions) produces clear fluid with the characteristics of cerebrospinal fluid.

Osteomata. Start from the nasal sinuses, usually from the frontal (Fig. 33.7); they are intensely hard and often large, producing great displacement of the globe.

Meningiomata. Apart from those originating in association with the optic nerve sheath (*vide infra*), generally arise in association with the intracranial meninges and invade the orbit secondarily causing a hyperostosis. The most typical are those arising from the lateral portion of the sphenoid ridge — slowly-growing tumours causing proptosis and visual failure by pressure on the optic nerve.

Haemopoietic tumours. These may occur — the various types of reticular tumour (lymphoma, lymphosarcoma, reticulo-sarcoma, Hodgkin's disease, etc.) and chloroma. Ocular changes in lymphomatous tumours include painless infiltration of the lids and a characteristic subconjunctival involvement with a smooth surface. Proptosis may occur due to deposits in the orbit itself or lacrimal gland. Most of the tumours are sensitive to radiation. In cases of suspected lymphoma a biopsy is indicated. A search should be made for an abnormal lymph node which may clinch the diagnosis. The histological appearance of orbital biopsy material falls into one of three broad categories — lymphoid hypoplasia which is benign and may require no treatment; unequivocal malignant lymphoma which should be substantiated by a peripheral blood picture, bone marrow aspiration and trephine, chest radiography, lymph angiogram and possible a whole body CT scan. If evidence of dissemination is found treatment is by chemotherapy. In children primary orbital lymphoma is rare and dissemination is likely so that treatment should initially be chemotherapy. In adults dissemination occurs in half the cases and radiotherapy alone is probably the best initial treatment. A tumour dose of 4000 rads in four weeks is given for histiocytic lymphoma. Cytotoxic therapy should be held in reserve for those cases which later show evidence of dissemination. In those cases which show indeterminate lymphocytic pathology treatment is by radiotherapy. Cavernous haemangiomata are not uncommon (Fig. 33.8).

Malignant tumours. Malignant tumours of the orbit are usually sarcomata, although carcinomata derived from the lacrimal gland (p. 324) or by extension from the nasal mucous membrane also occur. Rhabdomyosarcomata are extremely malignant tumours and occur in the first decade of life (Fig. 33.12). They arise from voluntary muscle and often produce a rapidly increasing proptosis. Extension occurs in all directions. Diagnosis is by biopsy wherein cross-striations in the tumour cells are pathognomatic. The treatment of rhabdomyosarcoma is a combination of chemotherapy and radiotherapy. Two injections of Vincristine, Cyclophosphamide and Actinomycin D are given at weekly intervals before radiotherapy. Radiotherapy is given to a dose of 5000 rads for five weeks during which Vincristine and Cyclophosphomide are administered weekly. After radiotherapy a combination of Vincristine, Cyclophosphomide and Doxorubicin is given three times weekly for a year or longer in those patients in whom metastases were detected.

Melanocytoma of the optic disc

Appears as a small deeply pigmented mass projecting

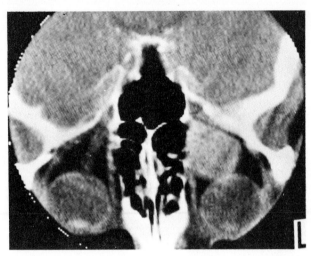

Fig. 33.8 Clearly defined rounded mass within the muscle cone typical of a cavernous haemangioma. (By courtesy of Glyn Lloyd.)

from the disc head and covering the adjacent retina with a feathery border. It produces no symptoms and remains static.

It is a benign tumour consisting of pigmented polyhedral cells.

Primary tumours of the optic nerve and its sheaths
These may be conveniently divided into two groups: 1. Ectodermal tumours of the nerve; gliomas. 2. Mesodermal tumours of the sheath of the nerve; meningiomas

Simple glial tumours derived from the astrocytes and oligidendroglial cells of the optic nerve are either a soli-

tary manifestation or a component of von Reckling hausen's neurofibromatosis. They are generally nonneoplastic and self-limiting with a good prognosis for life. They are more prevalent in childhood and probably congenital, the peak incidence being 2 – 5 years. They grow slowly extending over a large number of years and are treated conservatively. If they can be removed and are confined to the optic nerve there is a good prognosis for life. The neoplasm advances by extension along the nerve in a centripetal direction (Fig. 33.9). Once it reaches the chiasm the prognosis is poor. Enlargement of the optic canal is practically always present (Fig. 33.10). It is not however a reliable indicator of the

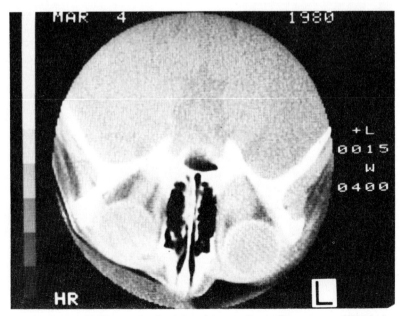

Fig. 33.9 Axial CT scan showing left optic nerve glioma. (By courtesy of Wright.)

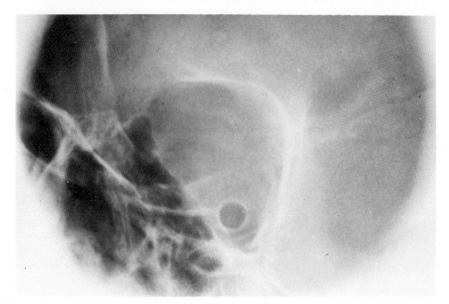

Fig. 33.10 Oblique radiograph of skull showing rounded enlargement of the optic canal typical of optic nerve glioma. (By courtesy of Wright.)

posterior extent of the tumour. There may be a place for radical surgery for a minority of patients in whom there is progressive growth without evidence of chiasmal involvement.

Primary orbital optic nerve meningiomas arise from the cap cells of the arachnoid around the intra-orbital portion of the optic nerve. Rarely meningiomatous tissue may extend from adjacent structures into the orbit in the sub-dural space of the optic nerve. C.T. scanners can show the orbital structures in both the axial and coronal planes and provide pictures which confirm the origin of the tumour (Fig. 33.11).

The predominant feature of optic nerve sheath meningiomas is early visual loss. Proptosis comes later and is often of a small degree. Tumours arising outside the dural sheath may cause considerable proptosis before compressing the optic nerve: the exception is an extra-dural tumour at the apex of the orbit.

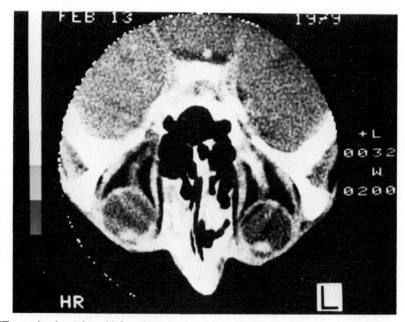

Fig. 33.11 Axial CT scan showing enlarged left optic nerve caused by secondary meningioma. (By courtesy of Wright.)

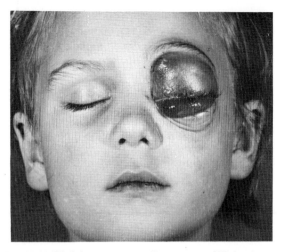

Fig. 33.12 Rhabdomyosarcoma. (By courtesy of Wybar.)

All patients present swollen or atrophic optic discs when first examined and in many cases optico-ciliary shunt vessels are present particularly if the meningioma of the optic nerve lies immediately behind the globe. Restriction of movement is common, particularly upwards when it is associated with a rise in intraocular pressure. Optic nerve meningiomas occur predominantly in middle-aged women. Patients with primary optic nerve meningiomas have a good prognosis because the tumours are peripheral, slow growing and isolated from the central nervous system. Patients with relatively good vision are left until it deteriorates and then the meningioma together with the optic nerve is removed. Biopsy or any surgery which transgresses the dura is to be avoided unless the rate of growth suggests a malignant type of meningioma when biopsy is indicated. If high resolution C.T. scans show a small anterior tumour and useful vision is retained the orbit may be explored and the lesion removed without endangering vision.

Secondary tumours

These also occur — carcinoma, hypernephroma, and in young children, sympathetic neuroblastoma; the parent growth of the last is usually in the adrenal medulla.

Malignant nasopharyngeal tumours

These form 0.4 % of all cases of cancer; 38 % of cases show ophthalmo-neurological symptoms, these being the earliest signs in 16% of cases. The fifth and sixth nerves are most frequently involved; more rarely the third, fourth and the optic nerve. Quadrantic and hemianopic lesions are rare, thus distinguishing these cases from lesions in the neighbourhood of the sella turcica. The presence of abducens paralysis, especially if associated with impairment of vision, Horner's syndrome or proptosis or enlargement of the cervical lymph nodes, should suggest a naso-pharyngeal growth. Treatment is by radiotherapy.

The lipodystrophies

These may give rise to tumour-like formations resulting from the reaction of the reticulo-endothelial system to the deposition of lipids — *diabetic exophthalmic dysostosis* (Hand – Schüller – Christian disease), *xanthomatosis*, etc.

The symptoms of most orbital tumours are similar; the differential diagnosis must frequently be made by biopsy.

Most orbital tumours cause proptosis, which is very rarely straight forwards except in the case of optic nerve tumours; this is an important diagnostic feature (Fig. 33.13). The proptosis is slowly progressive and (with the exception of the hæmopoietic tumours and sympathetic neuroblastomata) usually unilateral. The mobility of the eyeball is impaired in the direction towards the position of the tumour; diplopia is therefore common, while papillœdema may be present, especially with optic nerve tumours. Optic atrophy from pressure on the nerve occurs in the other forms. The tumour may be palpable by the finger inserted between the globe and the orbital wall. The lymphatic nodes are seldom affected.

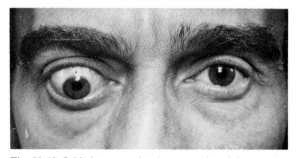

Fig. 33.13 Orbital tumour, showing proptosis and downward displacement of the globe

Careful examination of neighbouring parts — nose, antrum, mouth and especially the nasopharynx — must be made to determine whether the invasion of the orbit is secondary or whether the growth is primarily orbital. In all cases an X-ray examination should be made (vide supra).

Treatment. An exploratory operation and removal of a portion of the growth for microscopic examination may be a necessary preliminary to radical treatment. It may be feasible to remove dermoid cysts and some other benign tumours without injury to the globe, although its mobility is likely to be impaired in extensive operations. As already mentioned, many malignant orbital growths show little tendency to metastasis, so that their treatment may be more conservative than is usual in other parts of the body. Some tumours (particularly the reticular tumours) respond to radiational treatment and recurrences in the orbit or metastases should be treated by these means.

The majority, however, requires surgical excision. Three routes of approach with retention of the eye are available — an anterior orbitotomy, wherein an incision as for cellulitis (*q.v.*), made anteriorly at the orbital margin, provides access to the anterior half of the orbit; a lateral orbitotomy provides access to the deeper parts of the orbit and is a valuable exploratory procedure; while the apex of the orbit is best reached through a transfrontal (intracranial) approach. In the case of more malignant types of tumour their complete removal is imperative at all costs, and the eye, even if normal, may have to be sacrificed. In these cases, as well as in recurrence or in orbital extension of malignant intra-ocular growths (retinoblastoma, malignant melanoma of the uveal tract), it may be necessary to remove the whole contents of the orbit by exenteration.

In *lateral orbitotomy* (*Krönlein's operation*) a curved incision is made in the lateral two-third of the eyebrow, concentric with the superior and lateral orbital margin extending obliquely below the level of the lateral canthus over the zygomatic arch for about 4 cm. The bone is cut through at the upper and lower outer angles of the orbit with a Stryker saw and bone, muscle and skin are reflected backwards in one flap. The part of the orbit immediately posterior to the globe is thus freely exposed.

In *exenteration of the orbit* the lids may be retained if they are not implicated in the growth, but the free margins, carrying the cilia, should always be removed. If this is not done the lashes are troublesome when the lids become retracted into the orbit, as invariably follows. If the lids are removed the incision is carried through the skin at the margin of the orbit in its whole circumference. The orbital contents are separated from the walls by a periosteal elevator, so that they remain attached only at the apex of the orbit. The pedicle is then severed with strong scissors, or preferably by diathermy, thus avoiding hæmorrhage. At a later stage it may be advisable to apply split-skin grafts to the walls, since the lids and conjunctiva never afford sufficient epithelial covering, and the extension of the epithelium over so large a surface is a tedious process.

Endocrine exophthalmos

This is a puzzling condition the aetiology of which is not yet understood. Two types occur — a mild exophthalmos associated with thyrotoxicosis (exophthalmic goitre) and an extreme exophthalmos occurring in any state of thyroid activity, but usually in hypothyroidism, often after a thyroidectomy.

The cause of exophthalmos in either type is obscure. The retraction of the lid in thyrotoxicosis is due to contraction of Müller's muscle owing to the sensitising action of thyroxine on sympathomimetic receptors. The exophthalmos of exophthalmic ophthalmoplegia is due to œdema, lymphocytic infiltration and fibrosis of the orbital contents, particularly the extra-ocular muscles. These changes are probably due to a generalised disturbance of the endocrine system possibly associated with the thyrotropic hormone secreted by the anterior lobe of the pituitary gland which normally stimulates the thyroid gland to activity.

Exophthalmic goitre (*thyrotoxic exophthalmos, Graves's disease* or *Basedow's disease*). Includes in its symptomatology in addition to exophthalmos all the signs of thyrotoxicosis — tachycardia, muscular tremors and a raised basal metabolism. From the ocular point of view, the exophthalmos in the early stages may be unilateral but usually becomes bilateral. There is a peculiar stare with retraction of the upper eyelid, so that there is an unnatural degree of separation between the margins of the two lids (Dalrymple's sign) (Fig. 33.14). Normally, when the eye is directed downwards, the upper lid moves concordantly with it. In this disease the upper lid follows tardily or not at all (von Graefe's sign): this symptom is not always present and may occur in other forms of exophthalmos. There is diminished frequency of blinking and imperfect closure of the lids during the act (Stellwag's sign). There may be imperfect power of convergence (Möbius's sign), and often the skin of the eyelids shows pigmentation. Ophthalmoscopically, veins and arteries may be somewhat distended, but specific signs are absent. One or more of the cardinal symptoms may be absent. Recovery follows control of the thyrotoxic condition.

Exophthalmic ophthalmoplegia (*thyrotropic exophthalmos*). Usually this commences in middle age with insidious signs of proptosis and external ophthalmoplegia typically asymmetrically divided between the two eyes and involving preferentially limitation of upward

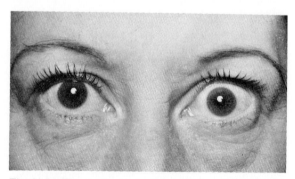

Fig. 33.14 Thyrotoxicosis, showing retraction of the upper lid and proptosis

movement. The ocular muscles are enormously swollen, pale, œdematous and infiltrated, giving rise to an irreducible exophthalmos which may easily result in the development of an exposure keratitis or even dislocation of the globe (Fig. 33.15). The disease runs a self-limited course characterised by intermissions and relapses, more or less unaffected by any kind of treatment, but eventually tends to spontaneous resolution which, however, is rarely complete.

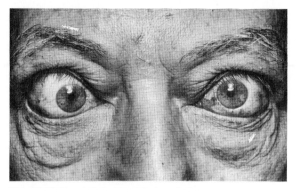

Fig. 33.15 Exophthalmic ophthalmoplegia

From the ophthalmological point of view the protection of the exposed cornea is of paramount importance; in less severe cases this is achieved by tarsorrhaphy (*q.v.*); in more severe cases a decompression of the orbit through the floor of the orbit by a Caldwell – Luc approach may be necessary especially if the optic nerve is threatened. Residual muscle palsies may require surgical adjustment.

Pulsating exophthalmos
This is generally due to arterio-venous aneurysm, the communication taking place between the internal carotid artery and the cavernous sinus. The eyeball is protruded and the blood vessels of the conjunctiva and lids are widely dilated. The angular vein and its branches near the inner canthus are very prominent, and they can be seen, or more easily felt, to pulsate synchronously with the arterial pulse since, owing to the arteriovenous communication, they are under arterial pressure. The patient complains of continual rumbling, as of a waterfall, and this can be heard on auscultation over the eye or orbit by the surgeon. The proptosis is diminished by steady pressure on the globe, and may be diminished or abolished by pressure on the common carotid artery of the same side, or sometimes only by pressure on the carotid of the opposite side also. Ophthalmoscopically, the veins of the retina are greatly distended: there may be papillœdema with defective vision, which may amount to complete blindness. There is often considerable pain from stretching of the branches of the fifth nerve.

The cause of the arterio-venous aneurysm is usually a severe blow or fall upon the head, and it is therefore commoner in men, but in most cases the walls of the artery are already degenerated. It may occur from atheromatous or syphilitic disease without discoverable traumatism, especially when it occurs in women. The exophthalmos in most cases subsides spontaneously. More commonly it increases, and may end in hæmorrhage or death from cerebral causes.

Treatment is conservative. If continuous pressure applied to the carotid artery stops the pulsation, ligation of the carotid may effect a cure, but recurrence of pulsation not in frequently occurs. Ligature of both internal and external carotid does not appear to give better results. The opposite carotid may also be tied, but this should not be done for some weeks after the first operation, owing to the risk of cerebral anaemia. This procedure also may fail to relieve the condition, and in these cases intracranial ligation proximally and distally to the aneurysm has been practised, an operation of considerable difficulty and danger.

Intermittent proptosis
Occasionally this occurs, generally when the head is depressed, enophthalmos not infrequently being present in the erect position. The proptosis is increased by pressure on the corresponding jugular vein. It is usually due to varicosity of the orbital veins and has been found to be caused by intracerebral arterio-venous communications.

Injuries of the orbit
Injuries to the soft parts usually arise from penetration of a foreign body which may be retained; the lids and eyeball are frequently implicated. The signs depend upon the particular structures injured. In most cases there is considerable hæmorrhage; as the blood does not find a ready exit proptosis may result and extravasation of blood under the conjuctiva and into the lids is common. Paralysis of the extrinsic muscles may be due to direct injury or to damage to the motor nerves. The optic nerve may be injured or severed with resultant atrophy. Avulsion of the disc, with the formation of a traumatic 'coloboma' or 'conus' of the disc, may occur, even without rupture of the sheath of the nerve. The eyeball may be perforated or contused or dislocated outside the lids. Retained foreign bodies are liable to set up suppuration and orbital cellulitis (*q.v.*).

A blow in the orbital region without the penetration of a foreign body may lead to an intra-orbital haemorrhage; this may occur from pressure with forceps at birth. It is to be noted that an orbital and subconjunctival hæmorrhage is a frequent sign of a fracture of the base of the skull. Dislocation of the globe forwards between the lids occurs most often when the blow is directed from the outer side where the orbital margin affords least protection; sight is not necessarily lost after such a dislocation.

Injuries to the bone most commonly affect the margin of the orbit but deep fractures may be caused by penetrating wounds or by severe contusions. Fractures near the orbital rim are easy to diagnose from the unevenness of the margin, sensitiveness to pressure, and sometimes crepitation. Deeper fractures may give rise to *emphysema* which may cause proptosis but is usually most evident in the lids. It is due to communication of the subcutaneous tissues with the nasal air sinuses so that air is forced into the tissues on blowing the nose, sneezing, straining, or coughing. The diagnostic signs are the considerable swelling and the peculiar soft crepitation on palpation.

In fractures of the orbital floor the globe may sink backwards and be depressed with a resultant troublesome diplopia (*traumatic enophthalmos*) (Fig. 33.16). It is important that blow-out fractures be accurately diagnosed at an early stage since the correction of the diplopia involves the insertion of a thin layer of silicone rubber between the periosteum and bone of the orbital floor after reducing the herniation of the soft tissues. Such fractures are diagnosed accurately by computerised coronal tomography which enables the entrapment of

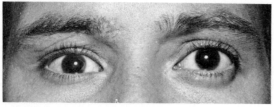

Fig. 33.16 Enophthalmos and downward displacement of the right eyeball due to a fracture of the floor of the orbit

the inferior rectus to be localised accurately.

Fractures of the base of the skull may involve one or both optic foramina, in which case the optic nerve may be injured or pulsating exophthalmos (*q.v.*) may ensue. Blindness without ophthalmoscopic signs may be caused in this manner probably as the result of a shearing force injuring the vessels entering the periphery of the nerve as it courses through the optic canal: atrophy of the disc follows in three to six weeks.

Gunshot wounds of the orbit without direct involvement of the eye frequently produce concussion changes which appear ophthalmoscopically as coarse tracks of white exudate in the retina and choroid, large blot-like hæmorrhages and multiple small choroidal tears. These resolve into densely scarred areas fringed with pigment, with finer pigmentary disturbances elsewhere in the fundus. The site may give an indication of the direction of the track of the missile and assist in localising a retained intracranial foreign body. Both eyes should be examined as the missile may have traversed both orbits.

Treatment. If there is a wound it must be cleansed and, if a foreign body is possibly retained, probed: it should be dusted with penicillin-sulphonamide powder and a prophylactic course of systemic antibiotic treatment given if indicated. Absorption of extravasated blood is often slow. The treatment of a retained foreign body depends upon its situation and the probability of subsequent infection. If the foreign body cannot be extracted with ease, a skiagram should be taken. If the position is such that serious manipulations would be necessary for its removal, and if there is evidence that the substance is aseptic, expectant treatment may be adopted. If suppuration occurs, the foreign body must be removed and the case treated as one of orbital cellulitis (*q.v.*).

Symptomatic diseases of the eye

34

Ocular manifestations of diseases of the nervous system

The ocular signs of nervous disease often appear superficially to be complicated and confusing but in most cases they are readily explained by the anatomy of the part of the nervous system involved. Even at the risk of some repetition the main ocular symptoms of these diseases will be summarised in this section without describing the diseases themselves.

Circulatory disorders

Intracranial aneurysms

Some of ophthalmological interest affect the circle of Willis, where they are usually congenital or the internal carotid artery (Fig. 34.1). They give rise to ophthalmic symptoms in three ways:

1. By mechanical pressure on neighbouring structures in their slow growth, causing symptoms characteristic of a tumour in the chiasmal region (q.v.).

2. Infraclinoid aneurysms produce symptoms by dilatation of the internal carotid artery within the cavernous sinus which affects the motor nerves to the eye and the ophthalmic and maxillary divisions of the trigeminal nerve. Expansion of the aneurysm gives rise to ophthalmoplegia as well as pain and paraesthesia in the face. A slowly progressive ophthalmoplegia overtakes the patient and pain is severe around the eye associated with corneal anaesthesia.

These aneurysms do not usually rupture but they may thrombose completely and thus cure spontaneously. Alternatively the artery may expand and produce erosion of the optic canal with compression of the optic nerve.

Ligation of the internal carotid is indicated provided digital compression produces no severe ischaemic symptoms.

3. Supraclinoid aneurysms suddenly rupture. They usually arise at the bifurcation of the internal carotid artery into the middle and anterior cerebral arteries. The majority of patients presenting rupture of such an aneurysm are middle-aged women.

There is a sudden onset with severe headache on one side of the head from meningeal irritation followed later by a third nerve palsy with pupillary dilatation. Death may occur from a subarachnoid haemorrhage or from bleeding into the brain tissue.

Subarachnoid haemorrhage is characterised by sudden violent head pain followed by photophobia and unconsciousness. Lumbar puncture shows fresh blood.

The ocular signs consist of loss of vision, sometimes swollen discs and exophthalmos. A subhyaloid haemorrhage may present at the posterior pole.

Vascular malformations of the nervous system

These are divided into four groups:

1. Capillary telangiectasis.
2. Cavernous angiomas.
3. Venous malformations.
4. Arteriovenous malformations.

Capillary telangiectasis are relatively common lesions generally found at necropsy. They are small and cause no symptoms. The pons is the commonest location for them.

Cavernous angiomas are uncommon lesions, though

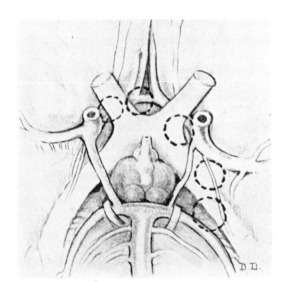

Fig. 34.1 The common sites of aneurysms in the chiasmal region. (By courtesy of Russell Brain.)

a potential source of bleeding. If they rupture there is severe intracranial haemorrhage. They are usually solitary and well-defined, often located on the surface of the cerebrum and can be removed surgically.

Venous malformations are commonly found in the spinal cord and meninges but often occur in the scalp and in the orbit. In the latter situation they cause intermittent exophthalmos, made worse on stooping. Histologically they are similar to arteriovenous malformations except that arterial structures are absent. They consist of multiple veins of varying calibre. They show up on a venous angiogram and are associated with raised intraocular pressure and eventually a secondary form of glaucoma.

Arteriovenous malformations are the commonest of the four groups. Grossly they appear as a tortuous mass or a 'bag of worms'. They are composed of arteries and veins of abnormal calibre and length. They are classified according to their arterial supply — from the pia, or from the dura, (the internal or external carotid artery or vertebral artery); or from both pia and dura. Carotid–cavernous fistulae involve a direct communication between the internal carotid arterial wall and the sinus itself. Such a fistula is a high-flow and high-pressure system which causes the arterialised blood to flow from the cavernous sinus forward into the ophthalmic veins in the orbit. This produces the classical signs and symptoms of severe ipsilateral headache, a homolateral carotid bruit, progressive exophthalmos, dilated and frequently pulsating episcleral blood vessels and varying degrees of ophthalmoloplegia. It responds to occlusion of the internal carotid artery. Seventy-five per cent of carotid – cavernous fistulae are regarded as traumatic and 25% spontaneous.

A cavernous sinus fistula or malformation is derived from the dural blood vessels in the cavernous sinus. The signs and symptoms associated with these dural shunts are essentially the same as those seen with classical carotid cavernous fistulae except they are more subtle. The dural arteriovenous shunts may be within the cavernous sinus or directly adjacent to it or they may involve a more distant sinus and subsequently drain into the cavernous sinus. They are probably due to a local congenital vascular malformation.

Symptoms arising are headache which is severe, unilateral often localised to the orbit, the temple or forehead Proptosis is minimal. Dilated conjunctival vessels are common and produce a red eye without pulsation. Raised intraocular pressure is common but mild. Unilateral VIth nerve palsy is a frequent finding. An objective bruit is found in half the cases. Dural arteriovenous fistulae may be associated with spontaneous choroidal detachments.

Because these lesions involve dural vessels they may be amenable to embolisation in selected cases. Catheterisation with embolisation of the feeding vessels by a transfemoral artery approach and the use of ground-up pieces of gel-foam may close the shunt.

Radiographic diagnosis requires complete selective cerebral angiography subtraction and magnification techniques (Figs 34.2 and 34.3)

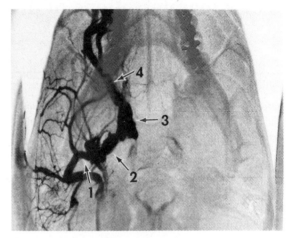

Fig. 34.2 Base view. The proximal portion of the middle meningeal vessel is dilated (arrow 1). A fistula communication is in the region of the foramen spinosum. A dilated vein (arrow 2) extends from the region of the foramen spinosum to the posterior portion of the cavernous sinus (arrow 3). The superior ophthalmic vein (arrow 4) fills in a retrograde direction (By courtesy of Costin.)

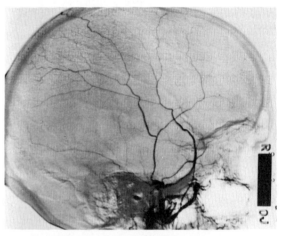

Fig. 34.3 After embolisation the middle meningeal and superficial temporal arteries fill normally. The fistula communication to the cavernous sinus has been occluded. (By courtesy of Costin.)

Cerebral haemorrhage and thrombosis

In the *occipital cortex* the posterior cerebral artery is usually involved; it supplies most of the occipital cortex and much of the temporal lobe. A lesion of this vessel thus causes a crossed homonymous hemianopia often with disturbances of the visuo-psychic areas (Fig. 24.1); the fixation area is usually spared owing to overlapping with the middle cerebral artery at the posterior pole (p. 231). Obstruction of the middle cerebral artery produces visual agnosia with a crossed homonymous field defect affecting preferentially the upper quadrants of the field by involvement of the optic radiations.

A lesion of the *frontal motor cortex* (Fig. 28.7) causes a conjugate deviation of the eyes away from the side of the lesion in the irritative stage, which is reversed in the paretic stage but the deviation is only apparent when the patient is asleep. A haemorrhage at the *internal capsule* produces a conjugate deviation of the head and eyes towards the side of the lesion with a contralateral hemiplegia. A haemorrhage into the *pons* (below the decussation of the corticofugal fibres) produces conjugate deviation of the head and eyes away from the side of the lesion, that is, towards the hemiplegic side and a palsy of horizontal conjugate gaze to the side of the lesion. The pupils are extremely small — an important diagnostic point in a comatose patient.

Obstruction of branches of the *basilar artery* in the brain-stem produces symptoms depending on the implication of the ocular motor nuclei and the pyramidal tracts.

Obstruction of the *posterior inferior cerebellar artery* gives rise to a characteristic clinical picture resulting from infarction of a wedge-shaped area on the lateral aspect of the medulla. In addition to vertigo, dysphagia, signs of cerebellar deficiency, and sensory disturbances due to trigeminal involvement, there is nystagmus and Horner's syndrome (miosis, enophthalmos and ptosis) on the affected side.

Hydrocephalus

In the *congenital* and the early acquired hydrocephalus of infancy, optic atrophy is not infrequently found. Papilloedema occurs only rarely in spite of the increased intracranial pressure, a fact doubtless due to the relief of pressure by the enlargement of the skull and the resiliency of the fontanelles and gaping sutures, as well as to the very gradual development. The eyeballs usually deviate downwards, and upward movements are restricted. (The 'setting-sun' syndrome.) Not infrequently there is considerable proptosis. Such children are lethargic, subject to fits, often blind with sluggish pupils and spastic diplegia.

The *acquired hydrocephalus* of later life, after the fontanelles and sutures have closed, can often only be diagnosed with certainty by encephalography or by computerised axial tomography. The cardinal signs of increased intracranial pressure — headache, vomiting and papilloedema — are present, and to these is often added ataxia of the cerebellar type. The cases are often diagnosed as intracranial tumours in which localising

signs are not infrequently absent or masked. Bitemporal hemianopia may give a clue to the true ætiology, being due to pressure on the chiasm and tracts by the bulging floor of the third ventricle. Defective vision due to post-neuritic atrophy may persist.

Infections

Meningitis

The N. meningitidis is a gram-negative aerobic and facultative anaerobic organism which forms a single coccus or occurs in pairs. It lives in the human nasopharynx. In *acute meningococcal (epidemic) cerebrospinal meningitis* papillitis is frequently present, never papillœdema; it is due to a descending infective perineuritis. In the early stages there is often kinetic strabismus or conjugate lateral deviation of the eyes. A characteristic sign is the widely open palpebral aperture, often associated with very infrequent blinking. Paralysis of the VIth nerve, usually unilateral, is commoner than that of the IIIrd, although divergent strabismus due to the latter cause has been frequently noted. Total IIIrd nerve paralysis is rare. The pupils vary, usually showing miosis in the early stages, mydriasis when coma sets in: loss of reaction to light is relatively rare. Metastatic endophthalmitis (*q.v.*) in children is an uncommon complication.

Sporadic acute basal meningitis may be associated with complete amaurosis with normal fundi and normal pupillary reactions, pointing to the action of toxins on the higher visual centres. The blindness may persist for many weeks after subsidence of other symptoms, but sight may be ultimately restored. *Chronic-basal meningitis* sometimes shows the same feature, but in these cases optic neuritis and post-neuritic atrophy may occur from secondary hydrocephalus and pressure of the distended third ventricle upon the chiasma and tracts or meningeal adhesions in the chiasmal region.

In the meningitis of *middle ear disease* papillitis or papillœdema is usually due to complications, such as. sinus thrombosis or cerebral abscess. When ocular paralysis occurs, the VIth nerve is usually affected, rarely the IIIrd (cf. Intracranial Abscess) The facial nerve is most frequently involved, the paralysis often causing lagophthalmos. Conjugate deviation of the eyes is not uncommon.

Chronic chiasmal arachnoiditis is a localised meningeal infection in the meninges around the chiasm and optic nerves; the ætiology is obscure although sepsis of the nasal sinuses or sarcoidosis may account for some cases. A primary optic atrophy usually develops bilaterally, with a central scotoma and irregular contraction of the visual fields, either concentrically or with bitemporal loss. The diagnosis from a pituitary tumour is based on negative radiological and other evidence and deformation of the chiasmal cistern on encephalography.

In *tuberculous meningitis* a moderate degree of papillitis is common (about 25%) and is generally bilateral. Miliary tubercles in the choroid are frequent and of great diagnostic importance. Until antibiotic therapy altered the almost invariably fatal prognosis of the condition, miliary choroidal tubercles were usually a terminal complication. There are often partial ocular pareses, usually of the IIIrd nerve, especially in the form of ptosis. Bilateral IIIrd paralysis is almost unknown, a point of distinction from syphilitic basal meningitis. Unilateral partial VIth nerve paralysis also occurs. Not infrequently there is a kinetic (not paralytic) conjugate deviation of the eyes and head to one side.

Encephalitis

Ocular palsies usually usher in an attack of *encephalitis lethargica*. Ptosis is the commonest feature, and other branches of the IIIrd nerve are especially involved. The muscles are usually only partially paralysed and generally recover. Diplopia is an early symptom, and nystagmus may be present. Papilloedema is rare and the pupils are usually normal. The general symptoms are lethargy, with great muscular debility and other signs of an acute general infection. The disease is often followed by Parkinsonian tremor (paralysis agitans), and in the later stages spasmodic conjugate deviation of the eyes occurs usually upwards (*oculogyric crises*) accompanied by synergic movements of the head and neck. Oculogyric crises may be relieved by benzedrine (up to 30 mg a day). They are sometimes a result of phenothiazine iodiosyncracy.

Acute *polioencephalitis* accounts for the not infrequent cases of paralytic squint following a febrile attack in young children. The VIth nerve is most often involved.

Syphilitic infections

Cerebral syphilis

This is the term usually applied to relatively early, direct syphilitic disease of the brain and meninges. It is due essentially to gummatous inflammation of the meninges and the walls of the cerebral blood vessels.

The chief form of brain syphilis is *basal gummatous meningitis*. It usually arises in the subarachnoid tissue in the region of the chiasm and spreads thence over the base of the brain. The optic nerves, chiasm, and tracts are generally involved. Papillitis, papilloedema, or postneuritic atrophy is frequently found (about 13% each), and is usually bilateral. Visual defects are very common, and consist of amblyopia, not infrequently amaurosis, and defects in the fields of vision. Of the latter, many cases show homonymous hemianopia from affection of one tract, fewer cases temporal hemianopia. Central scotoma and other signs of retrobulbar neuritis also occur.

The IIIrd nerve is paralysed in a third of the cases, less commonly the Vth and VIth, and least frequently the IVth. The IIIrd and VIth are often affected on both sides. The trigeminal paralysis is always unilateral and often causes neuroparalytic keratitis. Pupillary changes occur, dependent upon the IIIrd nerve lesions. In many cases the process is limited to a small area, oculomotor paralysis or an affection of the visual path being the only sign except headache. A very characteristic feature of basal gummatous meningitis is the inconstancy and variability of the symptoms, temporary and recurrent visual and oculomotor disturbances being very common.

Tabes dorsalis

Syphilitic Optic Atrophy (p. 229) occurs in about 10–20% of cases of locomotor ataxia. The disease is probably a primary interstitial neuritis arising as an extremely chronic exudative process from the pia and causing a secondary degeneration of the nerve fibres and their parent ganglion cells. The process usually becomes apparent first in the intracranial portion of the nerve distal to the chiasm. It is about twice as common in men as in women, most frequent between thirty and fifty years of age, and may precede the appearance of typical tabetic symptoms by some years. It is commonest in the preataxic stage. The onset is gradual, leading to total blindness in two to three years or more. Pallor of the disc may precede the failure of vision by a considerable period, never the reverse. The affection of one eye usually precedes that of the other by a few months.

The *fields* show progressive contraction, *pari passu* with the failure in central vision. It is rare for the failure of sight to commence with a central scotoma, thus differing from the onset in multiple sclerosis. Two types of field are met with: (1) general concentric shrinkage, the colour fields for red and green being lost early, and central vision much impaired; (2) irregular sectorial defects, which are sharply defined but gradually spread, although central vision may be good.

The characteristic *pupillary signs* include the so-called spinal miosis, the Argyll Robertson pupil reaction, inequality of the pupils, and distortion of the pupillary aperture. These signs are found in other diseases and are to be regarded as signs of syphilis of the central nervous system rather than as pathognomonic of tabes; their combination is of great diagnostic significance. Argyll Robertson pupils are found in 70% of tabetics and are almost invariably bilateral. Unequal pupils are found in 30% of tabetics, but are met with still more frequently in general paralysis. Ophthalmoplegia interna, i.e., paralysis of the sphincter pupillæ and the ciliary muscle, occurs in about 5% of tabetics and is generally unilateral. It is due to a lesion in the nucleus of the IIIrd nerve.

Paralyses of the extrinsic ocular muscles. This is common in tabes, occurring in about 20% of the cases. The order of frequency of the nerves affected is IIIrd (20%), VIth (13%), IVth (3%), external or total ophthalmoplegia (2%). It is characteristic of tabetic paralyses that they are partial pareses rather than paralyses, variable and transitory. The affection of the IIIrd nerve is always suggestive of a tabetic or syphilitic lesion. Total IIIrd nerve paralysis is rare in tabes, and isolated ptosis relatively common (4% of cases). The pareses of the ocular muscles nearly always occur in the pre-ataxic stage: when they occur at a later stage they are more likely to be permanent. They generally clear up rapidly, but show a marked tendency to recur. Nystagmus is rare, but the paresed muscles often give rise to jerky movements of the eyes which may be mistaken for nystagmoid jerks. Paralyses of associated movements (conjugate deviations) are very rare.

General paralysis of the insane (progressive paralysis, paralytic dementia)

This parasyphilitic disease is often accompanied by tabetic signs and symptoms which are due to lesions of the posterior tracts of the cord, identical with those in tabes (taboparalysis). The ocular symptoms are most common and unequivocal in these cases, and are to be attributed to the same causes.

The *pupillary* changes are most characteristic. In the early stages inequality is often accompanied by slight deformation in the shape of the pupil and irregularity of the pupillary margin is common. An Argyll Robertson reaction occurs in nearly half the cases. In about 5% of the cases the reactions both to light and convergence are lost, a condition which is rare in tabes and especially frequent in the juvenile form of general paralysis. The sensory reaction is very often lost with the light reaction. Spinal miosis is commoner in tabes, unequal pupils in general paralysis. Ophthalmoplegia interna is more rare in general paralysis.

Primary optic atrophy. Occurs in about 8% of cases showing the same type and course as in tabes. Like pupillary signs, it may precede the onset of the typical cerebral symptoms by a considerable period, especially in those cases which commence with tabetic symptoms.

Paralyses of the extrinsic ocular muscles. Occurs about half as frequently as in tabes, and have exactly the same characteristics, the IIIrd nerve being most frequently involved.

The demyelinating diseases

Multiple sclerosis (disseminated or insular sclerosis)

Lesions in the visual paths often occur in multiple sclerosis (50% of cases). Unlike the lesions of tabes, the medullary sheaths of the nerve fibres are especially attacked, the axis cylinders remaining relatively little affected. Hence, during the acute stage, defects in con-

ductivity are especially prominent; considerable variations succeed each other, and high degrees of functional restoration are possible. The optic nerves are most frequently attacked, with all the clinical signs of a typical retrobulbar neuritis, but patches of degeneration in the chiasm, optic tracts, or optic radiations may cause characteristic hemianopic or quadrantic changes in the fields.

The frequency of attacks of unilateral *retrobulbar neuritis* which clear up and recur, often many years before the disease becomes generalised, has already been noted (*q.v.*). They may clear up entirely but may be followed by irregular field defects — central scotomata, concentric contraction of the field and irregular peripheral defects, sometimes only for colours, and showing variations from time to time. Some degree of optic atrophy usually develops eventually, the appearance of which bears no relation to the functional defect, but permanent blindness almost never occurs.

Nystagmus occurs in 12% of cases, but nystagmoid jerks are much commoner (50% of cases). True nystagmus is a very important diagnostic sign since it is rare in other acquired diseases of the central nervous system. Both are probably due to central changes, and the latter show some analogy to the intention tremor so characteristic of multiple sclerosis.

Miosis is fairly common in this disease, and to a less degree inequality of pupils. Other pupillary abnormalities are rare.

Paralyses of the extrinsic ocular muscles are much less common than in tabes, and although resembling these in their partial and transitory nature, differ from them in that paralyses of associated movements are not uncommon. Unilateral inter-nuclear ophthalmoplegia with ataxic nystagmus indicates demyelination in the medial longitudinal fasiculus. Of individual nerves, the VIth is more often affected than the IIIrd, and total IIIrd nerve paralysis is never seen. Partial ophthalmoplegia externa also occurs, whereas ophthalmoplegia interna is unknown.

Neuromyelitis optic (Devic's disease)

In this association of bilateral optic neuritis with myelitis, the visual defect usually precedes the signs of myelitis. Its onset is sudden, but one eye may be affected a day or so before the other. Complete amaurosis generally supervenes rapidly. Sometimes there is an initial central scotoma, and there may be pain on moving the eyes, pointing to a retrobulbar neuritis. There is usually only slight neuritis, but considerable swelling of the disc has been seen. In cases which recover, the blindness passes off and good vision is restored. The site of the myelitis may be lumbar or dorsal. There are no signs of general meningitis, and the other cranial nerves escape.

Diffuse sclerosis (Schilder's disease)
This is characterised by a demyelination of the entire white matter of the cerebral hemispheres occurring in young people. The ocular symptoms appear early. Blindness is common, due to destruction of the optic radiations; optic neuritis or retrobulbar neuritis follows demyelination of the optic nerve. Ocular motor palsies and nystagmus are common.

Hereditary and degenerative diseases

Congenital oculo-motor ataxia
This is a diagnostic entity with a good prognosis. Patients make characteristic thrusting movements of the head opposite to the direction in which they wish their eyes to move. The beginning of the head movement is initiated by a blink, the head is turned considerably passed the target, such that the patient overshoots the target with the head, and following fixation on the target the head is then brought into line with regard to the target. The rapid head movements are thought to be related to the use of vestibular reflexes in changing the gaze position. Random eye movements are intact.

Chronic ophthalmoplegia of a progressive type, due to a myopathy of the ocular muscles, commences with ptosis or diplopia. In the course of months or years the degeneration spreads to all the ocular muscles of both sides, except that the intrinsic muscles often escape. Cases of isolated ophthalmoplegia of neurogenic origin are rare, but the condition is occasionally a precursor or symptom of tabes or general paralysis of the insane, rarely of multiple sclerosis. It may become associated later with bulbar symptoms; in these cases the internal musculature may be involved.

Hereditary ataxia (Friedreich's disease)
In this optic atrophy and paralyses of the ocular muscles are very rare. Nystagmoid jerkings of the eyes, very similar to those occurring in multiple sclerosis, are common, but visual symptoms are absent. The movements are probably due to the same lack of co-ordination which causes the other ataxic signs of the disease; they occur on voluntary movement, and are not usually present in passive fixation.

Status dysraphicus
This results from a defective or anomalous closure of the neural tube and may have various ocular implications. In *syringomyelia* cavities form around which secondary gliosis develops in the cervical and upper dorsal cord; in *syringobulbia* the process extends up to the medulla. The neural symptoms which develop between the ages of 20 and 40 include paralysis of the cervical sympathetic (Horner's syndrome), of the trigeminal and of various extra-ocular muscles.

Lipid dystrophies
The lipid dystrophies and their associated retinal lesions, and *hepato-lenticular degeneration* with the Kayser–Fleischer corneal ring have already been described (*q.v.*).

Ophthalmopegia caused by deficiencies and toxins
The chief exogenous poisons causing ophthalmoplegia are lead and ptomaines; the chief toxins, diphtheria and influenza. In *lead poisoning* the onset is slow and the intrinsic muscles are often involved. In *botulism*, due to food contaminated with *Cl. botulinum*, bilateral ophthalmoplegia interna, with or without ptosis, is typical but total ophthalmoplegia also occurs. In *diphtheria* isolated ocular palsies are common, but ophthalmoplegia externa is rare; the pupil often escapes, the ciliary muscle never. In *influenza* the palsies are similar, affecting the extrinsic and ciliary muscles, but usually not the pupil; the pupil, however, has been known to be affected without the ciliary muscle. In all cases recovery is common.

In *thiamine deficiency* (p. 372), frequently associated with alcoholism, the onset is sudden and accompanied by cerebral symptoms — headache, delirium, coma. Bilateral ophthalmoplegia externa occurs with or without ptosis, often followed by facial and bulbar paralyses with difficulty in speech and swallowing; the intrinsic muscles usually escape. Pathologically the condition is an *acute hæmorrhagic anterior polioencephalitis* (Wernicke). The prognosis is bad.

Intracranial tumours
Intracranial tumours (including neoplasms and such lesions as tuberculomata) produce two sets of symptoms.

1. Generalised symptoms of increased intracranial pressure — headache, vomiting, vertigo, convulsion, somnolence, alterations in the pulse, blood pressure and respiratory rhythm, papillœdema, and occasionally ocular palsies.

2. Focal signs owing to destruction of neighbouring structures, the ophthalmologically important of which are field defects and ocular pareses.

Papilloedema. This has already been discussed in this relation (*q.v.*). Precentral and temporo-sphenoidal tumours are nearly always associated with severe papillœdema, post-central tumours with moderate papillœdema, often of short duration. Of subcortical tumours about one-half cause papilloedema — as a rule, moderate and of short duration. Tumours of the optic thalamus and mid-brain are almost invariably associated with papilloedema of great severity. Cerebellar tumours are constantly and extracerebellar tumours usually accompanied by papilloedema of a grave character. Of pontine tumours, only about one-half give rise to papilloedema, and then only when neighbouring parts of the brain, especially the cerebellum, have become involved:

the papilloedema when it does develop is usually marked. Ventricular tumours cause a moderate papilloedema. There are two regions of the brain, the pons and the central white matter of the cerebral hemispheres, in which tumours usually develop without causing papilloedema.

Paralyses of the ocular muscles. Except for the lateral rectus, paralyses of the ocular muscles are rare as a sign of generalised pressure.

Focal signs. Prefrontal tumours, particularly meningiomata of the olfactory groove, are sometimes associated with a pressure-atrophy of the optic nerve on the side of the lesion due to direct pressure and a papillœdema on the other side due to generalised pressure (*Foster–Kennedy syndrome*).

Chiasmal and pituitary tumours. See p. 232.

Tumours of the temporal lobe. In 50% of cases these produce a characteristic crossed upper quadrantanopia, usually incongruous, being more accentuated in the ipsilateral field. This sign is due to pressure on the optic radiations. Visual hallucinations may occur owing to irritation of the visuo-psychic area. Downward pressure may involve the IIIrd nerve and the Vth, causing diminution of corneal sensitivity.

Tumours of the parietal lobe. These produce a crossed lower homonymous quadrantanopia from involvement of the upper fibres of the radiations, visual and auditory hallucinations, and an abnormal opto-kinetic response to the revolving drum.

Tumours of the occipital lobe. These present essentially visual symptoms. Typically there are crossed homonymous quadrantic or hemianopic defects extending up to the fixation point. Anteriorly situated tumours may cause a crescentic loss in the periphery in the opposite uniocular temporal field. Visual agnosia may also occur.

Tumours of the mid-brain. The localising signs of tumours in this region depend on involvement of the pyramidal tracts and ocular motor nerves. All of them may be associated with homonymous hemianopia owing to pressure on the optic tracts.

In the upper part of the mid-brain (*the colliculi and pineal gland*) the most characteristic sign is spasmodic contraction of the upper lid followed by ptosis, together with loss of conjugate movements upwards, sometimes followed by a similar failure of downward movement. There is light-near dissociation in that the pupil response to light is impaired as contrasted with the constriction obtained on testing the near reflex. There may be vertical nystagmus and adduction movements on attempted vertical gaze.

At an intermediate level in the *cerebral peduncles* the third nucleus becomes progressively involved. Ipsilateral ptosis and ultimately a complete IIIrd paralysis is associated with a contralateral hemiplegia involving a facial palsy of the upper neurone type (*Weber's syndrome*)

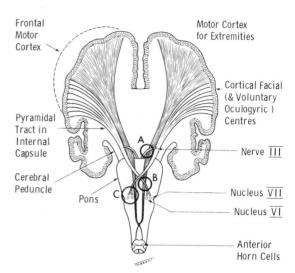

Fig. 34.4 The relation between the pyramidal tracts and the ocular motor nuclei. A. The site of a lesion causing Weber's syndrome (ipsilateral IIIrd paralysis and crossed hemiplegia of the face and body). B. The site of a lesion in the pons causing ipsilateral (upper neuron, i.e., without muscular atrophy) facial paralysis and contralateral hemiplegia which, on extension downwards, may involve abducens paralysis. C. The site of a lesion in the pons causing Foville's syndrome [ipsilateral abducens paralysis with loss of conjugate deviation to the same side, ipsilateral lower neurone facial palsy and contralateral (upper neurone) hemiplegia]

(Fig. 34.4). If the red nucleus is involved, tremor and jerky movements occur in the contralateral side of the body: this condition, combined with ipsilateral IIIrd nerve paralysis forms *Benedikt's syndrome.* If the lemniscus is involved there may be contralateral hemianaesthesia.

At a still lower level in the *pons* the same types of localising symptoms are found. In the upper part of the pons before the fibres to the facial nucleus have crossed, there is again a IIIrd paralysis with contralateral, hemiplegia and upper facial palsy. In the lower part of the pons the lateral rectus may be paralysed with a contralateral hemiplegia and an ipsilateral facial palsy (*Millard–Gubler's syndrome*) (Fig. 34.4); more commonly the VIth palsy is replaced by a loss of conjugate movement to the same side (*Foville's syndrome*). The Vth nerve may be paralysed causing loss of corneal sensation which is liable to cause neuroparalytic keratitis owing to the accompanying facial palsy, and implication of the VIIIth nerve may cause deafness. Miosis is rare.

Tumours of the auditory nerve, growing in the cerebello-pontine angle, give rise to a fairly characteristic syndrome with ocular signs. Corneal anæsthesia due to implication of the Vth nerve may be an early occurrence. Early tinnitus and deafness on one side is associated with cerebellar symptoms, among which nystagmus is common. The VIth nerve is usually involved, generally with paralysis of the lateral rectus only, rarely with paralysis of conjugate deviation. As might be expected, there is very often facial paralysis of the peripheral type, including the orbicularis palpebrarum.

Tumours of the cerebellum. Usually these cause nystagmus as well as marked papillœdema.

Congenital and development conditions

Oxycephaly (acrocephaly) is due to precocious union of certain cranial sutures: occipito-parietal and fronto-parietal (*turricephaly, tower skull*), or sagittal (*scaphocephaly*). Asynchronous fusion of the bones leads to a lopsided skull (*plagiocephaly*). The great wing of the sphenoid is displaced so that the orbit becomes shallow, causing some degree of proptosis. In the early stages there is papillœdema, but more commonly only the later stage of post-neuritic optic atrophy is seen. The amount of atrophy varies in degree. The papillœdema is probably due to increased intracranial pressure, owing to continued growth of the brain in a restricted space. Most of the patients are males. Acrocephaly may be associated with syndactylism (*Apert's disease*).

Congenital spastic diplegia (*Little's disease*)

This is a bilateral spastic paralysis present from birth, considered at one time to be due to meningeal hæmorrhage as a result of birth injury, is probably a degenerative cerebral process of obscure ætiology. With it may occur such ocular anomalies as optic atrophy, retinal degeneration, cataract, squint and internuclear palsies.

Head injury

Concussion injuries

Such injuries to the brain are frequently followed by haemorrhage, ususally subdural, often involving unconsciousness. The pupillary reactions are important since they may be the main diagnostic indication for operation in a patient in coma. At first the ipsilateral pupil is contracted; later, as intracranial pressure increases, this pupil dilates and does not react to light (*Hutchinson's pupil*); if pressure still increases, a similar phenomenon occurs in the other pupil. The presence of the dilated fixed pupil is a strong indication for cerebral decompression on the same side.

Fractures of the base of the skull

These commonly involve the cranial nerves. The most common complication is ipsilateral facial paralysis of the lower neurone type (22% of cases): the VIth (4%), IIIrd (2%), Vth (1.6%), and IVth (1%) follow in order of frequency. Fractures of the base sometimes involve the roof of the orbit but rarely traverse the optic foramen: occasionally both optic foramina are implicated. It may happen that the nerve is directly injured or compressed by hæmorrhage; more frequently, however, owing to the fact that the dura mater becomes the periosteum, the optic nerve is injured indirectly, probably by shearing involving laceration of the small meningeal vessels feeding it. If the injury is severe, in two to four weeks signs of primary optic atrophy appear and progress to total atrophy; in this event blindness is absolute and permanent. Papilloedema indicates haemorrhage into the nerve sheath and may occur from basal haemorrhage without fracture of the optic foramen; such cases have a serious prognosis. These injuries may cause concentric contraction of the field of vision, or quadrantic and other sectorial defects: a central scotoma is rare. Pigmentation in and around the disc may follow hæmorrhage into the sheath. The pupillary reactions vary and are not pathognomonic, but there is usually mydriasis on the side of the lesion.

35

Immunopathology of the eye

Immunopathology

The ability to mount a specific immune response to potentially harmful agents is confined to vertebrates and depends upon the presence of lymphoid tissue. Harmful agents which stimulate such a response (antigens) consist of exogenous micro-organisms or cells produced as a result of spontaneous genetic mutations.

Antigens are proteins of high molecular weight. Chemical substances may bind themselves to body proteins to form a complex which is antigenic as for example atropine used topically in the treatment of uveitis.

Most lymphocytes originate in the bone marrow during foetal growth and a proportion pass through the thymus where they are processed to respond to specific antigens and are known as T-lymphocytes. Neonatal thymectomy in mice leads to an inability to mount the cell-mediated response responsible for delayed hypersensitivity reactions and for tissue allograft rejection.

B-lymphocytes are processed by the bursa of Fabricius, a structure which has not been identified in humans. When processed they migrate to the periphery and are responsible for the cortical cells of lymph nodes and submucosal lymphoid tissue.

Immunologically competent B-lymphocytes and their plasma cell derivatives are endowed with the ability to form soluble globulins (antibodies) which combine with provocative antigens. There is a range of immunoglobulins which are classified according to their molecular structure.

Immunoglobulins

Immunoglobulin G — IgG is the smallest of the antibody molecules and is found in higher concentrations in the circulating plasma than other immunoglobulins. It is the principle source of humoral immunity against infective organisms.

Immunoglobulin A — IgA is present in normal plasma and is important in the defence of mucous membranes against infection and is the major antibody constituent of tears.

Immunoglobin M — IgM is the largest of the immunoglobulins. It does not normally leave the vascular compartment. It is chiefly involved in defence against bacteriaemia.

Immunoglobulin D — IgD is of little significance as an antibody in human disease.

Immunoglobulin E — On contact with an antigen, IgE precipitates the degranulation of mast cells with consequent release of histamine. This activity is responsible for the immediate hypersensitivity symptoms of asthma, hayfever and vernal conjunctivitis.

Exposure to an antigen leads to its uptake and processing by macrophages whereby it becomes recognisable. In a subsequent exposure the antigen is bound by receptors onto the surface of T-cells. When this happens the T-lymphocyte proliferates to produce daughter cells which exercise a cytolytic effect on cell-bound antigens by lymphokines.

B-lymphocytes require the co-operation of T-lymphocytes before they undergo transformation in response to antigenic stimulation. Once they are sensitised to antigens they transform themselves into plasma cells which are capable of secreting immunoglublins which enter into specific combination with antigens. When circulating antigens meet with such antibodies the combination activates a sequence of plasma proteins known as complement. Complement enhances the inflammatory response, promotes lysis of cell-bound antigens, and leads to direct neutralisation of the toxic properties of bacteria and the promotion of phagocytosis of the antigen itself.

Pathological immune mechanisms

Immunity confers protection from the effects of microbial invasion but this mechanism can sometimes go awry with resulting harmful effects to the tissues of the host. In such cases the reaction is called an allergic response or one of hypersensitivity and can arise from a persistence of the antigen or as a reaction to harmless substances such as house-dust, pollen, (Atopy) or as a harmful lymphoid response to self-antigens (autoimmunity or auto-allergy).

Hypersensitivity may be immediate or delayed. Immediate hypersensitivity is mediated by humoral antibodies and may occur in mucous membranes involving the immunoglobulin IgE or within the walls of blood vessels where antigen diffusing through the tissues meets immunoglobulins (IgG, IgM or IgA) passing out of the circulating blood, or within the circulating blood where antigen-antibody union may occur and initiate tissue damage in multiple sites.

Delayed hypersensitivity is mediated by cytotoxic T-lymphocytes and their lymphokines and reaches a maximum after 24 h.

Type 1 hypersensitivity (immediate hypersensitivity)
In this type of hypersensitivity the antibodies are IgE immunoglobulins. When the antigens at the body surface contact the immunoglobulin an enzyme reaction occurs in the cytoplasm of tissue cells to which the immunoglobulins IgE are bound. This results in the release of histamine and an eosinophil chemotactic factor.

In a generalised anaphylaxis antigen combines with specific IgE antibody in the circulating blood. This type of response may be produced by giving a small sensitising dose of antigen followed some weeks later by a larger intravenous dose. It gives rise to bronchiolar smooth muscle contraction and respiratory embarrassment and sometimes widespread vascular dilatation leading to shock as a result of the release of histamine. This is the type of reaction found occasionally in man following insect bites or the injection of Penicillin. In local anaphylaxis the combination of antigen or allergen such as dust and pollen with IgE antibody on body surfaces is associated with localised mast cell degranulation. In the skin this results in urticaria, in the nose allergic rhinitis, in the conjunctiva, vascular congestion and oedema.

Type II hypersensitivity (complement-dependent hypersensitivity)
Reactions include some forms of Hashimoto's thyroiditis and Goodpasture's syndrome. The antigen-antibody reaction concerns IgG and IgM antibodies and the cytotoxic effects are due to the activation of complement.

Type III hypersensitivity (immune-complex disease)
In Type III hypersensitivity the complement-mediated damage develops as a result of antibody combination with a diffusable antigen and its form depends upon whether the immune complex develops in the circulating blood or in the tissues.

An example of an acute circulating immune complex is serum sickness formed by the combination of soluble antigen in the form of heterologous serum protein with host IgG or IgM antibody in the circulating blood. In this condition there is excess antigen so that the resultant complex remains soluble and lesions develop in the walls of blood vessels and the perivascular tissues at points where the immune complexes gain access and the

lesions are mediated by the actions of activated complement.

Chronic circulating immune complex disease occurs as in systemic lupus erythematosis wherein antibodies are formed to a number of tissue components with immune complex deposition in the blood vessel walls. Disseminated vasculitis may be another example.

Arthus reaction
Acute localised immune complex disease occurs in Lepromatous leprosy wherein there are large numbers of degenerate leprosy bacilli in the tissues providing a soluble antigen which combines with circulating antibodies to form tender inflamed nodules in the skin and elsewhere. Chronic localised immune complex disease is due to persistence of antigen giving rise to an Arthus reaction in which the polymorpho-nuclear leucocyte infiltration characteristic of the acute lesion is replaced by a chronic inflammatory granulomata in some instances. Erythema nodosum associated with tuberculosis comes within this category as also does phacogenic uveitis.

Type IV delayed hypersensitivity
Type IV hypersensitivity is entirely due to the activity of T-dependent lymphocytes and clinically has a delayed onset. The skin reaction provoked by intradermal tuberculin as in the Mantoux Test is a good example. Individuals with specifically sensitised T-cells develop a zone of erythema and induration around the injection site maximal some 24–48 h later.

The caseous necrosis characteristic of tuberculous lesions in sensitised individuals is similarly attributable to T-cell cytocoxicity the damage being sustained principally by the phagocytic cells which have taken up the tubercle bacilli.

Cell-mediated hypersensitivity is a feature of graft rejection as is the immunological response to malignant tumours.

Type V hypersensitivity (stimulatory hypersensitivity)
An example of a stimulatory hypersensitivity concerns the long acting thyroid stimulator (LATS) which is a non-complement fixing IgG anti-thyroid antibody; on contact with specific sites on the membranes of thyroid cells activity is increased and excessive amounts of hormone are produced.

Finally, it must be understood that in any particular disease the types of sensitivity are often mixed.

Auto-immunity
Auto-immunity is a condition in which structural and functional damage is produced by the action of immunologically competent cells and antibodies against healthy tissue components. There is elevation of serum immunoglobulin levels with deposition of immunoglobu-

lins and immune complexes in the tissues. Round cell infiltration of the affected tissues due to T-lymphocytes is usual.

In auto-immune disease there should be a sustained auto-immune response with an identifiable antigen; it should be possible to elicit an auto-immune response in experimental animals and achieve passive transfer of the disease by inoculation with sera or lymphocytes. The auto-immune response should be susceptible to immunosuppression.

There are two broad groups of autoimmune diseases; those which are organ specific and the those which are not. Organ specific auto-immune disease has been described in relation to the thyroid, adrenal cortex, gastric and colonic mucosae, kidney, nervous system and myocardium. The affected organ is infiltrated by lymphocytes and plasma cells and circulating antibodies to organ specific antigens are demonstrable.

Non-organ specific auto-immune disease comprises the connective tissue disease group and includes systemic lupus erythematosis, rheumatoid arthritis and polyarteritis nodosa. The auto-antibodies themselves in these diseases probably cause little tissue damage and the injurious effect is a result of immune complex formation and consequent activation of complement. The initial stimulus is probably cryptogenic infection.

The typical immunological features of auto-immune disease are:
1. *Auto-antibodies* as for example the rheumatoid factor (IgM auto-antibody to the patients own IgG as found in rheumatoid arthritis) or the antinuclear factor (IgG immunoglobulin directed against deoxyribonucleoprotein as found in patients suffering from systemic lupus erythematosis)
2. *Fibrinoid necrosis* — the histological hallmark of connective tissue disease.
3. *Responsiveness* to immuno-suppressive drugs.

Immunological processes and the eye

Due to the avascularity of the cornea and the lens and the physiological selectivity of the blood/aqueous barrier as well as absence of lymphatic channels within the globe itself the eye has a privileged situation in regard to immunology.

Some examples of ocular hypersensitivity are:

Type I hypersensitivity (acute anaphylactic type)

Acute anaphylaxis is mediated chiefly by IgE. Systemic anaphylaxis such as follows the administration of Penicillin or the ingestion of certain foods in sensitised individuals may result in severe chemosis of the lids with generalised urticaria. Vernal conjunctivitis is believed to be a localised form of anaphylaxis since IgE has been demonstrated in tear fluid.

Type II hypersensitivity (complement-dependent type)

Antibodies which bind to antigens on cell surfaces may result in death of those cells due to activation of the lytic complement system or because of C3-mediated macrophage activity. In the eye an example of this type of reaction is destruction of a malignant melanoma of the choroid following exposure to autologous serum containing tumour-specific antibody.

Type III hypersensitivity (immune-complex type)

When the antibody and antigen present in tissue fluid or the circulating plasma combine the resulting complex activates components of the complement system with the development of inflammation and polymorphonuclear lymphocyte accumulation, tissue necrosis and vascular thrombosis. This mechanism may be responsible for some cases of recurrent uveitis in man.

Cell-mediated hypersensitivity (Type IV)

This delayed type of hypersensitivity is mediated by thymus-dependant lymphocytes. Manifestions of this type of hypersensitivity are seen in corneal graft rejection, helminth infestation of the retina, fungal infection of the choroid and conjunctivitis provoked by sensitisation to cosmetic eye preparations. It may play a part in sympathetic ophthalmitis, optic neuritis and possibly viral keratitis.

Transplantation or histocompatability antigens

Transplantation or histocompatability antigens are surface glycoproteins which occur on nucleated cells, platelets and reticulocytes. Small amounts are continuously released into the plasma and they are highly specific for each individual.

Originally they were referred to as HLA antigens because they were associated with human leucocytes and determined genetically at locus A (the first locus). This antigenic system is now known to involve more than one locus and the capital letters HLA are used to denominate the entire group. Indeed their development has been shown to be under the control of five adjacent loci (A, B, C, DR and D) on each of the pair of autosomal chromosomes 6.

In man there are probably 70 different transplantation or histocompatability antigens and it has been calculated that more than 300 million genetically different individuals can be formed by the known alleles of the HLA loci and of these more than 30 million will have recognisable combinations of antigens because some alleles at different loci are grouped together on the same chromosome more often than would be expected by chance, a tendency which is called 'linkage disequilibrium'.

To explain this altered frequency in the distribution of HLA antigens the existence of controlling genes has been suggested or alternatively a set of genes may be responsible for susceptibility or resistance to infection and may thus have acted as a protective mechanism in evolution towards survival. There is strong evidence to support a genetically determined mechanism for the association between HLA antigens and disease processes.

As an example, over 90% of patients with ankylosing spondylitis show the presence of HLA-B27 and a normal person who is positive for this antigen is 100 times more at risk of developing this disease than a B-27 negative person. The precise mechanism of HLA and disease susceptibility is still hypothetical. The table lists the diseases of ophthalmic importance which are associated with particular HLA antigens.

Apart from acute anterior uveitis, (HLA B27) optic neuritis (HLA DRw2 and HLA Dw2) and certain auto-immune diseases such as myasthenia gravis (HLA B8 and HLA DRw3) and thyrotoxicosis (HLA DW3 and HLA B8) there is little evidence of HLA association with eye disease but further evidence on this aspect of aetiology accumulates day by day. The finding of such an association can help in defining sub-groups of clinical disease, occasionally in clinical diagnosis, in defining individuals at risk from a disease (particularly in families) and in providing valuable information as a basis for further research on pathogenesis.

Table 35.1 Association of HLA with diseases of ophthalmic importance (RAHI)

Disease	Antigen	Frequency percentage		Relative risk
		Patients	Controls	
Behçet's disease	HLA B5	60	28	3.86
Vogt-Koyanagi-Harada syndrome	HLA Bw54	45	13	5.4
	HLA Dwa	67	16	10.5
Malignant melanoma of the choroid	HLA Aw32	11	3	4
Acute anterior uveitis	HLA B27	43	7	10
Diabetic retinopathy (juvenile)	B8 (without A1)	56	4	30*
Recurrent herpetic keratitis	B5	26	11	3
Cicatricial ocular pemphigoid	B12	45	20	3.2
Myasthenia gravis	HLA DRw3	32	17	2.3
	HLA B8	39	17	3.1
Thyrotoxicosis	HLA DW3	53	18	5.1
	HLA B8	44	18	3.6
Type I diabetes (juvenile)	HLA DRw3	27	17	1.8
	HLA DRw4	39	15	3.6
	HLA B8	32	16	2.5
Multiple sclerosis	HLA DRw2	41	22	2.5
	HLA Dw2	47	15	5
Ankylosing spondylitis	HLA B27	90	8	103.5
Reiter's disease	HLA B27	80	9	40.4
Rheumatoid arthritis	HLA DRw4	56	15	7.2
	HLA Dw4	60	12	11

* Normally, B8 is in linkage disequilibrium with A1. Presence of B8 alone in juvenile diabetes increases risk of retinopathy. (By courtesy of Rahi.)

SECTION 8

Preventive ophthalmology

The causes and prevention of blindness

The previous chapters have dealt chiefly with the diagnosis and treatment of already established diseases of the eye. An equally important branch of medical science is concerned with the prevention of disease, and although this aspect of ophthalmology has hitherto received less attention than it merits, it ought not to be ignored by the medical student or practitioner.

The most disastrous result of ocular disease, short of the relatively rare loss of life, is blindness. A study of the causes of blindness will enable the student to form a judgment as to the comparative danger of various ocular diseases.

The term 'blindness' implies inability to perceive light; but it is obvious that many people who yet retain some slight degree of visual capacity are helpless from the economic standpoint. In Great Britain therefore, for practical and statutory purposes, a definition is accepted as 'too blind to perform work for which eyesight is essential,' and the practical limits are taken to be a visual acuity of not more than 3/60 in the better eye or alternatively a visual field reduced to a small area around the fixation point. The Register of the Blind for England, compiled on this basis, shows that there are somewhat over 120 000 blind persons.

Statistics from other countries are not readily comparable, sometimes because they are incomplete and sometimes because of differences in the assessment of blindness. Thus while in Great Britain, for purposes of registration, vision of 3/60 or less is set as a standard, in the United States and Canada the limit is 20/200. It would seem, however, on the whole, that for Western Europe, North America, Australia and the Europeanized areas in Africa and Asia, the blindness rate is of the order of 200 per 100 000 of total population. In eastern Europe, India and the South Eastern Asian States, Japan, Central and South Africa, a rate of about twice this may be assumed. In the Middle East and North Africa the rate rises to the appalling figure of 800 per 100 000 and often above, due largely to trachoma and conjunctival infections and malnutrition. As an underestimate, statistics tend to lend to the conclusion that there are some ten million blind in the world today; a more correct figure would probably be twice or three times as high.

A sample analysis of statistics in the blind population in England and Wales shows that, of the total, approximately 60% are aged 70 years and over. The major causes are cataract, glaucoma, myopia and developmental and hereditary anomalies.

In the different age groups, different causes are operative.

1. In infants the vast majority of cases is due to congenital anomalies, particularly cataract, optic atrophy and buphthalmos.

2. In school age, some 60% of cases are due to congenital and developmental anomalies, and 10% to abiotrophic defects; a further 15% are due to neurological diseases.

3. In adult life (20–50 years) the developmental and abiotrophic defects account for 50% if myopia is included in this category; neurological diseases account for some 20%, and diabetes and trauma each 5%.

4. In late adult life (50–70 years) cataract and glaucoma become common causes of blindness, each of these and myopia and diabetes contributing 15% of the total.

5. In the elderly (70 and above) cataract and senile macular degeneration each accounts for 30%, glaucoma remains at 15%, while myopia, diabetes and cardiovascular diseases each accounts for about 5%.

During recent years there have been considerable changes in the incidence of the causes of blindness due largely to improvements in the control of infective conditions. This tendency has been most marked in the case of ophthalmia neonatorum, and consequently the number of blind in the early age groups has been lately much reduced. Thus the incidence of blindness was 37.0 per 100 000 school children aged 5–15 in 1923, and 21.3 in 1948. In 1922 the Board of Education in England, in a survey of 927 blind children in blind schools found that ophthalmia neonatorum was responsible for 30.4% of all cases of blindness; a parallel investigation twenty-two years later showed that ophthalmia neonatorum was responsible for not more than 9.2%. At the present day the disease has almost disappeared. The fall in the incidence of phlyctenular kerato-conjunctivitis, which used to account for 3.5% of blindness in children, has been equally great, a change due partly to the control of tuberculous milk and partly to better nutrition.

Retrolental fibroplasia provided an interesting interlude. In the late 1940s and early 1950s it accounted for an increasing incidence of bilateral blindness in infants, affecting the prematurely born. Since the administration of oxygen in the nursing of these children has been more strictly regulated it has almost disappeared.

On the other hand, there is no reason for believing that any one of the four major causes of blindness — cataract, glaucoma, myopia and the congenital, hereditary and developmental anomalies — is likely to have declined to any extent. In view of the fact that the population of England is ageing, and since 84% of the blind are in the age group of 50 years and over, there seems little ground for hoping that the number of blind is decreasing as a whole. Indeed, it seems reasonable to conclude that in a developed country a further substantial decline in the number of blind in the near future is unlikely, and that the major problems of blindness now present will remain the outstanding causes. Of these, cataract, and glaucoma are diseases of the ageing; myopia and congenital, hereditary and developmental anomalies affect the young and are essentially genetically determined. Genetic and geriatric problems relating to the two extremes of life are therefore the essential issues outstanding in the prevention of blindness in an advanced Western community; and unfortunately we have little real knowledge nor the ability to control these conditions. Of the major causes, glaucoma is essentially a matter of early diagnosis and treatment, while cataract is one of the availability of surgery, although this is sometimes not feasible in the age group wherein its incidence is highest.

Of the other less numerically important causes, the statistics of the blind in England and Wales show the following significant factors.

1. Syphilis is now a relatively minor cause of blindness.

2. The inflammatory diseases are of some importance, as is shown by the fact that iritis and iridocyclitis account for 4.7% of all cases, and nondescript choroidal lesions, some of them possibly inflammatory in origin, for another 1.7%.

3. 'Senile' fundus degenerations are a significant cause of blindness; 'senile' macular degeneration accounts for 6.4%.

4. Vascular lesions are also of significance. Diabetes contributes 1.8% and generalised vascular diseases 1.9%.

5. Optic atrophy as an ætiologically undiagnosed group contributes 3.5%, and nondescript corneal lesions 2.3% of all cases.

Industrial conditions may cause blindness, either by disease or accident. The chief diseases, such as poisoning (lead, derivatives of benzene, etc.), glass- and ironworkers' cataract, miners' nystagmus, etc., have already been discussed. Blindness due to industrial accidents is commonest among miners and in the engineering trades.

In Great Britain some indication of their frequency is given by the fact that injuries to the eyes occur in 5% of the injuries reported in factories, and in 4% of those occurring in construction work. Information on this subject is obtainable from the U.S.A. where conditions are essentially similar. It has been reliably estimated that 300 000 industrial eye accidents occur each year in that country, that is, an eye accident occurs every thirty seconds throughout every working day; every day of the working year 26 880 workers are idle because of eye injuries; each year 53 000 000 man-hours of work are lost thereby. As a result, each year approximately 1000 American workers lose the sight of one eye irreparably, and 100 more lose the sight of both.

More striking is the enormous economic loss entailed by relatively minor accidents, such as foreign bodies in the eye. Many of these could be entirely prevented by the use of appropriate guards, screens and goggles. These matters require special attention from factory medical officers.

37

The hygiene of vision

Apart from the conditions which seriously endanger the eyesight discussed briefly in the last chapter, there are many others which are liable to impair the efficiency of vision or the health of the individual. It is well known that the use of the eyes with uncorrected errors of refraction or muscle balance, or in unsuitable conditions of illumination, causes ocular discomfort (commonly known as 'eye-strain'), headaches, migraine, and general malaise. More serious disorders and diseases have been attributed by some to these causes. The exact pathology of 'eye-strain' is unknown, and the rationale of visual fatigue in the production of ocular and systemic disorders is largely a matter of conjecture. It is, in the first place, a safe principle to correct the ametropic eye by suitable spectacles. In the next place it is necessary to study the normal limits of adaptability of the eye to various conditions of illumination, and to use the knowledge thus obtained to prevent these limits being transgressed. When we bear in mind the evolution of the visual apparatus in man, and the immense increase in the amount and nature of the work which it is called upon to perform in modern civilised life, it is a considerable compliment to the adaptability of the human body that the eyes can usually meet the demands made upon them without complaint.

Errors of refraction

The correction of ametropia and gross errors of muscular imbalance by spectacles has already been discussed. It is evident that theoretically this correction should be made as early as possible, and especially before the increased visual strain of school life is encountered. In Great Britain much advance has been made in this direction in recent years, for the routine examination of the eyes of young school children ensures the discovery of serious errors; moreover, facilities for their correction and for the supply of suitable spectacles are now available. The most difficult problem in this connection is that of myopia, which has already been dealt with in Chapter 8. The most serious problem is the detection and treatment of amblyopia (Chap. 30) at an early

stage, for which reason alone the vision of all children should be tested at the earliest age practicable.

Illumination

Normal vision is capable of adaptation to very wide ranges of intensity and quality of illumination. Form vision is very defective under dark adaptation and with low intensities of illumination. As the intensity is increased and the eye becomes light-adapted, visual acuity increases — rapidly at first, and then only very slowly. The increase is proportional to the logarithm of the intensity of the illumination, so that successive doublings or treblings of the illumination cause only equal arithmetic increments of visual acuity as estimated by the distance at which a standard letter (1.25 mm square) can be read. Above 10 lumen/sq ft the increment becomes progressively less. For ordinary work this illumination suffices, but for fine work much higher values are desirable. At extremely high illuminations, visual acuity is diminished owing to glare.

There are many factors, however, which influence visual acuity besides the intensity of the light. Among these is the size of the pupils, but more important are the amount and character of the light falling upon peripheral areas of the retina. Thus, it is undesirable that there should be too great contrast between the areas under observation and surrounding areas; for example, self-luminous figures are very difficult to focus in complete darkness, especially in conditions of fatigue, as also is a television screen in a dark room. A brilliantly illuminated field of work in an otherwise dark room causes rapid alterations of adaptation which are deleterious. Hence a moderate amount of general illumination is preferable, and this has the additional advantage that it prevents the formation of very sharply defined shadows. On the other hand, it is important that there should be no glaring lights in the field of vision; such lights should be carefully shaded. Care, too, should be taken to avoid direct reflection of light into the eyes. Thus, in reading books printed on shiny paper, and in working on bright metals, if the source of light is in front of the eyes light is reflected directly into them. This light is useless for visual purposes, and indeed, diminishes the contrasts which are the basis of discrimination. Hence the source of light should be placed laterally and somewhat behind the worker preferably, for writing, to the left-hand side in right-handed people to avoid the shadow of the hand. Flickering lights should be avoided.

Various sources of light differ much in intensity and quality. The natural criterion is sunlight which we are accustomed to regard as white light. Sunlight, however, differs much in 'whiteness' and in intensity on different days, at different times of the day, and whether direct or diffuse. Owing to the adaptability of the eye it is difficult to judge the intensity of a given illumination. Measurements show that bright direct sunlight may give several thousand lumen/sq ft, and an illumination of several hundred lumen/sq ft on a well-placed desk is quite common. One great advantage of daylight is its diffusion; the illumination of a room usually comes, not directly from the sun, but from a considerable area of sky, and is reinforced by innumerable reflections from buildings and other objects. Sunlight is much richer in luminous radiation of short wavelength — blue and violet — than any artificial illuminants. Most modern illuminants have continuous spectra derived from incandescent solids; the higher the temperature the more nearly the energy-distribution of the spectrum approximates to that of sunlight. An approximation to diffuse daylight for purposes of matching colours, etc., can be obtained by suitable filters ('daylight lamps') and by fluorescent tubes. Incandescent gases — such as used in the mercury-vapour lamp — have line spectra; they therefore more nearly approximate monochromatic light.

Glare may be regarded as light in the wrong place. The more concentrated the light the more disturbing is the effect. Glare, therefore, varies rather with the intrinsic brilliancy of the light than with its intensity. Clear sky has a very low intrinsic brilliancy. A metal filament has an intrinsic brilliancy 350 times greater and an arc light 8000 times higher. The ratio of the intrinsic brilliancy of a source of light to that of the surrounding field should not exceed 100. In general, the eye works best when the object regarded is surrounded by a field illuminated to the same or slightly less degree. The illumination of the field must on no account be higher than that of the object. Glare is diminished in artificial interior illumination by the use of indirect lighting. In this method the light is reflected from the ceiling and suitably curved cornices, so that no direct light reaches the eye and shadows are almost eliminated. It is a restful but monotonous method of illumination and is quite unsuited for certain purposes. Thus, sewing is very difficult with it, especially the sewing of monochromatic material, because the threads of the texture throw no shadows, and consequently their discrimination is made very difficult. In semi-indirect lighting the use of opalescent bowls permits a certain amount of direct illumination.

Many modern illuminants emit a considerable amount of ultra-violet radiation, which may be deleterious. Most of this is absorbed by glass, so that the dangers arising

Table 37.1 Recommended minimum service values of illumination for different classes of visual task

Class of visual task	Examples	Minimum illumination (LUX)
Casual seeing	Locker rooms	100
Rough tasks with large detail	Heavy machinery assembly; stores	200
Ordinary tasks with medium size detail	Wood machining; general offices; general assembly	400
Fairly severe tasks with small detail	Food-can inspection; clothing, cutting and sewing; business machines; drawing offices	600
Severe prolonged tasks with small detail	Fine assembly and machining; hand-tailoring; weaving silk or synthetic fibres	900
Very severe prolonged tasks with very small detail	Hosiery mending; gauging very small parts; gem cutting	1300–2000
Exceptionally severe tasks (minute detail)	Watchmaking; inspection of very small instruments	2000–3000

In domestic activities the following are recommended:
Lounges — 200 lux
Reading — 400 lux
Sewing — 600 lux
Bed-head — 200 lux
Classrooms — 300; chalkboards — 400

from this cause are slight and have been much over-rated. It must be remembered, however, that globes also absorb an appreciable amount of the luminous energy; even clear glass globes absorb 5–15% and opal globes as much as 10–40%. The distribution of light from artificial sources varies greatly. It can be modified by the use of reflectors and prismatic (holophane) globes. Too little attention has hitherto been paid by architects and others to the position and characters of light sources from the hygienic point of view. It is of great importance in the lighting of factories and work-shops, and especially in that of schools. There has been great improvement in the lighting of schools, factories, shops, streets and houses of recent years, largely due to the work of the Illuminating Engineering Society, which has issued a schedule of Recommended Values of Illumination. The preceding table gives the general principles. On these lighting in Britain is based; American recommendations are considerably higher. The service value of illumination refers to the mean value throughout the life of the installation.

Reading and writing

Considering the vast importance of reading and writing in modern life it is surprising that they have been so little investigated by physiologists and ophthalmologists. The forms of printed types are derived from manuscripts, and have been modified for technical reasons. Further advance has been almost entirely empirical, and even in the best presses more care has been exercised in obtaining æsthetic effects than in fostering legibility.

If we consider ordinary Roman printed characters we find that all capital letters extend above the line. Of the small letters thirteen are short, nine extend above the line (ascending letters), and five below the line (descending letters). There are thus twice as many ascending as descending letters, and in an ordinary page of print it will be found that of the long letters about 85% are ascending and only 15% descending. Examination of the short letters shows that their most characteristic features are in the upper parts. Hence, in reading, attention is specially directed to the upper parts of the letters, as is strikingly demonstrated by covering the lower parts of a line of print with a card when the print is almost as legible as if it were uncovered; if, however, the upper halves of the letters are covered, it is almost, if not quite, impossible to read the print.

The ends of the lines of which letters are composed are commonly emphasised by means of serifs. These were doubtless introduced empirically, but the advantage in sharpness of definition has a physiological basis. They counteract irradiation, and hence the visibility of letters is improved if the serifs are triangular.

The tendency of type-founders has been to minimise the differences between letters, probably with a view to attaining regularity of line and uniformity in appearance. For example, round letters have been flattened laterally and square letters rounded. The loops of b, d, p, and q, have been equalised to o. If the lower parts of short letters are covered, the similarity in the topmost curves of a, c, e, o, s, of n and r, of h and b, or of n and p, is much greater in modern print than in some early samples.

Legibility is not determined solely by visibility in the physiological sense of the term. Thus, the emphasis of some lines in letters, which originated in the use of reeds and pens for writing, increases legibility whilst diminishing visibility. A child learning to read depends upon physiological visibility; hence there should be little difference between the breadth of the thick and slender strokes. As facility in reading is acquired, legibility is increased by diminishing the breadth of the slender strokes, and as smaller letters are used the diminution must be more rapid than that of the heavy strokes, so that the interspaces may not be unduly contracted. At the same time, the slender strokes must not transgress the limits of visibility at reading distance, and their distribution should be emphasised by suitably formed serifs. Hence, Jaeger small types are more legible than Snellen's.

The spacing of the letters and words has a considerable effect upon legibility. Here irradiation plays an important part. Roughly speaking, the interspaces between letters should be at least as broad as the blanks in m or n, but round letters like o and e should have slightly less interspace than square letters. Owing to irradiation the interspaces in general look larger than they really are, and two o's separated by a space look farther apart than two n's separated by the same space. Javal attributed a large part of the 'remarkable legibility of English books' to the shortness of most English words in comparison with German and the consequent multiplication of blank interspaces. Of course, the spacing of words, and to a less degree of letters, in ordinary printing is very largely haphazard as far as legibility is concerned, the main object of the printer being to obtain general uniformity of appearance with rigid equality in the lengths of the lines. There is some difference of opinion as to whether 'leading' or interlinear spacing is beneficial. Owing to the design of the blocks of type there is always a small space between the lower limits of descending and the upper limits of ascending letters, even without leading.

A line of print is read in a series of small jumps. At each pause a group of about ten letters is more or less accurately visualised; the movements are too rapid to allow visualisation whilst they are occurring. The number of leaps taken by the eye remains the same irrespective of the distance of the book, so long as this is consistent with legibility. A child reading makes more jumps in a line than the average, and the same applies to people reading a foreign language or correcting proofs. Attention is directed chiefly to the commencements of words, and words are not read by letters but by their general configuration. There is, therefore, a very important psychological factor involved in the act of reading, quite apart from the interpretation of the meaning of the words.

Enough has been said to show that reading is a highly complex act, and the rules which can at present be devised for the avoidance of strain and discomfort involve a multiplicity of factors which have not yet been satisfactorily correlated.

Handicrafts

The same visual principles as have been discussed above underlie the specific problems met with in many handicrafts and industrial processes. For some types of very fine work convex lenses bringing the near point to 8 or 9 inches from the eye, combined with appropriate prisms, bases in, magnify the retinal images and have been found to give much relief.

No attempt has been made in this Section to deal exhaustively with so extensive a subject as Preventive Ophthalmology, but it has been deemed advisable to indicate to the student how innumerable and complex are the applications of ophthalmology to everyday life.

APPENDIX 1
Moorfield's pharmacopoeia

CAUSTICS

Carbolic acid
    Liquefied phenol B.P.
    May be coloured by the addition of eosin 0.002%.

Iodine with potassium iodide spirit
    Iodine 7.0
    Potassium iodide 5.0
    Alcohol 90% .... to 100.0

EYE-DROPS

Acetylcysteine 2%, 5%, 10% & 20%
    2%, 5% and 10% strengths are prepared by dilution of
    the 20% solution with hypromellose (Alkaline) eye-
    drops. The pH is adjusted to 9.0 with 4% sodium
    hydroxide solution.

Adrenaline neutral 1% eye-drops
    Adrenaline base 1.1
    Boric acid 1.0
    Sodium borate 0.6
    Sodium metabisulphite 0.3
    Disodium edetate 0.1

    Ascorbic acid 0.2
    Hydroxypropylmethyl-cellulose 4500 .... 0.25
    Chlorhexidine acetate 0.005
    Distilled water .... to 100.0
    Also available containing 0.25% and 0.5% adrenaline.

Adrenaline eye-drops 0.01%
    Adrenaline solution 0.1% 10.0
    Sodium chloride 0.8
    Sodium metabisulphite 0.1
    Phenylmercuric nitrate 0.002
    Distilled water .... to 100.0

Alcian blue
    Alcian blue 1.0
    Phenylmercuric Nitrate 0.002
    Distilled water .... to 100.0

Alkaline eye-drops (Hypromellose B.P.C.)
    Hydroxypropylmethyl-cellulose 4500 .... 0.30
    Borax 0.19
    Boric acid 0.19
    Potassium chloride 0.37
    Sodium chloride 0.45
    Benzalkonium chloride 0.01
    Distilled water .... to 100.0

Amethocaine eye-drops
    Amethocaine eye-drops .... 0.25 or 1.0
Phenylmercuric acetate 0.002
Distilled water .... to 100.0

Amphotericin B eye-drops
    Amphotericin B 0.5
    Dextrose 5.0
    Thiomersal 0.004
    Distilled water .... to 100.0

Antazoline Co. eye-drops
    Antazoline hydrochloride 0.5
    Naphazoline nitrate 0.025
    Sodium chloride 0.84

Phenylmercuric nitrate 0.002
Distilled water .... to 100.0

Antrenyl eye-drops
see Oxyphenonium

Atropine eye-drops
Atropine sulphate .... 0.125 to 2.0
Phenylmercurie nitrate 0.002
Distilled water .... to 100.0
If no strength is specified 1.0% will be dispensed.

Bengal rose eye-drops
Bengal rose 1.0
Phenylmercuric acetate 0.002
Distilled water .... to 100.0

Benoxinate eye-drops (Novesine)
Benoxinate hydrochloride .... 0.2 to .04
Chlorhexidine acetate 0.01
Distilled water .... to 100.0

B.J.6. eye-drops
Sodium chloride 0.6
Sodium bicarbonate 0.45
Hydroxypropylmethyl-cellulose 4000 .... 0.25
Tween 80 .... 0.025
Chlorhexidine acetate 0.005
Distilled water .... to 100.0

Boric acid eye-drops
Boric acid 0.2
Chlorhexidine acetate 0.01
Distilled water .... to 100.0

Calcium sodium edetate eye-drops
Calcium sodium edetate   1.0, 5.0 or 10.0
Hydroxypropylmethyl-cellulose 4000 .... 1.0
Benzalkonium chloride 0.01
Distilled water .... to 100.0

Carbachol eye-drops
Carbachol .... 0.75 or 3.0
Benzalkonium chloride 0.01
Distilled water .... to 100.0

Chloramphenicol eye-drops B.P.C.
Chloramphenicol 0.5
Borax 0.3
Boric acid 1.5
Phenylmercuric acetate or nitrate 0.002
Distilled water .... to 100.0

Cocaine eye-drops
Cocaine hydrochloride .... 2.0 to 4.0

Chlorhexidine acetate 0.01
Distilled water .... to 100.0
The strength and quantity to be dispensed MUST be stated by the prescriber

Colomycin eye-drops
Colomycin 1.0
Sodium chloride 0.9
Distilled water .... to 100.0

Cyclopentolate eye-drops
Trade names Mydrilate; Cyclogyl.
This preparation contains cyclopentolate hydrochloride 0.5 or 1.0% w/v

Dexamethasone alc. eye-drops
Dexamethasone micronized 0.1
Hydroxypropylmethyl-cellulose 4000 .... 0.5
Benzalkonium chloride 0.01
Distilled water .... to 100.0
When dexamethasone eye-drops are prescribed the 0.1% suspension will be dispensed

Dexamethasone soluble 0.05% eye-drops
An isotonic solution containing 0.076% w/v of dexamethasone metasulphobenzoate (equivalent to 0.05% w/v of dexamethasone)

Dexamethasone soluble 0.1% eye-drops
An isotonic solution containing 0.152% w/v of dexamethosone metasulphobenzoate (equivalent to 0.1% w/v of dexamethosone)

Dexamethasone and framycetin eye-drops
An isotonic solution containing dexamethasone metasulphobenzoate 0.076% w/v (equivalent to dexamethasone 0.05% w/v) with framycetin sulphate 0.5% w/v

Disodium edetate eye-drops
Disodium edetate 0.38
Sodium acid phosphate hydrated 0.42
Sodium phosphate hydrated 1.43
Benzalkonium chloride 0.01
Distilled water .... to 100.0

Ecothiopate eye-drops (phospholine iodide)
Ecothiopate iodide .... 0.06 to 0.25
Chlorbutol 0.5
Mannitol 1.2
Boric acid 0.06
Sodium phosphate hydrated 0.026
Distilled water .... to 100.0

Eserine eye-drops
See Physostigmine eye-drops

Framycetin eye-drops
Framycetin sulphate 1.0
Phenylmercuric nitrate 0.002
Distilled water .... to 100.0

5-Fluoro-cytosine eye-drops
5-Fluorocytosine 1.0
Thiomersal 0.005
Distilled water .... to 100.0

Glycerin eye-drops
Glycerin 20.0
Phenylmercuric nitrate 0.002
Distilled water .... to 100.0

Heparin eye-drops
Heparin 1,000 units/ml in distilled water.

Homatropine eye-drops
Homatropine hydrobromide .... 1.0 or 2.0
Chlorhexidine acetate 0.01
Distilled water .... to 100.0

Homatropine and cocaine eye-drops
Cocaine hydrochloride 2.0
Homatropine hydrobromide 2.0
Chlorhexidine acetate 0.01
Distilled water .... to 100.0
This quantity to be dispensed MUST be stated by the
prescriber

Hydrocortisone eye-drops
An isotonic suspension 1.0% w/v of hydrocortisone
acetate

Hydrocortisone and neomycin eye-drops
An isotonic suspension containing 1.0% w/v of hydrocortisone acetate and 0.5% w/v of neomycin
sulphate

Hydroxypropylmethylcellulose eye-drops
Hydroxypropylmethyl-cellulose 4000 ..... 1.0 to 2.0
Sodium chloride 0.8
Benzalkonium chloride 0.01
Distilled water .... to 100.0
(For diagnostic contact lenses)

Hyoscine eye-drops
Hyoscine hydrobromide .... 0.25 to 0.5
Chlorhexidine acetate 0.01
Distilled water .... to 100.0
If no strength is specified 0.25% will be supplied

Hyoscine eye-drops 0.05%
Hyoscine hydrobromide 0.05
Chlorhexidine acetate 0.01
Distilled water .... to 100.0
For use in the refraction of children.
N.B. This concentration must not be exceeded.
Hyoscine is highly toxic for children.

Idoxuridine eye-drops
Idoxuridine 0.1
Sodium citrate 1.13
Citric acid 0.27
Benzalkonium chloride 0.01
Distilled water .... to 100.0

Cocaine N eye-drops
Adrenaline acid tartrate 0.18
Sodium metabisulphite 0.1
Cocaine hydrochloride 4.0
Neomycin sulphate 0.5
Chlorhexidine acetate 0.01
Distilled water .... to 100.0
The quantity to be dispensed MUST be stated by the
prescriber

Kanamycin eye-drops
Kanamycin 0.5
Boric acid 1.54
Borax 0.286
Phenylmercuric nitrate 0.002
Distilled water .... to 100.0

Lachesine eye-drops
Lachesine hydrochloride 1.0
Phenylmercuric nitrate 0.002
Distilled water .... to 100.0

Lignocaine eye-drops
Lignocaine hydrochloride 2.0
Chlorhexidine acetate 0.01
Distilled water .... to 100.0
May be used as an alternative to cocaine or ametho-
caine eye-drops.

L-Cysteine eye-drops
L-cysteine hydrochloride 0.1 to 0.3 molar concentration in isotonic solution containing benzalkonium
chloride 0.01%.

Methylcellulose eye-drops
Methylcellulose 20 .... 1.0 to 3.0
Phenylmercuric nitrate 0.002
Distilled water .... to 100.0

Methylcellulose alkaline eye-drops
Methylcellulose20 .... 0.5
Sodiumchloride.. 0.8
Sodiumbicarbonate 0.25
Polysorb 80 .... 0.025
Chlorhexidine acetate 0.005
Distilledwater .... to 100.0

Natamycin (pimaricin)
A 5% microcrystalline suspension adjusted to pH 6.5 to 7.0

Naphazoline eye-drops
Naphazoline nitrate 0.05
Sodium chloride 0.84
Phenylmercurie nitrate 0.004
Distilled water .... to 100.0

Neomycin eye-drops B.P.C.
Neomycin sulphate 0.5
Sodium phosphate hydrated 0.7
Sodium acid phosphate hydrated 0.7
Disodium edetate 0.01
Phenylmercuric nitrate 0.002
Distilled water .... to 100.0

Neutral adrenaline
see Adrenaline neutral

Novesine eye-drops
see Benoxinate

Novesine and fluorescein eye-drops
Benoxinate hydrochloride 0.3
Fluorescein sodium 0.125
Polyvinylpyrrolidone 1.0
Phenylmercuric nitrate 0.004
Distilled water .... to 100.0

Ocusol eye-drops
see Sulphacetamide and zinc

Oxyphenonium eye-drops (Antrenyl)
Oxyphenonium bromide .... 1.0 to 5.0
Chlorhexidine acetate 0.01
Distilled water .... to 100.0

Pimaricin eye-drop
see Natamycin

Penicillin eye-drops
Benzylpenicillin .... 5000 units
Sodium citrate .... 5 mg
Phenylmercuric nitrate .... 20 μg
Distilled water .... to 1.0 ml

Penicillin and streptomycin eye-drops strong
Benzylpenicillin .... 100,000 units
Streptomycin sulphate .... 0.1 g
Phenylmercuric nitrate .... 20 μg
Distilled water .... to 1.0 ml

Phenylephrine eye-drops
Phenylephrine hydrochloride 10.0
Sodium citrate 0.3
Sodium metabisulphite 0.5
Benzalkonium chloride 0.02
Distilled water .... to 100.0

Phospholine iodide eye-drops
see Ecothiopate

Physostigmine eye-drops (syn – Eserine eye-drops)
Physostigmine sulphate .... 0.25 to 1.0
Sodium metabisulphite 0.2
Ascorbic acid 0.1
Benzalkonium chloride 0.01
Distilled water .... to 100.0

Pilocarpine eye-drops B.P.C.
Pilocarpine hydrochloride .... 0.25 to 4.0
Benzalkonium chloride 0.01
Distilled water .... to 100.0

Pilocarpine and eserine eye-drops
Pilocarpine hydrochloride .... 2.0 to 4.0
Physostigmine sulphate .... 0.25 to 1.0
Sodium metabisulphite 0.2
Ascorbic acid 0.1
Benzalkonium chloride 0.01
Distilled water .... to 100.0

Polyvinylpyrrolidone eye-drops
Polyvinylprrolidone .... 0.5 to 1.0
Hydroxyethycellulose 0.5
Disodium edetate 0.1
Sodium acid phosphate hydrated 0.42
Sodium phosphate hydrated 1.43
Thiomersal 0.002
Distilled water .... to 100.0

Polyvinylpyrrolidone 0.5% alkaline eye-drops
Polyvinylpyrrolidone 0.5
Hydroxyethylcellulose 0.5
Disodium edetate 0.1
Sodium bicarbonate 1.0
Sodium chloride 0.6
Thiomersal 0.002
Distilled water .... to 100.0

Prednisolone eye-drops

Prednisolone sodium phosphate 0.31
Boric acid 0.3
Sodium borate 0.03
Disodium edetate 0.01
Phenylmercuric nitrate 0.004
Distilled water .... to 100.0
The standard strength supplied is 0.3%. Dilutions are available in 0.1%, 0.03%, 0.01%, 0.003%, 0.001% and 0.0003%.

Prednisolone Forte 1% eye-drops

Prednisolone sodium phosphate 1.0
Boric acid 0.3
Sodium borate 0.03
Disodium edetate 0.01
Phenylmercuric nitrate 0.004
Distilled water .... to 100.0
This strength will be supplied only on prescriptions specifying FORTE 1%.

Prednisolone and neomycin eye-drops

Prednisolone sodium phosphate   0.31
Neomycin sulphate 0.5
Boric acid 0.3
Sodium borate 0.3
Disodium edetate 0.01
Phenylmercuric nitrate 0.004
Distilled water .... to 100.0

Soframycin eyedrops

see Framycetin eye-drops

Streptomycin eye-drops

Streptomycin sulphate .... 5000 units
Phenylmercuric nitrate .... 20 μg
Distilled water .... to 1.0 ml.

Sucrose eye-drops

Sucrose .... 10.0 to 30.0
Phenylmercuric nitrate 0.002
Distilled water .... to 100.0

Sulphacetamide eye-drops

Sulphacetamide sodium .... 10.0, 20.0 or 30.0
Sodium metabisulphite 0.1
Phenylmercuric nitrate 0.002
Distilled water .... to 100.0

Sulphacetamide and zinc eye-drops

Sulphacetamide sodium 5.0
Zinc sulphate 0.1
Sodium carboxymethyl-cellulose 1.0
Phenylmercuric nitrate 0.004
Distilled water .... to 100.0

Zinc sulphate eye-drops

Zinc sulphate .... 0.125 to 0.25
Phenylmercuric nitrate 0.002
Distilled water .... to 100.0

Zinc and adrenaline eye-drops

Zinc sulphate 0.25
Adrenaline solution 1 in 1000 .... 5.0
Boric acid 2.0
Phenylmercuric nitrate 0.002
Distilled water .... to 100.0

EYE LOTIONS

Amphoteric lotion (universal lotion)

Potassium acid phosphate hydrated 7.0
Sodium phosphate hydrated 18.0
Distilled water 85.0

Saline eye lotion

Sodium chloride 0.57
Potassium chloride 0.02
Calcium chloride anhydrous 0.016
Distilled water .... to 100.0
This eye lotion is equivalent to $\frac{2}{3}$ strength Ringer solution.

Sodium bicarbonate eye lotion

Sodium bicarbonate 2.0
Distilled water .... to 100.0

EYE OINTMENTS

Atropine eye ointment

Atropine sulphate .... 0.5 to 2.0
Sterile eye ointment basis .... to 100.0

Chloramphenicol eye ointment

Chloramphenicol 1.0
Sterile eye ointment basis .... to 100.0

Framycetin eye ointment

Framycetin sulphate 0.5
Sterile eye ointment basis .... to 100.0

Idoxuridine eye ointment (Syn. I.D.U. eye ointment)

Idoxuridine micronised 0.5
Sterile eye ointment basis .... to 100.0

Neomycin eye ointment

Neomycin sulphate 0.5
Sterile eye ointment basis .... to 100.0

Penicillin eye ointment
Benzylpenicillin .... 5000 units
Sterile eye ointment basis .... to 1.0

Polymyxin and bacitracin eye ointment
Trade name: Polyfax eye ointment
Polymyxin B. sulphate .... 10 000 units

Zinc bacitracin .... 500 units
Sterile eye ointment basis .... to 1.0

Sulphacetamide eye ointment
Sulphacetamide sodium .... 6.0 to 10.0
Sterile eye ointment basis .... to 100.0

Tetracycline eye ointment
Trade name: Achromycin eye ointment
Tetracycline hydrochloride 1.0
Sterile eye ointment basis .... to 100.0

INJECTIONS

For anterior chamber injection
Anterior chamber irrigation — Ringer solution
Sodium chloride 0.86
Potassium chloride 0.03
Calcium chloride anhydrous 0.024
Distilled water .... to 100.0
Sterilize by autoclaving.

Pilocarpine injection (isotonic)
Pilocarpine nitrate 0.5
Sodium chloride 0.57
Potassium chloride 0.02
Calcium chloride anhydrous 0.016
Water for injection B.P. .... to 100.0
The injection, in 1 ml ampules, is sterilised by auto-
claving.

Injections for local anaesthesia and akinesia

Lignocaine hydrochloride injection
Lignocaine hydrochloride 2.0
Water for injection .... to 100.0

Sub-conjunctival injection doses
These are included for the guidance of prescribers only
Amphotericin B ....
Ampicillin ....
Benzylpenicillin ....
Benzylpenicillin and streptomycin
(crystamycin) ....

Betamethasone ....

Lignocaine and adrenaline injection
Lignocaine hydrochloride 2.0
Sodium chloride 0.45
Solution of adrenaline (1 in 1000) 1.0
Sodium metabisulphite 0.1
Water for injection .... to 100.0

Retrobulbar injections
All retrobulbar injections should be preceded by an
injection of lignocaine 2% or procaine 2%

Alcohol injection
Alcohol 40% v/v; 70% v/v or 90% v/v. Sterilised by
autoclaving in sealed ampoules.

Aminophylline injection
Aminophylline B.P. 500 mg in 2 ml

Tolazoline injection
Tolazoline hydrochloride 25 mg in 1 ml

Sub-conjunctival injection

Mydricaine No. 1
Procaine hydrochloride .... 3.0 mg
Atropine sulphate .... 0.5 mg
Boric acid .... 5.0 mg
Solution of adrenaline 1 in 1000 .... 0.06 ml
Sodium metabisulphite .... 0.3 mg
Water for injection .... to 0.3 ml

Dose: Children. Not to exceed 0.3 ml by subconjunctival injection.

Mydricaine No. 2
Procaine hydrochloride .... 6.0 mg
Atropine sulphate .... 1.0 mg
Boric acid .... 5.0 mg
Solution of adrenaline 1 in 1000 .... 0.12 ml
Sodium metabisulphite .... 0.3 mg
Water for injection .... to 0.3 ml

Dose: Adults. Not to exceed 0.3 ml by subconjunctival injection. To be used with caution in patients
under general anaesthesia.

150 to 300 μg maximum
125 mg in 0.5 ml normal saline
300 mg (500 000 u) in 0.5 ml lignocaine and adrenaline

300 mg benzylpenicillin and 500 μg streptomycin in 0.5
to 1.0 ml lignocaine and adrenaline

2 to 4 mg (0.5 to 1.0 ml)

Carbenicillin	125 mg in lignocaine and adrenaline
Cephaloridine	100 mg in 0.5 ml water for injection
Chloramphenicol	100 mg in lignocaine and adrenaline
Cloxacillin	100 mg in 0.5 ml lignocaine and adrenaline
Colomycin	8 mg in 0.5 ml lignocaine
Cortisone	10 mg with 1000 units hyalase
Framycetin	100 to 500 mg in 0.25 to 0.5 ml water for injection
Gentamicin	10 to 20 mg in lignocaine
Hydrocortisone	10 mg with 1000 units hyalase
Kanamycin	10 to 20 mg
Lincomycin	75 to 150 mg
Methicillin	500 mg in 0.5 ml normal saline
Methylprednisolone	10 to 20 mg
Neomycin	500 mg in adrenaline 1 in 5000. Toxic above 3G total dose
Polymyxin B	125 000 up to 200 000 ug in 0.5 ml. lignocaine and adrenaline
Spiramycin	10 to 20 mg
Streptomycin	250 mg in 0.5 ml lignocaine and adrenaline
Thiosporin	500 mg in 0.5 ml water for injection
Tobramycin	10 to 20 mg in lignocaine and adrenaline
Triamcinolone	10 to 20 mg
Vancomycin	25 mg in lignocaine and adrenaline

MISCELLANEOUS PREPARATIONS

Acetazolamide
Trade name: Diamox
Available as tablets 250 mg and sodium salt in vials of 500 mg for intramuscular and intravenous injection.
The dosage used in opthalmology is much higher than that used as a diuretic. In consequence, side-effects such as paraesthesia and drowsiness may appear and the dosage should be reduced to a minimum as early as possible

Dichlorphenamide tablets
Trade name: Daranide tablets 50 mg

Glycerin
For oral administration.
Dose: 1.5g/kg bodyweight
Supplied as 50% v/v solution

Mannitol
Dose: 1.8g/kg bodyweight by slow intravenous infusion. Risk of tissue necrosis if it enters tissues.

Urea
30% Urea in 10% dextrose
Dose: 1g (3 ml)/kg bodyweight by slow intravenous injection. Risk of tissue necrosis if it enters tissues

SOLUTIONS

For removal of calcium deposits

Sodium edetate	0.37
Sodium bicarbonate	0.1
Distilled water	to 100.0

For tattooing — artificial iris

Gold chloride solution

Gold chloride	4.0
Water injection	to 100.0

Artificial pupil

Platinum chloride solution

Platinum chloride	2.0
Water for injection	to 100.0

Hydrazine hydrate reducing solution

Hydrazine hydrate	2.0
Water for injection	to 100.0

PRESCRIBING AND POISONS REGULATIONS

Prescribing in the metric system

The formula of all tablets, capsules, lozenges, suppositories and injections of the British Pharamacopoeia, the British Pharmaceutical Codex and the British National Formulary are now expressed in the Metric System.

The abbreviation 'g' should be used for 'gram'.

When writing quantities of solids of less than 1 gram, the weight should be expressed in milligrams (mg)

Quantities of solid of less than 1 mg should be expressed as micrograms. This should, preferably be written in full but if an abbreviation is used, 'μg' should be employed

Prescribing for children

Doses of drugs for children should be calculated on a bodyweight basis.

Further information, if required, may be obtained from the Pharmacy or the drug manufacturer's data sheets.

Note that children are much more sensitive weight for weight than adults to certain drugs. These include morphine and its derivatives, choline esters and other parasympathetic stimulants

PRESCRIBING OF POISONS AND CONTROLLED DRUGS

The following brief notes are intended for the guidance of prescribers.

Schedule 1 poisons

Prescribing in hospital

May be prescibed only by a registered medical practitioner or dentist and the following details must be given for record purposes:
1. Name and address of patient (Hospital Number referring to Central Records will suffice in place of address.)
2. Quantity of poison and dose.
3. Prescriber's signature and date.

Prescribing in practice

Details required are as for hospital prescribing above.

Purchase

May be purchased without a prescription at the discretion of the pharmacist (i.e. the purchaser should be known to him or suitably vouched for). The buyer must sign the Poisons Book

Schedule 4 poisons

Schedule 4A
Prescribing in hospital
As for Schedule 1 above

Prescribing in practice

As for Schedule 1 in Hospital, and in addition the address of the prescriber must be given. The prescription may not be dispensed more than once except in accordance with an express direction on the prescription

Schedule 4B
Prescribing in hospital
As for Schedule 1 above

Prescribing in practice

The prescription must be dated by the prescriber and bear his usual signature

Records to be kept in the pharmacy

In hospital

Records to be kept for TWO years for both Schedule 1 and Schedule 4

In retail pharmacy

The pharmacist retains the prescription for Schedule 4 poisons when no longer valid for two years, full details being entered in the prescription book on each occasion on which the prescription is dispensed

MISUSE OF DRUGS ACTS

Prescribing in hospital

These drugs may only be prescribed by the medical practitioner in charge of the case. The prescription must be in writing on the patient's case sheet and must bear the following particulars:
1. Signature of the prescriber.
2. The date (this being added by the prescriber).
3. The name of the patient or the number of the case.
4. The name, dose and quantity of the drug.

Prescribing in practice

The prescription, in writing, must give the following particulars:
The usual signature of the prescriber.
The date (added by the prescriber).
The address of the prescriber.
The name and address of the patient.
The total amount of any B.P. or B.P.C. preparation

to be supplied and in any other case the total amount of the drug.

A prescription for a Controlled Drug may be dispensed once only unless it expressly states that it may, subject to the lapse of a specified interval or intervals, be supplied a second or third time. In any event it may not be dispensed on more than three occasions

Ordering and storage of stock on wards etc.

Drugs may only be supplied for stock on a written order signed by the sister or acting sister. This must be endorsed in the pharmacy and a copy kept by the sister. Precautions must be taken to prevent theft in transit. Drugs must be kept in a locked cupboard. They may only be used for patients in the particular ward or department

Records to be kept in the pharmacy

In hospital

Records to be kept for TWO years of the receipt and issue of all Controlled Drugs

In retail pharmacy

A prescription must be retained by the pharmacist even if 'repeats' are ordered

THERAPEUTIC SUBSTANCES ACT

Prescriptions for these preparations are valid only for one supply and within three months of the date of signing unless the number of times or the intervals over some other period than three months is specified.

The following particulars must be given:
1. Name and address of patient (hospital number referring to Central Records will suffice in place of address).
2. Quantity and dose.
3. Prescriber's signature and date.

METRIC AND IMPERIAL EQUIVALENTS

The following equivalents are prescribed by the Weights and Measures (Equivalents for dealing with drugs) Regulations 1964

Metric mg	*Metric* ug	*Imperial* gr
0.1	100	1/600
0.125	125	1/500
0.125	125	1/480
0.15	150	1/400
0.2	200	1/320
0.2	200	1/300
0.25	250	1/240
0.3	300	1/200
0.4	400	1/160
0.5	500	1/130
0.5	500	1/120
0.6	600	1/100
0.8	800	1/80
0.8	800	1/75

Metric mg	*Metric*	*Imperial* gr
1.0	0.001	1/60
1.25	0.00125	1/50
1.5	0.0015	1/40
2.0	0.002	1/30
2.5	0.0025	1/25
2.5	0.0025	1/24
3.0	0.003	1/20
4.0	0.004	1/15
5.0	0.005	1/12
6.0	0.006	1/10
7.5	0.0075	1/8
10	0.01	1/6
12.5	0.0125	1/5
15	0.015	1/4
20	0.02	1/3
25	0.025	2/5
30	0.03	1/2
40	0.04	3/5
50	0.05	3/4
60	0.06	1
75	0.075	1¼
100	0.1	1½
125	0.125	2
150	0.15	2½
200	0.2	3
250	0.25	4
300	0.3	5
400	0.4	6
450	0.45	7½
500	0.5	8
600	0.6	10
800	1.8	12
1000	1.0	15

THE APPLICATION OF HEAT TO THE EYE

Heat may be applied to the eye moist or dry. The best method for the application of *moist heat* is that of *hot bathing*. A pad of cotton wool is tied into the bowl of a wooden spoon. The wool is dipped into a bowl of hot water which can be replenished, and is then approximated to the closed eye. As soon as it has cooled sufficiently it is brought into contact with the closed lids. As soon as it ceases to feel hot the wool is again dipped in the hot water and the process repeated. The bathing is continued for ten to fifteen minutes, and then a pad of dry warm cotton wool is bandaged over the eye. The hot bathings may be repeated frequently.

An alternative is the application of *hot compresses*. These are large round pads of plain or boric lint, on one surface of which gutta-percha tissue is sewn. The compresses are placed in a cloth and immersed in boiling water; by keeping the ends of the cloth out of the water and turning them in opposite directions the excess of the water is wrung out without scalding the fingers. The compress is applied as hot as can be borne. It is at once covered with a large pad of hot cotton wool and bandaged into position.

Dry heat may be applied over long periods by means of an *electric eye pad*, an eye pad of gauze heated by incorporating in it a small electric resistance. An alternative method is by *medical diathermy*. An eye pad, composed of layers of cotton wool wrung out in warm saline and applied evenly to the closed lids, serves as one of the electrodes, the other being bound to the arm. The current is slowly increased until the desired amount of heat is attained. This is generally between 300 and 600 mA: it is maintained at this reading for five minutes and then slowly reduced to zero

VITAMINS

The following are the vitamins most important in ophthalmology, showing their natural sources, daily need, functions, and deficiency effects.

A. (Higher alcohol synthesised from carotene in the liver). *Carotene* from carrots, green vegetables; A from fat of fish, esp. liver — *cod liver oil, halibut oil* — egg yolk, milk: *corotene* 3 mg; A 3000 units: maintenance of healthy ectodermal structures (respiratory, alimentary, urinary, *conjunctival, corneal, retinal*); *production of visual purple*. Deficiency effects — dermatoses, demyelination, diminished resistance to infections; *xerosis, xerophthalmia, keratomalacia, night blindness*

B_1 (Thiamine, a pyramidine thiazole compound). From many foodstuffs, esp. lean pork, beans, peas, nuts, *whole* grain and flour, beef, *yeast*: 1 mg: carbohydrate metabolism. Deficiency effects — beri-beri, peripheral neuritis; *corneal and conjunctival dystrophy, retrobulbar neuritis*

B_2 or G. (Riboflavine). Same sources as B_1: 1 mg: oxygenation. Deficiency effects — glossitis and cheilosis; *vascularising keratitis*

Several other vitamins of the B group are now known but their precise importance is not yet fully determined

C. (Ascorbic or cevitamic acid). From fresh fruit and vegetables (destroyed by heating): 50 mg: Blood formation, osteogenesis, *lens metabolism*. Deficiency effects — scurvy, anæmia, osteoplasia; *conjunctival and retinal hæmorrhages, kerato-conjunctivitis.*

D. (Calciferol — isomer of ergosterol, formed by ultraviolet light on skin). From animal fats, esp. *cod liver oil and halibut oil;* sunshine: 1000 units, 0.025 mg: Ca and P metabolism. Deficiency effects — rickets, osteomalacia, dental caries, tetany; *cataract*

K. (Dimethylnaphthoquinone). From alfalfa: prothrombin formation

P. (Flavone). From citrous fruits: maintenance of health of capillaries. Deficiency effects of vitamins K and P — hæmorrhagic conditions

These vitamins have been isolated or synthesised, and are available in proprietary preparations. Deficiency should be counteracted as far as possible in the diet. Little harm seems to accrue from large doses, except in the case of hypercalcæmia from calciferol.

CARE OF INSTRUMENTS

Ophthalmic instruments should be kept in an air-tight glass cabinet, or when not constantly in use in velvet-lined cases.

All instruments may safely be sterilised before use by boiling in 3% sodium carbonate solution (*not* bicarbonate), made with *distilled* water. This procedure does not impair the cutting edges, but knives and scissors should not be boiled more than three to five minutes: this is simply sufficient if the surfaces are bright and free from tarnish, as they ought to be. If distilled water cannot be obtained the cutting instruments should be well soaked in 0.5% Hibitane in 70% spirit and then washed in sterile saline before use.

The instruments should be removed from the steriliser *immediately* before operating and used dry. *In no case must instruments be immersed in boric lotion*, since it tarnishes the steel.

It is safer to use the instruments dry as it is almost impossible to sterilise the skin of the hands efficiently, and if the instruments are wet, fluid from the fingers is liable to run along them into the eye. Dry sterilisation in a hot air oven offers many advantages — efficiency, the avoidance of damage to sharp cutting edges, and the possibility of the surgeon taking the instruments directly from the container in which they have been sterilised without handling by any other person. The points of knives should be dipped in sterile saline immediately before use to facilitate their passage through the tissues. While dry sterilisation is the best technique, its disadvantage is the time which it takes (1½ to 2 hours); for this reason in a busy hospital a separate set of instruments is required for each operation undertaken in a half-day.

The surgeon should wear a sterilised gown and also a mask containing a layer of cellophane covering the nose and mouth for all operations, as well as sterilised gloves whenever there is the possibility of the fingers' touching the surgical area

APPENDIX 2

Visual acuity transcription tables
For some decimals the distance at the examination has
to be altered from 6 to 5 m or from 20 to 15 feet

Decimal system	Snellen 6-m table	20-foot table	Resolution angle table
1.0	6/6	20/20	1.0
0.8	5/6	20/25	1.3
0.7	6/9	20/30	1.4
0.6	5/9	15/25	1.6
0.5	6/12	20/40	2.0
0.4	5/12	20/50	2.5
0.3	6/18	20/70	3.3
0.1	6/60	20/200	10.0

Index